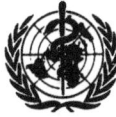

WORLD HEALTH ORGANIZATION

INTERNATIONAL AGENCY FOR RESEARCH ON CANCER

IARC MONOGRAPHS

ON THE

EVALUATION OF CARCINOGENIC

RISKS TO HUMANS

*Polychlorinated Dibenzo-***para***-dioxins and Polychlorinated Dibenzofurans*

VOLUME 69

This publication represents the views and expert opinions
of an IARC Working Group on the
Evaluation of Carcinogenic Risks to Humans,
which met in Lyon,

4–11 February 1997

1997

IARC MONOGRAPHS

In 1969, the International Agency for Research on Cancer (IARC) initiated a programme on the evaluation of the carcinogenic risk of chemicals to humans involving the production of critically evaluated monographs on individual chemicals. The programme was subsequently expanded to include evaluations of carcinogenic risks associated with exposures to complex mixtures, life-style factors and biological agents, as well as those in specific occupations.

The objective of the programme is to elaborate and publish in the form of monographs critical reviews of data on carcinogenicity for agents to which humans are known to be exposed and on specific exposure situations; to evaluate these data in terms of human risk with the help of international working groups of experts in chemical carcinogenesis and related fields; and to indicate where additional research efforts are needed.

This project is supported by PHS Grant No. 5-UO1 CA33193-15 awarded by the United States National Cancer Institute, Department of Health and Human Services. Additional support has been provided since 1986 by the European Commission.

©International Agency for Research on Cancer, 1997

IARC Library Cataloguing in Publication Data

Polychlorinated dibenzo-*para*-dioxins and polychlorinated dibenzofurans /
IARC Working Group on the Evaluation of
Carcinogenic Risks to Humans (1997 : Lyon,
France).

(IARC monographs on the evaluation of carcinogenic
risks to humans ; 69)

1. Polychlorinated dibenzo-*para*-dioxins – congresses 2. Polychlorinated
dibenzofurans – congresses I. IARC Working Group on the Evaluation of
Carcinogenic Risks to Humans II. Series

ISBN 92 832 1269 X   (NLM Classification: W 1)

ISSN 0250-9555

Distributed by IARC*Press* (Fax: +33 04 72 73 83 02; E-mail: press@iarc.fr)
and by the World Health Organization Distribution and Sales,
CH-1211 Geneva 27 (Fax: +41 22 791 4857)

PRINTED IN FRANCE

CONTENTS

NOTE TO THE READER

The term 'carcinogenic risk' in the *IARC Monographs* series is taken to mean the probability that exposure to an agent will lead to cancer in humans.

Inclusion of an agent in the *Monographs* does not imply that it is a carcinogen, only that the published data have been examined. Equally, the fact that an agent has not yet been evaluated in a monograph does not mean that it is not carcinogenic.

The evaluations of carcinogenic risk are made by international working groups of independent scientists and are qualitative in nature. No recommendation is given for regulation or legislation.

Anyone who is aware of published data that may alter the evaluation of the carcinogenic risk of an agent to humans is encouraged to make this information available to the Unit of Carcinogen Identification and Evaluation, International Agency for Research on Cancer, 150 cours Albert Thomas, 69372 Lyon Cedex 08, France, in order that the agent may be considered for re-evaluation by a future Working Group.

Although every effort is made to prepare the monographs as accurately as possible, mistakes may occur. Readers are requested to communicate any errors to the Unit of Carcinogen Identification and Evaluation, so that corrections can be reported in future volumes.

IARC WORKING GROUP ON THE EVALUATION OF CARCINOGENIC RISKS TO HUMANS: POLYCHLORINATED DIBENZO-*PARA*-DIOXINS AND POLYCHLORINATED DIBENZOFURANS

Lyon, 4–11 February 1997

LIST OF PARTICIPANTS

Members[1]

P. Bannasch, Department of Cytopathology, German Cancer Research Center, Im Neuenheimer Feld 280, Postfach 101949, 69120 Heidelberg, Germany

H. Becher, Division of Epidemiology, German Cancer Research Center, Im Neuenheimer Feld 280, Postfach 101949, 69120 Heidelberg, Germany

P.A. Bertazzi, Institute of Occupational Health, Clinica del Lavoro 'Luigi Devoto', University of Milan, via San Barnaba 8, 20122 Milan, Italy

L.S. Birnbaum, Experimental Toxicology Division (MD-66), National Health and Environmental Effects Research Laboratory, US Environmental Protection Agency, Research Triangle Park, NC 27711, United States

S. Cordier, Unit of Epidemiological and Statistical Research on the Environmental and Health, INSERM - U 170, 16 avenue Paul Vaillant Couturier, 94807 Villejuif, France

Y. Dragan, Department of Oncology, McArdle Laboratory for Cancer Research, University of Wisconsin Medical School, 1400 University Avenue, Madison, WI 53706, United States

M. Kogevinas, Department of Epidemiology and Public Health, Institut Municipal d'Investigació Mèdica, IMIM, Universitat Autònoma de Barcelona, c/Doctor Aiguader 80, 08003 Barcelona, Spain

V.V. Khudoley, Laboratory of Genetic Toxicology and Ecology, N.N. Petrov Research Institute of Oncology, Pesochny-2, Leningradskaja 68, 289646 St Petersburg, Russian Federation

G.W. Lucier, Environmental Toxicology Program, National Institute of Environmental Health Sciences, PO Box 12233, MD A3-O2, Research Triangle Park, NC 27709, United States (*Chairman*)

---

[1] Unable to attend: S.H. Safe, Department of Veterinary Physiology and Pharmacology, College of Veterinary Medicine, Texas A&M University, College Station, TX 77843-4466, United States

J. Nagayama, Laboratory of Environmental Health Sciences, School of Health Sciences, Kyushu University, 3-1-1 Maidashi, Higashi-ku, Fukuoka 812, Japan

S.S. Olin, Risk Science Institute, International Life Sciences Institute, 1126 Sixteenth Street NW, Washington DC 20036, United States

O. Päpke, ERGO Forschungsgesellschaft mbH, Albert-Einstein-Ring 7, 22761 Hamburg, Germany

L. Poellinger, Department of Cell and Molecular Biology, Medical Nobel Institute, Karolinska Institutet, 171 77 Stockholm, Sweden

A. Poland, McArdle Laboratory for Cancer Research, University of Wisconsin, 1400 University Avenue, Madison, WI 53706, United States

C. Rappe, Institute of Environmental Chemistry, University of Umeå, 901 87 Umeå, Sweden (*Vice-Chairman*)

W.J. Rogan, National Institute of Environmental Health Sciences, PO Box 12233, Research Triangle Park, NC 27709, United States

C. Schlatter, Institute of Toxicology, Swiss Federal Institute of Technology, Schoren-strasse 16, 8603 Schwerzenbach/Zürich, Switzerland

D. Schrenk, Institute of Toxicology, University of Tübingen, Wilhelmstrasse 56, 72074 Tübingen, Germany

A.H. Smith, University of California, Berkeley, School of Public Health, Earl Warren Hall, Berkeley, CA 94720-7360, United States

R. Stahlmann, Institute of Toxicology and Embryonal Pharmacology, Free University of Berlin, Garystrasse 5, 14195 Berlin, Germany

J.R. Startin, Central Science Laboratory, Room 06GA04, Sand Hutton, York YO4 1LZ, United Kingdom

K. Steenland, Centers for Disease Control, National Institute for Occupational Safety and Health, 4676 Columbia Parkway, Cincinnati, OH 45226-1998, United States

M.H. Sweeney, National Institute for Occupational Safety and Health, Education and Information Division, Mailstop C-15, 4676 Columbia Parkway, Cincinnati, OH 45226-1988, United States

M. Van den Berg, Environmental Toxicology Group, Research Institute of Toxicology, University of Utrecht, PO Box 80176, 3508 TD Utrecht, The Netherlands

S. Watanabe, Department of Nutrition and Epidemiology, Tokyo University of Agriculture, 1-1-1, Sakuragaoka, Setagaya-ku, Tokyo 156, Japan

Representatives/Observers

Representative of the National Cancer Institute

S. Hoar Zahm, National Cancer Institute, EPN 418, 6130 Executive Boulevard, Rockville, MD 20892-7364, United States

American Industrial Health Council

R.S. Greenberg, Medical University of South Carolina, 171 Ashley Avenue, Charleston, SC 29425, United States

European Centre for Ecology and Toxicology of Chemicals

L.J. Bloemen, Dow Europe SA, Epidemiology and Biochemical Research, Addock Center, PO Box 48, 4530 AA Terneuzen, The Netherlands

Japanese National Institute of Health Science

R. Hasegawa, Division of Toxicology, Biological Safety Research Center, National Institute of Health Sciences, 1-18-1 Kamiyoga, Setagaya-ku, Tokyo 158, Japan

WHO Centre for Environment and Health

F.X.R. van Leeuwen, WHO Centre for Environment and Health, PO Box 10, 3730 AA De Bilt, The Netherlands

Secretariat

R. Black, Unit of Descriptive Epidemiology
P. Boffetta, Unit of Environmental Cancer Epidemiology
J. Cheney (*Editor*)
M. Friesen, Unit of Gene Environment Interactions
P. Hainaut, Unit of Mechanisms of Carcinogenesis
E. Kramarova, Unit of Descriptive Epidemiology
V. Krutovskikh, Unit of Multistage Carcinogenesis
N. Malats, Unit of Environmental Cancer Epidemiology
C. Malaveille, Unit of Endogenous Cancer Risk Factors
D. McGregor, Unit of Carcinogen Identification and Evaluation (*Responsible Officer*)
D. Mietton, Unit of Carcinogen Identification and Evaluation
D. Parkin, Unit of Descriptive Epidemiology
C. Partensky, Unit of Carcinogen Identification and Evaluation (*Technical Editor*)
J. Rice, Unit of Carcinogen Identification and Evaluation (*Head of Programme*)
S. Ruiz, Unit of Carcinogen Identification and Evaluation
J. Vena, Unit of Environmental Cancer Epidemiology
J. Wilbourn, Unit of Carcinogen Identification and Evaluation

Secretarial assistance

M. Lézère
J. Mitchell
S. Reynaud

PREAMBLE

IARC MONOGRAPHS PROGRAMME ON THE EVALUATION OF CARCINOGENIC RISKS TO HUMANS[1]

PREAMBLE

1. BACKGROUND

In 1969, the International Agency for Research on Cancer (IARC) initiated a programme to evaluate the carcinogenic risk of chemicals to humans and to produce monographs on individual chemicals. The *Monographs* programme has since been expanded to include consideration of exposures to complex mixtures of chemicals (which occur, for example, in some occupations and as a result of human habits) and of exposures to other agents, such as radiation and viruses. With Supplement 6 (IARC, 1987a), the title of the series was modified from *IARC Monographs on the Evaluation of the Carcinogenic Risk of Chemicals to Humans* to *IARC Monographs on the Evaluation of Carcinogenic Risks to Humans*, in order to reflect the widened scope of the programme.

The criteria established in 1971 to evaluate carcinogenic risk to humans were adopted by the working groups whose deliberations resulted in the first 16 volumes of the *IARC Monographs series*. Those criteria were subsequently updated by further ad-hoc working groups (IARC, 1977, 1978, 1979, 1982, 1983, 1987b, 1988, 1991a; Vainio *et al.*, 1992).

2. OBJECTIVE AND SCOPE

The objective of the programme is to prepare, with the help of international working groups of experts, and to publish in the form of monographs, critical reviews and evaluations of evidence on the carcinogenicity of a wide range of human exposures. The *Monographs* may also indicate where additional research efforts are needed.

The *Monographs* represent the first step in carcinogenic risk assessment, which involves examination of all relevant information in order to assess the strength of the available evidence that certain exposures could alter the incidence of cancer in humans. The second step is quantitative risk estimation. Detailed, quantitative evaluations of epidemiological data may be made in the *Monographs*, but without extrapolation beyond

[1] This project is supported by PHS Grant No. 5-UO1 CA33193-15 awarded by the United States National Cancer Institute, Department of Health and Human Services. Since 1986, the programme has also been supported by the European Commission.

the range of the data available. Quantitative extrapolation from experimental data to the human situation is not undertaken.

The term 'carcinogen' is used in these monographs to denote an exposure that is capable of increasing the incidence of malignant neoplasms; the induction of benign neoplasms may in some circumstances (see p. 17) contribute to the judgement that the exposure is carcinogenic. The terms 'neoplasm' and 'tumour' are used interchangeably.

Some epidemiological and experimental studies indicate that different agents may act at different stages in the carcinogenic process, and several different mechanisms may be involved. The aim of the *Monographs* has been, from their inception, to evaluate evidence of carcinogenicity at any stage in the carcinogenesis process, independently of the underlying mechanisms. Information on mechanisms may, however, be used in making the overall evaluation (IARC, 1991a; Vainio *et al.*, 1992; see also pp. 23–25).

The *Monographs* may assist national and international authorities in making risk assessments and in formulating decisions concerning any necessary preventive measures. The evaluations of IARC working groups are scientific, qualitative judgements about the evidence for or against carcinogenicity provided by the available data. These evaluations represent only one part of the body of information on which regulatory measures may be based. Other components of regulatory decisions may vary from one situation to another and from country to country, responding to different socioeconomic and national priorities. **Therefore, no recommendation is given with regard to regulation or legislation, which are the responsibility of individual governments and/or other international organizations.**

The *IARC Monographs* are recognized as an authoritative source of information on the carcinogenicity of a wide range of human exposures. A survey of users in 1988 indicated that the *Monographs* are consulted by various agencies in 57 countries. About 4000 copies of each volume are printed, for distribution to governments, regulatory bodies and interested scientists. The Monographs are also available from the International Agency for Research on Cancer in Lyon and via the Distribution and Sales Service of the World Health Organization.

3.   SELECTION OF TOPICS FOR MONOGRAPHS

Topics are selected on the basis of two main criteria: (a) there is evidence of human exposure, and (b) there is some evidence or suspicion of carcinogenicity. The term 'agent' is used to include individual chemical compounds, groups of related chemical compounds, physical agents (such as radiation) and biological factors (such as viruses). Exposures to mixtures of agents may occur in occupational exposures and as a result of personal and cultural habits (like smoking and dietary practices). Chemical analogues and compounds with biological or physical characteristics similar to those of suspected carcinogens may also be considered, even in the absence of data on a possible carcinogenic effect in humans or experimental animals.

The scientific literature is surveyed for published data relevant to an assessment of carcinogenicity. The IARC information bulletins on agents being tested for carcinogenicity (IARC, 1973–1996) and directories of on-going research in cancer epidemiology (IARC, 1976–1996) often indicate exposures that may be scheduled for future meetings. Ad-hoc working groups convened by IARC in 1984, 1989, 1991 and 1993 gave recommendations as to which agents should be evaluated in the IARC Monographs series (IARC, 1984, 1989, 1991b, 1993).

As significant new data on subjects on which monographs have already been prepared become available, re-evaluations are made at subsequent meetings, and revised monographs are published.

4. DATA FOR MONOGRAPHS

The *Monographs* do not necessarily cite all the literature concerning the subject of an evaluation. Only those data considered by the Working Group to be relevant to making the evaluation are included.

With regard to biological and epidemiological data, only reports that have been published or accepted for publication in the openly available scientific literature are reviewed by the working groups. In certain instances, government agency reports that have undergone peer review and are widely available are considered. Exceptions may be made on an ad-hoc basis to include unpublished reports that are in their final form and publicly available, if their inclusion is considered pertinent to making a final evaluation (see pp. 23–25). In the sections on chemical and physical properties, on analysis, on production and use and on occurrence, unpublished sources of information may be used.

5. THE WORKING GROUP

Reviews and evaluations are formulated by a working group of experts. The tasks of the group are: (i) to ascertain that all appropriate data have been collected; (ii) to select the data relevant for the evaluation on the basis of scientific merit; (iii) to prepare accurate summaries of the data to enable the reader to follow the reasoning of the Working Group; (iv) to evaluate the results of epidemiological and experimental studies on cancer; (v) to evaluate data relevant to the understanding of mechanism of action; and (vi) to make an overall evaluation of the carcinogenicity of the exposure to humans.

Working Group participants who contributed to the considerations and evaluations within a particular volume are listed, with their addresses, at the beginning of each publication. Each participant who is a member of a working group serves as an individual scientist and not as a representative of any organization, government or industry. In addition, nominees of national and international agencies and industrial associations may be invited as observers.

6. WORKING PROCEDURES

Approximately one year in advance of a meeting of a working group, the topics of the monographs are announced and participants are selected by IARC staff in consultation with other experts. Subsequently, relevant biological and epidemiological data are collected by the Carcinogen Identification and Evaluation Unit of IARC from recognized sources of information on carcinogenesis, including data storage and retrieval systems such as MEDLINE and TOXLINE.

For chemicals and some complex mixtures, the major collection of data and the preparation of first drafts of the sections on chemical and physical properties, on analysis, on production and use and on occurrence are carried out under a separate contract funded by the United States National Cancer Institute. Representatives from industrial associations may assist in the preparation of sections on production and use. Information on production and trade is obtained from governmental and trade publications and, in some cases, by direct contact with industries. Separate production data on some agents may not be available because their publication could disclose confidential information. Information on uses may be obtained from published sources but is often complemented by direct contact with manufacturers. Efforts are made to supplement this information with data from other national and international sources.

Six months before the meeting, the material obtained is sent to meeting participants, or is used by IARC staff, to prepare sections for the first drafts of monographs. The first drafts are compiled by IARC staff and sent, before the meeting, to all participants of the Working Group for review.

The Working Group meets in Lyon for seven to eight days to discuss and finalize the texts of the monographs and to formulate the evaluations. After the meeting, the master copy of each monograph is verified by consulting the original literature, edited and prepared for publication. The aim is to publish monographs within six months of the Working Group meeting.

The available studies are summarized by the Working Group, with particular regard to the qualitative aspects discussed below. In general, numerical findings are indicated as they appear in the original report; units are converted when necessary for easier comparison. The Working Group may conduct additional analyses of the published data and use them in their assessment of the evidence; the results of such supplementary analyses are given in square brackets. When an important aspect of a study, directly impinging on its interpretation, should be brought to the attention of the reader, a comment is given in square brackets.

7.   EXPOSURE DATA

Sections that indicate the extent of past and present human exposure, the sources of exposure, the people most likely to be exposed and the factors that contribute to the exposure are included at the beginning of each monograph.

Most monographs on individual chemicals, groups of chemicals or complex mixtures include sections on chemical and physical data, on analysis, on production and use and on occurrence. In monographs on, for example, physical agents, occupational exposures and cultural habits, other sections may be included, such as: historical perspectives, description of an industry or habit, chemistry of the complex mixture or taxonomy.

Monographs on biological agents have sections on structure and biology, methods of detection, epidemiology of infection and clinical disease other than cancer.

For chemical exposures, the Chemical Abstracts Services Registry Number, the latest Chemical Abstracts Primary Name and the IUPAC Systematic Name are recorded; other synonyms are given, but the list is not necessarily comprehensive. For biological agents, taxonomy and structure are described, and the degree of variability is given, when applicable.

Information on chemical and physical properties and, in particular, data relevant to identification, occurrence and biological activity are included. For biological agents, mode of replication, life cycle, target cells, persistence and latency and host response are given. A description of technical products of chemicals includes trades names, relevant specifications and available information on composition and impurities. Some of the trade names given may be those of mixtures in which the agent being evaluated is only one of the ingredients.

The purpose of the section on analysis or detection is to give the reader an overview of current methods, with emphasis on those widely used for regulatory purposes. Methods for monitoring human exposure are also given, when available. No critical evaluation or recommendation of any of the methods is meant or implied. The IARC publishes a series of volumes, *Environmental Carcinogens: Methods of Analysis and Exposure Measurement* (IARC, 1978–93), that describe validated methods for analysing a wide variety of chemicals and mixtures. For biological agents, methods of detection and exposure assessment are described, including their sensitivity, specificity and reproducibility.

The dates of first synthesis and of first commercial production of a chemical or mixture are provided; for agents which do not occur naturally, this information may allow a reasonable estimate to be made of the date before which no human exposure to the agent could have occurred. The dates of first reported occurrence of an exposure are also provided. In addition, methods of synthesis used in past and present commercial production and different methods of production which may give rise to different impurities are described.

Data on production, international trade and uses are obtained for representative regions, which usually include Europe, Japan and the United States of America. It should not, however, be inferred that those areas or nations are necessarily the sole or major sources or users of the agent. Some identified uses may not be current or major applications, and the coverage is not necessarily comprehensive. In the case of drugs, mention of their therapeutic uses does not necessarily represent current practice nor does it imply judgement as to their therapeutic efficacy.

Information on the occurrence of an agent or mixture in the environment is obtained from data derived from the monitoring and surveillance of levels in occupational environments, air, water, soil, foods and animal and human tissues. When available, data on the generation, persistence and bioaccumulation of the agent are also included. In the case of mixtures, industries, occupations or processes, information is given about all agents present. For processes, industries and occupations, a historical description is also given, noting variations in chemical composition, physical properties and levels of occupational exposure with time and place. For biological agents, the epidemiology of infection is described.

Statements concerning regulations and guidelines (e.g., pesticide registrations, maximal levels permitted in foods, occupational exposure limits) are included for some countries as indications of potential exposures, but they may not reflect the most recent situation, since such limits are continuously reviewed and modified. The absence of information on regulatory status for a country should not be taken to imply that that country does not have regulations with regard to the exposure. For biological agents, legislation and control, including vaccines and therapy, are described.

8.   STUDIES OF CANCER IN HUMANS

(a)   Types of studies considered

Three types of epidemiological studies of cancer contribute to the assessment of carci-nogenicity in humans — cohort studies, case–control studies and correlation (or ecolo-gical) studies. Rarely, results from randomized trials may be available. Case series and case reports of cancer in humans may also be reviewed.

Cohort and case–control studies relate individual exposures under study to the occur-rence of cancer in individuals and provide an estimate of relative risk (ratio of incidence or mortality in those exposed to incidence or mortality in those not exposed) as the main measure of association.

In correlation studies, the units of investigation are usually whole populations (e.g., in particular geographical areas or at particular times), and cancer frequency is related to a summary measure of the exposure of the population to the agent, mixture or exposure circumstance under study. Because individual exposure is not documented, however, a causal relationship is less easy to infer from correlation studies than from cohort and case–control studies. Case reports generally arise from a suspicion, based on clinical experience, that the concurrence of two events — that is, a particular exposure and occurrence of a cancer — has happened rather more frequently than would be expected by chance. Case reports usually lack complete ascertainment of cases in any population, definition or enumeration of the population at risk and estimation of the expected number of cases in the absence of exposure. The uncertainties surrounding interpretation of case reports and correlation studies make them inadequate, except in rare instances, to form the sole basis for inferring a causal relationship. When taken together with case–control and cohort studies, however, relevant case reports or correlation studies may add materially to the judgement that a causal relationship is present.

Epidemiological studies of benign neoplasms, presumed preneoplastic lesions and other end-points thought to be relevant to cancer are also reviewed by working groups. They may, in some instances, strengthen inferences drawn from studies of cancer itself.

(b)   Quality of studies considered

The Monographs are not intended to summarize all published studies. Those that are judged to be inadequate or irrelevant to the evaluation are generally omitted. They may be mentioned briefly, particularly when the information is considered to be a useful supplement to that in other reports or when they provide the only data available. Their inclusion does not imply acceptance of the adequacy of the study design or of the analysis and interpretation of the results, and limitations are clearly outlined in square brackets at the end of the study description.

It is necessary to take into account the possible roles of bias, confounding and chance in the interpretation of epidemiological studies. By 'bias' is meant the operation of factors in study design or execution that lead erroneously to a stronger or weaker association than in fact exists between disease and an agent, mixture or exposure circumstance. By 'confounding' is meant a situation in which the relationship with disease is made to appear stronger or weaker than it truly is as a result of an association between the apparent causal factor and another factor that is associated with either an increase or decrease in the incidence of the disease. In evaluating the extent to which these factors have been minimized in an individual study, working groups consider a number of aspects of design and analysis as described in the report of the study. Most of these considerations apply equally to case–control, cohort and correlation studies. Lack of clarity of any of these aspects in the reporting of a study can decrease its credibility and the weight given to it in the final evaluation of the exposure.

Firstly, the study population, disease (or diseases) and exposure should have been well defined by the authors. Cases of disease in the study population should have been identified in a way that was independent of the exposure of interest, and exposure should have been assessed in a way that was not related to disease status.

Secondly, the authors should have taken account in the study design and analysis of other variables that can influence the risk of disease and may have been related to the exposure of interest. Potential confounding by such variables should have been dealt with either in the design of the study, such as by matching, or in the analysis, by statistical adjustment. In cohort studies, comparisons with local rates of disease may be more appropriate than those with national rates. Internal comparisons of disease frequency among individuals at different levels of exposure should also have been made in the study.

Thirdly, the authors should have reported the basic data on which the conclusions are founded, even if sophisticated statistical analyses were employed. At the very least, they should have given the numbers of exposed and unexposed cases and controls in a case–control study and the numbers of cases observed and expected in a cohort study. Further tabulations by time since exposure began and other temporal factors are also important. In a cohort study, data on all cancer sites and all causes of death should have been given, to reveal the possibility of reporting bias. In a case–control study, the effects of investigated factors other than the exposure of interest should have been reported.

Finally, the statistical methods used to obtain estimates of relative risk, absolute rates of cancer, confidence intervals and significance tests, and to adjust for confounding should have been clearly stated by the authors. The methods used should preferably have been the generally accepted techniques that have been refined since the mid-1970s. These methods have been reviewed for case–control studies (Breslow & Day, 1980) and for cohort studies (Breslow & Day, 1987).

(c)   Inferences about mechanism of action

Detailed analyses of both relative and absolute risks in relation to temporal variables, such as age at first exposure, time since first exposure, duration of exposure, cumulative exposure and time since exposure ceased, are reviewed and summarized when available. The analysis of temporal relationships can be useful in formulating models of carcino-genesis. In particular, such analyses may suggest whether a carcinogen acts early or late in the process of carcinogenesis, although at best they allow only indirect inferences about the mechanism of action. Special attention is given to measurements of biological markers of carcinogen exposure or action, such as DNA or protein adducts, as well as markers of early steps in the carcinogenic process, such as proto-oncogene mutation, when these are incorporated into epidemiological studies focused on cancer incidence or mortality. Such measurements may allow inferences to be made about putative mechanisms of action (IARC, 1991a; Vainio et al., 1992).

(d)   Criteria for causality

After the quality of individual epidemiological studies of cancer has been summarized and assessed, a judgement is made concerning the strength of evidence that the agent, mixture or exposure circumstance in question is carcinogenic for humans. In making its judgement, the Working Group considers several criteria for causality. A strong asso-ciation (a large relative risk) is more likely to indicate causality than a weak association, although it is recognized that relative risks of small magnitude do not imply lack of causality and may be important if the disease is common. Associations that are replicated in several studies of the same design or using different epidemiological approaches or under different circumstances of exposure are more likely to represent a causal relation-ship than isolated observations from single studies. If there are inconsistent results among investigations, possible reasons are sought (such as differences in amount of exposure), and results of studies judged to be of high quality are given more weight than those of studies judged to be methodologically less sound. When suspicion of carcino-genicity arises largely from a single study, these data are not combined with those from later studies in any subsequent reassessment of the strength of the evidence.

If the risk of the disease in question increases with the amount of exposure, this is considered to be a strong indication of causality, although absence of a graded response is not necessarily evidence against a causal relationship. Demonstration of a decline in risk after cessation of or reduction in exposure in individuals or in whole populations also supports a causal interpretation of the findings.

Although a carcinogen may act upon more than one target, the specificity of an asso-ciation (an increased occurrence of cancer at one anatomical site or of one morphological type) adds plausibility to a causal relationship, particularly when excess cancer occurrence is limited to one morphological type within the same organ.

Although rarely available, results from randomized trials showing different rates among exposed and unexposed individuals provide particularly strong evidence for causality.

When several epidemiological studies show little or no indication of an association between an exposure and cancer, the judgement may be made that, in the aggregate, they show evidence of lack of carcinogenicity. Such a judgement requires first of all that the studies giving rise to it meet, to a sufficient degree, the standards of design and analysis described above. Specifically, the possibility that bias, confounding or misclassification of exposure or outcome could explain the observed results should be considered and excluded with reasonable certainty. In addition, all studies that are judged to be methodologically sound should be consistent with a relative risk of unity for any observed level of exposure and, when considered together, should provide a pooled estimate of relative risk which is at or near unity and has a narrow confidence interval, due to sufficient population size. Moreover, no individual study nor the pooled results of all the studies should show any consistent tendency for relative risk of cancer to increase with increasing level of exposure. It is important to note that evidence of lack of carcinogenicity obtained in this way from several epidemiological studies can apply only to the type(s) of cancer studied and to dose levels and intervals between first exposure and observation of disease that are the same as or less than those observed in all the studies. Experience with human cancer indicates that, in some cases, the period from first exposure to the development of clinical cancer is seldom less than 20 years; latent periods substantially shorter than 30 years cannot provide evidence for lack of carcinogenicity.

9.   STUDIES OF CANCER IN EXPERIMENTAL ANIMALS

All known human carcinogens that have been studied adequately in experimental animals have produced positive results in one or more animal species (Wilbourn et al., 1986; Tomatis et al., 1989). For several agents (aflatoxins, 4-aminobiphenyl, azathioprine, betel quid with tobacco, BCME and CMME (technical grade), chlorambucil, chlornaphazine, ciclosporin, coal-tar pitches, coal-tars, combined oral contraceptives, cyclophosphamide, diethylstilboestrol, melphalan, 8-methoxypsoralen plus UVA, mustard gas, myleran, 2-naphthylamine, nonsteroidal oestrogens, oestrogen replacement therapy/steroidal oestrogens, solar radiation, thiotepa and vinyl chloride), carcinogenicity in experimental animals was established or highly suspected before epidemiological studies confirmed the carcinogenicity in humans (Vainio et al., 1995). Although this association cannot establish that all agents and mixtures that cause cancer in experimental animals also cause cancer in humans, nevertheless, **in the absence of adequate data on humans, it is biologically plausible and prudent to regard agents and mixtures for which there is sufficient evidence (see p. 24) of carcinogenicity in experimental animals as if they presented a carcinogenic risk to humans.** The possibility that a given agent may cause cancer through a species-specific mechanism which does not operate in humans (see p. 25) should also be taken into consideration.

The nature and extent of impurities or contaminants present in the chemical or mixture being evaluated are given when available. Animal strain, sex, numbers per group, age at start of treatment and survival are reported.

Other types of studies summarized include: experiments in which the agent or mixture was administered in conjunction with known carcinogens or factors that modify carcinogenic effects; studies in which the end-point was not cancer but a defined precancerous lesion; and experiments on the carcinogenicity of known metabolites and derivatives.

For experimental studies of mixtures, consideration is given to the possibility of changes in the physicochemical properties of the test substance during collection, storage, extraction, concentration and delivery. Chemical and toxicological interactions of the components of mixtures may result in nonlinear dose–response relationships.

An assessment is made as to the relevance to human exposure of samples tested in experimental animals, which may involve consideration of: (i) physical and chemical characteristics, (ii) constituent substances that indicate the presence of a class of substances, (iii) the results of tests for genetic and related effects, including genetic activity profiles, DNA adduct profiles, proto-oncogene mutation and expression and suppressor gene inactivation. The relevance of results obtained, for example, with animal viruses analogous to the virus being evaluated in the monograph must also be considered. They may provide biological and mechanistic information relevant to the understanding of the process of carcinogenesis in humans and may strengthen the plausibility of a conclusion that the biological agent under evaluation is carcinogenic in humans.

(a) Qualitative aspects

An assessment of carcinogenicity involves several considerations of qualitative importance, including (i) the experimental conditions under which the test was performed, including route and schedule of exposure, species, strain, sex, age, duration of follow-up; (ii) the consistency of the results, for example, across species and target organ(s); (iii) the spectrum of neoplastic response, from preneoplastic lesions and benign tumours to malignant neoplasms; and (iv) the possible role of modifying factors.

As mentioned earlier (p. 11), the *Monographs* are not intended to summarize all published studies. Those studies in experimental animals that are inadequate (e.g., too short a duration, too few animals, poor survival; see below) or are judged irrelevant to the evaluation are generally omitted. Guidelines for conducting adequate long-term carcinogenicity experiments have been outlined (e.g., Montesano *et al.*, 1986).

Considerations of importance to the Working Group in the interpretation and evaluation of a particular study include: (i) how clearly the agent was defined and, in the case of mixtures, how adequately the sample characterization was reported; (ii) whether the dose was adequately monitored, particularly in inhalation experiments; (iii) whether the doses and duration of treatment were appropriate and whether the survival of treated animals was similar to that of controls; (iv) whether there were adequate numbers of animals per group; (v) whether animals of both sexes were used; (vi) whether animals were allocated randomly to groups; (vii) whether the duration of observation was adequate; and (viii) whether the data were adequately reported. If available, recent data on the incidence of specific tumours in historical controls, as well as in concurrent controls, should be taken into account in the evaluation of tumour response.

When benign tumours occur together with and originate from the same cell type in an organ or tissue as malignant tumours in a particular study and appear to represent a stage in the progression to malignancy, it may be valid to combine them in assessing tumour incidence (Huff et al., 1989). The occurrence of lesions presumed to be preneoplastic may in certain instances aid in assessing the biological plausibility of any neoplastic response observed. If an agent or mixture induces only benign neoplasms that appear to be end-points that do not readily undergo transition to malignancy, it should nevertheless be suspected of being a carcinogen and requires further investigation.

(b) Quantitative aspects

The probability that tumours will occur may depend on the species, sex, strain and age of the animal, the dose of the carcinogen and the route and length of exposure. Evidence of an increased incidence of neoplasms with increased level of exposure strengthens the inference of a causal association between the exposure and the development of neoplasms.

The form of the dose–response relationship can vary widely, depending on the particular agent under study and the target organ. Both DNA damage and increased cell division are important aspects of carcinogenesis, and cell proliferation is a strong determinant of dose–response relationships for some carcinogens (Cohen & Ellwein, 1990). Since many chemicals require metabolic activation before being converted into their reactive intermediates, both metabolic and pharmacokinetic aspects are important in determining the dose–response pattern. Saturation of steps such as absorption, activation, inactivation and elimination may produce nonlinearity in the dose–response relationship, as could saturation of processes such as DNA repair (Hoel et al., 1983; Gart et al., 1986).

(c) Statistical analysis of long-term experiments in animals

Factors considered by the Working Group include the adequacy of the information given for each treatment group: (i) the number of animals studied and the number examined histologically, (ii) the number of animals with a given tumour type and (iii) length of survival. The statistical methods used should be clearly stated and should be the generally accepted techniques refined for this purpose (Peto et al., 1980; Gart et al., 1986). When there is no difference in survival between control and treatment groups, the Working Group usually compares the proportions of animals developing each tumour type in each of the groups. Otherwise, consideration is given as to whether or not appropriate adjustments have been made for differences in survival. These adjustments can include: comparisons of the proportions of tumour-bearing animals among the effective number of animals (alive at the time the first tumour is discovered), in the case where most differences in survival occur before tumours appear; life-table methods, when tumours are visible or when they may be considered 'fatal' because mortality rapidly follows tumour development; and the Mantel-Haenszel test or logistic regression, when occult tumours do not affect the animals' risk of dying but are 'incidental' findings at autopsy.

In practice, classifying tumours as fatal or incidental may be difficult. Several survival-adjusted methods have been developed that do not require this distinction (Gart *et al.*, 1986), although they have not been fully evaluated.

10. OTHER DATA RELEVANT TO AN EVALUATION OF CARCINOGENI-CITY AND ITS MECHANISMS

In coming to an overall evaluation of carcinogenicity in humans (see pp. 23–25), the Working Group also considers related data. The nature of the information selected for the summary depends on the agent being considered.

For chemicals and complex mixtures of chemicals such as those in some occupational situations and involving cultural habits (e.g., tobacco smoking), the other data considered to be relevant are divided into those on absorption, distribution, metabolism and excretion; toxic effects; reproductive and developmental effects; and genetic and related effects.

Concise information is given on absorption, distribution (including placental transfer) and excretion in both humans and experimental animals. Kinetic factors that may affect the dose–response relationship, such as saturation of uptake, protein binding, metabolic activation, detoxification and DNA repair processes, are mentioned. Studies that indicate the metabolic fate of the agent in humans and in experimental animals are summarized briefly, and comparisons of data from humans and animals are made when possible. Comparative information on the relationship between exposure and the dose that reaches the target site may be of particular importance for extrapolation between species. Data are given on acute and chronic toxic effects (other than cancer), such as organ toxicity, increased cell proliferation, immunotoxicity and endocrine effects. The presence and toxicological significance of cellular receptors is described. Effects on reproduction, teratogenicity, fetotoxicity and embryotoxicity are also summarized briefly.

Tests of genetic and related effects are described in view of the relevance of gene mutation and chromosomal damage to carcinogenesis (Vainio *et al.*, 1992). The adequacy of the reporting of sample characterization is considered and, where necessary, commented upon; with regard to complex mixtures, such comments are similar to those described for animal carcinogenicity tests on p. 18. The available data are interpreted critically by phylogenetic group according to the end-points detected, which may include DNA damage, gene mutation, sister chromatid exchange, micronucleus formation, chromosomal aberrations, aneuploidy and cell transformation. The concentrations employed are given, and mention is made of whether use of an exogenous metabolic system *in vitro* affected the test result. These data are given as listings of test systems, data and references; bar graphs (activity profiles) and corresponding summary tables with detailed information on the preparation of the profiles (Waters *et al.*, 1987) are given in appendices.

Positive results in tests using prokaryotes, lower eukaryotes, plants, insects and cultured mammalian cells suggest that genetic and related effects could occur in mammals. Results from such tests may also give information about the types of genetic effect produced and about the involvement of metabolic activation. Some end-points described are clearly genetic in nature (e.g., gene mutations and chromosomal aberrations), while others are to a greater or lesser degree associated with genetic effects (e.g., unscheduled DNA synthesis). In-vitro tests for tumour-promoting activity and for cell transformation may be sensitive to changes that are not necessarily the result of genetic alterations but that may have specific relevance to the process of carcinogenesis. A critical appraisal of these tests has been published (Montesano *et al.*, 1986).

Genetic or other activity manifest in experimental mammals and humans is regarded as being of greater relevance than that in other organisms. The demonstration that an agent or mixture can induce gene and chromosomal mutations in whole mammals indicates that it may have carcinogenic activity, although this activity may not be detectably expressed in any or all species. Relative potency in tests for mutagenicity and related effects is not a reliable indicator of carcinogenic potency. Negative results in tests for mutagenicity in selected tissues from animals treated *in vivo* provide less weight, partly because they do not exclude the possibility of an effect in tissues other than those examined. Moreover, negative results in short-term tests with genetic end-points cannot be considered to provide evidence to rule out carcinogenicity of agents or mixtures that act through other mechanisms (e.g., receptor-mediated effects, cellular toxicity with regenerative proliferation, peroxisome proliferation) (Vainio *et al.*, 1992). Factors that may lead to misleading results in short-term tests have been discussed in detail elsewhere (Montesano *et al.*, 1986).

When available, data relevant to mechanisms of carcinogenesis that do not involve structural changes at the level of the gene are also described.

The adequacy of epidemiological studies of reproductive outcome and genetic and related effects in humans is evaluated by the same criteria as are applied to epidemiological studies of cancer.

Structure–activity relationships that may be relevant to an evaluation of the carcinogenicity of an agent are also described.

For biological agents — viruses, bacteria and parasites — other data relevant to carcinogenicity include descriptions of the pathology of infection, molecular biology (integration and expression of viruses, and any genetic alterations seen in human tumours) and other observations, which might include cellular and tissue responses to infection, immune response and the presence of tumour markers.

11. SUMMARY OF DATA REPORTED

In this section, the relevant epidemiological and experimental data are summarized. Only reports, other than in abstract form, that meet the criteria outlined on p. 11 are considered for evaluating carcinogenicity. Inadequate studies are generally not summarized: such studies are usually identified by a square-bracketed comment in the preceding text.

(a) Exposure

Human exposure to chemicals and complex mixtures is summarized on the basis of elements such as production, use, occurrence in the environment and determinations in human tissues and body fluids. Quantitative data are given when available. Exposure to biological agents is described in terms of transmission, and prevalence of infection.

(b) Carcinogenicity in humans

Results of epidemiological studies that are considered to be pertinent to an assessment of human carcinogenicity are summarized. When relevant, case reports and correlation studies are also summarized.

(c) Carcinogenicity in experimental animals

Data relevant to an evaluation of carcinogenicity in animals are summarized. For each animal species and route of administration, it is stated whether an increased incidence of neoplasms or preneoplastic lesions was observed, and the tumour sites are indicated. If the agent or mixture produced tumours after prenatal exposure or in single-dose experiments, this is also indicated. Negative findings are also summarized. Dose–response and other quantitative data may be given when available.

(d) Other data relevant to an evaluation of carcinogenicity and its mechanisms

Data on biological effects in humans that are of particular relevance are summarized. These may include toxicological, kinetic and metabolic considerations and evidence of DNA binding, persistence of DNA lesions or genetic damage in exposed humans. Toxicological information, such as that on cytotoxicity and regeneration, receptor binding and hormonal and immunological effects, and data on kinetics and metabolism in experimental animals are given when considered relevant to the possible mechanism of the carcinogenic action of the agent. The results of tests for genetic and related effects are summarized for whole mammals, cultured mammalian cells and nonmammalian systems.

When available, comparisons of such data for humans and for animals, and particularly animals that have developed cancer, are described.

Structure–activity relationships are mentioned when relevant.

For the agent, mixture or exposure circumstance being evaluated, the available data on end-points or other phenomena relevant to mechanisms of carcinogenesis from studies in humans, experimental animals and tissue and cell test systems are summarized within one or more of the following descriptive dimensions:

(i) Evidence of genotoxicity (structural changes at the level of the gene): for example, structure–activity considerations, adduct formation, mutagenicity (effect on specific genes), chromosomal mutation/aneuploidy

(ii)   Evidence of effects on the expression of relevant genes (functional changes at the intracellular level): for example, alterations to the structure or quantity of the product of a proto-oncogene or tumour-suppressor gene, alterations to metabolic activation/-inactivation/DNA repair

(iii)   Evidence of relevant effects on cell behaviour (morphological or behavioural changes at the cellular or tissue level): for example, induction of mitogenesis, compensatory cell proliferation, preneoplasia and hyperplasia, survival of premalignant or malignant cells (immortalization, immunosuppression), effects on metastatic potential

(iv)   Evidence from dose and time relationships of carcinogenic effects and interactions between agents: for example, early/late stage, as inferred from epidemiological studies; initiation/promotion/progression/malignant conversion, as defined in animal carcinogenicity experiments; toxicokinetics

These dimensions are not mutually exclusive, and an agent may fall within more than one of them. Thus, for example, the action of an agent on the expression of relevant genes could be summarized under both the first and second dimensions, even if it were known with reasonable certainty that those effects resulted from genotoxicity.

12. EVALUATION

Evaluations of the strength of the evidence for carcinogenicity arising from human and experimental animal data are made, using standard terms.

It is recognized that the criteria for these evaluations, described below, cannot encompass all of the factors that may be relevant to an evaluation of carcinogenicity. In considering all of the relevant scientific data, the Working Group may assign the agent, mixture or exposure circumstance to a higher or lower category than a strict interpretation of these criteria would indicate.

(a)   Degrees of evidence for carcinogenicity in humans and in experimental animals and supporting evidence

These categories refer only to the strength of the evidence that an exposure is carcinogenic and not to the extent of its carcinogenic activity (potency) nor to the mechanisms involved. A classification may change as new information becomes available.

An evaluation of degree of evidence, whether for a single agent or a mixture, is limited to the materials tested, as defined physically, chemically or biologically. When the agents evaluated are considered by the Working Group to be sufficiently closely related, they may be grouped together for the purpose of a single evaluation of degree of evidence.

(i)   Carcinogenicity in humans

The applicability of an evaluation of the carcinogenicity of a mixture, process, occupation or industry on the basis of evidence from epidemiological studies depends on the variability over time and place of the mixtures, processes, occupations and industries. The Working Group seeks to identify the specific exposure, process or activity which is considered most likely to be responsible for any excess risk. The evaluation is focused as narrowly as the available data on exposure and other aspects permit.

The evidence relevant to carcinogenicity from studies in humans is classified into one of the following categories:

Sufficient evidence of carcinogenicity: The Working Group considers that a causal relationship has been established between exposure to the agent, mixture or exposure circumstance and human cancer. That is, a positive relationship has been observed between the exposure and cancer in studies in which chance, bias and confounding could be ruled out with reasonable confidence.

Limited evidence of carcinogenicity: A positive association has been observed between exposure to the agent, mixture or exposure circumstance and cancer for which a causal interpretation is considered by the Working Group to be credible, but chance, bias or confounding could not be ruled out with reasonable confidence.

Inadequate evidence of carcinogenicity: The available studies are of insufficient quality, consistency or statistical power to permit a conclusion regarding the presence or absence of a causal association, or no data on cancer in humans are available.

Evidence suggesting lack of carcinogenicity: There are several adequate studies covering the full range of levels of exposure that human beings are known to encounter, which are mutually consistent in not showing a positive association between exposure to the agent, mixture or exposure circumstance and any studied cancer at any observed level of exposure. A conclusion of 'evidence suggesting lack of carcinogenicity' is inevitably limited to the cancer sites, conditions and levels of exposure and length of observation covered by the available studies. In addition, the possibility of a very small risk at the levels of exposure studied can never be excluded.

In some instances, the above categories may be used to classify the degree of evidence related to carcinogenicity in specific organs or tissues.

(ii) *Carcinogenicity in experimental animals*

The evidence relevant to carcinogenicity in experimental animals is classified into one of the following categories:

Sufficient evidence of carcinogenicity: The Working Group considers that a causal relationship has been established between the agent or mixture and an increased incidence of malignant neoplasms or of an appropriate combination of benign and malignant neoplasms in (a) two or more species of animals or (b) in two or more independent studies in one species carried out at different times or in different laboratories or under different protocols.

Exceptionally, a single study in one species might be considered to provide sufficient evidence of carcinogenicity when malignant neoplasms occur to an unusual degree with regard to incidence, site, type of tumour or age at onset.

Limited evidence of carcinogenicity: The data suggest a carcinogenic effect but are limited for making a definitive evaluation because, e.g., (a) the evidence of carcinogenicity is restricted to a single experiment; or (b) there are unresolved questions regarding the adequacy of the design, conduct or interpretation of the study; or (c) the agent or mixture increases the incidence only of benign neoplasms or lesions of uncertain neoplastic potential, or of certain neoplasms which may occur spontaneously in high incidences in certain strains.

Inadequate evidence of carcinogenicity: The studies cannot be interpreted as showing either the presence or absence of a carcinogenic effect because of major qualitative or quantitative limitations, or no data on cancer in experimental animals are available.

Evidence suggesting lack of carcinogenicity: Adequate studies involving at least two species are available which show that, within the limits of the tests used, the agent or mixture is not carcinogenic. A conclusion of evidence suggesting lack of carcinogenicity is inevitably limited to the species, tumour sites and levels of exposure studied.

(b)   *Other data relevant to the evaluation of carcinogenicity and its mechanisms*

Other evidence judged to be relevant to an evaluation of carcinogenicity and of sufficient importance to affect the overall evaluation is then described. This may include data on preneoplastic lesions, tumour pathology, genetic and related effects, structure–activity relationships, metabolism and pharmacokinetics, physicochemical parameters and analogous biological agents.

Data relevant to mechanisms of the carcinogenic action are also evaluated. The strength of the evidence that any carcinogenic effect observed is due to a particular mechanism is assessed, using terms such as weak, moderate or strong. Then, the Working Group assesses if that particular mechanism is likely to be operative in humans. The strongest indications that a particular mechanism operates in humans come from data on humans or biological specimens obtained from exposed humans. The data may be considered to be especially relevant if they show that the agent in question has caused changes in exposed humans that are on the causal pathway to carcinogenesis. Such data may, however, never become available, because it is at least conceivable that certain compounds may be kept from human use solely on the basis of evidence of their toxicity and/or carcinogenicity in experimental systems.

For complex exposures, including occupational and industrial exposures, the chemical composition and the potential contribution of carcinogens known to be present are considered by the Working Group in its overall evaluation of human carcinogenicity. The Working Group also determines the extent to which the materials tested in experimental systems are related to those to which humans are exposed.

(c)   *Overall evaluation*

Finally, the body of evidence is considered as a whole, in order to reach an overall evaluation of the carcinogenicity to humans of an agent, mixture or circumstance of exposure.

An evaluation may be made for a group of chemical compounds that have been evaluated by the Working Group. In addition, when supporting data indicate that other, related compounds for which there is no direct evidence of capacity to induce cancer in humans or in animals may also be carcinogenic, a statement describing the rationale for this conclusion is added to the evaluation narrative; an additional evaluation may be made for this broader group of compounds if the strength of the evidence warrants it.

The agent, mixture or exposure circumstance is described according to the wording of one of the following categories, and the designated group is given. The categorization of an agent, mixture or exposure circumstance is a matter of scientific judgement, reflecting the strength of the evidence derived from studies in humans and in experimental animals and from other relevant data.

Group 1 — The agent (mixture) is carcinogenic to humans.
The exposure circumstance entails exposures that are carcinogenic to humans.

This category is used when there is *sufficient evidence* of carcinogenicity in humans. Exceptionally, an agent (mixture) may be placed in this category when evidence in humans is less than sufficient but there is *sufficient evidence* of carcinogenicity in experimental animals and strong evidence in exposed humans that the agent (mixture) acts through a relevant mechanism of carcinogenicity.

Group 2

This category includes agents, mixtures and exposure circumstances for which, at one extreme, the degree of evidence of carcinogenicity in humans is almost sufficient, as well as those for which, at the other extreme, there are no human data but for which there is evidence of carcinogenicity in experimental animals. Agents, mixtures and exposure circumstances are assigned to either group 2A (probably carcinogenic to humans) or group 2B (possibly carcinogenic to humans) on the basis of epidemiological and experimental evidence of carcinogenicity and other relevant data.

Group 2A — The agent (mixture) is probably carcinogenic to humans.
The exposure circumstance entails exposures that are probably carcinogenic to humans.

This category is used when there is *limited evidence* of carcinogenicity in humans and sufficient evidence of carcinogenicity in experimental animals. In some cases, an agent (mixture) may be classified in this category when there is inadequate evidence of carcinogenicity in humans and *sufficient evidence* of carcinogenicity in experimental animals and strong evidence that the carcinogenesis is mediated by a mechanism that also operates in humans. Exceptionally, an agent, mixture or exposure circumstance may be classified in this category solely on the basis of limited evidence of carcinogenicity in humans.

Group 2B — The agent (mixture) is possibly carcinogenic to humans.
The exposure circumstance entails exposures that are possibly carcinogenic to humans.

This category is used for agents, mixtures and exposure circumstances for which there is *limited evidence* of carcinogenicity in humans and less than *sufficient evidence* of carcinogenicity in experimental animals. It may also be used when there is *inadequate evidence* of carcinogenicity in humans but there is *sufficient evidence* of carcinogenicity in experimental animals. In some instances, an agent, mixture or exposure circumstance for which there is *inadequate evidence* of carcinogenicity in humans but *limited evidence* of carcinogenicity in experimental animals together with supporting evidence from other relevant data may be placed in this group.

Group 3 — The agent (mixture or exposure circumstance) is not classifiable as to its carcinogenicity to humans.

This category is used most commonly for agents, mixtures and exposure circumstances for which the evidence of carcinogenicity is inadequate in humans and inadequate or limited in experimental animals.

Exceptionally, agents (mixtures) for which the evidence of carcinogenicity is inadequate in humans but sufficient in experimental animals may be placed in this category when there is strong evidence that the mechanism of carcinogenicity in experimental animals does not operate in humans.

Agents, mixtures and exposure circumstances that do not fall into any other group are also placed in this category.

Group 4 — The agent (mixture) is probably not carcinogenic to humans.

This category is used for agents or mixtures for which there is *evidence suggesting lack of carcinogenicity* in humans and in experimental animals. In some instances, agents or mixtures for which there is *inadequate evidence* of carcinogenicity in humans but *evidence suggesting lack of carcinogenicity* in experimental animals, consistently and strongly supported by a broad range of other relevant data, may be classified in this group.

References

Breslow, N.E. & Day, N.E. (1980) *Statistical Methods in Cancer Research*, Vol. 1, *The Analysis of Case–Control Studies* (IARC Scientific Publications No. 32), Lyon, IARC

Breslow, N.E. & Day, N.E. (1987) *Statistical Methods in Cancer Research*, Vol. 2, *The Design and Analysis of Cohort Studies* (IARC Scientific Publications No. 82), Lyon, IARC

Cohen, S.M. & Ellwein, L.B. (1990) Cell proliferation in carcinogenesis. *Science*, **249**, 1007–1011

Gart, J.J., Krewski, D., Lee, P.N., Tarone, R.E. & Wahrendorf, J. (1986) *Statistical Methods in Cancer Research*, Vol. 3, *The Design and Analysis of Long-term Animal Experiments* (IARC Scientific Publications No. 79), Lyon, IARC

Hoel, D.G., Kaplan, N.L. & Anderson, M.W. (1983) Implication of nonlinear kinetics on risk estimation in carcinogenesis. *Science*, **219**, 1032–1037

Huff, J.E., Eustis, S.L. & Haseman, J.K. (1989) Occurrence and relevance of chemically induced benign neoplasms in long-term carcinogenicity studies. *Cancer Metastasis Rev.*, **8**, 1–21

IARC (1973–1996) *Information Bulletin on the Survey of Chemicals Being Tested for Carcinogenicity/Directory of Agents Being Tested for Carcinogenicity*, Numbers 1–17, Lyon

IARC (1976–1996)
Directory of On-going Research in Cancer Epidemiology 1976. Edited by C.S. Muir & G. Wagner, Lyon

Directory of On-going Research in Cancer Epidemiology 1977 (IARC Scientific Publications No. 17). Edited by C.S. Muir & G. Wagner, Lyon

Directory of On-going Research in Cancer Epidemiology 1978 (IARC Scientific Publications No. 26). Edited by C.S. Muir & G. Wagner, Lyon

Directory of On-going Research in Cancer Epidemiology 1979 (IARC Scientific Publications No. 28). Edited by C.S. Muir & G. Wagner, Lyon

Directory of On-going Research in Cancer Epidemiology 1980 (IARC Scientific Publications No. 35). Edited by C.S. Muir & G. Wagner, Lyon

Directory of On-going Research in Cancer Epidemiology 1981 (IARC Scientific Publications No. 38). Edited by C.S. Muir & G. Wagner, Lyon

Directory of On-going Research in Cancer Epidemiology 1982 (IARC Scientific Publications No. 46). Edited by C.S. Muir & G. Wagner, Lyon

Directory of On-going Research in Cancer Epidemiology 1983 (IARC Scientific Publications No. 50). Edited by C.S. Muir & G. Wagner, Lyon

Directory of On-going Research in Cancer Epidemiology 1984 (IARC Scientific Publications No. 62). Edited by C.S. Muir & G. Wagner, Lyon

Directory of On-going Research in Cancer Epidemiology 1985 (IARC Scientific Publications No. 69). Edited by C.S. Muir & G. Wagner, Lyon

Directory of On-going Research in Cancer Epidemiology 1986 (IARC Scientific Publications No. 80). Edited by C.S. Muir & G. Wagner, Lyon

Directory of On-going Research in Cancer Epidemiology 1987 (IARC Scientific Publications No. 86). Edited by D.M. Parkin & J. Wahrendorf, Lyon

Directory of On-going Research in Cancer Epidemiology 1988 (IARC Scientific Publications No. 93). Edited by M. Coleman & J. Wahrendorf, Lyon

Directory of On-going Research in Cancer Epidemiology 1989/90 (IARC Scientific Publications No. 101). Edited by M. Coleman & J. Wahrendorf, Lyon

Directory of On-going Research in Cancer Epidemiology 1991 (IARC Scientific Publications No.110). Edited by M. Coleman & J. Wahrendorf, Lyon

Directory of On-going Research in Cancer Epidemiology 1992 (IARC Scientific Publications No. 117). Edited by M. Coleman, J. Wahrendorf & E. Démaret, Lyon

Directory of On-going Research in Cancer Epidemiology 1994 (IARC Scientific Publications No. 130). Edited by R. Sankaranarayanan, J. Wahrendorf & E. Démaret, Lyon

Directory of On-going Research in Cancer Epidemiology 1996 (IARC Scientific Publications No. 137). Edited by R. Sankaranarayanan, J. Wahrendorf & E. Démaret, Lyon

IARC (1977) *IARC Monographs Programme on the Evaluation of the Carcinogenic Risk of Chemicals to Humans*. Preamble (IARC intern. tech. Rep. No. 77/002), Lyon

IARC (1978) *Chemicals with* Sufficient Evidence *of Carcinogenicity in Experimental Animals* — IARC Monographs *Volumes 1–17* (IARC intern. tech. Rep. No. 78/003), Lyon

IARC (1978–1993) *Environmental Carcinogens. Methods of Analysis and Exposure Measurement*:

Vol. 1. *Analysis of Volatile Nitrosamines in Food* (IARC Scientific Publications No. 18). Edited by R. Preussmann, M. Castegnaro, E.A. Walker & A.E. Wasserman (1978)

Vol. 2. *Methods for the Measurement of Vinyl Chloride in Poly(vinyl chloride), Air, Water and Foodstuffs* (IARC Scientific Publications No. 22). Edited by D.C.M. Squirrell & W. Thain (1978)

Vol. 3. *Analysis of Polycyclic Aromatic Hydrocarbons in Environmental Samples* (IARC Scientific Publications No. 29). Edited by M. Castegnaro, P. Bogovski, H. Kunte & E.A. Walker (1979)

Vol. 4. *Some Aromatic Amines and Azo Dyes in the General and Industrial Environment* (IARC Scientific Publications No. 40). Edited by L. Fishbein, M. Castegnaro, I.K. O'Neill & H. Bartsch (1981)

Vol. 5. *Some Mycotoxins* (IARC Scientific Publications No. 44). Edited by L. Stoloff, M. Castegnaro, P. Scott, I.K. O'Neill & H. Bartsch (1983)

Vol. 6. *N-Nitroso Compounds* (IARC Scientific Publications No. 45). Edited by R. Preussmann, I.K. O'Neill, G. Eisenbrand, B. Spiegelhalder & H. Bartsch (1983)

Vol. 7. *Some Volatile Halogenated Hydrocarbons* (IARC Scientific Publications No. 68). Edited by L. Fishbein & I.K. O'Neill (1985)

Vol. 8. *Some Metals: As, Be, Cd, Cr, Ni, Pb, Se, Zn* (IARC Scientific Publications No. 71). Edited by I.K. O'Neill, P. Schuller & L. Fishbein (1986)

Vol. 9. *Passive Smoking* (IARC Scientific Publications No. 81). Edited by I.K. O'Neill, K.D. Brunnemann, B. Dodet & D. Hoffmann (1987)

Vol. 10. *Benzene and Alkylated Benzenes* (IARC Scientific Publications No. 85). Edited by L. Fishbein & I.K. O'Neill (1988)

Vol. 11. *Polychlorinated Dioxins and Dibenzofurans* (IARC Scientific Publications No. 108). Edited by C. Rappe, H.R. Buser, B. Dodet & I.K. O'Neill (1991)

Vol. 12. *Indoor Air* (IARC Scientific Publications No. 109). Edited by B. Seifert, H. van de Wiel, B. Dodet & I.K. O'Neill (1993)

IARC (1979) *Criteria to Select Chemicals for* IARC Monographs (IARC intern. tech. Rep. No. 79/003), Lyon

IARC (1982) *IARC Monographs on the Evaluation of the Carcinogenic Risk of Chemicals to Humans*, Supplement 4, *Chemicals, Industrial Processes and Industries Associated with Cancer in Humans* (IARC Monographs, Volumes 1 to 29), Lyon

IARC (1983) *Approaches to Classifying Chemical Carcinogens According to Mechanism of Action* (IARC intern. tech. Rep. No. 83/001), Lyon

IARC (1984) *Chemicals and Exposures to Complex Mixtures Recommended for Evaluation in IARC Monographs and Chemicals and Complex Mixtures Recommended for Long-term Carcinogenicity Testing* (IARC intern. tech. Rep. No. 84/002), Lyon

IARC (1987a) *IARC Monographs on the Evaluation of Carcinogenic Risks to Humans*, Supplement 6, *Genetic and Related Effects: An Updating of Selected* IARC Monographs *from Volumes 1 to 42*, Lyon

IARC (1987b) *IARC Monographs on the Evaluation of Carcinogenic Risks to Humans*, Supplement 7, *Overall Evaluations of Carcinogenicity: An Updating of* IARC Monographs *Volumes 1 to 42*, Lyon

IARC (1988) *Report of an IARC Working Group to Review the Approaches and Processes Used to Evaluate the Carcinogenicity of Mixtures and Groups of Chemicals* (IARC intern. tech. Rep. No. 88/002), Lyon

IARC (1989) *Chemicals, Groups of Chemicals, Mixtures and Exposure Circumstances to be Evaluated in Future IARC Monographs, Report of an ad hoc Working Group* (IARC intern. tech. Rep. No. 89/004), Lyon

IARC (1991a) *A Consensus Report of an IARC Monographs Working Group on the Use of Mechanisms of Carcinogenesis in Risk Identification* (IARC intern. tech. Rep. No. 91/002), Lyon

IARC (1991b) *Report of an Ad-hoc* IARC Monographs *Advisory Group on Viruses and Other Biological Agents Such as Parasites* (IARC intern. tech. Rep. No. 91/001), Lyon

IARC (1993) *Chemicals, Groups of Chemicals, Complex Mixtures, Physical and Biological Agents and Exposure Circumstances to be Evaluated in Future* IARC Monographs, *Report of an ad-hoc Working Group* (IARC intern. Rep. No. 93/005), Lyon

Montesano, R., Bartsch, H., Vainio, H., Wilbourn, J. & Yamasaki, H., eds (1986) *Long-term and Short-term Assays for Carcinogenesis — A Critical Appraisal* (IARC Scientific Publications No. 83), Lyon, IARC

Peto, R., Pike, M.C., Day, N.E., Gray, R.G., Lee, P.N., Parish, S., Peto, J., Richards, S. & Wahrendorf, J. (1980) Guidelines for simple, sensitive significance tests for carcinogenic effects in long-term animal experiments. In: *IARC Monographs on the Evaluation of the Carcinogenic Risk of Chemicals to Humans*, Supplement 2, *Long-term and Short-term Screening Assays for Carcinogens: A Critical Appraisal*, Lyon, pp. 311–426

Tomatis, L., Aitio, A., Wilbourn, J. & Shuker, L. (1989) Human carcinogens so far identified. *Jpn. J. Cancer Res.*, **80**, 795–807

Vainio, H., Magee, P.N., McGregor, D.B. & McMichael, A.J., eds (1992) *Mechanisms of Carcinogenesis in Risk Identification* (IARC Scientific Publications No. 116), Lyon, IARC

Vainio, H., Wilbourn, J.D., Sasco, A.J., Partensky, C., Gaudin, N., Heseltine, E. & Eragne, I. (1995) Identification of human carcinogenic risk in *IARC Monographs. Bull. Cancer*, **82**, 339–348 (in French)

Waters, M.D., Stack, H.F., Brady, A.L., Lohman, P.H.M., Haroun, L. & Vainio, H. (1987) Appendix 1. Activity profiles for genetic and related tests. In: *IARC Monographs on the Evaluation of Carcinogenic Risks to Humans*, Suppl. 6, *Genetic and Related Effects: An Updating of Selected IARC Monographs from Volumes 1 to 42*, Lyon, IARC, pp. 687–696

Wilbourn, J., Haroun, L., Heseltine, E., Kaldor, J., Partensky, C. & Vainio, H. (1986) Response of experimental animals to human carcinogens: an analysis based upon the IARC Monographs Programme. *Carcinogenesis*, **7**, 1853–1863

THE MONOGRAPHS

POLYCHLORINATED DIBENZO-*para*-DIOXINS

These substances were considered by previous working groups, in February 1977 (IARC, 1977a) and March 1987 (IARC, 1987a). Since that time, new data have become available and these have been incorporated in the monograph and taken into consideration in the evaluation.

1. Exposure Data

1.1 Chemical and physical data

1.1.1 *Nomenclature and molecular formulae and weights*

Chemical Abstracts Service (CAS) names and synonyms, CAS Registry numbers, molecular formulae and molecular weights for dibenzo-*para*-dioxin and selected polychlorinated dibenzo-*para*-dioxins (PCDDs) are presented in **Table 1**. The tetra-, penta, hexa- and hepta-chlorinated compounds are referred to here as TCDDs, PeCDDs, HxCDDs and HpCDDs or collectively as, for example, Cl_4–Cl_7 CDDs or hepta/octa-CDDs.

1.1.2 *Structural formulae*

The general structure of the PCDDs is shown in **Table 2**. Any or all of the eight hydrogen atoms of dibenzo-*para*-dioxin can be replaced with chlorine, giving rise to 75 possible chlorinated dibenzo-*para*-dioxin structures. All of the 75 are referred to as congeners (members of a like group) of one another and congeners having the same number of chlorines are isomers. The term 'dioxins' has been widely used to refer to the PCDDs and often the polychlorinated dibenzofurans (PCDFs) as well (Liem & van Zorge, 1995), although it is technically incorrect (Clement, 1991) and is not so used in this monograph.

1.1.3 *Chemical and physical properties*

Knowledge of basic chemical and physical properties is essential to understanding and modelling environmental transport and fate as well as pharmacokinetic and toxicological behaviour. The most important parameters for the PCDDs appear to be water solubility, vapour pressure, and octanol/water partition coefficient (K_{ow}). The ratio of vapour pressure to water solubility yields the Henry's Law constant for dilute solutions of organic compounds, an index of partitioning for a compound between the vapour and aqueous solution phases (Mackay *et al.*, 1991). Chemical and physical properties of selected PCDDs are presented in **Table 3**.

Table 1. Nomenclature, molecular formulae, and molecular weights of dibenzo-dioxin and chlorinated derivatives

CAS Reg. No. (Deleted CAS Nos)	CAS name and synonyms[a]	Molecular formula	Molecular weight
262-23-4	**Dibenzo[*b,e*][1,4]dioxin**; Dibenzodioxin; dibenzo-[1,4]dioxin; dibenzo-*para*-dioxin; diphenylene dioxide; oxanthrene; phenodioxin; DD	$C_{12}H_8O_2$	184.2
33857-26-0	**2,7-Dichlorodibenzo[*b,e*][1,4]dioxin**; 2,7-dichloro-dibenzo-*para*-dioxin; 2,7-DCDD; 2,7-dichlorodibenzo-dioxins; 2,7-diCDD	$C_{12}H_6Cl_2O_2$	253.0
1746-01-6 (56795-67-6)	**2,3,7,8-Tetrachlorodibenzo[*b,e*][1,4]dioxin**; D48; dioxin; TCDBD; TCDD; 2,3,7,8-TCDD; 2,3,7,8-tetra-chlorodibenzo-1,4-dioxin; 2,3,7,8-tetrachlorodibenzo-*para*-dioxin; 2,3,7,8-tetraCDD	$C_{12}H_4Cl_4O_2$	321.98
40321-76-4	**1,2,3,7,8-Pentachlorodibenzo[*b,e*][1,4]dioxin**; D54; 1,2,3,7,8-PeCDD; 1,2,3,7,8-PnCDD; 1,2,3,7,8-penta-chlorodibenzo-*para*-dioxin; 1,2,3,7,8-pentachloro-dibenzodioxin; 2,3,4,7,8-pentachlorodibenzo-*para*-dioxin; 2,3,4,7,8-pentachlorodibenzodioxin; 1,2,3,7,8-pentaCDD	$C_{12}H_3Cl_5O_2$	356.42
39227-28-6	**1,2,3,4,7,8-Hexachlorodibenzo[*b,e*][1,4]dioxin**; D66; 1,2,3,4,7,8-hexachlorodibenzodioxin; 1,2,3,4,7,8-hexa-chlorodibenzo-*para*-dioxin; 1,2,3,4,7,8-hexachloro-dibenzo[1,4]dioxin; 1,2,3,4,7,8-HxCDD; 1,2,3,4,7,8-hexaCDD	$C_{12}H_2Cl_6O_2$	390.87
57653-85-7	**1,2,3,6,7,8-Hexachlorodibenzo[*b,e*][1,4]dioxin**; D67; 1,2,3,6,7,8-hexachlorodibenzodioxin; 1,2,3,6,7,8-hexa-chlorodibenzo-*para*-dioxin; 1,2,3,6,7,8-hexachloro-dibenzo[1,4]dioxin; 1,2,3,6,7,8-HxCDD; 1,2,3,6,7,8-hexaCDD	$C_{12}H_2Cl_6O_2$	390.87
19408-74-3	**1,2,3,7,8,9-Hexachlorodibenzo[*b,e*][1,4]dioxin**; D70; 1,2,3,7,8,9-hexachlorodibenzodioxin; 1,2,3,7,8,9-hexa-chlorodibenzo-*para*-dioxin; 1,2,3,7,8,9-hexachloro-dibenzo[1,4]dioxin; 1,2,3,7,8,9-HxCDD; 1,2,3,7,8,9-hexaCDD	$C_{12}H_2Cl_6O_2$	390.87
35822-46-9	**1,2,3,4,6,7,8-Heptachlorodibenzo[*b,e*][1,4]dioxin**; D73; 1,2,3,4,6,7,8-heptachlorodibenzodioxin; heptachloro-dibenzo-*para*-dioxin; 1,2,3,4,6,7,8-heptachlorodibenzo-*para*-dioxin; 1,2,3,4,6,7,8-heptachlorodibenzo[1,4]dioxin; 1,2,3,4,6,7,8-HpCDD; 1,2,3,4,6,7,8-heptaCDD	$C_{12}HCl_7O_2$	425.31
3268-87-9	**Octachlorodibenzo[*b,e*][1,4]dioxin**; D75; OCDD; octa-chlorodibenzo-*para*-dioxin; 1,2,3,4,6,7,8,9-octachloro-dibenzo-*para*-dioxin; 1,2,3,4,6,7,8,9-octachlorodibenzo-[1,4]dioxin; octaCDD	$C_{12}Cl_8O_2$	460.76

[a] Names in bold letters are the Chemical Abstracts Service (CAS) names

Table 2. Dibenzo-*para*-dioxin structural formula and numbers of chlorinated isomers

Formula

No. of chlorines (x + y)	No. of isomers
1	2
2	10
3	14
4	22
5	14
6	10
7	2
8	1
Total	75

Table 3. Chemical and physical properties of dibenzo-*para*-dioxin and selected chlorinated derivatives[a]

Chemical	Melting point (°C)	Water solubility (mg/L) at 25 °C	Vapour pressure (Pa) at 25 °C	Henry's Law constant (Pa × m³/mol)	log K_{ow}
Dibenzo-*para*-dioxin	122–123	0.87	5.5×10^{-2}	11.70	4.30
2,7-DCDD	209–210	3.75×10^{-3}	1.2×10^{-4}	8.10	5.75
2,3,7,8-TCDD	305–306	1.93×10^{-5}	2.0×10^{-7}	3.34	6.80
1,2,3,7,8-PeCDD	240–241		5.8×10^{-8}		6.64
1,2,3,4,7,8-HxCDD	273–275	4.42×10^{-6}	5.1×10^{-9}	1.08	7.80
1,2,3,6,7,8-HxCDD	285–286		4.8×10^{-9}		
1,2,3,7,8,9-HxCDD	243–244		6.5×10^{-9}		
1,2,3,4,6,7,8-HpCDD	264–265	2.40×10^{-6}	7.5×10^{-10}	1.27	8.00
OCDD	325–326	0.74×10^{-7}	1.1×10^{-10}	0.68	8.20

[a] From Rordorf (1987); Sijm *et al.* (1989); Mackay *et al.* (1991)

Limited research has been carried out to determine physical and chemical properties of PCDDs. The tetra- through octa-chloro congeners with 2,3,7,8-chlorination (sometimes referred to as laterally substituted PCDDs) have received the most attention, with 2,3,7,8-TCDD being the most intensively studied compound. Of the large number of possible congeners, only the 2,3,7,8-chlorinated compounds and a few others are available commercially, and synthesis and separation can be both time-consuming and difficult. Some of the PCDD congeners have not yet been prepared in pure form. The PCDDs are intentionally prepared only for research purposes.

The concept of toxic equivalency factors (TEFs) was developed by several agencies and national and international organizations (Ahlborg *et al.*, 1988; Safe, 1990; Ahlborg *et al.*, 1992a) to aid the interpretation of the complex database and in the evaluation of the risk of exposure to mixtures of structurally related PCDDs and PCDFs. TEF values are derived by evaluating the potency of each PCDD and PCDF isomer relative to that of 2,3,7,8-tetrachlorodibenzo-*para*-dioxin (2,3,7,8-TCDD). TEFs are order-of-magnitude estimates that are based on the evaluation of all available information, including binding to the Ah receptor (see Section 4.3.1) and other in-vitro responses as well as in-vivo effects ranging from enzyme induction to tumour formation (Ahlborg *et al.*, 1992a).

The concentrations of all the individual PCDDs and PCDFs in a mixture may be converted into one value of toxic equivalents (TEQs), as follows:

$$TEQ = \Sigma \, (TEF \times concentration)$$

Toxicologists have widely adopted the set of TEFs shown in **Table 4** (I-TEFs, also adopted by NATO (North Atlantic Treaty Organization)). Other sets of TEFs have been used in the past (e.g., BGA (German), Nordic, Swiss, Eadon (American)), but TEQs calculated with these TEFs normally do not differ from those based on I-TEFs by more than a factor of 2 (Ahlborg *et al.*, 1988; Rappe *et al.*, 1993).

Table 4. I-TEFs for 2,3,7,8-substituted PCDDs[a]

Congener	I-TEF
2,3,7,8-TCDD	1
1,2,3,7,8-PeCDD	0.5
1,2,3,4,7,8-HxCDD	0.1
1,2,3,6,7,8-HxCDD	0.1
1,2,3,7,8,9-HxCDD	0.1
1,2,3,4,6,7,8-HpCDD	0.01
OCDD	0.001
All other PCDDs	0

[a]From Ahlborg *et al.* (1992a)
I-TEF, international toxic equivalency factor

1.1.4   *Methods of analysis*

The analysis of environmental and biological samples for PCDDs and PCDFs has presented a major challenge for analytical chemists and has catalysed the development of new and improved methods and equipment with applications to many other problems in environmental chemistry. The challenge in PCDD/PCDF analysis arises from several factors. First, these compounds are usually present at very low levels in environmental samples, requiring methods with detection limits several orders of magnitude lower than those for other environmental contaminants. In addition, the toxicities of the various PCDD/PCDF congeners differ dramatically, so that for a proper risk assessment, individual PCDD and PCDF isomers must be selectively determined, often in the presence of other isomers and congeners. Interference between congeners and with other chlorinated compounds in the matrix can cause serious analytical difficulties. The widespread occurrence of these compounds in the environment has required the development of methods for many different media and sample types.

Progress in the analytical chemistry of the PCDDs and PCDFs over the past 30 years has been remarkable (Buser, 1991; Clement, 1991; de Jong & Liem, 1993). In the 1960s and early 1970s, the principal method of analysis was packed column gas chromatography (GC) with electron capture detection (ECD), and detection limits were in the parts-per-million (ppm; µg/g or mg/kg) to parts-per-billion (ppb; ng/g or µg/kg) range. Most work during this period focused on the determination of levels of 2,3,7,8-TCDD as a contaminant in herbicides and other industrial chemicals, and PCDDs and PCDFs were frequently not detected in environmental samples due to the lack of sensitivity and specificity of the methods.

Beginning in the 1970s, mass spectrometry (MS) was used, first by direct injection of samples and extracts, to reduce interferences and confirm the presence of 2,3,7,8-TCDD (Baughman & Meselson, 1973a,b). Soon, the advantages of MS as a detection method with GC were recognized, and GC-MS became the analytical method of choice for PCDDs and PCDFs in environmental and biological samples (Hass & Friesen, 1979; Rappe, 1984a; Crummett *et al.*, 1986). Advances in sample clean-up procedures, gas chromatographic separations with fused silica capillary columns and GC-MS systems in the 1970s and 1980s and the availability of appropriate calibration standards have made it possible now to identify and quantify individually all of the 2,3,7,8-substituted PCDDs and PCDFs at ng/kg concentrations or lower in most matrices (Clement & Tosine, 1988; Buser, 1991; Clement, 1991). However, these methods for ultra-trace analysis remain complex and difficult, and considerable variability still exists among laboratories in their capabilities and skill in performing these analyses (Stephens *et al.*, 1992).

Guidelines and methods of analysis have been proposed or established by a number of international and national governmental organizations and agencies. Examples include IARC Scientific Publications No. 108 (Rappe *et al.*, 1991a), recommendations from a workshop convened by the Community Bureau of Reference of the Commission of the European Union (Maier *et al.*, 1994) and United States Environmental Protection Agency Methods (United States Environmental Protection Agency, 1986, 1995, 1996a).

(a)   *General considerations*

The recognition by toxicologists of the extreme toxicity and biological activity of some PCDD/PCDF congeners has generated the requirement for highly sensitive and specific analytical methods. Method development has been directed primarily at the quantitative determination of the seven PCDDs and 10 PCDFs with chlorine at the 2, 3, 7 and 8 positions on the aromatic rings (see **Table 2** in this monograph as well as Table 2 in PCDF monograph). The remaining 68 PCDDs and 125 PCDFs can seriously interfere with the determination of the 2,3,7,8-substituted congeners. In addition, the pattern of congeners in an environmental sample can provide clues as to the source of the PCDDs/-PCDFs. The larger number of isomers with four or five chlorines (see **Table 1**) makes isomer-specific analysis more difficult in the tetra- and penta-substituted series (Rappe, 1984a; Buser, 1991; Clement, 1991).

Ultra-trace PCDD/PCDF analyses can require sample enrichment by a few thousand-fold to a million-fold or more before GC-MS determination. Co-extracted, interfering compounds may be present in the sample at much higher levels than the PCDDs and PCDFs, necessitating sophisticated matrix-specific clean-up techniques as well as highly selective separation and detection methods (Clement & Tosine, 1988; Buser, 1991; de Jong & Liem, 1993).

Two different strategies have been applied in PCDD/PCDF analyses. In the first approach, the objective is to recover all PCDDs and PCDFs in a single fraction by a containment-enrichment procedure, and then to analyse this fraction for all congeners by high-resolution GC-MS. In this approach, congener distribution patterns can be obtained that may help to identify sources of the PCDDs/PCDFs. The second approach focuses on separation of isomers during sample preparation and purification (e.g., by including reversed-phase and normal-phase high-performance liquid chromatography (HPLC) steps in the clean-up procedures) and results in multiple fractions that may be analysed for one or more congeners. This approach has often been applied to the determination of a specific congener, such as 2,3,7,8-TCDD (Rappe, 1984a; Buser, 1991).

Analyte standards for calibration are essential in ultra-trace analysis, and by the mid-1980s an adequate set of labelled and unlabelled PCDDs and PCDFs had become commercially available. Although not all of the 210 PCDD and PCDF congeners are available, all of the 2,3,7,8-substituted congeners can be purchased in crystalline form or in solution. These congeners are also available fully ^{13}C-labelled, and some are available fully labelled with [37]Cl. Analysis of environmental and biological samples requires the use of these standards for method development, to monitor recoveries and for isotope-dilution or other GC-MS analyses. It would be desirable to have available natural-matrix certified reference materials to verify spiked-sample recoveries based on calibration standards, but few are currently available (Rappe, 1984a; Clement & Tosine, 1988; Alvarez, 1991; Clement, 1991; Schimmel *et al.*, 1994; Maier *et al.*, 1995).

PCDD and PCDF determinations are frequently required for incinerator emissions (flue gases, fly ash, bottom ash and aqueous effluents), soils, sediments and sludges, air (vapour and particulates), water, biological samples of all types and chemical products. At present, typical detection limits of methods used for biological samples are in the

1 ng/kg range; lower detection limits are possible for some media, such as ambient air (in the low femtogram [10^{-15} g]/m^3 range) and drinking-water (as low as 0.01 pg/L), and higher detection limits (µg/kg range) are often adequate for chemical products (Buser, 1991; de Jong & Liem, 1993).

The analysis of PCDDs and PCDFs in environmental and biological samples can be considered to proceed in five stages, each of which must be carefully controlled and optimized to ensure reliable data: (1) sampling, (2) extraction, (3) clean-up, (4) separation and (5) quantification. Each of these stages is discussed briefly in the following sections. Reviews and guidelines have been published for various environmental and biological matrices (Buser, 1991; Maier *et al.*, 1994). The following comments are based on these reviews and the other references cited. In the subsequent text and tables, methods are indicated by the system presented in **Table 5**. In the text, this information is given as '(analytical method...)', using these abbreviations.

Table 5. Abbreviations for descriptions of analytical methods[a]

A	HRGC (high-resolution gas chromatography)
a	LRGC (low-resolution gas chromatography)
B	HRMS (high-resolution mass spectrometry)
C	LRMS (low-resolution mass spectrometry)
I	Isomer-specific polar column, e.g., SP 2330/31
O	Other than isomer-specific nonpolar column, e.g., DB-5
N	No information
S	Sophisticated clean-up, e.g., multicolumn, use of all ^{13}C-labelled 2,3,7,8-substituted standards
R	Reduced clean-up
W	WHO-accepted laboratory. The laboratory has fulfilled the requirements for interlaboratory studies of determination of PCDDs/PCDFs in biological material, organized by WHO (Stephens *et al.*, 1992; WHO, 1996).

[a]Descriptions usually have four elements: gas-chromatographic resolution (A or a), mass-spectrometric resolution (B or C), isomer-specificity of GC column (I or O) and clean-up (S or R). Any one or more of these may have no information (N).

(*b*) *Sampling*

The sampling protocols for PCDD and PCDF analyses depend on the type of sample, the level of PCDDs/PCDFs and potential interferences in the sample, the detection limit of the method, the requirements of the analysis, and the specific situations encountered. As with most ultra-trace analyses, sample size, homogeneity, storage and handling and the avoidance of contamination are important considerations.

Samples should be protected from light and heat. Although PCDDs and PCDFs are generally quite stable, they are prone to photolysis, especially in solution. The less chlorinated congeners tend to photolyse more rapidly than those with more chlorine substituents (ECETOC, 1992).

Contamination of samples is a serious problem. Potential sources of contamination include sampling equipment and containers, solvents and reagents, adsorbents, glassware, other samples and even laboratory tissue wipes, floor-cleaning solutions and cigarette smoke (Albro, 1979; Patterson *et al.*, 1990).

Samples to characterize incinerator emissions may include grab samples of fly ash (from electrostatic precipitators) and bottom ash (or slag), aqueous effluents from gas-scrubbing equipment and flue gases and particulates. Stack sampling is carried out iso-kinetically, collecting particulates on filters (e.g., glass fibres) and volatiles by cooling and trapping in impingers or on adsorbent resins. Collection efficiencies are checked by introducing isotope-labelled PCDDs and PCDFs into the sampling train (Ozvacic, 1986; ECETOC, 1992; United States Environmental Protection Agency, 1995). For measurement of flue gases of municipal waste incinerators operating with emissions below 0.1 ng I-TEQ/m^3 (European Union Directive; see Section 1.5), certain modifications in the sampling and analytical procedures are necessary, as described by Ball and Düwel (1996) and Bröker (1996).

PCDD and PCDF levels in air (particles and gases) are normally determined by collecting high-volume samples (up to 1000 m^3 over a 24-h period) on glass fibre/polyurethane foam filters (Tondeur *et al.*, 1991). For samples of, say, 1500 m^3 collected over several days, the filters should be spiked before sampling with ^{13}C-labelled standards to demonstrate possible sampling losses (Tysklind *et al.*, 1993).

PCDDs and PCDFs have very low solubilities in water, with solubility decreasing with increasing number of chlorine substituents. However, they tend to adsorb strongly onto fine particles suspended in water, so water samples must include suspended particulates and cannot be subsampled after collection unless they are first micro-filtered and the water and fine particulates are analysed separately. Small to medium sample volumes (1–5 L) can be extracted directly, but larger volumes needed for ultra-trace analysis are preconcentrated on sorbent resins (e.g., XAD-2) or a polyurethane filter (Ryan, 1991; Luksemburg, 1991).

Soils and sediments are sampled with core samplers at the surface (top 5–10 cm) and sometimes at lower depths. Often, several core samples are pooled for composite analysis (500–1000 g), based on a sampling grid for investigation of soil contamination in an area. Samples are air-dried, sieved (to remove debris), mixed and homogenized before extraction (Kleopfer *et al.*, 1985; Solch *et al.*, 1985; de Jong *et al.*, 1993; Fortunati *et al.*, 1994).

Biological samples should be deep frozen (–20 °C or lower) until analysed to prevent enzymatic or microbiological alterations. Choice of sampling procedures depends on the tissue and species; for example, usually only small samples of human fat are available, whereas larger samples of ecological species (e.g., fish) or foods normally can be obtained. Tissue samples may be ground with anhydrous sodium sulfate or silica gel and homogenized before extraction (Stanley *et al.*, 1985; Norstrom & Simon, 1991; Patterson *et al.*, 1991; Olsson, 1994).

In discussing problems associated with the variation in biological samples, Bignert *et al.* (1994) noted that large numbers of samples are generally required to define spatial or temporal trends or differences between various ecological matrices with respect to the concentrations of PCDDs and PCDFs.

(c)   Extraction

^{13}C-Labelled internal standards are added before extraction and clean-up to determine recoveries and to allow correction for losses during work-up. Homogenized samples are sometimes digested to destroy the sample matrix and free any trapped PCDDs/PCDFs before extraction (e.g., hydrochloric acid treatment of fly ash and some soil/sediment samples). However, alkaline saponification at elevated temperatures (which has some-times been used with fatty samples) is not recommended, as it can cause decomposition of PCDDs and PCDFs (Albro, 1979; Ryan *et al.*, 1989a). For chlorophenols and chloro-phenoxyacetic acid herbicides, initial separation of the (neutral) PCDDs and PCDFs is often accomplished by partitioning with alkali (Buser, 1991; United States Environmental Protection Agency, 1996a).

Extraction procedures and solvents vary widely, depending on the type of sample and method of clean-up and analysis. Extraction of PCDDs/PCDFs into solvent may be accomplished by simple dissolution, shaking, blending, ultrasonic treatment or Soxhlet extraction. For example, fats and oils may be dissolved directly in dichloromethane, and water samples may be extracted with dichloromethane, toluene or hexane. Particulates filtered from water or resin-sorbed water samples may require Soxhlet extraction with toluene or benzene. Incinerator flue gases (adsorbed on polyurethane foam) and fly or bottom ash are usually Soxhlet-extracted with toluene or benzene. For soils, sediments and sludges, sequential Soxhlet extractions with different and/or mixed solvents (acetone/hexane, toluene, benzene, dichloromethane) are sometimes required.

Many different extraction procedures and solvents have been used with biological samples, such as fish and animal tissues, human tissues and vegetation. Multi-laboratory comparison studies with fish tissues and porcine fat, human blood and adipose tissue and human and cow's milk suggest that acceptable recoveries can be obtained with a variety of extraction methods (Clement & Tosine, 1988; Patterson *et al.*, 1990; Stephens *et al.*, 1992; Schimmel *et al.*, 1994).

Supercritical fluid extraction (SFE) using carbon dioxide is a new technique, which has been used for extraction of PCDDs and PCDFs. Alexandrou *et al.* (1992) have used it for extraction of solid samples such as fly ash and paper pulp, and also for aqueous matrices such as pulp mill effluents. More recently van Bavel *et al.* (1996) have demonstrated the use of SFE in the extraction of biological samples, including human adipose tissue.

(d)   Clean-up

The objective of the clean-up procedures is to purify and prepare the extract for final separation and quantification. Such procedures remove co-extracted compounds that may interfere in the GC-MS analysis. The extent of clean-up required is determined by the analytical objectives (number of congeners to be quantified), the matrix and the sophistication of the GC-MS system.

Clean-up is normally accomplished by column chromatography through a series of columns, sometimes followed by HPLC. Pretreatment to remove large quantities of co-extractives may be necessary for some samples. Pretreatment may include acid or base washing; elution through multilayer columns containing silica gel impregnated with sulfuric acid, sodium hydroxide and silver nitrate (de Jong *et al.*, 1993); or gel permeation chromatography to remove lipids and other compounds of high molecular weight (Norstrom & Simon, 1991).

Column chromatography of extracts on alumina removes chlorinated benzenes, poly-chlorinated biphenyls (PCBs) and terphenyls, and higher chlorinated diphenyl ethers in a first fraction (2% dichloromethane in *n*-hexane); PCDDs and PCDFs are then recovered from the column with 50% dichloromethane in *n*-hexane. This treatment also removes the polychlorinated 2-phenoxyphenols (predioxins) that can undergo thermal ring closure in the gas chromatograph to form PCDDs (Buser, 1991).

Since the mid-1980s, a two-column procedure (Smith *et al.*, 1984a) has come into extensive use. Extracts are first chromatographed on activated carbon with dichloro-methane to separate planar compounds (including PCDDs and PCDFs, which are retained) from non-planar compounds. The planar compounds are removed from the carbon column by reverse elution with toluene and then chromatographed on alumina to separate the PCDDs and PCDFs from other planar contaminants (e.g., non-*ortho*-substi-tuted PCBs, polychloronaphthalenes). The method has been adapted and validated for complex biological samples in a semi-automated format (with additional clean-up steps) (Patterson *et al.*, 1990; Turner *et al.*, 1991).

HPLC also has found extensive application in PCDD/PCDF analysis in recent years (Clement & Tosine, 1988). It has been used principally for isomer-specific quantification of 2,3,7,8-TCDD and/or the other toxic PCDD/PCDF congeners. It is also used to supplement other clean-up methods for difficult samples.

Bergqvist *et al.* (1993) have described the use of a polyethylene semipermeable membrane in a nondestructive method for the reduction of lipid in analyses of PCDDs and PCDFs in environmental biological samples. This allows the analysis of samples with total size of 500 g.

Many other clean-up methods have been reported for environmental and biological matrices. The extent of clean-up required for a given sample depends on a number of factors, as noted above. Even with elaborate clean-up procedures, the final fractions may still contain chlorinated contaminants that need to be considered in the separation and quantification steps.

(e)   *Separation*

The final separation of PCDDs and PCDFs from residual contaminants and into the individual congeners is almost invariably performed by high-resolution GC (HRGC). In the 1960s and 1970s, GC with packed columns (low-resolution GC (LRGC)) allowed separation into groups of isomers (e.g., separation of the TCDDs as a group from the

PeCDDs), but the resolution was inadequate for separation of the isomers within a group (e.g., separation of the 22 isomeric TCDDs). In the mid-1970s, glass capillary columns were first used with PCDDs and PCDFs and were found to offer much better separation of isomers and improved sensitivity. The special skills required to prepare these columns, however, initially restricted their use to a limited number of laboratories. Thus, the commercial development of prepared glass capillary columns, especially the introduction of flexible, stable, reproducible fused silica columns around 1980, was one of the most important advances in environmental PCDD/PCDF analysis (Clement & Tosine, 1988; Clement, 1991).

The HRGC columns used for PCDD/PCDF analysis range from 15 to 60 m in length with inner diameters in the range of 0.22–0.35 mm. They are often referred to as wall-coated open-tubular (WCOT) columns, as the inner wall of the column is uniformly coated with a thin film (0.15–0.25 μm) of a silicone (stationary phase) that accomplishes the separations. Many different stationary phases have been used in PCDD/PCDF analyses. In general, non-polar stationary phases (e.g., alkyl/aryl siloxanes) efficiently separate PCDD/PCDF mixtures into groups with the same numbers of chlorines (all TCDDs and TCDFs, all PeCDDs and PeCDFs, etc.), while polar stationary phases (e.g., cyanosilicones) distinguish between the isomers within a group. Frequently, separate analyses using more than one column are required to ensure adequate separation of congeners, for example, a short to medium-length, non-polar (SE-54 or DB-5) column and a longer polar (Silar 10C or SP 2330) column (Clement & Tosine, 1988). A workshop convened by the Community Bureau of Reference of the Commission of the European Union recently recommended the use of a single, nonpolar column (e.g., DB-5) for samples containing only 2,3,7,8-substituted PCDDs and PCDFs, and both a non-polar and a polar column (e.g., SP 2331, CPSIL 88) for samples which also contain PCDDs/PCDFs with chlorine at other positions (Maier *et al.*, 1994). Since higher terrestrial vertebrates tend to accumulate selectively the 2,3,7,8-substituted congeners, satisfactory analyses of biological samples from farm animals and humans are often achieved on non-polar columns alone (de Jong *et al.*, 1993).

Gas chromatographic retention times are compared with those of authentic standards of the various PCDD and PCDF isomers (^{13}C-labelled or unlabelled) for tentative isomer identification. Confirmation of identity and quantification are accomplished by mass spectrometry.

(f)   Quantification

Although a few early studies used GC with ECD to quantify PCDDs and PCDFs, modern practice depends almost exclusively on mass spectrometric detection with selected ion monitoring (SIM) of two or more ions from the isotopic group of molecular ions. This allows the use of stable-isotope-labelled internal standards, provides selectivity against coextracted endogenous compounds and many other contaminants and allows congeners with different degrees of chlorination to be quantified separately (Clement & Tosine, 1988). Monitoring of the exact masses of the ions at high mass spectometer resolution provides additional selectivity (Lamparski *et al.*, 1991; Tondeur & Beckert, 1991).

The advantages and disadvantages of various mass spectrometric methods for PCDDs and PCDFs have been extensively reviewed and discussed in recent years (Clement & Tosine, 1988; Buser, 1991; de Jong & Liem, 1993) and are therefore not reviewed here. Either low-resolution mass spectrometry (LRMS) or high-resolution mass spectrometry (HRMS) can provide adequate data, if it has been demonstrated by the analyst that 'the entire analytical procedure exhibits a sufficient sensitivity and specificity with regard to concentration levels of the PCDD/F and the matrix composition' (Maier *et al.*, 1994). Most analysts agree that HRMS, although not essential, is preferable. The monitoring of additional fragment ions or use of collision-induced dissociation and tandem MS can provide additional selectivity for confirmation or resolution of specific analytical diffi-culties but, in practice, are seldom used.

Electron impact ionization is most commonly used for PCDD/PCDF analyses. Negative-ion chemical ionization is very sensitive for the highly chlorinated congeners but is not suitable for lower congeners such as 2,3,7,8-TCDD and may be difficult to use quantitatively because of its marked dependence on operating conditions (Buser, 1991; Maier *et al.*, 1994).

Some differences in the relative abundances of ion fragments from different isomers have been observed (Buser & Rappe, 1978), but do not provide a means of unambi-guously differentiating between isomers; this requires chromatographic separation by GC and/or by prior fractionation (Hagenmaier *et al.*, 1986; Lamparski *et al.*, 1991).

Quantification of PCDDs and PCDFs is accomplished by SIM comparisons of the responses for sample components with those of internal standards, usually ^{13}C-labelled 2,3,7,8-substituted PCDDs. Calibration standards are used to determine detector response for the various congeners and to confirm its linearity in the concentration range of the samples. Careful attention to quality control and quality assurance procedures is essential for the successful analysis of PCDDs and PCDFs at ultra-trace levels (Mitchum & Donnelly, 1991).

1.2   Formation and destruction

PCDDs can be formed by a number of different reactions including synthetic chemical, thermal, photochemical and biochemical; analogous pathways can be used for their destruction. PCDDs already present in reservoir sources such as sediments, soil and sewage sludge are significant contributors to current environmental levels.

1.2.1   *Formation of PCDDs*

(a)   *Chemical reactions*

(i)   *Chlorophenoxyacetic acid herbicides* (referred to hereafter as phenoxy herbicides)

The phenoxy herbicide 2,4,5-trichlorophenoxyacetic acid (2,4,5-T) (see IARC, 1977b, 1986a, 1987b) was introduced in the late 1940s, and its use was maximal in the 1960s and 1970s. After that time, it was phased out in most European countries and the United States of America. 2,4,5-Trichlorophenol (TCP) (see IARC, 1979a, 1986b, 1987c) is the key intermediate in the production of 2,4,5-T. PCDDs, primarily 2,3,7,8-TCDD, were formed during the production of TCP from 1,2,4,5-tetrachlorobenzene.

Depending on the temperature control and purification efficiency, levels of 2,3,7,8-TCDD in commercial products vary greatly. For example, levels of 2,3,7,8-TCDD in drums of the herbicide Agent Orange (a 1 : 1 mixture of the *n*-butyl esters of 2,4,5-T and 2,4-dichlorophenoxyacetic acid (2,4-D); see IARC, 1977c) stored in the United States and in the Pacific before 1970 were between 0.02 and 47 mg/kg (analytical method N). Nearly 500 samples were analysed and the mean value was 1.98 mg/kg (Young *et al.*, 1978; Young, 1983). Since Agent Orange was formulated as a 1 : 1 mixture of the butyl esters of 2,4,5-T and 2,4-D, the levels of 2,3,7,8-TCDD in individual preparations of 2,4,5-T manufactured and used in the 1960s could have been as high as 100 mg/kg (Rappe & Buser, 1981).

Rappe *et al.* (1978a) reported that in other samples of Agent Orange (as well as in 2,4,5-T formulations produced in Europe and the United States in the 1950s and 1960s), 2,3,7,8-TCDD was the dominant PCDD/PCDF contaminant. Only minor amounts of other PCDDs were found, primarily lower chlorinated PCDDs, in samples of Agent Orange (analytical method AC). The concentrations of 2,3,7,8-TCDD have been reported for 2,4,5-T formulations used in Scandinavia (**Table 6**) and New Zealand (**Table 7**).

Table 6. Concentrations of 2,3,7,8-TCDD (mg/kg) in Scandinavian 2,4,5-trichloro-phenoxyacetic acid and ester formulations

Sample	Source	2,3,7,8-TCDD
2,4,5-T acid	1952, Sweden	1.10
2,4,5-T ester	Unknown, Sweden	0.50
2,4,5-T ester	Unknown, Sweden	< 0.05
2,4,5-T ester	1960, Sweden	0.40
2,4,5-T ester	1962, Finland	0.95
2,4,5-T ester	1966, Finland	0.10
2,4,5-T ester	1967, Finland	< 0.05
2,4,5-T ester	1967, Finland	0.22
2,4,5-T ester	1967, Finland	0.18
2,4,5-T acid	1964, USA	4.8
2,4,5-T acid	1969, USA	6.0

From Rappe *et al.* (1978a); Norström *et al.* (1979); Rappe & Buser (1981)

**Table 7. Average concentrations
of 2,3,7,8-TCDD (µg/kg) in
2,4,5-T produced in New
Zealand**

Year	2,3,7,8-TCDD
1971	950
1972	470
1973	47
1974	33
1975	24
1976	27
1977	31
1978	22
1979	13
1980	14
1981	7.3
1982	8.5
1983	5.3
1984	5.9
1985	4.7

From Smith & Pearce (1986)

As a result of governmental regulations, efforts were made by producers during the 1970s to minimize the formation of 2,3,7,8-TCDD during the production of 2,4,5-T. In the 1980s, all producers claimed that their products contained less than 0.1 mg/kg 2,3,7,8-TCDD (Rappe & Buser, 1981). During production, TCP is separated from 2,3,7,8-TCDD by one or two distillations, which results in 2,3,7,8-TCDD being concentrated in the still-bottom residues. Up to 1 g/kg 2,3,7,8-TCDD in such residues has been reported (Kimbrough *et al.*, 1984; analytical method N).

Sixteen samples of 2,4-D esters and amine salts from Canada were analysed for the presence of PCDDs. Eight of nine esters and four of seven amine salts were found to be contaminated, with esters showing significantly higher levels (210–1752 µg/kg) than salts (20–278 µg/kg) (analytical method AC). The TCDD isomer observed was the 1,3,6,8-isomer, verified using a synthetically prepared standard (Cochrane *et al.*, 1982). On the other hand, Schecter *et al.* (1993a) found no 2,3,7,8-TCDD at a detection limit of 0.02 µg/kg in one 2,4-D sample of Russian origin. Higher chlorinated PCDDs were found in this sample at < 1 µg/kg (I-TEQ for PCDDs/PCDFs, 0.2 µg/kg). Although 2,3,7,8-TCDD is not expected to be a contaminant in 2,4-D, Hagenmaier (1986) reported that one German 2,4-D formulation contained 6.8 µg/kg 2,3,7,8-TCDD (analytical method ACS).

No data were available to the Working Group on the analysis of samples of the herbicide 4-chloro-2-methylphenoxyacetic acid (MCPA) for 2,3,7,8-TCDD or other PCDDs. [However, it is not expected that PCDDs would be formed during the production of MCPA, based on the starting materials and production route.]

(ii) *Hexachlorophene*

The bactericide hexachlorophene (see IARC, 1979b) is prepared from TCP. Due to additional purification, the level of 2,3,7,8-TCDD in this product is usually below 0.03 mg/kg (WHO, 1989) (analytical method AC). Ligon and May (1986) reported 4.7 µg/kg 2,3,7,8-TCDD in one hexachlorophene sample; Baughman and Newton (1972) found 3.8 and 0.5 µg/kg in two samples. The use of hexachlorophene in cosmetics has been banned in the European Union (Her Majesty's Stationery Office, 1989).

(iii) *Chlorophenols*

Due to occupational and environmental risks, the use of chlorophenols has now been phased out in most European countries and in a few countries outside Europe. Chlorophenols have been used extensively since the 1950s as insecticides, fungicides, mould inhibitors, antiseptics and disinfectants. In 1978, the annual world production was estimated to be approximately 150 000 tonnes (Rappe *et al.*, 1979a). The most important use of 2,4,6-tri-, 2,3,4,6-tetra- and pentachlorophenol (PCP) and their salts is for wood preservation. PCP is also used as a fungicide for slime control and in the manufacture of paper pulp, and for a variety of other purposes such as in cutting oils and fluids, for tanning leather and in paint, glues and outdoor textiles (Rappe *et al.*, 1978b). **Table 8** summarizes a number of analyses of the levels of PCDDs in commercial chlorophenol formulations.

Table 8. Levels of PCDDs in commercial chlorophenols (mg/kg)

	2,4,6-Tri-chlorophenol	2,3,4,6-Tetra-chlorophenol	Pentachlorophenol	
			Sample A	Sample B
TCDDs	–	0.7	< 0.02	< 0.1
PeCDDs	< 0.3	5.2	< 0.03	< 0.1
HxCDDs	< 0.5	9.6	10	8
HpCDDs	< 0.2	5.6	130	520
OCDD	–	0.7	210	1 380

From Rappe (1979a)

Buser and Bosshardt (1976) reported the results of a survey of the PCDD and PCDF content of PCP and its sodium salt from commercial sources in Switzerland (analytical method AC). On the basis of the results, the samples could be divided into two groups: a first series with generally low levels (HxCDD, < 1 mg/kg) and a second series with much higher levels (HxCDD, > 1 mg/kg) of PCDDs. Samples with high PCDD levels also had high levels of PCDFs. The ranges of the combined levels of PCDDs and PCDFs were 2–16 and 1–26 mg/kg, respectively, for the first series of samples and 120–500 and 85–570 mg/kg, respectively, for the second series of samples. The levels of OCDD were as high as 370 mg/kg; this congener dominated the PCDD content of the samples.

Miles *et al.* (1985) analysed HxCDDs in PCP samples from five different manufacturers in Canada using an isomer-specific analytical method (analytical method ACI).

The study included both free PCP and sodium salts. Total HxCDDs in PCP samples ranged from 0.66 to 38.5 mg/kg while, in the sodium salts, levels between 1.55 and 16.3 mg/kg were found. The most abundant HxCDD isomer in free PCP was the 1,2,3,6,7,8-isomer; however, in the sodium salts, the 1,2,3,6,7,9- and 1,2,3,6,8,9-HxCDD pair was the most abundant, probably due to different routes of synthesis.

Hagenmaier (1986) reported that 2,3,7,8-TCDD could be detected in PCP formulations from Germany and the United States at concentrations of 0.21–0.56 µg/kg (analytical method ABS). 1,2,3,7,8-PeCDD was found in these formulations at higher concentrations (0.9–18 µg/kg; analytical method ABS) (Hagenmaier & Brunner, 1987).

(iv) *Chlorodiphenyl ether herbicides*

Yamagishi *et al.* (1981) reported on the occurrence of PCDDs and PCDFs in the Japanese commercial diphenyl ether herbicides primarily used in rice fields: 1,3,4-trichloro-2-(4-nitrophenoxy)benzene (CNP), 2,4-dichloro-1-(4-nitrophenoxy)benzene (Nitrofen; NIP; see IARC, 1983) and 2,4-dichloro-1-(3-methoxy-4-nitrophenoxy)-benzene (chlomethoxynil; X-52). The total TCDD content was 140–170 mg/kg in CNP, 0.38 mg/kg in NIP and 0.03 mg/kg in X-52. Very few synthetic standards were used, but the major TCDDs identified were the 1,3,6,8- and 1,3,7,9- isomers, the expected impurities in the starting material 2,4,6-trichlorophenol (2,4,6-TCP). No 2,3,7,8-TCDD was detected in these samples.

(v) *Hexachlorobenzene*

Hexachlorobenzene (see IARC, 1979c) used to be applied for the control of wheat bunt and fungi. Villanueva *et al.* (1974) analysed three commercial hexachlorobenzene preparations and identified OCDD in the range of 0.05–211.9 mg/kg (analytical method C).

(vi) *Pulp bleaching*

During the 1950s, free chlorine gas was introduced for the bleaching of pulp in pulp and paper mills. In 1986–87, it was first reported that bleaching pulp using free chlorine gas produced 2,3,7,8-TCDD (Rappe *et al.*, 1987a). A survey performed in 1987 in the United States showed that the concentrations of 2,3,7,8-TCDD in bleached pulp ranged from undetectable (at a detection limit of 1 ng/kg) up to 51 ng/kg, with a median concentration of 4.9 ng/kg and a mean of 13 ng/kg (Gillespie & Gellman, 1989).

New technology has been developed for pulp bleaching using chlorine dioxide (elemental chlorine-free, ECF) or non-chlorinated reagents (total chlorine-free, TCF). No 2,3,7,8-TCDD was found in ECF- or TCF-bleached pulp (detection limit, 0.03 ng/kg) (analytical method ABS) (Rappe & Wågman, 1995).

(vii) *Dyes and pigments*

Williams *et al.* (1992) analysed a series of dioxazine dyes and pigments (Blue 106, Blue 108 and Violet 23) from Canada. OCDD was detected in all samples (analytical method ACS) in the range of 23 µg/kg–42 mg/kg, with the highest concentrations in three samples of Blue 106.

(*b*) *Thermal reactions*

(i) *Incineration of municipal waste*

Olie *et al.* (1977) reported the occurrence of PCDDs and PCDFs in fly ash from three municipal incinerators in the Netherlands. Their results indicated the presence of up to 17 PCDD peaks, but isomer identification and quantification were not possible due to the lack of synthetic standards. Buser *et al.* (1978a) studied fly ash from a municipal incinerator and an industrial heating facility in Switzerland. In the former, the total level of PCDDs was 0.2 mg/kg. In the industrial incinerator fly ash, the level was 0.6 mg/kg.

In 1986, a working group of experts convened by the World Health Organization Regional Office for Europe (WHO/EURO, 1987) reviewed the available data on emissions of PCDDs from municipal solid-waste incinerators. They concluded that, because of their high thermal stability, PCDDs were destroyed only after adequate residence times (> 2 s) at temperatures above 800 °C. Total emissions of PCDDs from tests on municipal solid-waste incinerators were reported to range between a few and several thousand ng/m^3 dry gas at 10% carbon dioxide. The WHO working group prepared a table giving a range of estimated isomer-specific emissions for those isomers of major concern with respect to municipal solid-waste incinerators operating under various conditions (**Table 9**).

The emissions tabulated in column 1 are those which the working group considered to be achievable in modern, highly controlled and carefully operated plants in use in 1986. The results given in column 1 are not representative of emissions that might be expected from such plants during start-up or during occasional abnormal conditions. Emission levels listed in column 2 were considered by the working group to be indicative of the upper limit of emissions from modern municipal solid-waste incinerators. These plants might experience such emissions during start-up or during occasional abnormal conditions, although some of the data reviewed have shown that the figures in column 2 should not be considered to be an absolute maximum. However, most plants existing in 1986, if carefully operated, will have had PCDD emissions in the range between columns 1 and 2. The highest values for municipal solid-waste incinerators (column 3) were obtained by multiplying the values in column 2 by a factor of 5. Emission levels that were reported to the working group from all tests and under all circumstances were no greater than these values. Generally, these emission levels are associated with irregular or unstable operating conditions, high moisture content of the municipal solid waste, or low combustion or afterburner temperatures. Of special importance is the observation that the emission of 1,2,3,7,8-PeCDD normally exceeds the emission of 2,3,7,8-TCDD by a factor of 3–10.

During the second half of the 1980s and 1990, regulatory agencies in several countries, such as Sweden, Germany and the Netherlands, announced strict regulations for municipal solid-waste incinerators. The European Union value is 0.1 ng I-TEQ per m^3 (European Union, 1994) (see column 4, **Table 9**). This directive has resulted in the introduction of modern air pollution control devices and, together with improved burning conditions, has led to a decrease in PCDD emissions from municipal solid-waste incinerators, which had been considered to be major sources.

Table 9. Estimated range of emissions of PCDDs from municipal solid-waste (MSW) and municipal sewage sludge (MSS) incinerators

| | Emissions from MSW combustion (ng/m³) | | | | Emissions from MSS combustion (ng/m³) |
	Achievable with modern plants with no gas cleaning (1)	Maximum from average operation (2)	High emissions[a] (3)	Achievable with modern plants with gas cleaning[b] (4)	Most probably highest emissions (5)
2,3,7,8-TCDD	0.1	1.5	7.5	0.01	0.1
1,2,3,7,8-PeCDD	0.3	14	70	0.03	0.3
1,2,3,4,7,8-HxCDD	0.2	31	155	0.02	0.2
1,2,3,6,7,8-HxCDD	0.6	56	280	0.05	0.6
1,2,3,7,8,9-HxCDD	0.4	20	100	0.04	0.4

From WHO/EURO (1987) excepted when noted
[a] Values obtained by multiplying values in column 2 by a factor of 5
[b] Adapted from ECETOC (1992)

(ii) *Incineration of sewage sludge*

Sludge from municipal waste-water treatment plants may be incinerated after being dehydrated. The WHO working group in 1986 reviewed the available data from municipal sewage sludge incinerators and found that PCDD and PCDF emissions from this type of plant were generally lower than emissions from municipal solid-waste incinerators (see **Table 9**, column 5) (WHO/EURO, 1987).

(iii) *Incineration of hospital waste*

Doyle *et al.* (1985) claimed that the incomplete combustion of certain hospital wastes containing halogenated compounds could produce high emission of PCDDs. They found the mean levels of total PCDDs to be 69 ng/m^3, but no isomer-specific data were given. Data cited by the United States Environmental Protection Agency indicate that flue gas emissions from hospital waste incinerators are in the range 10–100 ng I-TEQ/m^3, higher than the levels achievable with modern municipal solid-waste incinerators (United States Environmental Protection Agency, 1994; Thomas & Spiro, 1995). [The Working Group noted that, due to smaller emission volumes, the overall emissions from hospital waste incinerators are generally lower than those from municipal solid-waste incinerators.]

(iv) *Incineration of polyvinyl chloride (PVC)*

The formation of PCDDs during the combustion of PVC (see IARC, 1979d) is a controversial issue. However, the incineration conditions appear to be quite important. On the basis of laboratory experiments, Christmann *et al.* (1989a) considered PVC to be an important source of PCDDs/PCDFs. However, experiments performed in incinerators showed the effect of PVC on the formation of PCDDs/PCDFs to be minimal (Frankenhaeuser *et al.*, 1993; Wikström *et al.*, 1996).

(v) *Combustion of wood*

Schatowitz *et al.* (1994) measured PCDD/PCDF emissions from small-scale laboratory studies of combustion of wood and household waste (analytical method ABS). The results (in ng I-TEQ/m^3) are summarized in **Table 10**. Data on PCDDs and PCDFs are not separated.

Table 10. PCDD/PCDF emissions from wood and household waste combustion

Fuel	Furnace	(ng I-TEQ/m^3)
Beech wood sticks	Fireplace	0.064
Beech wood sticks	Stick wood boiler	0.019–0.034
Wood chips	Automatic chip furnace	0.066–0.214
Uncoated chipboard	Automatic chip furnace	0.024–0.076
Waste wood chips	Automatic chip furnace	2.70–14.42
Household waste	Household stove, closed	114.4

From Schatowitz *et al.* (1994)

(vi) *Automobile emissions*

Hagenmaier *et al.* (1990a) reported on the automobile exhaust emissions of PCDDs/-PCDFs and the lower chlorinated congeners and brominated analogues. The results of four representative experiments using leaded gasoline, unleaded gasoline with or without catalytic converters, and diesel fuel (analytical method ABS) are summarized in **Table 11**.

Table 11. PCDDs from automobile emissions (pg/m³)

	Leaded gasoline	Unleaded gasoline	Unleaded gasoline with catalytic converter	Diesel engine
TCDDs	595	84	3.7	1.9
2,3,7,8-TCDD	16.7	0.5	0.21	0.40
PeCDDs	436	93	3.3	1.0
1,2,3,7,8-PeCDD	55.5	3.7	0.21	0.46
HxCDDs	244	59	3.4	1.2
1,2,3,4,7,8-HxCDD	24.5	3.2	0.31	< 0.26
1,2,3,6,7,8-HxCDD	27.1	3.3	0.45	< 0.26
1,2,3,7,8,9-HxCDD	24.1	3.4	0.40	< 0.26
HpCDDs	152	18	5.0	4.5
1,2,3,4,6,7,8-HpCDD	65.7	7.8	1.97	2.24
OCDDs	65	34	21.9	22.4
I-TEQ pg/m³	141.5	9.8	0.93	1.20
I-TEQ pg/L fuel	1 083.3	50.7	7.20	23.60

From Hagenmaier *et al.* (1990a)

(c) *Photochemical reactions*

It was reported by Nilsson *et al.* (1974) that chlorinated 2-phenoxyphenols (pre-dioxins) could be converted to PCDDs by a photochemical cyclization reaction. More recently, Vollmuth *et al.* (1994) reported on the photochemical dimerization of chloro-phenols yielding OCDD. The most important photochemical reaction, however, is photo-chemical dechlorination resulting in transformation of PCDDs to lower chlorinated compounds. Kieaitwong *et al.* (1990) reported that 2,3,7,8-TCDD could be identified among the products of photochemical dechlorination of OCDD.

(d) *Biochemical reactions*

Öberg *et al.* (1990) showed that chlorinated phenols could be transformed *in vitro* to PCDDs by peroxidase-catalysed oxidation. It was also demonstrated, using ¹³C-labelled PCP, that HpCDDs and OCDDs could be formed in sewage sludge (Öberg *et al.*, 1993).

1.2.2   *Destruction of PCDDs*

Although PCDDs generally are considered to be very stable, they can undergo a series of chemical degradation reactions. Peterson and Milicic (1992) reported the degradation of a series of PCDDs using a mixture of potassium hydroxide in polyethylene glycol. Oku *et al.* (1995) also reported the successful destruction of PCDDs using sodium or potassium hydroxide in the new solvent 1,3-dimethyl-2-imidazolidinone.

Thermal degradation of PCDDs occurs at temperatures above 800 °C and at residence times of longer than 2 s (WHO/EURO, 1987), but the conditions required for thermal degradation are matrix-dependent.

Hosoya *et al.* (1995) showed that 2,3,7,8-TCDD can be decomposed successfully by photochemical reactions with a hydrophobic octadecylsilylated-silica gel used as the solid support. Conversely, Vollmuth and Niessner (1995) reported no significant degradation of PCDDs by ultraviolet radiation, ozone or a combination of the two.

Adriaens *et al.* (1995) reported on the biologically mediated reductive dechlorination of HxCDDs in sediments using inocula derived from contaminated environments.

1.3 Occurrence

All tissue concentrations reported in this section are lipid-based (as ng/kg fat), unless otherwise stated.

1.3.1 *Occupational and accidental exposures to PCDDs*

(a) *Occupational exposures*

(i) *Exposure during production of TCP, 2,4,5-T and PCP*

Germany: In November 1953, an uncontrolled decomposition reaction occurred in an enclosed TCP production facility of BASF at Ludwigshafen, Germany. 2,3,7,8-TCDD was formed during the reaction and contaminated the autoclave section of the building. Employees were exposed to 2,3,7,8-TCDD contaminant during subsequent clean-up and repair activities (Zober *et al.*, 1990; Zober & Päpke, 1993). Analysis of a sample of adipose tissue collected in 1984 from one of the exposed workers showed a 2,3,7,8-TCDD concentration of 100 ng/kg wet weight adipose tissue (Nygren *et al.*, 1986). Zober and Päpke (1993) later analysed samples of autopsy tissues collected from four cases 35–39 years after the same accident. In all samples, the concentrations of most PCDDs were in the normal range, with the exception of 2,3,7,8-TCDD, the concentrations of which were much higher (see **Table 12**; analytical method ACS). Measurements of the blood concentration of 2,3,7,8-TCDD were performed in 1988 in 138 men whose first contact with PCDDs occurred within one year of the accident (Zober *et al.*, 1994). Current values were extrapolated back to the time of exposure. The geometric mean concentrations ranged from 1118 ng/kg in group with severe chloracne to 148 ng/kg in group with no chloracne. Background blood levels of 2,3,7,8-TCDD in the plant were ≤ 5 ng/kg. Ott *et al.* (1993) reported on the concentrations of 2,3,7,8-TCDD in blood lipids of these workers sampled between 1988 and 1992, 35–39 years after the accident. The geometric mean value was 15.4 ng/kg. [Back-calculation to the time of the accident, using a 2,3,7,8-TCDD half-life of seven years, gives an estimated blood lipid concentration of 480 ng/kg. If the normal German background concentration in 1990 is first subtracted, the estimate is approximately 400 ng/kg.]

Table 12. Post-mortem concentrations of 2,3,7,8-TCDD (ng/kg fat) in autopsy samples from four individuals involved in the 1953 BASF accident

	Blood	Adipose[a]	Liver	Kidney	Brain
Case 1	255	171	178	198	36
Case 2	32	34	28	–	7
Case 3	7482[b]	13 563	13 563	11 195	2457
Case 4	448	648	550	–	–

From Zober & Päpke (1993)

[a] German background concentration, 5 ng/kg

[b] Significant weight loss before death may have resulted in increased levels of 2,3,7,8-TCDD in blood and other tissues, especially in Case 3. Eight months before death, blood concentration for Case 3 was 518 ng/kg (compared with 7482 ng/kg at autopsy); Case 3 lost 20–25 kg in body weight in the eight months before death. Case 2 showed a smaller effect but in the same direction (blood concentration, 17 ng/kg at 5 months before death; 7–10 kg weight loss). Case 4 had a blood level of 590 ng/kg 10 months before death, and no subsequent weight loss was reported. No data were available for Case 1.

Päpke *et al.* (1992) analysed in 1988–91 the blood of 12 workers exposed during production of TCP. Concentrations of 2,3,7,8-TCDD were approximately 100 times higher than those in a group of background controls, while the concentrations of the higher chlorinated PCDDs were lower in exposed workers than in controls, but not significantly. In blood from 20 workers exposed to PCDDs during production of PCP, the concentrations of OCDD, 1,2,3,4,6,7,8-HpCDD and 2,3,7,8-derived HxCDDs were much higher in the exposed workers than in controls (see **Table 13**).

Table 13. Concentrations of PCDDs in human blood (ng/kg fat) during production of chlorophenols in Germany

	TCP (n = 12)	PCP (n = 20)	Control (n = 102)
2,3,7,8-TCDD	331.8	4.5	3.6
1,2,3,7,8-PeCDD	10.7	28.3	13.8
All 2,3,7,8-substituted HxCDDs	34.5	398.8	78.9
1,2,3,4,6,7,8-HpCDD	44.3	2 514.1	92.4
OCDD	428.9	33 191.5	610.3

From Päpke *et al.* (1992)

TCP, 2,4,5-trichlorophenol; PCP, pentachlorophenol

Flesch-Janys *et al.* (1996a) studied 48 workers (45 men and 3 women) from a Boehringer-Ingelheim plant in Hamburg manufacturing a range of herbicides. The blood of these workers was sampled twice (for 43 workers) or three times (for 5 workers). The mean time between the end of employment and the first blood sampling was 5.4 years (median, 2.0 years), and the mean time between first and last blood sampling was 5.6 years (median, 6.3 years) (analytical method AB). The results are given in **Table 14**. In the first sampling, the median concentration of 2,3,7,8-TCDD was 84.1 ng/kg (range, 15.6–300.2 ng/kg). The corresponding values for the second sampling are: median, 48.9 ng/kg (range, 7.7–277.9 ng/kg). More measurements from the Boehringer plant and two other German plants (the BASF plant in Ludwigshafen (this cohort was different from the accident-exposed group) and a Bayer plant in Ingelheim (Becher *et al.*, 1996)) were also performed (summarized in Kogevinas *et al.*, 1997). The 190 subjects from the Boehringer plant showed mean estimated concentrations at the end of employment of 141 ng/kg 2,3,7,8-TCDD (range, 3–2252 ng/kg). In the BASF plant, 20 subjects showed mean 2,3,7,8-TCDD values of 401.7 ng/kg (range, 23–1935 ng/kg), while 19 workers at the Bayer plant had a mean level of 3.2 ng/kg (range, 1.3–6.5 ng/kg).

Table 14. Concentrations of PCDDs (ng/kg fat) in blood of workers at a German herbicide plant (Boehringer-Ingelheim plant)

	No.[a]	First blood sample[b]		Last blood sample[c]	
		Median	Range	Median	Range
2,3,7,8-TCDD	48	84.1	15.6–300.2	48.9	7.7–277.9
1,2,3,7,8-PeCDD	40	51.1	27.2–251.2	35.9	13.2–190.3
1,2,3,4,7,8-HxCDD	41	83.2	25.6–746.9	51.3	18.7–559.7
1,2,3,6,7,8-HxCDD	40	354.7	127.7–2939	255.8	101.6–2493
1,2,3,7,8,9-HxCDD	39	88.2	29.3–680.8	39.5	17.6–288.3
1,2,3,4,6,7,8-HpCDD	26	641.2	310.5–5152	234.5	94.2–1526
OCDD	32	2 526	1356–17 566	1 288.5	842–10 395
TEQ[d]	45	191.9	43.1–767.2	115.3	29.4–500.4

From Flesch-Janys *et al.* (1996a)
[a] Number of persons whose levels exceeded upper background concentrations at all points in time
[b] Mean, 5.4 years after end of employment
[c] Mean, 5.6 years after the first blood sample
[d] German TEQ (total PCDDs/PCDFs)

United States: The largest study in the United States of workers assigned to production of substances contaminated with 2,3,7,8-TCDD was conducted by the United States National Institute for Occupational Safety and Health (Fingerhut *et al.*, 1991a). A more detailed technical report of this study is also available (Fingerhut *et al.*, 1991b). This 12-plant study included the Nitro, WV, plant of Monsanto and the Midland, MI, plant of Dow. The cohort was constructed after a review of personnel records at plants producing chemicals known to be contaminated with 2,3,7,8-TCDD (principally TCP and 2,4,5-T). The cohort included most workers in the United States likely to have been exposed to 2,3,7,8-TCDD in chemical manufacturing; these were 5000 men with work records showing assignment to a production or maintenance job in a process involving 2,3,7,8-TCDD contamination, as well as an additional 172 men without work history records but known to have been exposed based upon inclusion in a prior cross-sectional medical study by Suskind and Hertzberg (1984) at the Nitro, WV, plant. These latter 172 men and an additional 30 men in the United States National Institute for Occupational Safety and Health study lacked sufficient work history information to permit their inclusion in more detailed analyses by duration of exposure. Follow-up was conducted through 1987. Serum 2,3,7,8-TCDD levels, available for 253 cohort members at two plants (different from the Nitro and Midland plants), measured in 1987 averaged a mean of 233 ng/kg, compared with 7 ng/kg for a group of 79 unexposed workers. The mean level was 418 ng/kg for 119 workers exposed for more than one year. All workers had last been exposed 15–37 years earlier. Extrapolation to the date of last employment of these workers, assuming a 7.1-year half-life for 2,3,7,8-TCDD elimination, indicated a mean serum level at that time of 2000 ng/kg (highest level, 32 000 ng/kg). The correlation between extrapolated serum 2,3,7,8-TCDD levels and duration of exposure was 0.72 (Fingerhut *et al.*, 1991b).

Sweden: Littorin *et al.* (1994) analysed blood from five workers at a factory in Sweden where 2,4-D, MCPA, 2-(4-chloro-2-methylphenoxy)propanoic acid (MCPP) and 2,4,6-trichlorophenol (Saracci *et al.*, 1991) had been formulated, but where production had ceased in 1979, and that of five referents. [2,4,5-T was not produced at this site.] The results are given in **Table 15**. The concentrations of all PCDDs were high, especially that of 1,2,3,7,8-PeCDD, which was unexpectedly found to be higher than that of 2,3,7,8-TCDD. However, a leachate sample from the factory also contained a higher level of 1,2,3,7,8-PeCDD.

Austria: Neuberger *et al.* (1991) reported mean blood levels of 389 ng/kg 2,3,7,8-TCDD (range, 98–659 ng/kg) in TCP and 2,4-D production workers with chloracne exposed about 17 years earlier.

Netherlands: Hooiveld *et al.* (1996a) took blood samples in 1993 from 48 persons occupationally exposed to phenoxy herbicides, chlorophenols (and the contaminant 2,3,7,8-TCDD) in 1955–85 in a chemical factory where an accident occurred in 1963. The geometric mean levels of 2,3,7,8-TCDD were 22.9 ng/kg in men who worked in the main production unit and 87.2 in subjects exposed as a result of the accident.

(ii)   *Exposure during handling and spraying of 2,4,5-T*

Nygren *et al.* (1986) reported analyses of adipose tissue from 31 persons in Sweden, 13 of whom were exposed to phenoxy herbicides and 18 of whom were unexposed controls. Of the exposed persons, 11 had neoplastic diseases; in controls, six persons had cancer, giving a total of 17 cancer patients and 14 persons without cancer. No difference was found between exposed and unexposed or between cancer patients and persons without cancer (see **Table 16**; analytical method ACS).

Table 15. Blood plasma concentrations of PCDDs in five phenoxy herbicide/chlorophenol production workers and five referents in Sweden

Analyte	Plasma concentration (ng/kg fat)				
	Workers		Referents		p value[a]
	Mean[b]	Range	Mean[b]	Range	
PCDDs					
2,3,7,8-TCDD	17	9.1–37	2.0	0.7–3.3	0.008
1,2,3,7,8-PeCDD	22	14–33	6.9	4.0–10	0.008
1,2,3,4,7,8-HxCDD	4.5	2.7–6.9	2.4	0.8–4.4	0.2
1,2,3,6,7,8-HxCDD	43	28–58	28	10–39	0.2
1,2,3,7,8,9-HxCDD	18	8.8–27	7.5	2.0–13	0.1
1,2,3,4,6,7,8-HpCDD	87	33–120	43	7.9–78	0.06
OCDD	750	400–1300	280	110–440	0.02
I-TEQ	56	30–94	21	8.2–34	0.02

From Littorin *et al.* (1994)
[a] Wilcoxon's rank sum test for unpaired samples (two-tail)
[b] Values below the detection limit were set at half that concentration.

In another study in Sweden including 20 non-Hodgkin lymphoma patients and 17 controls, Hardell *et al.* (1996) reported no significant differences in the concentrations of PCDDs and PCDFs in adipose tissue (see also Section 2.2.2(*b*)).

Professional pesticide applicators involved in ground-level spraying of 2,4,5-T in New Zealand are claimed to be the group most heavily exposed to agricultural use of 2,4,5-T in the world (Smith *et al.*, 1992a). Many of the applicators sprayed for more than six months per year and some were spraying for more than 20 years. Measurements of 2,3,7,8-TCDD in blood serum of nine of these workers (**Table 17**) gave arithmetic means of 53.3 ng/kg for the exposed group and 5.6 ng/kg for a group of matched controls (ratio, 9.5). For all other congeners, the ratio between the levels in the exposed group and the controls was below 1.5.

Military personnel in Viet Nam: The Viet Nam Experience Study is described by its authors as a 'multidimensional assessment of the health of Viet Nam veterans (Centers for Disease Control Vietnam Experience Study, 1988a,b,c,d). This study was designed to examine effects among men who served in the United States armed forces in Viet Nam, where Agent Orange (see Section 1.2.1(*a*)(i)) was widely sprayed as a herbicide and defoliant (Operation Ranch Hand). The study population was a random sample of men who enlisted in the United States Army from 1965 through 1971, whose military occupational status was other than 'duty soldier', who enlisted for a single term with a minimum of 16 weeks' active duty and who were discharged at pay grades of E-1 to E-5. The controls were selected from among veterans enlisting during the same period but whose duty station was the United States, Germany or Korea. Participation involved

Table 16. Concentrations of PCDDs in human adipose tissue (ng/kg wet weight) from persons exposed to phenoxy herbicides in Sweden

Compound	Mean value (n = 31)	Range	Exposed		Unexposed		Cancer patients		Controls (without cancer)	
			Mean (n = 13)	Range	Mean (n = 18)	Range	Mean (n = 17)	Range	Mean (n = 14)	Range
2,3,7,8-TCDD	3	0–9	2	0–9	3	2–6	3	2–9	3	2–6
1,2,3,7,8-PeCDD	10	3–24	6	3–24	9	4–18	9	4–24	9	3–18
1,2,3,6,7,8-HxCDD	15	3–55	19	8–55	12	3–18	18	3–55	12	8–18
1,2,3,7,8,9-HxCDD	4	3–5	5	3–13	4	3–5	4	3–13	4	3–5
1,2,3,4,6,7,8-HpCDD	97	12–380	104	20–380	85	12–176	100	12–380	85	20–168
OCDD	414	90–763	398	90–763	421	98–679	408	90–620	421	182–763

From Nygren et al. (1986)

completion of a telephone survey of current and past health status by 7924 veterans who served in Viet Nam and 7364 veterans who served outside Viet Nam. A random subsample of 2940 Viet Nam and 1972 non-Viet Nam veterans participated in the health evaluation component.

Table 17. Levels of PCDDs in serum of nine 2,4,5-T applicators and nine matched control subjects in New Zealand

Congener	Average level (ng/kg fat ± SE)[a]		Ratio[b]
	Applicator	Matched control	
2,3,7,8-TCDD	53.3 ± 16.1	5.6 ± 1.1	9.5
1,2,3,7,8-PeCDD	12.4 ± 1.1	8.8 ± 0.7	1.4
1,2,3,4,7,8-HxCDD	6.8 ± 0.5	5.7 ± 0.4	1.2
1,2,3,6,7,8-HxCDD	28.6 ± 5.1	23.3 ± 4.9	1.2
1,2,3,7,8,9-HxCDD	9.9 ± 0.9	8.2 ± 0.6	1.2
1,2,3,4,6,7,8-HpCDD	121.9 ± 28.5	119.4 ± 18.4	1.0
OCDD	788.6 ± 82.3	758.7 ± 92.8	1.0

From Smith *et al.* (1992a)

[a] Values are adjusted for total lipids in serum.

[b] Ratio, average for applicators/average for matched control subjects

Investigators in the Centers for Disease Control Veterans Health Studies (1988; see **Table 18**) studied serum levels of 2,3,7,8-TCDD among 646 Viet Nam veterans who were ground combat troops during 1967–68 in areas heavily sprayed with Agent Orange. Also studied were 97 veterans who did not serve in Viet Nam. The mean serum level was 4 ng/kg for each group, as measured in 1987. There was no correlation between serum levels of 2,3,7,8-TCDD and service in areas of Viet Nam ranked by level of presumed intensity of spraying based on military records, or between serum levels and self-reported levels of exposure to Agent Orange. Only two Viet Nam veterans had levels above 20 ng/kg (25 and 45 ng/kg). This study did not include Viet Nam veterans who served in the Air Force spraying of Agent Orange (the Operation Ranch Hand veterans), nor members of the Army Chemical Corps which also sprayed Agent Orange. There are data indicating that these specific groups (especially Ranch Hand veterans) had significant levels of exposure to PCDDs above background.

One of the largest epidemiological studies of United States military personnel stationed in Viet Nam is being conducted by the United States Air Force. The study population consists of Air Force personnel who served in Operation Ranch Hand units in Viet Nam from 1962 to 1971 and who were employed in the dissemination of Agent Orange through aerial spraying. Comparisons included Air Force personnel who flew or maintained C-130 aircraft in south-east Asia during the same period. The study design includes a series of cross-sectional medical studies conducted at five-year intervals

Table 18. Serum levels of 2,3,7,8-TCDD in United States veterans who served in Viet Nam and elsewhere in 1987

Place of service	No.	Mean ± SD (ng/kg)	Percentile				
			25th	50th	75th	90th	95th
Non-Viet Nam	97	4.1 ± 2.3	2.8	3.8	4.9	7.2	9.2
Viet Nam	646	4.2 ± 2.6	2.8	3.8	5.1	6.8	7.8

From Centers for Disease Control Veterans Health Studies (1988)

beginning with the baseline study in 1982 (1045 exposed, 1224 unexposed). Two follow-up evaluations were conducted in 1985 (1016 exposed, 1293 unexposed) and 1987 (995 exposed, 1299 unexposed). Each cross-sectional study included comprehensive physical and psychological evaluations. In the 1982 baseline and 1985 and 1987 follow-up studies, exposure was based on the comparison of the Ranch Hand group versus the comparison group. An additional analysis estimated the approximate exposure (low, medium or high) for the Ranch Hand group by using historical military data and herbicide procurement and usage records (Roegner *et al.*, 1991).

The Air Force Ranch Hand veterans (Wolfe *et al.*, 1990) (see **Table 19**) tested in 1987 and exposed during 1962–71 (*n* = 888) had a median of 12.4 ng/kg serum 2,3,7,8-TCDD compared with a median of 4.2 ng/kg for comparison subjects (*n* = 856) who were Air Force personnel not exposed to herbicides. The highest levels were for non-flying enlisted personnel (*n* = 407), with a median of 23.6 ng/kg. Air Force Ranch Hand veterans sprayed approximately 88–90% (Thomas & Kang, 1990) of the Agent Orange applied in Viet Nam, with application from airplanes. The remaining 10–12% was sprayed by the Army Chemical Corps which applied the herbicide around the perimeter of bases either from the ground or from helicopters. Kahn *et al.* (1988) studied 2,3,7,8-TCDD serum levels in a sample of 10 heavily exposed Viet Nam veterans and matched controls. The two highest levels were found in Army Chemical Corps personnel (approximately 75 and 180 ng/kg. It should be noted that both Ranch Hand veterans and Army Chemical Corps veterans sprayed other herbicides (Agent White or Agent Blue) besides Agent Orange, although few other herbicides were contaminated with PCDDs (Thomas & Kang, 1990). These data suggest that, although some Ranch Hand subjects were exposed to very high levels of 2,3,7,8-TCDD, most had lower exposures.

Nygren *et al.* (1988) analysed adipose tissue and blood samples collected 15–20 years after military service from 27 men, 10 of whom were heavily exposed during their service in Viet Nam, 10 of whom had marginal exposure during service and served as Viet Nam controls and seven veterans who did not serve in Viet Nam and were used as 'era' controls. The results are summarized in **Table 20**. The only difference in the mean values was for 2,3,7,8-TCDD, for which the arithmetic mean for the heavily exposed group is approximately 8–10 times higher than that for controls. The highest level found was 213 ng/kg. In another report from the same study group, Gochfeld *et al.* (1989)

found a good correlation ($r = +0.89$) between the concentrations of 2,3,7,8-TCDD in blood and adipose tissue.

Table 19. Serum 2,3,7,8-TCDD levels (ng/kg) in Ranch Hand and control veterans

Stratum	Ranch Hand veterans			Comparison subjects		
	No.	Median	Range	No.	Median	Range
Flying officers (pilot)	247	7.3	0.0–42.6	239	4.7	0.0–18.5
Flying officers (navigator)	63	9.3	1.1–35.9	53	4.5	2.2–7.9
Nonflying officers	19	6.6	3.1–24.9	11	4.3	0.0–6.0
Flying enlisted personnel	152	17.2	0.0–195.5	137	4.0	0.0–12.7
Nonflying enlisted personnel	407	23.6	0.0–617.7	416	3.9	0.0–54.8
All personnel	888	12.4	0.0–617.7	856	4.2	0.0–54.8

From Wolfe *et al.* (1990)

(iii) *Exposure to PCDDs at incinerators*

The levels of PCDDs in blood from 11 workers at a Swedish hazardous waste incinerator fell within the range of the normal background (Rappe *et al.*, 1992). The same result was reported by Bolm-Audorff *et al.* (1994) for 31 workers at three hazardous waste incinerators in Germany.

Böske *et al.* (1995) analysed 37 blood samples of employees at a municipal solid-waste incinerator. They reported that no increased concentrations could be attributed to professional activities by the donors. Similarly, Päpke *et al.* (1993a) found normal I-TEQ values in 10 blood samples from workers employed at municipal solid-waste incinerators in Germany.

In order to determine occupational exposure of employees in three hazardous waste incinerators, 25 workplace air measurements were analysed (Päpke *et al.*, 1994a). The highest concentration measured was 3.79 pg I-TEQ/m^3, corresponding to 7.6% of the German occupational technical exposure limit (TRK) of 50 pg I-TEQ/m^3 (see Section 1.5). All the sampling took place during a normal working day at the plants.

The exposure situation can change quite drastically when repair works are carried out at hazardous waste incinerators and/or during welding, cutting and burning of metals (Menzel *et al.*, 1996), which can lead to exceptionally high concentrations. Outside of hazardous waste incinerators, high concentrations can also occur at demolition sites where steel constructions and machines are burned. The TRK value was exceeded by factors of 2–24 in the cases observed. All air samples were taken by personal sampling.

Table 20. Concentrations of PCDDs in blood plasma of exposed and unexposed groups of United States Army veterans (ng/kg fat)

Isomers	Arithmetic means						Geometric means		
	Exposed Viet Nam veterans		Viet Nam controls		Era controls[a]		Exposed Viet Nam veterans	Viet Nam controls	Era controls
	Mean	SEM[b]	Mean	SEM	Mean	SEM	Mean	Mean	Mean
2,3,7,8-TCDD	46.2	19.1	6.6	0.9	4.6	0.9	15.7	5.9	3.9
1,2,3,7,8-PeCDD	13.7	2.5	14.3	2.3	14.4	2.3	11.7	12.9	13.3
1,2,3,4,7,8-HxCDD	15.5	2.7	12.0	2.8	8.8	2.2	13.2	8.5	7.0
1,2,3,6,7,8-HxCDD	124	10.7	108	25.5	96.3	30.3	120	80.6	73.8
1,2,3,7,8,9-HxCDD	21.6	4.0	11.5	2.1	11.1	4.8	16.9	8.7	6.8
1,2,3,4,6,7,8-HpCDD	201	19.2	157	28.2	139	51.1	194	137	108
OCDD	1 582	461	1 118	356	1 120	406	1 204	618	709

From Nygren et al. (1988)

[a] Era controls are veterans who served outside Viet Nam during the period of the Viet Nam conflict

[b] SEM, standard error of mean

(iv) *Exposure in paper and pulp mills*

Exposure to PCDDs and PCDFs among workers in paper and pulp mills appears not to be significantly higher than among referents outside the paper industry, even among those workers thought to have the most opportunity for exposure (those exposed to the effluent of the bleaching process).

The United States National Institute for Occupational Safety and Health (Mouradian *et al.*, 1995) conducted air and wipe sampling in a paper mill and measured PCDD and PCDF levels in the sera of 46 workers (14 with low potential exposure, 32 with high potential exposure) and in 16 community residents who served as referents. While some low levels of PCDD and PCDF were detected in the air, there were no differences in serum PCDD and PCDF levels between referents, 'low-exposure' workers and 'high-exposure' workers, all of whom showed normal low levels. For 2,3,7,8-TCDD, the respective medians were 1.8, 1.9 and 1.9 ng/kg, while the median PCDD/PCDF total I-TEQs were 19.1, 21.2 and 18.1 ng/kg for each group, respectively. Regression analyses indicated that occupational exposure was not a significant predictor of serum I-TEQ levels, but consumption of local fish, age and body mass index were predictors. A number of workers had a long history in the plant and would have been expected to have higher serum levels if occupational exposure was significant.

Rosenberg *et al.* (1994) found similar results for workers in a Finnish paper mill. They measured serum levels of PCDDs and PCDFs in 14 workers from the bleaching area, 20 workers from the paper mill and 14 controls who worked in areas of the mill without contact with paper or bleach. There were no significant differences in lipid-adjusted PCDD/PCDF concentrations between the three groups (median PCDD/PCDF total I-TEQs, 52.7, 54.7 and 47.0 ng/kg, respectively) and results for all three groups were similar to background concentrations for men not occupationally exposed. There were some significant differences in levels of 2,3,7,8-TCDD (medians, 4.9, 2.4 and 3.3 ng/kg, respectively) and of 2,3,7,8-TCDF (medians, 2.9, 1.5 and 1.6 ng/kg, respectively), with workers in the bleaching areas having the highest levels. However, levels of these congeners did not differ from background levels for workers not exposed occupationally. The authors indicated that workers ate locally caught fish one to two times a week and that fish consumption may have influenced the results.

(v) *Exposure in steel mills*

PCDDs and PCDFs have been investigated in the work environment in steel mills in Sweden by Antonsson *et al.* (1989). Values for air samples at points close to a furnace, an overhead crane and a crane cabin ranged between 0.80 and 14 pg Nordic TEQ/m^3.

From these results, a daily intake of PCDDs/PCDFs was estimated to be 5–10% of the maximum limit of admissible daily intake (ADI; 35 pg/kg per week).

(b) *Population exposure due to industrial accident*

In an accident on 10 July 1976 at the ICMESA plant at Seveso, Italy, a runaway reaction led to a blow-out of a TCP production reactor. The chemical cloud that emerged from the reactor entrained nearly 2900 kg of organic matter, including at least 600 kg of sodium trichlorophenate and an amount of 2,3,7,8-TCDD which is still being evaluated [probably of the order of several kilograms]. The visible part of the cloud rose up to about 50 m, subsequently subsided and fell back to the earth, but was wind-driven over a wide area. Within less than 2 h after the accident, chemicals settled on the ground as far as 6 km south of the factory, or were dispersed by wind streams. Plants, domestic animals and birds were seriously affected, many dying within a few days of the accident [probably due to chemicals other than 2,3,7,8-TCDD]. About 10 days after the accident, 2,3,7,8-TCDD was found in samples of various types collected near the factory (Bertazzi & di Domenico, 1994). As a first step, information on the location of toxic and patho-logical events was used to draw an approximate diagram of the contaminated area. This was confirmed by chemical monitoring of 2,3,7,8-TCDD in the soil carried out under emergency conditions. Within five weeks of the accident, the area was subdivided into Zones A, B and R in descending order of 2,3,7,8-TCDD contamination and toxicological risk levels. The borderline between Zones A and B was set at average 2,3,7,8-TCDD concentrations in the soil of ≤ 50 $\mu g/m^2$; the boundaries between Zones A and B and Zone R were fixed where the average contamination was ≤ 5 $\mu g/m^2$. Zone R included the remaining territory where detectable levels of 2,3,7,8-TCDD (formally ≥ 0.75 $\mu g/m^2$) were found. Soil levels are further described in Section 1.3.2.

From Zone A, over 730 inhabitants were evacuated. Zones B and R were subjected to area-specific hygiene regulations including prohibition of farming, consumption of local agricultural products and keeping poultry and other animals. All persons residing in these zones at the time of the accident, as well as all the newborn and new residents in the subsequent 10-year period, were considered to have been exposed. Three exposure categories were formed, corresponding to the zone of residence of the subjects at the time of the accident or later entry into the area. As a reference, the population of 11 muni-cipalities surrounding the contaminated area was adopted (Bertazzi et al., 1993).

Mocarelli et al. (1990) reported analyses of 19 non-randomly selected samples of blood collected in 1976 from persons living in Zone A (**Table 21**) (analytical method ACS). Of these persons, 10 had chloracne of type 3 or 4 (see Section 4.2.1(a)) and nine had no chloracne. The persons with chloracne in general had higher concentrations than persons without chloracne, but high concentrations were also found in the healthy group. The 2,3,7,8-TCDD level of 56 000 ng/kg fat is the highest ever reported.

Recently, blood measurements of 2,3,7,8-TCDD were performed in persons randomly sampled from the most contaminated areas (Zones A and B), and in members of the population adopted as reference in the epidemiological investigations (Landi et al., 1996). Preliminary results were reported. In the six persons from Zone A, the median value was 71.5 ng/kg (extrapolation back to 1976 assuming a half-life of 7.1 years gave a value of 388.7 ng/kg); in the 52 inhabitants in Zone B, the corresponding values were 12.5 ng/kg and 77.6 ng/kg, while in the 52 subjects from the reference population, the median value was 5.5 ng/kg. Women consistently had higher levels of 2,3,7,8-TCDD than men in all three areas.

Table 21. Concentrations of 2,3,7,8-TCDD in the blood[a] of individuals from Zone A, Seveso

Age in 1976	Chloracne type[b]	2,3,7,8-TCDD (ng/kg fat)
4	Type 4	56 000
2	Type 4	27 800
6	Type 4	26 400
4	Type 4	26 000
8	Type 3	17 300
6	Type 4	15 900
11	Type 4	12 100
10	Type 3	7 420
5	Type 3	1 690
16	Type 3	828
15	None	10 400
38	None	9 140
27	None	6 320
71	None	5 560
39	None	4 540
41	None	3 730
55	None	3 050
46	None	2 650
50	None	1 770

From Mocarelli *et al.* (1990)
[a] Blood samples were collected in 1976
[b] Types 3 and 4 are the most severe chloracne

(c)   *Summary table*

Table 22 summarizes data from the major cohorts of populations highly exposed to 2,3,7,8-TCDD occupationally or as a result of accidents. Estimates of mean or median exposures, or in one case a range of individual exposures, are presented as reported in the cited publications. When tissue concentrations were measured, concentrations at the time of exposure estimated in the cited publications, or back-calculated by the Working Group based on a seven-year half-life, are also given.

1.3.2   *Environmental occurrence*

I-TEQ values are for PCDDs and PCDFs combined.

(a)   *Air*

PCDD/PCDF levels in air have been reported for many countries during the last 10 years. Due to the enormous amount of information, only a selection of representative data are summarized below. For detailed information, see Appendix 1 (Table 1).

Table 22. Estimated exposures to 2,3,7,8-TCDD (ng/kg blood lipid) of selected study populations

Study	Date(s) or duration of exposure	Date of sampling	No. of workers	Mean measured 2,3,7,8-TCDD blood concentration	Back-calculated to exposure date
Industrial workers					
BASF (Germany) (Ott et al., 1993)	1953 (accident)	1988–92	138	15.4 (geom.)	geom. mean: [~ 400][a] (1008: estimated cumulative concentration at time of exposure in workers with severe chloracne)
Boehringer-Ingelheim (Germany) (Flesch-Janys et al., 1995, 1996a; Kogevinas et al., 1997)	13.1 years Mean of 5.4 years after end of exposure Mean of 11.0 years after end of employment	1985–94	48 48 (same 48 as above)	84.1 (median) 48.9 (median)	141 (3–2252) (measured levels for the total cohort)
USA (Fingerhut et al., 1991a,b)	1987 (15–37 years after employment) > 1 year of exposure		253 (from 2 of 12 plants) 119	233 418	~ 2000 (mean) 32 000 (max.)
Netherlands (Hooiveld et al., 1996a,b)	1955–1985 (factory A)	1993	48	22.9 (production) (geom.) 87.2 (1963 accident) (geom.)	geom. mean: 286 (17–1160) 1434 (301–3683)
Handling and spraying of 2,4,5-T					
Ranch Hand/ US Viet Nam veterans (Nygren et al., 1988)	Late 1960s	1984–85	9	46.3 (arith.) 15.7 (geom.)	[~ 180][a] [~ 60][a]
Ranch Hand/ US Viet Nam veterans (Wolfe et al., 1990)	Late 1960s	1987	888	12.4 (median)	[~ 50][a]

Table 22 (contd)

Study	Date(s) or duration of exposure	Date of sampling	No. of workers	Mean measured 2,3,7,8-TCDD blood concentration	Back-calculated to exposure date
Handling and spraying of 2,4,5-T (contd)					
New Zealand (Smith et al., 1992a)	1953–88 (mean duration of exposure, 16 years)	1988	9	53.3	~ 300 (in 1970)
Seveso accident					
Mocarelli et al. (1990)	1976	1976	19 (zone A)	828–56 000 (range of individuals)	
Landi et al. (1996)	1976	[1992–93]	6 (zone A)	61.5 (mean) 71.5 (median)	333.8 388.7
			52 (zone B)	16.8 (mean) 12.5 (median)	111.4
			52 (outside)	5.3 (mean) 5.5 (median)	77.6

[a]Values in [ ] calculated by the Working Group

(i)   *Australia*

Taucher *et al.* (1992) reported PCDD/PCDF data from four sites in Sydney. The levels found in urban areas (0.016–0.062 pg I-TEQ/m^3) were similar to those from the northern hemisphere. There seemed to be a dose similarity with profiles obtained from combustion sources.

(ii)   *Austria*

The first systematic approach (Moche & Thanner, 1996a) to monitor ambient air concentrations of PCDDs/PCDFs in Austria was started in 1992. Within and in the vicinity of Vienna, Graz, Linz and Steyregg, 100 samples were taken during a whole year. The values generally ranged in the summer and winter period between 0.022–0.041 and 0.050–0.222 pg I-TEQ/m^3, respectively. The winter PCDD/PCDF values at Graz (south of the city centre on the grounds of a garden nursery) were approximately 0.22 pg I-TEQ/m^3 and were clearly above the levels found at Vienna and Linz.

(iii)   *Belgium*

Wevers *et al.* (1992) compared PCDD/PCDF concentrations in air in a vehicle tunnel near Antwerp with local ambient air. The I-TEQ values in tunnel air were two to three times higher than those in ambient (background) air. Wevers *et al.* (1993) also reported values from six sampling locations across Flanders (Belgium) in the neighbourhood of typical emission sources. The values found ranged between 0.018 and 0.379 pg I-TEQ/m^3.

(iv)   *Canada*

Measurement of PCDDs/PCDFs in ambient air in south-west Ontario have been presented by Bobet *et al.* (1990) for two sampling stations: downtown Windsor and Walepole Island Indian Reserve. No isomer-specific analyses were reported. Concentrations measured at the Walepole station in 1988 were 4–20 times lower than those in Windsor. In the 13 samples collected in Windsor, the mean level of OCDD was 2.12 pg/m^3 with a maximum of 7.09 pg/m^3. The mean for total HpCDD was 1.19 pg/m^3. At both stations, the majority of the PCDDs detected comprised hepta- and octa-chlorinated congeners. The tetra- and penta-CDDs were not found above detection limit (0.1 pg/m^3) at either station.

Additional data for Ontario were measured in 1988 in Dorset and on Toronto Island by Steer *et al.* (1990a). The highest levels were mainly for OCDD: Toronto Island, 0.3–0.8 pg/m^3; Dorset, 0.1–7 pg/m^3. No other isomer-specific data were reported.

Samples collected in the vicinity of a cement kiln were reported by Reiner *et al.* (1995). The values found were lower than the average values found in air samples taken on Toronto Island. All levels were considerably lower than the Ontario Ministry of Environment and Energy guideline of 5 pg/m^3.

Steer *et al.* (1990b) reported elevated PCDD and PCDF air levels in connection with a fire at a disposal site containing some 14 million tyres. Sampling sites were changed as required to provide samples near the fire (1 km downwind) and samples at the limit of the evacuation zone (3 km downwind). The highest total I-TEQ of 2.5 pg/m^3 measured represents 50% of the provincial interim guideline of 5 pg/m^3 (annual average).

(v) Germany

Bruckmann and Hackhe (1987) reported 21 ambient air measurements in Hamburg. The sampling was performed at sites with wide differences in air quality (e.g., at a dump site, residential area, industrial area, highway tunnel, close to a highway, vicinity of Hamburg). The values were between < 0.1 pg and 2.2 pg/m^3 expressed in German TEQs. The main sources of the PCDDs/PCDFs detected were thermal processes (industry, traffic and probably home heating facilities). Using more sophisticated analytical techniques, Rappe *et al.* (1988) analysed 13 Hamburg samples not only for the 2,3,7,8-substituted isomers but also for all single isomers separated on SP 2331 GC.

Between 1985 and 1986, 18 sites in North-Rhine-Westphalia were sampled to quantify PCDDs/PCDFs in ambient air (Kirschmer, 1987). For the Rhine-Ruhr area, mean values for total PCDDs and PCDFs at 11 sampling sites were 3.2 pg/m^3 and 5.5 pg/m^3, respectively. 2,3,7,8-TCDD was not detected in any sample (detection limit, 0.1 pg/m^3).

Christmann *et al.* (1989b) analysed 22 air samples originating from Berlin, Gelsen-kirchen and Recklinghausen. Usually, PCDD/PCDF levels were in the lower pg/m^3 (0.02–0.4 pg German TEQ/m^3). In one indoor air sample, the TEQ value was increased, due to the application of PCP as wood preservative, up to 2.6 pg/m^3.

Measurements in kindergartens with PCP-treated wood have been reported by Päpke *et al.* (1989a). The mean of 15 measurements was 0.696 pg German TEQ/m^3 (range, 0.018–2.46).

In 1990, at six sites located in Hessen, average ambient air PCDD/PCDF concentrations (calculated as I-TEQ) of between 0.048 pg/m^3 (rural reference site) and 0.146 pg/m^3 (industrial sites combined) were determined (König *et al.*, 1993). At five locations, a distinct annual cycle of PCDD/PCDF concentrations was observed, with relatively low concentrations in summer and increasing concentrations towards the winter months. On the other hand, the ratio of total PCDF to total PCDD levels showed a maximum in summer because of a comparatively larger decrease in PCDD towards the summer months. The annual average distribution of PCDD/PCDF homologue groups was similar at all six sites. The contributions of PCDF homologues to the total tetra- to octa-CDD/CDF content decreased with increasing degree of chlorination, whereas that of PCDD homologues increased with increasing degree of chlorination. For each homo-logous group, the contribution of congeners with a 2,3,7,8-chlorine substitution pattern was similar.

Towara *et al.* (1993) analysed the distribution of airborne PCDDs/PCDFs in relation to particle size. Particle sizes from < 0.15 to > 4.05 μm were grouped into five categories; the patterns of PCDDs/PCDFs detected were very similar for all five categories. Hence, particle-mediated transport and deposition should be similar for all PCDD/PCDFs.

Data on PCDDs/PCDFs in ambient air have recently been reported by Wallenhorst *et al.* (1995) for Baden-Württemberg. In rural areas, total concentrations were 0.015–0.020 pg I-TEQ/m^3. In urban areas, the concentrations were 0.07–0.08 pg I-TEQ/m^3. PCDD/PCDF concentrations in total air decreased from city centre to suburban areas and the surrounding areas.

Annual mean concentrations of PCDDs/PCDFs in the ambient air of four cities in North-Rhine-Westphalia were measured at the same locations in 1987–88 and again in 1993–94 (Hiester *et al.*, 1995). Over this period, the annual average PCDD/PCDF concentrations decreased from 0.130 to 0.040 pg I-TEQ/m^3 in Cologne (69%), from 0.332 to 0.124 pg I-TEQ/m^3 in Duisburg (63%), from 0.204 to 0.076 pg I-TEQ/m^3 in Essen (63%) and from 0.224 to 0.120 pg I-TEQ/m^3 in Dortmund (46%). This decrease can be related to actions taken since 1989.

A similar situation has been shown for Hamburg by Friesel *et al.* (1996). Monitoring of ambient air and deposition demonstrated decreases of about 70% and 20% respectively in PCDD/PCDF concentrations in air (pg I-TEQ/m^3) and deposition flux (pg I-TEQ/m^2 per day). Ambient air concentrations decreased from 0.108 in 1990 and 0.037 in 1993 to 0.036 in 1995; deposition decreased from 16 in 1990 to 11 in 1993 but rose to 13 in 1995. The fact that the reduction in ambient air concentrations has been much greater than the reduction in emissions may be attributed to long-range transport and to smaller diffuse sources not yet identified.

The atmospheric levels of PCDDs/PCDFs in both the gas and particle phase were measured continuously over one year (1992–93) at seven sites on the outskirts of Augsburg (Hippelein *et al.*, 1996; Swerev *et al.*, 1996) and at a rural site 15 km from the city. The PCDD/PCDF levels were about two times higher at the sampling points on the edge of the city than at the remote location. There was a pronounced temporal variability in total air concentrations, levels in winter being nine times higher than those in summer. The gas/particle partitioning was characterized by higher gaseous fraction for more volatile compounds and higher ambient temperatures. It was concluded that the ambient air concentrations of the PCDDs/PCDFs are determined by local and regional emissions, with seasonal (winter) sources contributing the vast majority of the emission fluxes.

Rabl *et al.* (1996) reported PCDD/PCDF measurements in relation to distance of 1.3, 2.0 and 3.3 km from a supposed local major emission source in Bavaria (a municipal waste incinerator at Schwandorf). The PCDD/PCDF concentrations were quite similar at each distance. At emission concentrations of 1–10 pg I-TEQ/m^3 from the incinerator, no influence of the waste incineration plant could be found.

(vi) *Japan*

Isomer-specific analyses of PCDD/PCDFs and other chlorinated components in ambient air have been reported by Sugita *et al.* (1993, 1994). The concentrations of PCDDs/PCDFs were higher in winter than in summer. Ranges were 0.469–1.427 pg I-TEQ/m^3 in summer and 0.294–2.990 pg I-TEQ/m^3 in winter. Coplanar and mono-*ortho* PCBs were present at concentrations about 10 times higher than those of 2,3,7,8-substituted PCDDs/PCDFs. PCDFs accounted for about 70% of the total toxic equivalents, PCDDs for 20% and the sum of both types of PCBs for 10%.

Similar findings have been presented by Kurokawa *et al.* (1994). At three different sites, values were highest in winter. Coplanar PCBs contributed about 11% to the total TEQ. In winter, most of the PCDDs/PCDFs were found in the particle phase.

(vii) *The Netherlands*

van Jaarsveld and Schutter (1993) estimated (air calculation models) emissions of PCDDs/PCDFs to the atmosphere in various parts of north-western Europe on the basis of emission factors combined with production quantities. Atmospheric residence times were calculated for different particle sizes. Small particles, carrying more than 50% of total PCDDs/PCDFs, have residence times of the order of three days, while very large particles (diameter, > 20 μm) reside only a few hours in the atmosphere. Comparison of predicted PCDD/PCDF levels in ambient air with available measurements showed fairly good agreement.

Ambient air measurements of PCDDs/PCDFs in The Netherlands have been performed by Bolt and de Jong (1993). Particulate-bound PCDD/PCDF levels in air around a municipal waste incinerator ranged between 0.015 ± 0.005 and 0.125 ± 0.025 pg I-TEQ/m^3. Congener profiles were very similar in all wind directions and were well correlated with the incinerator emissions.

(viii) *Norway*

Oehme *et al.* (1991) reported on the determination of PCDDs/PCDFs in air at the inlet and outlet of a longitudinally ventilated tunnel with separate tubes for each traffic direction. The varying percentage of heavy-duty vehicles made it possible to differentiate between factors for light-duty vehicles (LDVs) and heavy-duty (diesel) vehicles (HDDVs). Depending on driving conditions, the estimated emission factors were of the order of 0.04–0.5 ng Nordic TEQ/km for LDVs and 0.8–9.5 ng/km for HDDVs. On a volume basis, the values ranged between 0.097 and 0.98 pg Nordic TEQ/m^3. A typical ambient air concentration for central Oslo was 0.04 pg Nordic TEQ/m^3.

First measurements for PCDDs/PCDFs in Arctic air have been reported recently by Schlabach *et al.* (1996). The sampling was performed in spring and summer of 1995 in Spitzbergen. The values of two samples were 0.0023 and 0.0011 pg I-TEQ/m^3.

(ix) *Poland*

The first results for PCDDs/PCDFs in ambient air were published by Grochowalski *et al.* (1995). Two measurements performed in winter 1995 in Cracow — a heavily industrialized city — gave values of 0.95 pg I-TEQ/m^3 (market square) and 11.95 pg I-TEQ/m^3 (crossroads), respectively. OCDD and OCDF were reported at 280 and 220 pg/m^3, respectively.

(x) *Russian Federation*

Khamitov and Maystrenko (1994) reported ambient air levels, sampled in Ufa, of between 0.2 and 0.5 pg I-TEQ/m^3. Levels of isomers were measured by Kruglov *et al.* (1996) in two air samples originating from an industrial city during an accidental oil fire.

(xi) *Slovakia*

As part of the TOCOEN (Toxic Compounds in the Environment) project, Holoubek *et al.* (1991) reported I-TEQ values in ambient air from former Czechoslovakia. The samples — collected in industrial and urban areas in 1990 — showed a wide range of PCDD/PCDF contamination, from none detected to 6.3 pg I-TEQ/m^3.

(xii) *Spain*

Ambient air samples associated with municipal waste incinerators, chemical industry, traffic and urban air ranged between 0.05 and 0.55 pg I-TEQ/m^3. Surprisingly high levels of OCDF (126.8 pg/m^3) were found near a municipal waste incinerator, while OCDD was reported at only 5.7 pg/m^3. Levels of highly chlorinated PCDDs and PCDFs correlated poorly (Abad *et al.*, 1996).

(xiii) *Sweden*

Rappe *et al.* (1989a) analysed nine ambient air samples taken in winter in 1986 in Rörvik and in Gothenburg under various atmospheric conditions. The results demonstrated that the contribution to the total *air* burden in Gothenburg from local sources during periods with good ventilation seems to be of secondary importance. The isomeric patterns of PCDDs/PCDFs among all samples were very similar. There was also a striking similarity in the isomeric pattern for TCDFs and PeCDFs in the particulate samples, automobile exhaust and emissions from municipal waste incinerators. The results strongly indicated that the general background of PCDDs and PCDFs in airborne particulates has its origin in various types of incineration processes, including automobile exhaust.

(xiv) *United Kingdom*

Data on PCDD/PCDF air concentrations have been monitored in three major cities (London, Manchester and Cardiff) and a busy industrial town (Stevenage) from the beginning of 1991 to the end of 1992 (Clayton *et al.*, 1993). Levels of total 2,3,7,8-substituted PCDDs and PCDFs, other isomers and the total I-TEQ for the four sites have been reported. Concentrations of the 2,3,7,8-substituted PCDDs are mainly associated with the HpCDDs and OCDD, the OCDD accounting for over 76% of the total 2,3,7,8-substituted PCDDs. The tetra-, penta- and hexa-chlorinated congeners were generally below detection limits. Higher values were found in winter than in summer. The mean values for about 43 single measurements for each site were between 0.039 and 0.102 pg I-TEQ/m^3.

Dyke and Coleman (1995) reported PCDD/PCDF measurements before, during and after 'bonfire night' at Oxford. Bonfire night (5 November) is an annual event during which it is customary in England to set off fireworks and light bonfires. An increase in PCDD/PCDF concentrations by approximately a factor of four occurred during the period of bonfire night.

(xv) *United States*

The results of a baseline study on PCDDs/PCDFs in the ambient atmosphere have been published (Eitzer & Hites, 1989). Between 1985 and 1987, 55 samples were taken at three sites in Bloomington, IN, and a set of samples was also taken in the Trout Lake, WI, area, a much more rural area than Bloomington. In ambient air, consistency was seen in the isomer pattern within each group of congeners with the same number of chlorine substituents, but overall levels of the various groups had somewhat more variation. Some of this variation was related to the atmospheric temperatures, with more of the lower chlorinated congeners found in the vapour phase at higher temperatures. No isomer-specific concentrations (except for OCDD) were reported. The mean OCDD values for Bloomington and the Trout Lake area were 0.89 pg/m^3 and 0.16 pg/m^3, respectively.

Smith *et al.* (1989, 1990a,b), analysed downwind and upwind ambient air samples around the industrial area of Niagara Falls, for PCDDs/PCDFs. One location, predominantly downwind of Niagara Falls, showed a variety of patterns and a wide concentration range of PCDDs/PCDFs (0.07–53 pg Eadon TEQ/m^3). The upwind 'control' location results showed lower concentrations of PCDDs and PCDFs and less variable patterns. In nearly all samples, HpCDDs and OCDD were found at ranges from not detected to 5.43 pg/m^3 and from 1.36 to 8.88 pg/m^3, respectively.

PCDDs and PCDFs were measured in ambient air samples collected in Ohio in 1987 by Edgerton *et al.* (1989). No 2,3,7,8-TCDD was detected in any of the samples at a detection limit of less than 0.24 pg/m^3. Using a chemical mass balance model applied to PCDD/PCDF congener group profiles, major potential sources of these compounds to the atmosphere in Ohio were determined to be municipal solid waste and sewage sludge combustion plants.

Hahn *et al.* (1989) reported on pre-operational background ambient air levels of PCDDs/PCDFs around two modern municipal waste incinerators. In addition, workplace air levels inside one facility (Hillsborough County, FL) were measured to evaluate the potential exposure of employees. The levels of PCDDs/PCDFs and heavy metals were similar to ambient levels outside the facility before the facility began operation.

The concentrations of PCDDs and PCDFs in ambient air of several sites in metropolitan Dayton, OH, have been determined (Tiernan *et al.*, 1989). Total PCDDs detected in industrial areas ranged from 1.6 to 11.2 pg/m^3, and the corresponding total PCDFs ranged from 0.62 to 11.7 pg/m^3. No PCDDs or PCDFs were found in rural regions, typical average detection limits being on the order of 0.02–0.17 pg/m^3. Approximately 50% of the total PCDD/PCDFs in the ambient air samples collected consisted of 2,3,7,8-chlorine-substituted congeners.

Airborne concentrations of PCDDs/PCDFs in office buildings and in corresponding ambient air in Boston, MA, were measured by Kominsky and Kwoka (1989). Twelve of the 16 samples were collected inside the buildings and four were collected at the ambient air intake plenums of the buildings. The distribution of total PCDD congeners was quite similar to corresponding surface wipe samples. In all 20 samples, it was possible to detect OCDD.

PCDD/PCDF concentrations in ambient air in winter at Bridgeport, the largest city in Connecticut, have been analysed by Hunt and Maisel (1990). The Connecticut Department of Environmental Protection has proposed an ambient air quality standard for PCDDs/PCDFs expressed in 2,3,7,8-TCDD equivalents on an annualized basis of

1.0 pg/m^3. In order to ensure that this standard is satisfied, it is required that ambient monitoring for each of the 2,3,7,8-substituted PCDD/PCDF isomers be conducted in the vicinity of each municipal solid-waste incinerator on both a pre-operational and post-operational basis. The report described the pre-operational measurements in the autumn and winter of 1987–88 in the vicinity of a municipal solid-waste incinerator. The TCDFs were the major PCDF class found. 1,2,3,4,6,7,8-HCDF was the predominant PCDF of toxicological significance. HxCDDs, HpCDDs and OCDD were the predominant PCDD congeners, and 1,2,3,4,6,7,8-HpCDD the predominant PCDD isomer of toxicological significance. In winter months, PCDDs/PCDFs are almost exclusively particulate-associated. Comparison of pre- and post-operational ambient PCDD/PCDF concentrations in the vicinity of the incinerator during winter showed similar levels and profiles for both periods.

Maisel and Hunt (1990) presented data on PCDDs/PCDFs in a 'typical' ambient air sample from Los Angeles, CA, including isomer-specific concentrations. Ambient PCDD/PCDF burdens for a Connecticut coastal location ($n = 27$, urban, winter), a southern Californian location ($n = 34$, urban) and a central Minnesota location ($n = 16$, rural) were 0.092, 0.091 and 0.021 pg I-TEQ/m^3, respectively.

A comprehensive programme for measurement of airborne toxic agents, designed to establish baseline concentrations of atmospheric PCDDs/PCDFs in the South Coast Air Basin (California), involved nine sampling sessions between December 1987 and March 1989 at eight different locations (Hunt & Maisel, 1992). The PCDD/PCDF congener profiles from most of the sample examined strongly suggested the influence of combustion sources. 1,2,3,4,6,7,8-HpCDD was the most prevalent PCDD after OCDD. The most toxic congener, 2,3,7,8-TCDD, was below the 10–20 fg/m^3 detection limit for most of the ambient air samples.

Ten years after the Binghamton State Office Building transformer incident in 1981 (see PCDF monograph, Section 1.2.1(b)(viii)), Schecter and Charles (1991) presented data on PCDDs/PCDFs in the air. In 1981–82, airborne samples contained levels of 352 pg Eadon TEQ/m^3 at the transformer site. In 1986, nine years into clean up, levels of 74 pg/m^3 TEQ were recorded. The guidelines for reoccupancy of the building were reported to be 14 pg TEQ/m^3 for renovation workers and 10 pg TEQ/m^3 for office workers.

The levels of airborne PCDDs/PCDFs in the area of the Columbus Municipal Waste-to-Energy facility in Columbus, OH, were reported by Lorber et al. (1996a). This facility, the largest single source of PCDDs/PCDFs identified in the literature (1992, 984 g I-TEQ per year; 1994, 267 g I-TEQ per year), ceased operation in December 1994. Air concentrations in the city were higher in 1994 when the facility was operating than after it shut down: in March and April 1994, the levels were 0.067 and 0.118 pg I-TEQ/m^3, respectively, compared with 0.049 pg I-TEQ/m^3 in June 1995 after the facility had closed.

Also in Ohio, air in the vicinity of the Montgomery County north and south municipal waste incinerators was analysed for PCDD/PCDFs (Riggs et al., 1996). PCDD levels in September 1995 were similar to those in the same area in 1988, but PCDF levels were much lower. At one site, the TEQ of PCDDs/PCDFs in ambient air was about a factor of 10 lower in 1995 than in 1988.

(b) Water (see Appendix 1, Table 2)

Because of the complex cycling and partitioning of PCDDs/PCDFs in the aquatic environment and the difficulty of analysis, adequate sampling and analysis methods have become available only over the past decade.

PCDDs and PCDFs are highly lipophilic and thus have an affinity for particulate organic carbon (Webster *et al.*, 1986). Knowledge of their partitioning between the sedimentary, colloidal, dissolved, organic and even vapour phases remains limited, largely because of the difficulty of measuring these compounds in solution.

PCDDs partition between particulate and dissolved fractions. Material that passes through a filter of 0.45 μm or 0.2 μm pore size is commonly defined as dissolved. The major problem with this definition is that colloidal particles (suspended solid particles of < 0.2 μm diameter) and other macromolecules pass through such filters and are included in the 'dissolved' phase. However, colloids and 'dissolved' organics may function as 'small particles' in terms of the mechanisms of PCDD/PCDF uptake by biological systems (Broman *et al.*, 1991, 1992).

(i) Canada

A survey of drinking-water supplies in the Province of Ontario was initiated in 1983 to determine the extent of their contamination with PCDDs/PCDFs (Jobb *et al.*, 1990). A total of 49 water supplies were examined. Water supplies in the vicinity of chemical industries and pulp and paper mills were sampled up to 20 times. Detection limits were in the low ppq (pg/L) range for all tetra- to octa-CDDs/CDFs. From 399 raw and treated water samples, only 37 positive results were reported. OCDD was detected in 36 of these samples, at values of 9–175 pg/L. 2,3,7,8-TCDD was not detected in any sample.

Muir *et al.* (1995) analysed water and other matrices downstream from a bleached kraft pulp mill on the Athabasca River (Alberta) in 1992. The 'dissolved phase' and the suspended particulates from continuous centrifuged samples were analysed for 41 PCDDs and PCDFs ranging from mono- to octachloro-substituted congeners. Most PCDD congeners (including 2,3,7,8-TCDD) were undetectable (< 0.1 pg/L) in the centrifugate.

(ii) Finland

High concentrations (70–140 μg/L) of total chlorophenols were found in drinking-water and 56 000–190 000 μg/L in ground water close to a sawmill in southern Finland. No data on PCDDs/PCDFs were reported. Due to their presence in commercial chlorinated phenols used, exposure of the population to PCDDs/PCDFs could not be excluded. No increased PCDD/PCDF concentrations were found in milk samples from mothers who had used the contaminated water (Lampi *et al.*, 1990).

(iii) *Germany*

Götz *et al.* (1994) reported an analysis of dissolved and particle-bound PCDDs/-PCDFs in the River Elbe. Samples upstream of Hamburg (Bunthaus) showed total values of 3.15 pg I-TEQ, while downstream in Blankenese values of 1.21 pg I-TEQ were found. More than 98% of the I-TEQ concentration in the water was particle-bound.

(iv) *Japan*

Seawater from Japanese coastal areas has been analysed. Adequate detection limits were achieved by use of a pre-concentration system, applied to 2000 L coastal seawater, resulting in the detection of almost all 2,3,7,8-substituted PCDDs and PCDFs. Values between < 5 and 560 fg/L were found (Matsumura *et al.*, 1994, 1995).

Hashimoto *et al.* (1995a) reported data on two seawater samples taken in 1990 near Matsuyama and Misaki. Only hepta- and octa-CDDs were detected (0.1–2.5 pg/L) but no PCDFs.

Drinking-water samples including home tap-water and well-water collected in 1991 in Shiga and Osaka Prefectures were analysed for PCDDs/PCDFs. The levels were in the low ppq (pg/L) or less in all samples analysed. The total daily intake of PCDDs/PCDFs via drinking-water was estimated to be only 0.00086–0.015% of that via food (Miyata *et al.*, 1992, 1993).

(v) *New Zealand*

A national Organochlorine Programme, including monitoring for PCDDs/PCDFs in water, was initiated in 1995. Samples were collected from 13 rivers at 16 sites during the period January to March 1996. No PCDDs/PCDFs were detected in any of the 16 composite samples. Limits of detection for the tetra-, penta- and hexa-chlorinated congeners were typically 1 pg/L or less. The I-TEQs were in the range of 0.25–2.4 pg/L, with a mean of 0.97 pg/L. The approximate 10-fold range of TEQ values determined for these samples is a result of variation in the detection limits in the analyses rather than any inherent differences in the samples. In calculating TEQs, half the detection limits were taken for non-detectable congeners (Buckland *et al.*, 1996).

(vi) *Russian Federation*

Ignatieva *et al.* (1993) found a level of 8.0 pg/L of total PCDDs in water from the Angara River, the only river that emerges from Lake Baikal.

Data on PCDD/PCDF concentrations in various river water samples were reported by Khamitov and Maystrenko (1995): Belaja River, 1.7–6.0 pg/L; Ufa River, 0.6–1 pg/L ; Inzer River, 1.8 pg/L; Zilim River, 0.2 pg/L. In contrast, drinking-water from the Ufa River was reported to be contaminated in 1990 with 0.5–1.0 pg/L. [It was not apparent from the paper whether the values were I-TEQs or total PCDDs/PCDFs].

Smirnov *et al.* (1996) reported values for PCDDs/PCDFs in the Ufa River at totals of 0.13–0.20 µg/L. 'Emergency' situations, where the concentration of PCDDs/PCDFs in river or tap-water exceeds the 'permissible' level (0.02 ng/L) by 10 to 100 times were stated to occur on a regular basis.

Fedorov (1993) reported on levels of PCDDs/PCDFs in various matrices (soil, sediments, air and water) near or at sites of some Russian chemical plants. In the spring of 1991, the drinking-water at Ufa, after cleaning, was found to be contaminated with 0.14 ng/L 1,2,3,6,7,8-HxCDD. Especially high concentrations of 28–167 pg/L 2,3,7,8-TCDD were measured in April 1992 in samples of Ufa drinking-water from four different water sources.

(vii) *Spain*

Sludge from drinking-water treatment plants was analysed by Rivera *et al.* (1995). Because of the high level of pollution in water from the Llobregat River, a combination of several treatment processes, including prechlorination, activated carbon and post-chlorination, is applied. The sludge from two treatment plants has been reported to be contaminated at levels of 5.59 and 2.74 ng I-TEQ/kg, respectively.

(viii) *Sweden*

Rappe *et al.* (1989b, 1990a) analysed surface and drinking-water with very low detection limits. At very low detection limits, most 2,3,7,8-substituted PCDDs and PCDFs were detected in all samples. 2,3,7,8-TCDD was found in most water samples, but at extremely low levels, between 0.0031 pg/L for river water and 0.0005 pg/L for drinking-water. This is at or below the lower level in the United States Environmental Protection Agency guideline of 0.0013 pg/L for this compound.

(ix) *United States*

Results of a survey conducted in 1986 for PCDDs/PCDFs and other pollutants in finished water systems throughout New York State were described by Meyer *et al.* (1989). The finding of OCDD is unsure, as it has been detected at 1 pg/L in blanks. Except for a trace of OCDF detected in one location, no other PCDDs or PCDFs were detected in any of 19 other community water systems surveyed.

Storm-water samples were collected from two outfalls that discharge into San Francisco Bay, CA, and represent sources of run-off from areas with different dominant land uses. The samples from the outfall located close to Oakland had higher values (mean, 21 pg I-TEQ/L) than samples from the city of Benicia located at the north of San Francisco Bay (mean, 3.5 pg I-TEQ/L) (Paustenbach *et al.*, 1996).

(c) *Soil* (see Appendix 1, Table 3)

(i) *Australia*

In 1990, surface soil samples from the Melbourne metropolitan area were analysed for PCDDs/PCDFs and other compounds (Sund *et al.*, 1993). A surface sample from Werribee Farm treatment complex paddock, where cattle graze on land that is used for filtration of sewage, contained the highest concentration (520 ng I-TEQ/kg). Samples of other origins contained between 0.09 and 8.2 ng I-TEQ/kg. Detection limits ranged from 0.08 to 24 ng/kg.

Levels of PCDDs/PCDFs in soil samples from conservation areas following bush fires have been reported by Buckland *et al.* (1994). Samples were collected (2 cm deep) six weeks after the fires were extinguished. The total PCDD/PCDF levels in the unburned conservation area samples were 1.1, 7.2 and 7.7 µg/kg (3.1, 8.7 and 10.0 ng I-TEQ/kg). The total PCDD/PCDF levels in the burnt conservation area samples were 1.3, 2.0 and 27.8 µg/kg (2.2, 3.0 and 36.8 ng I-TEQ/kg). The total PCDDs/PCDFs in the single Sydney metropolitan area sample was 22.3 µg/kg (42.6 ng I-TEQ/kg). The results of this limited survey indicate that bush fires have not had a major impact on the levels of PCDDs/PCDFs in conservation area soil.

(ii) *Austria*

Around a densely populated industrial urban area (Linz), soils from grassland and forest areas were analysed for PCDDs/PCDFs and PCBs (Weiss *et al.*, 1993, 1994). The concentrations of PCDDs/PCDFs were higher in soils near chemical and/or steel plants. The highest PCDD/PCDF concentration in grassland soil (I-TEQ, 14.4 ng/kg) was measured near a hospital refuse incineration plant.

Riss *et al.* (1990) compared PCDD/PCDF levels in soil, grass, cow's milk (see Section 1.3.2(*d*)(i)), human blood and spruce needles in an area of PCDD/PCDF contamination through emissions from a metal reclamation plant (Brixlegg, Tyrol). Soil concentrations were highest near the plant and in the main wind direction, and decreased in all directions with increasing distance. The highest concentration found corresponds to 420 ng German TEQ/kg. The level of 40 ng/kg TEQ (which has been proposed as an upper limit for agricultural use) was exceeded in an area reaching 600 m from the plant in the main wind directions. Milk samples from farms with meadows in the contaminated area contained TEQ levels of PCDDs/PCDFs ranging from 13.5 to 37.0 ng/kg fat, which were considerably higher than that of 3.6 ng/kg in the control sample from Kossen/Tyrol. About 50% of the TEQ of the contaminated milk was accounted for by 2,3,7,8-TCDD (normally about 10%). Because of the elevated PCDD/PCDF levels in cow's milk, blood plasma from two farmers who drank milk from their own cows was analysed for PCDDs/PCDFs. One had significantly elevated blood levels (see **Table 25**).

Determinations of PCDDs and PCDFs in soil samples from rural, urban and industrial sites in Salzburg state (Boos *et al.*, 1992) gave I-TEQ values generally in the low ng/kg range. Six samples contained PCDDs/PCDFs. Levels exceeding 5 ng German TEQ/kg, above which limit the cultivation of certain vegetables is restricted, but none exceeded 40 ng TEQ/kg, which would exclude the cultivation of any plants. Including in the calculation undetected congeners at 50% of the detection limit would lead to seven samples exceeding the lower limit. The lowest level found was 0.1 ng TEQ/kg.

(iii) *Belgium*

Topsoil samples were collected at six locations in Flanders, and analysed isomer-specifically [not in tables reported] for PCDDs/PCDFs (Van Cleuvenbergen *et al.*, 1993). Concentrations in the 0–3-cm soil fraction, averaged for each location, ranged from 2.1 ng/kg at a rural location to 8.9 ng/g (both as I-TEQ) in an industrialized area.

(iv) *Brazil*

Krauss *et al.* (1995) analysed PCDDs/PCDFs and PCBs in forest soils from Brazil. The I-TEQ values found in four areas are presented in Appendix 1 (Table 4). In the Amazon basin the PCDD/PCDF concentrations of soil were close to the detection limits. In industrial regions around Rio de Janeiro and São Paulo, highly contaminated soils with I-TEQ values between 11 and 654 ng/kg were found.

(v) *Canada*

Soil in the vicinity of a large municipal refuse incinerator was analysed for PCDDs/PCDFs. Fourteen locations, which included three control sites, were sampled in 1983 (McLaughlin *et al.*, 1989; Pearson *et al.*, 1990). In nearly all samples, OCDD was detected. The measurements were not isomer-specific. As expressed by the authors, the results showed that PCDDs/PCDFs emitted from the incinerator (Suaru, Hamilton) since 1973 had not accumulated in surface soil in the vicinity of the plant (McLaughlin *et al.*, 1989). Concentrations of PCDDs/PCDFs in soils near refuse and sewage sludge incinerators and in remote rural and urban locations (no 2,3,7,8-substituted isomers, exclusively OCDD and in some cases OCDF) were measured. In nearly all cases, total hepta-CDD and OCDD were most abundant. No evidence of any source-related airborne deposition of PCDDs/PCDFs in the soil around a sewage sludge incinerator in Scarborough was identified.

In 97 soil samples analysed for PCDDs/PCDFs, no clear connection between emission sources and levels of these components in soil or food was found by Birmingham (1990). Levels, patterns and quantities of I-TEQ in soils from various sources were analysed. The mean and standard deviation for I-TEQ, expressed in ng/kg, were: rural soils ($n = 30$), 0.4 ± 0.6; urban soils ($n = 47$), 11.3 ± 21.8; industrial soils ($n = 20$), 40.8 ± 33.1. Using the worst-case scenario, an infant consuming urban soil containing the mean plus three standard deviations (77 ng I-TEQ/kg) would ingest less than one tenth of the tolerable daily intake (see Section 1.5).

In 1989, soils were sampled in areas of cleared forest in New Brunswick, where 2,4-D/2,4,5-T herbicide was applied in one or more application at 3–10 lbs/acre (3.3–11 kg/ha) between 1956 and 1965. Residues of 2,3,7,8-TCDD were detected at up to 20 ng/kg in the upper 5 cm of soil. Residues were also found at greater depths at lower concentrations at one test site. 2,3,7,8-TCDF was not found in soil samples from sprayed or unsprayed areas (Hallett & Kornelsen, 1992).

(vi) *China*

Wu *et al.* (1995) published results for two soil samples, originating from the Ya-Er lake area where chemical plants which produce chlorine compounds have discharged much waste water into the sea. The two samples contained hexachlorobenzene at levels of 35 and 38 mg/kg, respectively, but only very low levels of PCDDs/PCDFs. Sediment samples originating from the same area contained maximal levels of 136.6 μg OCDD/kg and 797 ng I-TEQ/kg.

(vii) *Czech Republic*

2,3,7,8-TCDD contamination was measured in more than 100 soil samples (0–20 cm depth) from a factory that produced mainly sodium 2,4,5-trichlorophenoxyacetate, sodium pentachlorophenolate, PCP and TCP, starting in 1965 (Zemek & Kocan, 1991). 2,3,7,8-TCDD levels ranged from undetectable to 29.8 µg/kg. Samples from residential and agricultural areas in Neratovice showed levels between undetectable and 100 ng/kg. Soil samples collected at a distance of 50–80 m from the plant contained levels between undetectable and 60 ng/kg 2,3,7,8-TCDD.

(viii) *Finland*

Soils at sites where wood preservatives had been used (Sandell & Tuominen, 1993) contained high levels of PCDDs/PCDFs. The dominant congeners were 1,2,3,6,7,8-HxCDD, 1,2,3,4,6,7,8-HpCDD, OCDD, 1,2,3,4,7,8-HxCDF, 1,2,3,6,7,8-HxCDF, 2,3,4,6,7,8-HxCDF, 1,2,3,4,6,7,8-HpCDF and OCDF. In the surface layers (0–20 cm), I-TEQ values ranging from 1.7–85 µg/kg were found.

Assmuth and Vartiainen (1995) reported on further soil samples from sites where wood preservatives like 2,3,4,6-tetrachlorophenol, PCP and 2,4,6-TCP have been used. High concentrations (maximum value, 90 µg I-TEQ/kg; mean, 19 µg I-TEQ/kg) were found. PCDDs/PCDFs were distributed heterogeneously between soil layers, the concentrations in topsoil samples being generally lower. Concentrations of PCDDs/PCDFs were unrelated to the chlorophenol contents in the soil samples. Hexa-, hepta- and octa-CDFs were the dominant congeners in concentration.

(ix) *Germany*

In soils contaminated with motor oils and re-refined oils, Rotard *et al.* (1987) found PCDDs at µg/kg levels. No PCDFs were detected.

An analytical programme to detect contaminants in soil samples at the site of a herbicide plant in Hamburg that closed in 1984 was presented by Schlesing (1989) and Jürgens and Roth (1989). In total, 2652 soil samples deriving from 196 borings were investigated. The highest value reported (presumably a production residue stored on site) reached at a depth of 2 m was 0.7 mg 2,3,7,8-TCDD/kg. Even at depths of 7 and 9 m, values for 2,3,7,8-TCDD of 391 and 41.8 µg/kg, respectively, were found.

The fate of polychlorinated aromatics was studied in the vicinity of a former copper smelter (Rastatt) and a former cable pyrolysis plant (Maulach) that both closed in 1986. Contamination with PCDDs/PCDFs from stack emissions in samples taken within a radius of 100 m from the source at 0–30 cm in depth reached 29 µg I-TEQ/kg soil (Hagenmaier *et al.*, 1992; She & Hagenmaier, 1996). Comparing homologue and isomer concentrations of samples collected in 1981, 1987 and 1989 (same sites, same depths, same sampling method), no significant difference in either homologue pattern or isomer pattern could be detected. Vertical migration of PCDDs/PCDFs in highly contaminated soil is very slow and more than 90% of the compounds were found in the top 10 cm three years after the sources of emission were closed. Within the limits of analytical accuracy (± 20%), there was no indication of appreciable loss of PCDDs/PCDFs by vertical migration, evaporation or decomposition over a period of eight years, which underlines the persistence of these compounds in the soil.

The distribution of PCDDs/PCDFs in soil around a hazardous waste incinerator at Schwabach was analysed by Deister and Pommer (1991). The highest values were 20.7 and 4.4 ng German TEQ/kg (350 m from the chimney) at depths of 0–2 cm and 0–30 cm, respectively.

Unger and Prinz (1991) found that levels of PCDD/PCDF contamination of soils decreased with increasing distance from a road. The highest values were 23–44.8 ng I-TEQ/kg between 0.1 and 1 m from the road. The number of cars per day on a certain road influenced the PCDD/PCDF levels found.

The finding of PCDDs and especially PCDFs in surface gravel of playgrounds and sports fields (*Kieselrot*) is described in Section 1.3.2(*c*) of the monograph on PCDFs in this volume (see also **Table 25** in this monograph).

Concurrence of farmers' and municipal interests has led to the widespread use of sewage sludge fertilization in West Germany. In 1988, 608 thousand tonnes (dry weight) of sewage sludge, 25% of the total German production, was spread on 360 000 hectares of farmland (McLachlan & Hutzinger, 1990). A survey of 43 samples from 28 German waste-water treatment plants found PCDD/PCDF concentrations between 28 and 1560 ng German TEQ/kg dry weight (Hagenmaier *et al.*, 1985). This compares with the German recommendation for unlimited agricultural use of soil of 5 ng TEQ/kg. McLachlan and Reissinger (1990) analysed soil samples from north-eastern Bavaria with different sludge fertilization histories. The relationship observed between the length of sewage sludge use and PCDD/PCDF concentrations showed clearly that PCDDs/PCDFs accumulate in the soil. The TEQ level was 4.5 times higher in soil that had been fertilized for the previous 10 years than in soil that had had no sludge fertilization. It was 11 times higher in field soil and 18 times higher in meadow soil that had been fertilized for 30 years. The homologue pattern of the fertilized soils lay between that of unfertilized soil and that of the sludge. Similar results on the influence of sewage sludge on PCDD/PCDF levels in soil have been found by Hembrock-Heger (1990) and Albrecht *et al.* (1993).

On the other hand, as observed also in air and food, PCDD/PCDF levels in sewage sludge are generally declining. Ilic *et al.* (1994) found mean I-TEQ values in sewage sludge of 39 ng/kg (dry matter) in 1991 and 28 ng/kg (dry matter) in 1992.

Fürst *et al.* (1993) studied PCDDs/PCDFs in cow's milk in relation to their levels in grass and soil. The contamination levels in soil did not influence the PCDD/PCDF levels in cow's milk, as had been suspected. Even soil levels of up to 30 ng I-TEQ/kg were not associated with elevated PCDD/PCDF levels in cow's milk. However, increasing levels in grass were associated with slightly higher levels in milk.

Levels of PCDDs/PCDFs in soil and atmospheric deposition in an agricultural area in the south-east of Hamburg, adjacent to an industrial area, were measured (Sievers *et al.*, 1993). Soil samples were collected at 62 sites at a maximum depth of 15 cm. The PCDD/PCDF contents ranged from 1.7 to 684 ng I-TEQ/kg with a median of 18 ng/kg. Elevated soil levels were observed in the vicinity of a former chemical plant (up to

159 ng I-TEQ/kg) and along the banks of tributaries of the River Elbe (up to 684 ng I-TEQ/kg), where until the 1950s the land was regularly flooded during winter time.

Rotard *et al.* (1994) examined background levels of PCDDs/PCDFs in soils in Germany at sites outside industrial and urban regions. Elevated levels were found in the topsoil layers of forest. PCDD/PCDF levels found in ploughland and grassland samples were considerably lower, with means of 2 ng I-TEQ/kg. The isomer profiles for air and forest soil samples showed striking coincidence.

Little is known about PCDD/PCDF contamination of soils in the former German Democratic Republic. Kujawa *et al.* (1995) analysed 49 soil samples of rural origin. Only total I-TEQ levels of PCDDs/PCDFs were reported. The authors compared data for samples originating from the western and eastern parts of Germany (see Appendix 1, Table 5).

(x)   *Italy*

Following the Seveso accident in 1976, soil levels of 2,3,7,8-TCDD were determined in the Zones A, B and R established around the ICMESA plant (see Section 1.3.1(b)). Since 2,3,7,8-TCDD concentrations detected in Zone A ranged over more than four orders of magnitude (from < 0.75 $\mu g/m^2$ to > 20 mg/m^2), the zone was broken down into subzones A_1–A_8, each characterized by a somewhat lower range of 2,3,7,8-TCDD levels (di Domenico & Zapponi, 1986). Mean concentrations of 2,3,7,8-TCDD in the soil in September 1976 in Zones A_1–A_8 were 1600, 2500, 130, 260, 120, 91, 12 and < 5 $\mu g/m^2$, respectively. The mean concentrations in Zones B and R in 1976–77 were 3.4 and ~0.5 $\mu g/m^2$, respectively. Tolerable limits for land (soil), housing interiors, equipment and other matrices and items were set by regional law. The risk areas — namely Zones A, B and R — were defined by taking into account the 2,3,7,8-TCDD levels detected predominantly in the 7-cm topsoil layer, and therefore the 'surface density' unit $\mu g/m^2$ was extensively used, the unit surface being defined as a 1-m square with a 7-cm thickness. 2,3,7,8-TCDD surface densities were converted to the more common ng/kg concentration units by multiplying by an average factor of 8. The following limits were obtained for the different risk areas and matrices (Bertazzi & di Domenico, 1994): farmable land, < 0.75 $\mu g/m^2$ (< 6 ng/kg); non-farmable land, ≤ 5 $\mu g/m^2$ (≤ 40 ng/kg); limit of evacuation, > 50 $\mu g/m^2$ (> 400 ng/kg); and, for comparison, outdoor surfaces of buildings, ≤ 0.75 $\mu g/m^2$; indoor surfaces of buildings, ≤ 0.01 $\mu g/m^2$.

di Domenico *et al.* (1993a) reported on the occurrence of PCDDs/PCDFs and PCBs in the general environment in Italy. Sampling was carried out in five regions, at or slightly above sea level ($n = 10$), at an altitude of 800–1300 m ($n = 11$) and in caves normally not visited by the general public ($n = 6$). All sampling sites were far from an urban or industrial setting, at least 5 km from towns or villages, and the soil was collected from top to 7-cm depth. PCDD/PCDF levels were between 0.10 and 4.3 ng I-TEQ/kg in open areas and between 0.057 and 0.12 ng I-TEQ/kg in samples from caves.

(xi) *Japan*

Very few data have been reported on Japanese soils. Nakamura *et al.* (1994) found PCDD/PCDF levels in soils of 271 and 49.6 ng I-TEQ/kg (two agricultural fields) and 42.4 ng I-TEQ/kg (urban field).

(xii) *Jordan*

Alawi *et al.* (1996a) described the concentration of PCDDs/PCDFs in the Jordanian environment in a preliminary study on a municipal landfill site with open combustion near Amman. Six samples were collected from locations distributed over the area of the landfill. The concentrations measured in soil samples ranged from 8.2 to 1470 ng German TEQ/kg dry weight.

(xiii) *The Netherlands*

van Wijnen *et al.* (1992) measured PCDD/PCDF levels in 20 soil samples collected from areas in the vicinity of Amsterdam where it was known that small-scale (illegal) incineration of scrap wire and scrap cars might have resulted in contamination with PCDDs/PCDFs. At certain spots, the illegal incineration resulted in strongly increased soil levels of PCDDs/PCDFs, ranging between 60 and 98 000 ng I-TEQ/kg dry matter. Nine samples had PCDD/PCDF levels (far) above the so-called 'level of concern' of 1000 ng/kg dry matter proposed by Kimbrough *et al.* (1984) for soil contamination with 2,3,7,8-TCDD in Times Beach, Missouri (USA).

At the Volgermeerpolder hazardous waste site, 10 years after all dumping activities ceased, the concentrations of the most toxic PCDD/PCDF congeners in topsoil and eel determined in 1994 fell within the same range as was found in 1981–84, indicating that the contamination circumstances had remained basically unaltered (Heida *et al.*, 1995).

(xiv) *Russian Federation*

Soil samples taken near plants where products such as chlorophenol, TCP and 2,4-D had been produced had 2,3,7,8-TCDD levels in the range of 900–40 000 ng/kg (Pervunina *et al.*, 1992).

Some information on ecological problems in Russia caused by PCDD/PCDF emissions from other chemical industry facilities is available (Fedorov, 1993). In 1990, at a chemical fertilizer plant in Chapaevsk, the soil near the section for PCP production contained 18.7 μg 2,3,7,8-TCDD/kg. It should be noted that the major PCDD/PCDF isomers formed in PCP production are OCDD, OCDF and HpCDDs. Soil originating from Chapaevsk farming areas (1991–92) contained between 0.2 and 68 ng 2,3,7,8-TCDD/kg. In Ufa, close to a TCP production plant, values of between 8000 and 40 000 ng 2,3,7,8-TCDD/kg have been reported.

In the Bashkortostan Republic, the main sources of environmental contamination with PCDDs/PCDFs are chemical plants in Ufa and Sterlitamak, which have manufactured organochlorine products including the pesticides 2,4,5-T and 2,4-D for more than 40 years. Soil samples taken in urban areas of Ufa and Sterlitamak, had PCDD/PCDF concentrations of 1–20 ng I-TEQ/kg, which did not exceed the norms for Russia. High concentrations of PCDDs/PCDFs were detected in industrial zones not far from chemical and oil/chemical plants of Ufa, ranging between 280 and 980 ng I-TEQ/kg. In the majority of farm regions, PCDD/PCDF content in soil was reported to be between 0.01 and 0.13 ng I-TEQ/kg and did not exceed the permissible level of 10 ng/kg (Khamitov & Maystrenko, 1995). [It was not apparent from the paper whether the values reported were I-TEQs or total PCDD/PCDFs.]

(xv) Spain

Near a clinical waste incinerator in Madrid, PCDD/PCDF levels in soil samples (0–5 cm) from 16 sites indicated slight contamination by these pollutants (Gonzáles et al., 1994; Jiménez et al., 1996a). The highest levels were found at points located between 400 and 1200 m from the incinerator but there was no relation between PCDD/-PCDF levels and the prevailing wind direction. The analytical data for PCDDs/PCDFs and the distribution of the PCDD/PCDF homologues and the 2,3,7,8-substituted congeners failed to reveal whether this plant was the only source responsible for the soil contamination detected.

Schuhmacher et al. (1996) analysed soil samples in the vicinity of a municipal solid-waste incinerator in Tarragona. The highest PCDD/PCDF level (0.84 ng I-TEQ/kg) was found at a distance of 750 m from the incinerator.

(xvi) Sweden

PCDDs/PCDFs in soil and digested sewage sludge from Stockholm were analysed (Broman et al., 1990). The contribution of PCDDs/PCDFs from sewage sludge to the total soil level was compared with the contribution from two non-point emission sources, i.e., road traffic and the urban area of the city of Stockholm. The data reported (based on the Nordic TEF model) are not based on dry matter but on organic weight, making it difficult to compare the data obtained with other published data. The mean concentration in four sludge samples was 79 ng TEQ/kg organic weight. Soil samples taken close to major roads varied between 13 and 49 ng TEQ/kg organic weight and soil samples which were not taken close to major roads varied between 9 and 32 ng TEQ/kg organic weight. The results indicate that both traffic and the urban area influence PCDD/PCDF concentrations in arable soil. Fertilization with sludge (1 tonne dry weight/hectare and year) raised the initial soil concentration of PCDDs/PCDFs in the fields by approximately 2–3%.

(xvii) Switzerland

Soil samples were collected at 33 sites in the northern part of Switzerland (Rheinfelden to Wallbach) (Gälli et al., 1992). Concentrations of PCDDs/PCDFs in the topsoil ranged from 0.7 to 26.8 ng German TEQ/kg. Eighty per cent of the samples had concentrations < 5 ng TEQ/kg, slightly above the background level of ~ 1 ng TEQ/kg in rural areas.

(xviii) Taiwan

Since 1966, waste electric wires and/or magnetic cards have been incinerated directly on site during reclamation of metals, especially copper, silver and gold, in Taiwan. Surface soil samples from six sites at which these open incinerations took place were analysed for PCDDs/PCDFs (Huang *et al.*, 1992). All samples were contaminated, with total PCDD levels ranging from undetectable to 540 ng/kg and total PCDF levels of 1.8– 310 ng/kg. Only the samples from the incineration sites with waste electric wire were heavily polluted.

Soong and Ling (1996) found exceptionally high PCDD/PCDF levels in soil samples collected from a PCP manufacturing facility located in the southern part of Taiwan (maximum, 1357 µg I-TEQ/kg) five years after operation had ceased.

(xix) *United Kingdom*

PCDD/PCDF levels in archived soil samples collected from the same semi-rural plot in south-east England between 1846 and the present were determined by Kjeller *et al.* (1990, 1991). Atmospheric deposition is known to have been the only source of PCDDs/PCDFs to the site. PCDDs/PCDFs were present in all the samples. Generally, the total PCDD/PCDF concentration began to increase in the early twentieth century from about 30 ng/kg in the 1850s to the 1890s to about 90 ng/kg in the 1980s.

A comprehensive study of British soils to measure the background contamination with PCDDs/PCDFs was performed by Creaser *et al.* (1989), who analysed 77 topsoil samples (0–5 cm) from points of a 50 km grid covering England, Wales and Scotland. Mean concentrations for a reduced data-set were in the range of 9.4 ng/kg for total TCDDs to 191 ng/kg for OCDD.

In a further study by Creaser *et al.* (1990), soil samples from five British cities (London, Birmingham, Leeds, Sheffield and Port Talbot) were analysed for PCDDs/-PCDFs. The mean levels were significantly higher than those from rural and semi-urban locations. The concentrations of the lower PCDD and PCDF congener groups show the greatest increase. By principal component analysis, it was deduced that combustion processes, such as coal burning and municipal waste incineration, are the main sources of PCDDs/PCDFs in these soils.

Stenhouse and Badsha (1990) presented baseline concentrations for PCDDs/PCDFs and PCBs around a site proposed for a chemical waste incinerator near Doncaster. The values were between 3 and 20 ng I-TEQ/kg, indicating that the area had relatively low contamination with these components and may be comparable with a rural environment.

Biomass burning is known to constitute a highly dispersed source of PCDDs/PCDFs (Levine, 1992). Walsh *et al.* (1994) monitored soils before and after straw field fires and assessed the degree and nature of formation/destruction and transformation processes occurring during biomass burning. PCDD/PCDF concentrations of post-burn soils showed a slight relative reduction with respect to the corresponding pre-burn soils at three burnings. This reduction may be attributed to the high temperature achieved during the burn, leading to vaporization and destruction of PCDDs/PCDFs in the surface layer of soil. The overall I-TEQ for PCDDs/PCDFs decreased after the straw fire, with a decrease in concentration of 2,3,7,8-TCDD and an increase in that of OCDD.

Foxall and Lovett (1994) analysed soil samples from South Wales, Pantec district, where the major industries used to be coal mining, iron and steel production, aluminium smelting and glass manufacturing. Current industries involve steel rolling, automotive engineering, pharmaceuticals and others. Forty-two samples from 32 sites were analysed by eight national or international laboratories. The total PCDD/PCDF levels show considerable variation between sampling sites, with a mean of 66 ng I-TEQ/kg and a median of 10.5 ng I-TEQ/kg (range, 2.5–1745 ng I-TEQ/kg). The maximal concentration in soil was found at a site near a chemical water incinerator.

PCDD/PCDF contamination on land around a chemical waste incinerator has been described (Holmes *et al.*, 1995; Sandalls *et al.*, 1996). After 1991 during a routine surveillance, high PCDD/PCDF concentrations were detected in the milk of cows grazing within 2 km of a chemical factory in Bolsover, Derbyshire, which had produced 2,4,5-TCP. As a follow-up, PCDDs/PCDFs were measured in soil samples taken up to 5 km from the factory. The samples were taken from 46 sites where the soil had remained undisturbed for many years. As in flue gas at the incinerator, total TCDD was always found to be prominent in soil and was selected as a marker for assessment purposes. Within 1 km of the factory, the concentration of total TCDDs in soil was up to 9400 ng/kg, and even 4–5 km away several hundred ng/kg were found. The authors concluded that the special distribution pattern of PCDDs on surrounding land implicated the chemical factory as the likely source since the soil samples showed a congener ratio pattern not resembling that found in a United Kingdom background survey.

(xx) *United States*

In 1971, 29 kg of 2,3,7,8-TCDD-contaminated chemical sludge were mixed with waste oils and used as a dust suppressant at sites in 10 counties of Missouri. Kimbrough *et al.* (1977) described an epidemiological and laboratory investigation of a poisoning outbreak that involved three riding arenas and killed 57 horses and numerous other animals. The outbreak was traced to the spraying of the arenas with the contaminated oil containing TCP, PCBs and hexachloroxanthene. The 2,3,7,8-TCDD levels in the soil samples ranged up to 33 mg/kg. The presence of hexachloroxanthene in most of the contaminated sites, although at levels varying considerably from site to site and also within sites, implicates a hexachlorophene producer as the source (Kleopfer *et al.*, 1985).

Nestrick *et al.* (1986) measured levels of 2,3,7,8-TCDD in samples taken at various sites at a major chemical plant in Midland, MI, in the city of Midland and in other industrialized areas in the United States. Within the chemical plant, certain areas had localized elevated levels (above 5 µg/kg) 2,3,7,8-TCDD in the surface soil (Appendix 1, Table 6). In the zone immediately surrounding the Midland plant, most 2,3,7,8-TCDD soil levels were below 1000 ng/kg, but many times higher than those found in other industrialized urban areas, suggesting that the chemical plant was a primary source of 2,3,7,8-TCDD found in the immediate environment. The data for other US cities are summarized in Appendix 1 (Table 7).

Reed *et al.* (1990) measured PCDD/PCDF levels at Elk River, Minnesota, before operation of an electric generating station by powered refuse-derived fuel. The area was semi-rural without industry. The soil data reflect generally low background concentrations of PCDDs/PCDFs, with surprisingly high values for OCDD (ranging from 340 to 3300 ng/kg).

Concentrations of PCDDs/PCDFs in 36 soil samples from eight counties in southern Mississippi were reported by Rappe *et al.* (1995) and Fiedler *et al.* (1995). The selected sampling sites were not directly influenced by human activities, such as heavy traffic or dust. Controlled burning is a common practice in southern Mississippi, and potential sites were not excluded when traces of former fires could be seen. The sampling depth was 5 cm. Most Cl_4–Cl_8 PCDDs/PCDFs were detected in all samples. 2,3,7,8-TCDD was identified in 17 of the 36 samples at a detection limit of 0.02–0.05 ng/kg dry weight. The highest concentration was 22.6 ng I-TEQ/kg in a sample from Perry County. In some cases, surprisingly high values for OCDD were found (13–15 µg/kg) (see Appendix 1, Table 8). The source of these high levels is not known but the authors suggested a non-anthropogenic origin.

The Columbus Municipal Waste-to-Energy facility in Columbus, OH, began operation in 1983. In 1992 it was reported to be the largest known single source of PCDD/-PCDF emissions. Emission was reduced from 984 g I-TEQ/year in 1992 to 267 g/year in 1994. Soil was monitored for PCDDs/PCDFs at the plant site, directly off-site in the predominant wind direction (four samples), at 14 sites in the city of Columbus and 28 miles away from Columbus in a rural setting (Lorber *et al.*, 1996b). The high PCDD/PCDF levels in the four samples taken close to the facility (average, 356 ng I-TEQ/kg) suggest direct soil contamination due to the operation of the plant (stack emission and/or on site ash handling). The congener profile seen in the stack emission was very similar to those observed in the soil samples taken at the plant. The background soil concentrations of 1–2 ng I-TEQ/kg are consistent with other measurements in North America and elsewhere.

(xxi) *Viet Nam*

During the Second Indo-China War, the south of Viet Nam was sprayed with herbicides contaminated with 2,3,7,8-TCDD (see Section 1.3.1(*a*)(ii)). Matsuda *et al.* (1994) measured the persisting levels of 2,3,7,8-TCDD in soils. To assess background concentration in soil, five samples were collected in Hanoi, where the herbicides had not been sprayed and no 2,3,7,8-TCDD has been found. Contrary to expectation, 2,3,7,8-TCDD was detected in only 20 out of 106 south Vietnamese samples analysed. The levels of 2,3,7,8-TCDD detected in 14/54 samples from Tay Ninh Province, South Viet Nam, ranged between 1.2 and 38.5 ng/kg dry weight (mean, 14.0 ng/kg). The results suggest that most of the sprayed material has been leached and ultimately drained towards the sea and/or to the soil subsurface during the rainy season.

(*d*)   Food

It is estimated that intake from food consumption accounts for well over 90% of the body-burden of PCDDs and PCDFs in the general human population (Gilman *et al.*, 1991; Travis & Hattemer-Frey, 1991).

Over the last decade a number of studies of foods have appeared, but several are of only limited usefulness because of low sensitivity. The results from Canadian studies of meat collected in 1980 were published by Ryan *et al.* (1985a), but the lower chlorinated congeners were not detected. Firestone *et al.* (1986) published the results of analyses for the higher chlorinated PCDDs in various foods collected in the United States by the Food and Drug Administration in a five-year period beginning in 1979; lower chlorinated PCDDs including 2,3,7,8-TCDD were not determined. Stanley and Bauer (1989) analysed composites of selected foods collected from San Francisco and Los Angeles, CA, including salt-water fish, freshwater fish, beef chicken, pork, cow's milk and eggs. The analytical methods and quality control were rigorous but the limits of detection were somewhat higher than those obtained in some other recent studies and few measurable residues were found. Birmingham *et al.* (1989) analysed samples of beef, pork, chicken, eggs, milk, apples, peaches, potatoes, tomatoes and wheat from Ontario (Canada). Some samples were found to contain detectable concentrations of the higher chlorinated congeners but no Cl_4 or Cl_5 PCDDs or PCDFs were detected. The data from this study are available only on a whole sample rather than a lipid-adjusted basis.

Studies by Beck *et al.* (1987, 1989a) of foods available in Berlin, Germany, were based on analysis of 12 random purchases of foods (chicken, eggs, butter, pork, red fish, cod, herring, vegetable oil, cauliflower, lettuce, cherries and apples) and of eight samples of cow's milk. The analysis used high-resolution mass spectrometry and achieved very high sensitivity, so that most of the congeners with a 2,3,7,8-substitution pattern were detected in most of the samples. Fürst *et al.* (1990) concentrated on fatty foods and foods of animal origin in a study involving over 100 individual samples from the North-Rhine Westphalia area of Germany, but with slightly lower sensitivity. Fürst *et al.* (1992a) subsequently reported further analysis of milk and dairy products which made use of more sensitive high-resolution mass spectrometry, but detailed congener-specific results were not published.

A comprehensive assessment of Dutch foodstuffs was reported by Liem *et al.* (1991a,b). The sampling scheme was designed after considering the individual consumption data of approximately 6000 individuals from 2200 families over a two-day period. Animal fat and liver from six different types of animal were collected from slaughter houses, and cereal products, cow's milk, dairy products, meat products, nuts, eggs, fish and game from retail sources. In each of these groups, duplicate collection of samples was carried out in each of four Dutch regions and proportional pooling was performed to provide a pair of duplicate samples for each group and region, and one national composite sample from the four regional pools. Analysis was by high-resolution mass spectrometry and achieved high sensitivity. Liem *at al.* (1991c) also reported the analysis of 200 samples of cow's milk obtained from the vicinity of municipal solid-waste incinerators and other potential PCDD/PCDF sources in the Netherlands.

Results are available from a study of composite samples from the UK Total Diet Study (TDS) (Ministry of Agriculture, Fisheries and Food, 1995; Wright & Startin, 1995; Wearne *et al.*, 1996; see **Table 23**). In this scheme, retail samples of 115 specified food items are purchased at two-week intervals from different locations in the United Kingdom, prepared as for consumption, then combined into one of 20 food groups in proportions representing the relative importance of the retail foods in the average British diet. Concentrations of PCDDs and PCDFs were determined in archived TDS samples of fatty foods and bread collected in 1982 and 1992. For each food group, the material analysed was a composite of samples from all 24 locations included in the TDS that year. Fruit, vegetables and other non-fatty foods were not analysed. The determinations used high-resolution mass spectrometry and met appropriate acceptance criteria (Ambidge *et al.*, 1990).

Table 23. Concentrations of PCDDs/PCDFs (ng I-TEQ/kg whole food) in Total Diet Study samples collected in 1982 and 1992 in the United Kingdom

Food group	PCDDs/PCDFs (ng I-TEQ/kg)	
	1982	1992
Bread	0.02	0.03
Other cereals	0.13	0.17
Carcass meat	0.49	0.13
Offal	1.6	0.59
Meat products	0.32	0.08
Poultry	0.50	0.13
Fish	0.41	0.21
Oils and fats	1.3	0.20
Eggs	0.92	0.17
Milk	0.16	0.06
Milk products	1.2	0.16

From Wearne *et al.* (1996)

Several studies of food items from Viet Nam, Russian Federation and the United States have been reported by Schecter *et al.* (1989a, 1990a, 1994a), who worked with various analytical laboratories of good repute. Most of the data relate to individual samples. In the study of food in the United States, 18 samples of dairy products, meat and fish from a supermarket in upstate New York were analysed (Schecter *et al.*, 1994a). A more recent study (Schecter *et al.*, 1996a) of 100 food items combined by type has not been fully reported, but led to estimates of intake close to those of the earlier study. A more comprehensive investigation of concentrations in beef in the United States has been reported by Ferrario *et al.* (1996).

Several studies have been conducted of foods in the Japanese diet, but some doubt must be attached to the results. Ono *et al.* (1987) reported the analysis of vegetables, cooking oils, cereals, fish, pork, beef, poultry and eggs collected in Matsuyame in 1986. In contrast to other studies, the dominant congeners in the fish and animal samples were generally not those with 2,3,7,8-substitution, suggesting that the results do not reflect biologically incurred residues but some other form of contamination. OCDD (which is normally the congener of highest concentration) was not consistently found and it is possible that the alkaline saponification procedure used for some samples resulted in dechlorination of OCDD and distortion of the congener profile. Other studies by

Takizawa and Muto (1987) and by Ogaki *et al.* (1987) also employed alkaline saponification and the reports do not include congener-specific results.

Relevant data are summarized in Appendix 1 (Tables 9–18). The data included have been selected to meet a number of criteria, including relevance to dietary intake rather than environmental monitoring, and adequate detection limits and appropriate analytical methodology. Some exceptions have, however, been made and some data that are available only as summed I-TEQs have been included where they seem to be of value. Additionally, the results included were either available on a lipid basis or could be so converted using either reported fat contents or reasonable assumptions. Some additional results omitted from the tables are discussed below. All concentrations quoted are lipid-adjusted unless otherwise stated.

Most of the summed I-TEQ concentrations included in the tables have been re-calculated using I-TEF values and assuming that congeners that were not detected were present at the full value of the detection limit. Obviously, however, this was not possible where detection limits were not reported (indicated as 'ND') or where the original author's calculations were used.

(i) *Background exposure*

Vegetables

Studies on uptake from soil, which have been reviewed (Kew *et al.*, 1989), are not entirely consistent but it is generally accepted that systemic uptake through the roots and translocation within plants is virtually absent in most species. Some members of the *Cucurbitaceae* family, however, have been shown to take up PCDDs and PCDFs from soil, leading to a uniform concentration of about 20 ng I-TEQ/kg dry mass in the above-ground parts of plants grown in soil containing 148 ng I-TEQ/kg (Hülster *et al.*, 1994).

Apart from localized contamination, PCDD and PCDF concentrations in fruit and vegetables have usually been found to be immeasurably small. In the survey of food-stuffs available in West Berlin (Beck *et al.*, 1989a), five vegetable samples were analysed (including cauliflower, lettuce, cherries and apples) and PCDDs and PCDFs were not found, subject to a detection limit of 0.01 ng/kg for each isomer. Similarly PCDDs and PCDFs were not detected to any significant extent in vegetable samples from the Total Diet Survey schemes in the United Kingdom (Ministry of Agriculture, Fisheries and Food, 1992) or in Canada (Birmingham *et al.*, 1989).

A number of studies have dealt with vegetable oils. Beck *et al.* (1989a), Fürst *et al.* (1990) and Liem *et al.* (1991a,b) have all reported that the concentrations of PCDDs and PCDFs were below the limit of detection, apart from some low levels of the hepta- and octa-chlorinated congeners.

Cow's milk

The detection of PCDDs and PCDFs in cow's milk was first reported by Rappe *et al.* (1987b) in samples from Switzerland. In retail milk from Bern and Bowil (a location remote from potential PCDD sources), several PCDDs were identified although concentrations were close to the detection limit. The congeners found were exclusively 2,3,7,8-substituted.

Data from this and subsequent reports on levels of PCDDs in milk are given in Appendix 1 (Table 9; summarized in Table 10).

Data on levels in cow's milk from various locations are dominated by European samples from the late 1980s and early 1990s. The data show a mean concentration of 2.3 ng I-TEQ/kg with a range of 0.26–10.0 ng I-TEQ/kg. Concentrations of 2,3,7,8-TCDD, 1,2,3,7,8-PeCDD and 1,2,3,4,7,8-HxCDD are all within a range of 0.13–2.3 with means of about 0.6–0.7 ng/kg. Levels of 1,2,3,6,7,8-HxCDD are somewhat greater, with a mean of 2.0 ng/kg and range of 0.3–8.9 ng/kg. [The concentration of 1,2,3,7,8,9-HxCDD found in Spanish milk (Ramos *et al.*, 1996) is dubious; the other results give a mean of 0.58 ng/kg.] Measured concentrations of HpCDD and OCDD are frequently unreliable due to the confounding influence of laboratory contamination and other analytical difficulties, but are greater than those of the Cl_4–Cl_6 congeners.

The data of Fürst *et al.* (1993) (see Section 1.3.2(*c*)(ix)) imply that the pathway air → grass → cow is more important than the pathway soil → grass → cow. The carry-over factors for PCDD/PCDF congeners between grass and milk differ significantly. While 2,3,7,8-TCDD showed the highest carry-over factor, OCDD was accumulated less by a factor of almost 40.

In addition to the tabulated data, Stanley and Bauer (1989) reported the analysis of eight composite samples from the United States, but most PCDDs and PCDFs were not detected and the detection limits were slightly higher than typical background concentrations found in other studies. LaFleur *et al.* (1990) reported 0.002 ng 2,3,7,8-TCDD/kg in milk used in a study of migration of PCDDs from milk cartons, but did not analyse higher congeners. Glidden *et al.* (1990) have also reported that these congeners were not detectable in milk that had not been packaged in paperboard cartons.

Dairy products

Reported concentrations of PCDDs and PCDFs in dairy products are given in Appendix 1 (Table 11) and Appendix 2 (Table 4) and, as expected, are similar to those in milk when expressed on a fat basis. In milk products, the mean summed I-TEQ concentration for PCDDs together with PCDFs (calculated assuming non-detected congeners to be present at the full value of the detection limit) is about 2.4 ng I-TEQ/kg (range, 0.8 to 8 ng I-TEQ/kg fat). [The Working Group noted that this is a conservative estimate; the true concentrations may be lower in some cases but most of the studies considered achieved excellent sensitivity, and other assumptions would lead to fairly small changes in the mean.] As with milk, data from UK Total Diet Survey samples show a considerable decrease from 1982 to 1992 (Wright & Startin, 1995; Wearne *et al.*, 1996).

Meat

Reported data for various meats and meat products, shown in Appendix 1 (Table 12; summarized in Table 13), indicate a mean concentration of 2,3,7,8-TCDD which is also about 0.5 ng/kg fat, but with a range of about two orders of magnitude. Concentrations of the other congeners tend to be a little higher than in milk — between 1.5 and 5 ng/kg for PeCDD and HxCDD isomers, 62 ng/kg for HpCDDs and 350 ng/kg for OCDD. Ranges are again rather large and are widest for OCDD (a factor of 250). In TEQ terms, the average concentration is about 6.5 ng I-TEQ/kg.

Beck et al. (1989a) found concentrations in the range of 1.65–2.59 ng I-TEQ/kg for beef, lamb and chicken but a much lower concentration (0.28 ng I-TEQ/kg) in pork. Similar results were reported by Fürst et al. (1990); concentrations in beef, lamb, chicken and in canned meat were in the range 2.4–3.7 ng I-TEQ/kg while PCDDs and PCDFs other than OCDD were not detected in pork. Fürst found a rather higher average concentration of 7.7 ng I-TEQ/kg in veal, that is presumably due to the high early-life input from milk.

Similar concentrations were found in beef, mutton and chicken from the Netherlands where the range was 1.6–1.8 ng I-TEQ/kg (Liem et al., 1991b). Again a rather lower level of 0.42 ng I-TEQ/kg was found in pork. This study also included horse and goat fat, in which higher concentrations of 14 and 4.2 ng I-TEQ/kg, respectively, were found. Liver from these animals was also analysed and the concentrations, on a fat basis, were 2–10-fold higher than in the corresponding animal fat.

The limited number of reported measurements of levels in animal liver from food distribution channels show a tendency to higher concentrations in I-TEQ terms (6–60 ng I-TEQ/kg). Concentrations of HpCDD and OCDD especially are relatively large, with maxima approaching 1 µg/kg for the former and exceeding 4 µg/kg for the latter congener.

LaFleur et al. (1990) examined samples of canned corned beef hash, ground beef, beef hot dogs and ground pork available in the United States for 2,3,7,8-TCDD and 2,3,7,8-TCDF. The former was found in all the beef samples at concentrations between 0.03 and 0.35 ng/kg but was not detected in pork.

Schecter et al. (1994a) more recently reported on a number of individual samples of retail meat products from the United States. The concentrations in four different samples of beef and beef products spanned a wide range from 0.04 to 1.5 ng I-TEQ/kg on a whole sample basis. Cooked ham contained 0.03 ng I-TEQ/kg, while a single pork chop contained 0.26 ng I-TEQ/kg and a sample of lamb sirloin 0.41 ng I-TEQ/kg. A very low level of 0.04 ng I-TEQ/kg was found in a sample of chicken.

Concentrations in samples from widely separated locations in the Soviet Union ranged from 0.2–6 ng I-TEQ/kg in beef, pork and sausage (see Appendix 1, Table 12).

Poultry

The rather limited data (Appendix 1, Table 14) on poultry meat suggest typical concentrations of the same order of magnitude as those in other animal products, apart from the rather greater concentrations found in two samples from Viet Nam (Schechter et al., 1989a). The UK Total Diet Survey (Wright & Startin, 1995) shows a marked decrease between 1982 and 1992.

Eggs

Although the 2,3,7,8-substituted PCDD/PCDF congeners predominate in eggs, other congeners are observed to a greater extent than in other animal-derived foods. There have been relatively few studies of contamination in eggs at the retail level, but the limited data in Appendix 1 (Table 15) show reasonable agreement between samples from the Netherlands, Germany, Spain and the United Kingdom (1992 Total Diet Survey sample). In terms of I-TEQ concentrations for PCDDs and PCDFs, the British results show a decrease from 1982 to 1992 of nearly a factor of 5.

Earlier results of 0.22 and 0.16 ng I-TEQ/kg whole egg found in two egg composites from the UK Total Diet Survey from 1988 (Ministry of Agriculture, Fisheries and Food, 1992) and an average of 0.2 ng TEQ/kg whole egg in samples from Norway (Faerden, 1991) are also consistent, assuming a fat content of 10%.

In the United States, the data of Stephens *et al.* (1995) point to a similar background level in eggs from chickens fed on commercial formulations to that in Europe, whereas in eggs from free-range birds with access to moderately contaminated soils, concentrations were as much as 100-fold higher than in commercial eggs.

In the Canadian data, only higher chlorinated congeners were detected in eggs, but an average concentration of 0.59 ng I-TEQ/kg was used for dietary intake calculations (Birmingham *et al.*, 1989).

Two chicken's eggs from Viet Nam had concentrations of 0.55 and 1.62 ng I-TEQ/kg whole egg while PCDDs and PCDFs were not detected in a single sample of duck eggs (Olie *et al.*, 1989).

Lovett *et al.* (1996) reported 1.2 ng I-TEQ/kg fresh mass in chicken eggs from rural sites in Wales, 0.6 ng I-TEQ/kg in bantam hen eggs and 0.7 ng I-TEQ/kg in duck eggs. [Assuming 10% as a typical fat content, these seem much too high.]

Fish

Although PCDDs and PCDFs are usually present in aquatic systems only at very low levels, bioaccumulation of the 2,3,7,8-substituted congeners can result in significant concentrations in fish. As with animals, the 2,3,7,8-substituted congeners dominate the congener pattern found in fish, although this is not true of crustaceans and shellfish (Oehme *et al.*, 1989). Since different species occupy quite different trophic positions, large differences in PCDD and PCDF concentrations are to be expected.

Data from studies of food fish are shown in Appendix 1 (Table 16; summarized in Table 17). Average concentrations of 2,3,7,8-TCDD and of 1,2,3,7,8-PeCDD are about an order of magnitude greater than in foods of animal origin.

A study of cod and herring from the seas around Sweden has been reported (Bergqvist *et al.*, 1989). Herring from the Baltic were found to have PCDD/PCDF concentrations in the range of 6.7–9.0 ng I-TEQ/kg wet weight, while considerably lower concentrations of 1.8–3.4 ng I-TEQ/kg were found in fish from the west coast of Sweden. de Wit *et al.* (1990) also demonstrated higher levels in fish from the Baltic Sea.

Takayama *et al.* (1991) reported data on coastal and marketing fish from Japan. The means for these two groups were 0.87 and 0.33 ng I-TEQ/kg, respectively, on a wet weight basis.

A number of studies have dealt with contamination of fish in the North American Great Lakes and rivers in the Great Lakes Basin (Harless *et al.*, 1982; O'Keefe *et al.*, 1983; Ryan *et al.*, 1983; Stalling *et al.*, 1983; Fehringer *et al.*, 1985), which have been among the most severely contaminated in the United States. An extensive survey of 2,3,7,8-TCDD in fish from inland waters in the United States has also been conducted (Kuehl *et al.*, 1989) and over 25% of all samples were found to be contaminated at or above the detection limit, which varied between 0.5 and 2.0 ng/kg. Concentrations in excess of 5.0 ng/kg were found in 10% of samples and the highest level was 85 ng/kg. Samples collected near sites of discharge from pulp and paper mills had a higher frequency of 2,3,7,8-TCDD contamination than other samples. More recently, Firestone *et al.* (1996) summarized the results of monitoring for 2,3,7,8-TCDD in the edible portion of fish and shellfish from various United States waterways since 1979. Analyses of 1623 test samples indicated that 2,3,7,8-TCDD residues in fish and shellfish were not widespread but rather were localized in areas near waste sites, chlorophenol manufacturers and pulp and paper mills. The levels in aquatic species from these sites have been declining steadily. No 2,3,7,8-TCDD (limit of detection and confirmation, 1–2 ng/kg) has been found in recent years in aquatic species from most Atlantic, Pacific and Gulf of Mexico sites and Great Lakes other than Lake Ontario and Saginaw Bay (Lake Huron).

There are rather fewer data on retail samples of the major food species and the ranges of reported results are wider than for animal products. Two recent studies of composite samples of sea fish, formulated to represent national average dietary habits in the United Kingdom and the Netherlands, showed considerable differences for all congeners (see Appendix 1, Table 16) (Liem *et al.*, 1991b; Ministry of Agriculture, Fisheries and Food, 1995). The available data lead to averages of about 5 ng/kg for 2,3,7,8-TCDD, 1,2,3,7,8-PeCDD and 1,2,3,6,7,8-HxCDD, with lower concentrations of 1,2,3,4,7,8-HxCDD and 1,2,3,7,8,9-HxCDD and rather higher ones of HpCDDs and OCDD. The mean total concentration of 25 ng I-TEQ/kg has a larger contribution from PCDFs than that for animal products (see Appendix 1, Table 17).

In addition to the tabulated results, data from the United Kingdom from eight retail samples, including plaice, mackerel, herring, cod, skate and coley, gave a mean of 0.74 ng/kg and a range of 0.15–1.84 ng TEQ/kg on a wet weight basis (Startin *et al.*, 1990), but fat contents were not determined.

In contrast to the extensive North American measurements on fish caught in specific locations, there is little information documenting the levels in the general food supply there, apart from the results reported by Schecter *et al.* (1994a) who found 0.02 and 0.03 ng I-TEQ/kg in haddock fillets, 0.023 ng I-TEQ/kg in a cod fillet and in a perch fillet, and 0.13 ng I-TEQ/kg in crunchy haddock. Fat contents were not measured. These levels are rather lower than those typical in Europe but relate to a very restricted sampling base.

The very limited reported data on fish oils (used, for example, as dietary supplements) are consistent with the lipid-based concentrations reported in fish.

Other foods

Table 18 in Appendix 1 gives PCDD concentrations that have been found in some other commodities and products. Bread was included in the UK TDS as it is a staple item in most people's diet and also because fat is usually used in preparing the dough. Many of the congeners were not detected but detection limits varied so that the upper-bound total I-TEQ concentration appears to increase in the more recent pooled sample. [The summations are almost certainly a considerable overestimate of true concentrations.]

Various studies of cooked foods and prepared dishes have been reported; concentrations of PCDDs found were broadly similar to those in individual commodities.

[The Working Group noted that the available data on food show that average PCDD/PCDF concentrations in animal fats consumed in the diet in different industrialized regions are similar, even for different continents.]

Data from a UK study (Wearne *et al.*, 1996) in which a comparison was made of composites of various fatty food composites taken from Total Diet Study (TDS) samples from 1982 and 1992 show a considerable decrease in PCDD/PCDF levels over this decade (**Table 23**). Results obtained separately on a small number of individual TDS samples from 1988, while less robust, support this finding (Ministry of Agriculture, Fisheries and Food, 1995).

Fürst and Wilmers (1995) have reported a decrease of nearly 25% in PCDD/PCDF levels in cow's milk and milk products collected from all 30 dairies in North Rhine–Westphalia in Germany in 1994 compared to 1990.

(ii)   *Foods from contaminated areas*

Vegetables

The outer surface of root crops can obviously become contaminated by soil contact; low concentrations of PCDDs and PCDFs have been measured in root crops such as carrots and potatoes grown in contaminated soils but were largely absent if the vegetables were peeled (Facchetti *et al.*, 1986; Hülster & Marschener, 1993).

Surface-borne PCDD and PCDF contamination of foliage and fruits may include contributions from direct deposition of airborne particulates and from absorption of vapour-phase contaminants from the air, including those which are attributable to evaporation from the soil (Reischl *et al.*, 1989). In apples and pears grown on highly contaminated soil, Müller *et al.* (1993) found total concentrations of PCDDs and PCDFs (including non-2,3,7,8-substituted congeners) in the range of 1–4 ng/kg. Peeling removed most of the PCDD and PCDF contamination, although washing was not effective.

In studies of field-grown vegetables, measurable amounts of PCDDs/PCDFs have generally been found only in areas where a specific contamination problem was known to exist. Concentrations of 2,3,7,8-TCDD of 100 ng/kg were detected in the peel of fruits grown on soils contaminated in the Seveso incident, but not in the flesh (Wipf *et al.*, 1982). Investigations in the vicinity of a wire reclamation incinerator showed contamination of leaf vegetables at concentrations of 5–10 ng I-TEQ/kg and rather less in fruits (Prinz *et al.*, 1990).

Cows' milk

A number of studies have demonstrated the localized influence of incinerators and other sources on PCDD/PCDF concentrations in cow's milk (**Table 24**). Thus, Rappe *et al.* (1987b) found between about 8 and 12 ng I-TEQ/kg in the milk of individual cows grazing near municipal solid-waste incinerators and a chlorinated chemical production site in Switzerland.

More recently, in surveillance around incinerators in the Netherlands, levels up to 13.5 ng I-TEQ/kg in cow's milk were found (Liem *et al.*, 1991c). The highest PCDD concentrations were usually found within about 2 km of the source.

Schmid and Schlatter (1992) analysed milk from sites near waste incineration, metal recycling and other industrial facilities in Switzerland, where the PCDD/PCDF levels were reported to be two- to four-fold greater than in commercial samples.

In the United Kingdom, Startin *et al.* (1990) found between 3 and 6.2 ng I-TEQ/kg for PCDDs/PCDFs in milk from farms near an incinerator and close to a densely populated and industrialized area, compared with the mean for rural background areas of 1.1 ng I-TEQ/kg. In 1990, concentrations of 40 and 42 ng I-TEQ/kg were found in milk from two farms near Bolsover in Derbyshire, while milk from 30 other farms in the region contained an average of 4.3 ng I-TEQ/kg (range, 1.8–12.5) (Harrison *et al.*, 1996). In contrast to the results discussed above where the proportions of different congeners were fairly similar to those in background samples, milk from Bolsover showed a distinctive pattern dominated by 2,3,7,8-TCDD, 1,2,3,7,8-PeCDD and 1,2,3,4,7,8-/1,2,3,6,7,8-HxCDD.

Riss *et al.* (1990) investigated contamination caused by a metal reclamation plant at Brixlegg in Austria and found PCDD/PCDF levels in two samples of cow's milk giving 55 and 69 ng I-TEQ/kg.

(iii) *Human intake levels from food*

Birmingham *et al.* (1989) estimated the daily intake of PCDDs and PCDFs from food for Canadian adults to be 92 pg I-TEQ, the main contributors being milk and dairy products, beef and eggs. Beck *et al.* (1989a) and Fürst *et al.* (1990) estimated West German exposure to be 93.5 and 85 pg German TEQ/day, respectively. Both groups concluded that intake was derived about equally from milk, meat and fish.

The estimates above were derived by multiplying average concentration in foods and average food consumption statistics. An alternative approach using a database of food consumption data for 5898 individuals was applied by Theelen *et al.* (1993) to estimate intakes in the Netherlands. This showed a median adult intake of about 70 pg I-TEQ/day.

In the United Kingdom, both approaches have been applied to estimating intakes in 1982 and 1992 (Wearne *et al.*, 1996). Using the average consumption method, estimated intakes of PCDDs and PCDFs were [240 pg TEQ/day] in 1982 and [69 pg TEQ/day] in 1992. Based on seven-day consumption records for over 2000 adults, mean intake

Table 24. Concentrations of PCDDs reported in cow's milk from contaminated areas

Reference	Origin	Sample year	No.	PCDD concentration (ng/kg fat)[a]							I-TEQ[b] PCDD/PCDF
				TCDD 2378	PeCDD 12378	HxCDD 123478	123678	123789	HpCDD 1234678	OCDD	
Riss et al. (1990)	Austria, Tyrol, Brixlegg (metal reclamation)	1988	1	17.8	24.5	3.7	11.2	9.4	5.6	NR	[54.6]
			1	18.5	25.3	5.4	14.5	3.6	17.1	NR	[69.1]
Rappe et al. (1987b)	Switzerland, Hunzenschwil (SE from MSWI)	NR	1	[1.1]	[5.59]	[5.15]	[6.49]	[3.8]	[5.82]	[6.26]	[11.8]
	Switzerland, Rheinfelden (Cl compound manuf.)	NR	1	[0.60]	[<2.87]	[<4.01]	[<6.02]	[<3.15]	[12.0]	[16.9]	[7.53]
	Switzerland, Suhr (SW from MSWI)	NR	1	[1.2]	[<2.71]	[4.42]	[5.05]	[<2.52]	[<3.0]	[<5.05]	[8.38]
Startin et al. (1990)	UK, incinerator	1989	1	[0.85]	[1.2]	0	[2.58]	[0.83]	[1.7]	[6.45]	[3.04]
			1	[0.9]	[1.95]	0	[2.15]	[<1.78]	[1.73]	[7.75]	[4.07]
	UK, urban/industrial	1989	1	[2.03]	[1.05]	0	[1.58]	[0.4]	[1.63]	[8.05]	[6.24]
			1	[1.08]	[0.48]	0	[0.6]	[<0.75]	[4.15]	[6.4]	[3.71]
Harrison et al. (1996)	UK, Derbyshire (Cl compound manuf.) (Farm A) (4% fat assumed)	1990	1	[24.5]	[18.75]		[45]	[13.3]	[4.5]	[15]	[44.7]
Eitzer (1995)	USA, Connecticut (incineration) (4% fat assumed)	1993	12	[0.38]	[0.17]	[0.65]	[0.58]	[0.23]	[3]	[42.5]	[0.82]

NR, not reported; MSWI, municipal solid-waste incinerator

[a] When concentrations were given by the authors on whole milk basis, they have been recalculated on lipid basis by the Working Group.

[b] Summed TEQ concentrations recalculated by the Working Group where possible assuming congeners that were not detected were present at the full value of the limit of detection

estimates were made of 250 pg TEQ/day in 1982 and 88 pg TEQ/day in 1992. The decrease in intake was attributed partly to the decrease in the concentration of PCDDs and PCDFs (on a fat basis) in foods, and partly to changes in dietary habits and a decrease in the average fat content of the foods consumed between 1982 and 1992.

1.4   Human tissue measurements (see **Table 25**)

This section considers exclusively populations without exposure to PCDDs through occupation or industrial accidents.

PCDDs and PCDFs are found ubiquitously in human tissues. The concentrations in humans are higher in industrialized countries than in non-industrialized countries, now being about 15 ng I-TEQ/kg lipid and normally below 10 ng I-TEQ/kg lipid, respectively. These values are several orders of magnitude lower than those observed in accidentally and/or occupationally exposed individuals. In general, no significant differences in tissue levels have been found between people living in urban and rural areas. Extreme consumption of certain foods or normal consumption of highly contaminated foods may result in higher body burden, but only in some special circumstances does the increase exceed a factor of about 5.

Human milk is both a useful matrix for biological monitoring and an important food. Data on levels of PCDDs in human milk are therefore presented in some detail in a separate table, organized by country and discussed separately (see Section 1.4.2).

With a very few exceptions, only 2,3,7,8-substituted congeners are found in human tissue samples. A general observation for human background contamination is that OCDD is the most abundant isomer, followed by the 2,3,7,8-substituted hepta- and hexa-chloro-congeners. 2,3,7,8-TCDD is normally less abundant than PeCDD.

All values reported in this section are given on a lipid content basis. The concentrations are reported in µg/kg extractable fat (if not expressed otherwise).

1.4.1   *Blood and tissue samples*

(*a*)   *Austria*

For comparison with an exposed group of 2,4,5-T production workers, Neuberger *et al.* (1991) reported 2,3,7,8-TCDD blood concentrations in men with low or no occupational exposure to 2,3,7,8-TCDD. The range and median for the group were < 5–23 and 13 ng/kg, respectively.

Samples of milk from cows grazing in the vicinity of a metal reclamation plant showed significantly higher PCDD/PCDF levels than control samples. In the blood of two farmers in the same area, increased levels of certain isomers were found. The highest value (one sample) was found for 1,2,3,7,8-PeCDD at 780 ng/kg (Riss *et al.*, 1990).

(*b*)   *Canada*

Ryan *et al.* (1985b) reported that adipose tissue from 23 older subjects (> 60 years old) who had died in Ontario hospitals in 1979–81 contained an average of 11 ng/kg 2,3,7,8-TCDD.

Table 25. Concentrations of PCDDs in human samples from the general population

Reference	Origin; sample description (and no.)	Coll. period	Anal. meth.	PCDD concentration (ng/kg fat)							I-TEQ PCDD/PCDF
				TCDD 2378	PeCDD 12378	HxCDD 123478	123678	123789	HpCDD 1234678	OCDD	
Austria											
Neuberger et al. (1991)	Blood	90	BSI (med.)								
	Occup. physicians (2)			16 (8–24)	—				—	—	
	MWI plant										
	External workers (11)			15 (< 5–23)	—	—	—	—	—	—	
	External referents (6)			13 (< 5–23)	—	—	—	—	—	—	
Riss et al. (1990)	Brixlegg; blood from (1)	88	CSN	55.0	780	40	412	ND	32.5	—	
	farmer (1)			13.1	92.4	6.4	242	ND	116	—	
Canada											
Ryan et al. (1985b)	Adipose;	79–81	BSIW								
	Kingston^a (13)			12.4 ± 5.8	—	—	—	—	—	—	
	Ottawa^a (10)			8.6 ± 4.4	—	—	—	—	—	—	
Ryan et al. (1985c)	Adipose;		BSIW								
	Québec (5)	72		ND^b	12.5 (4 pos.)	—	42.6	—	83.6	756	
	(10)	76		5.4 (5 pos.)	11.6	—	63.1	—	70.7	628	
	British Columbia (5)	72		10.7	21.7	—	180	—	444	1355	
	(10)	76		7.5 (3 pos.)	11.6	—	117	—	160	1304	
	Maritimes (10)	76		5.3 (7 pos.)	8.3	—	64.0	—	82.1	572	
	Ontario (6)	76		6.1 (5 pos.)	6.1	—	40.3	—	116	528	
	Prairies (10)	76		12.7 (1 pos.)	13.3	—	97.9	—	247	843	
	E. Ontario^a (10)	80		10.0 ± 4.9	13.2 ± 4.0	—	90.5 ± 38.9	—	116 ± 41.8	611 ± 226	
LeBel et al. (1990)	Adipose;		BSO								
	Ontario (76)	84		11.2 ± 7.8	23.7 ± 11.5	—	172.4 ± 74.1	22.1 ± 9.2	231.7 ± 181	1037 ± 712	65.9 ± 31.5
				(1.4–49.1)	(3.4–65.7)		(31.2–533.8)	(6.9–53.2)	(69.5–1242)	(194–5024)	(10.9–184)
	Kingston^a (13)	79–81	BSO	19.5	27.5	—	212.3	31.7	342.3	1627	88.3
	Ottawa^a (10)			8.7	22.0	—	178.5	20.9	244.9	1154	61.6
Teschke et al. (1992)	British Columbia; adipose, residents of forest industry region (41)	90–91	CSO	4.2 (1.8–9.2)	14 (4.1–26)	15 (2.8–33)	137 (33–313)	17 (6.0–39)	136 (42–300)	500 (67–1333)	29.1 (8.4–56.4)

Table 25 (contd)

Reference	Origin: sample description (and no.)	Coll. period	Anal. meth.	PCDD concentration (ng/kg fat)							I-TEQ PCDD/PCDF
				TCDD 2378	PeCDD 12378	HxCDD 123478	123678	123789	HpCDD 1234678	OCDD	
China											
Ryan et al. (1987)	Shanghai; Adipose	84	BSOW								
	LC, 58% (1)			<2						<10	
	LC, 50% (1)			<2						<10	
	LC, 73% (1)			<2						70	
	LC, 73% (1)			<2	5.3		15		18	122	
	LC, 70% (1)			<2			9.6		27	373	
	LC, 73% (1)			<2			9.5		<2	63	
	LC, 72% (1)			<2	6.5		19		<2	59	
	LC, 76% (1)			<2							
Schecter (1994)	Blood, general population;	92	BSOW (pool)								
	Age 15–19 y (50)			<1.2	1.6	1.8	4.3	1.7	11.6	104.1	4.8
	Age over 40 y (50)			<1.2	3.1	3.8	4.9	2.6	17.5	117.0	5.7
Finland											
Rosenberg et al. (1995)	Plasma, general population; Age 41 (28–60)	89–90	BSTW	4.1 (1.3–10)	17 (7.0–45)	4 (1.8–6.1)	150 (87–216)	12 (5.8–26)	132 (36–317)	804 (369–1745)	49 (20–99)
France											
Huteau et al. (1990a)	Paris; adipose tissue (8)	<90	BSO	10.3 (6 pos.) (2.9–23)	9.8 (1 pos.)	5.7 (2 pos.) (4.9–6.4)	46.7 (7 pos.) (28.6–61.6)	11.0 (2 pos.) (8.6–13.3)	164 (7 pos.) (80.4–232)	624 (8 pos.) (362–887)	
Germany											
Beck et al. (1989b)	Hamburg; adipose (20)	86	BSTW	7.2 (1.5–1.8)	21 (8.8–48)	19 (8.7–29)	89 (35–129)	12 (5.8–20)	101 (39–216)	591 (212–1061)	56 (18–122)
Thoma et al. (1990)	Munich	<89	BSO								
	Adipose (28)			8.0 (2.6–18)	16.4 (7.7–40.4)		94.7 (35.7–178.2)		107 (35.1–246)	373 (117–789)	
	Liver (28)			16.4 (1.0–88.9)	20.1 (7.3–58.7)		166.8 (56.4–615.1)		1002 (95.7–3463)	4416 (473–15259)	
	Adipose, infants (8)			3.0 (<1–7.0)	5.4 (1.4–13.1)		25.5 (4.5–68.8)		27.1 (11.8–51.1)	104.9 (55.3–180)	

Table 25 (contd)

Reference	Origin; sample description (and no.)		Coll. period	Anal. meth.	PCDD concentration (ng/kg fat)							I-TEQ PCDD/PCDF
					TCDD 2378	PeCDD 12378	HxCDD 123478	123678	123789	HpCDD 1234678	OCDD	
Germany (contd)												
Schecter et al. (1991a)	Whole blood	(4)	< 90		4.0	17.5		109	9.8	185	761	69
	Adipose	(4)	< 90		5.1	21.5		101	8.1	153	653	69
Päpke et al. (1992)	General population; blood	(102)	89–90	BSOW	3.6 (0.6–9.1)	13.8 (2.1–39.0)	1.9 (1.0–33.0)	54.6 (15.0–124)	10.6 (0.5–71.0)	92.4 (19.0–280)	610 (145–1524)	40.8 (11.6–93.5)
Kieselrotstudie (1991)	General population; blood	(56)	91	BSOW	4.5 (ND–12)	17.3 (6.7–43)	16.9 (3.6–38)	54.5 (18–110)	11.4 (4.7–23)	98.3 (30–210)	565 (180–1100)	44.4 (16.9–98)
Päpke et al. (1993b)	General population; blood	(44)	92	BSOW	3.7 (1.0–8.8)	8.3 (2.8–20.8)	10.2 (3.6–19.4)	35.5 (7.5–99.0)	5.9 (1.8–15.8)	56.7 (16.7–159)	462 (126–1267)	26.0 (12–61)
Schrey et al. (1992)	General population; blood	(95)	91	BSOW	4.62 (1.2–12)	18.0 (5.6–44)	16.3 (3.9–38)	45.9 (12–110)	9.26 (2.9–22)	87.2 (21–210)	446 (140–950)	42.7 (11.2–114)
Päpke et al. (1994b)	General population; blood	(70)	93	BSOW	3.2 (0.5–8.7)	7.2 (3.5–16.0)	7.9 (3.4–21.8)	28.9 (9.5–71.4)	5.4 (0.5–13.8)	46.9 (13.6–143)	389 (99.9–945)	21.7 (10.3–48.8)
Päpke et al. (1996)	General population; blood	(134)	94	BSOW	2.9 (1.0–7.8)	6.3 (1.6–15.4)	6.9 (ND–22)	26.7 (5.3–62.2)	4.9 (1.3–11.9)	45.3 (8.6–115.8)	370 (90.3–949)	19.1 (5.2–43.9)
	Age 18–71 y	(139)	97	BSOW	2.3 (ND–4.9)	5.9 (1.7–12.1)	5.7 (2.0–15.7)	22.6 (3.7–60.3)	3.8 (1.5–11.1)	33.0 (9.5–93.5)	293 (106–664)	16.1 (7.3–33.6)
	Age 18–30 y	(47)			2.1 (1.0–4.3)	4.8 (1.7–9.8)	5.0 (2.0–15.7)	16.8 (3.7–33.6)	3.6 (1.8–6.7)	34.0 (9.8–56.7)	278 (108–530)	131 (7.3–13.1)
	Age 31–42 y	(48)			2.2 (ND–4.4)	5.9 (2.5–11)	5.7 (2.3 (10.5)	24.4 (8.6–42.5)	3.9	33.2 (12.4–79.4)	310 (114–597)	16.3 (7.9–22.3)
	Age 43–71 y	(44)			2.8 (ND–4.9)	7.0 (3.6–12.1)	6.5 (2.8–11.4)	26.7 (6.8–60.3)	3.9 (1.9–11.1)	31.5 (9.5–93.5)	280 (106–664)	19.1 (10.1–336)
Wittsiepe et al. (1993)	Marsberg; vicinity of copper smelter, blood	(56)	91	BSOW	4.6 (ND–12)	19.4 (6.7–80)	16.3 (5.3–51)	57.9 (19–110)	11 (3.4–31)	93.2 (18–248)	666 (120–1770)	52.7 (22.1–231)
Körner et al. (1994)	Mammary tumour tissue	(7)		BSO	7.8 (5.1–11.7)	16.5 (11.4–26.2)		86.5 (41–121)		128 (72–183)	608 (186–1361)	50.1 (27.4–76.0)
Wuthe et al. (1990)	Metal reclamation plant neighbourhood; blood	(22)	89	BSOW	3.4 (1.3–6.2)	12.4 (2.9–21)		59.2 (29.7–118)		83.5 (23–238)	506 (176–2126)	31.0 (16.1–80.4)

Table 25 (contd)

Reference	Origin; sample description (and no.)	Coll. period	Anal. meth.	PCDD concentration (ng/kg fat)							I-TEQ PCDD/PCDF
				TCDD 2378	PeCDD 12378	HxCDD 123478	123678	123789	HpCDD 1234678	OCDD	
Germany (contd)											
Wuthe et al. (1993)	One woman; blood (1)	92	BSOW	2.2	5.7		31.3		41.1	229	
Ewers et al. (1994)	Allotment gardeners; blood (21)	92	BSOW	5.8 (2.4–14)	17 (11–26)		69 (37–110)		83 (20–150)	390 (270–680)	44.3 (29.2–81.1)
Beck et al. (1994)	Infants, 3–23 months	<93	BSOW								
	Adipose tissue (8)			1.1 (<0.2–3.9)	4.5 (0.4–14)	2.9 (0.3–9.2)	14 (2.1–37)	3.4 (0.8–9.5)	18 (5.1–57)	114 (43–341)	11 (2.1–36)
	Liver (8)			1.4 (<1–4.6)	5.0	6.5	19 (3.0–54)	5.7	115 (20–396)	1221 (375–2916)	28 (4.7–88)
	Spleen (8)			2.2 (<1–<10)	5.5 (1.1–20)	11 (1.6–50)	24 (<5–113)	4.9 (0.8–18)	76 (16–236)	166 (107–281)	20 (4.3–77)
	Thymus (8)			3.4 (<1–7.5)	4.4 (<2–<15)	5.6 (2.4–<15)	15 (7.5–24)	4.6 (1.5–<15)	60 (19–155)	782 (446–1500)	19 (8.4–39)
	Brain (8)			–	–	–	–	–	–	–	< 1
Jödicke et al. (1992)	Infant, 3 months; stool (1)	91	BSO	< 2	< 5	< 5	36.7	< 5	152	1367	13.6
Welge et al. (1992)	Mother's milk (2)			1.0–2.1	4.6–5.3	3.8–4.2	25.4–31.4	2.8–3.0	26.7–29.7	104–118	14.6–18.6
Welge et al. (1993)	Blood	92	BSOW								
	Vegetarians (24)			3.4 (1.2–5.4)	14.1 (6.5–25)	12.3 (4.6–23)	36.0 (17–66)	6.8 (3.7–12)	70.2 (32–120)	447 (180–1100)	32.6 (14.6–52.9)
	Non-vegetarians (24)			3.6 (1.2–11)	15.5 (5.8–43)	14.7 (5.4–36)	39.9 (18–110)	8.3 (2.9–22)	80.0 (24–160)	456 (150–950)	34.3 (14.3–98.0)
Abraham et al. (1995a)	Mother's blood (3)	93–94	BSOW	[1.6]	[4.5]	[4.2]	[18.3]	[3.1]	[26.2]	[367]	[12.4]
	Placenta (3)			[2.7]	[4.5]	[2.5]	[8.7]	[1.7]	[11.7]	[114]	[11.1]
	Umbilical cord (3)			[< 1.0]	[2.6]	[2.6]	[8.9]	[1.8]	[9.0]	[93.6]	[6.5]
	Meconium (1)			[1.4]	[3.2]	[2.5]	[9.9]	[2.2]	[12.2]	[152]	[7.7]
Guam											
Schecter et al. (1992)	Guam Island; whole blood (10)	89	BSOW	2.6	14.7	8.3	62.1	15.5	163	749	28

Table 25 (contd)

Reference	Origin; sample description (and no.)	Coll. period	Anal. meth.	TCDD 2378	PeCDD 12378	HxCDD 123478	123678	123789	HpCDD 1234678	OCDD	I-TEQ PCDD/PCDF
Japan											
Ryan (1986)	Adipose;	84	BSIW								
	Age 21 y; LC, 43% (1)			ND	–		70		–	560	
	Age 33 y; LC, 37% (1)			ND	–		146		–	650	
	Age 46 y; LC, 67% (1)			9.7	–		90		–	1600	
	Age 55 y; LC, 80% (1)			5.5	–		61		–	2400	
	Age 64 y; LC, 71% (1)			3.2	–		66		–	860	
	Age 70 y; LC, 56% (1)			8.0	–		84		–	2100	
	Mean; LC, 59%			6.6	–		86		–	1360	
Ono et al. (1986)	Cancer patients; adipose (13)	85	CSF	9 (6–18)	15 (3–36)	8 (5–14)	70 (26–220)	12 (4–44)	77 (29–180)	230 (25–1100)	
Ogaki et al. (1987)	Adipose;	<84	CRI								
	Big city (9)			13 (2.7–33)	22 (1.6–45)		130 (64–290)		190 (27–840)	2000 (130–10000)	
	Rural town (3)			8.1 (6.4–11)	23 (15–30)		34 (20–58)		27 (13–40)	660 (160–1400)	
	(5)			15 (9.3–25)	18 (12–32)		77 (40–160)		58 (27–87)	250 (160–390)	
Hirakawa et al. (1991)	Controls; adipose (8)	<91	BSI	3 (1–5)	14 (4–18)	–	70 (21–130)	–	–	563 (180–1330)	17 (5–24)
Muto et al. (1991)	Cancer patients;	84–86	CSF								
	Lung (5)			2	9.3	4.1	3.8	6.2	112	249	
	Liver (5)			2.2	31.5	8.1	31.6	4.9	78.1	165	
	Kidney (5)			1.7	11.5	1.2	18.8	3.7	12.4	17.3	
	Pancreas (5)			1.2	37.4	123	62.7	16.8	25.2	39.9	
	Spleen (5)			ND	84.0	11.4	67.5	1.2	113	243	
	Gonad (5)			2.7	25.3	5.7	36.7	1.0	23.2	110	
	Gall-bladder (5)			ND	11.0	ND	1.5	ND	90.3	132	
	Muscle (5)			ND	17.0	6.2	18.0	1.5	304	344	
Masuda (1996)	Control; serum	91–92	BSIW	3.1	[9.2]	[4.3]	[38.8]	[8.3]	[46]	[1140]	[26]

Table 25 (contd)

Reference	Origin; sample description (and no.)		Coll. period	Anal. meth.	PCDD concentration (ng/kg fat)							I-TEQ PCDD/PCDF
					TCDD 2378	PeCDD 12378	HxCDD 123478	123678	123789	HpCDD 1234678	OCDD	
Netherlands												
van Wijnen et al. (1990)	Fetus; liver	(4)	<90	BSTW	0.23	0.09	0.09	0.29	0.07	1.03	8.8	
	Infant not nursed											
	Liver	(1)			0.03	0.07	0.04	0.16	0.03	0.29	3.87	
	Fat	(1)			3.4	2.13	ND	7.07	ND	12.3	87.4	
	Infant nursed											
	Liver	(1)			0.29	0.58	0.49	2.77	0.52	6.84	67.9	
	Fat	(1)			3.98	6.93	3.18	29.98	2.95	10.0	105.1	
	Placenta	(1)			0.26	0.53	0.21	0.42	0.08	0.59	4.22	
New Zealand												
Smith et al. (1992a)	Control group for 2,4,5-T applicators; serum		88	BSTW	5.6 ± 1.1	8.8 ± 0.7	5.7 ± 0.4	23.3 ± 4.9	8.2 ± 0.6	119 ± 18.4	759 ± 93	
Norway												
Johansen et al. (1996)	Blood		93	BSO								
	Controls	(10)			3.6	5.9	2.4	14.7	4.3	54.1	478	2.1[i]
					(0.2–7.0)	(0.5–10.6)	(0.9–3.4)	(2.7–24.5)	(0.6–7.3)	(10–179)	(52–951)	
	Moderate crab intake	(15)			7.7	17.3	8.0	27.6	8.6	45.5	336	60.8[g]
					(3–13.6)	(6.9–34.8)	(ND–30.1)	(13.1–48.2)	(ND–43.5)	(21–77)	(157–440)	
	High crab intake	(9)			11.0	28.3	10.8	39.1	9.9	33.3	267	109.6[i]
					(6.3–22.4)	(15.4–45)	(4.0–17.4)	(16.9–63.7)	(5.9–20.9)	(17–64)	(104–363)	
Russian Federation												
Schecter et al. (1992)	Whole blood		88–89	BSOW (pool)								
	Baikalsk	(8)			3.7	4.7	4.7	6.3	2.0	9.6	57	18
	St Petersburg	(60)			4.5	9.3	2.1	8.5	2.4	14	89	17
Spain												
Jiménez et al. (1995)	Madrid, unexposed; serum	(11)	93	BSO	1.52 ± 1.19	4.09 ± 0.91	2.75 ± 1.18	32.6 ± 12.4	5.81 ± 2.67	71.5 ± 34.7	397 ± 174	
					(0.61–3.9)	(2.25–5.71)	(1.55–5.10)	(18.8–57.2)	(2.01–11.4)	(32.5–137.2)	(117–690)	
Gonzaléz et al. (1997)	Mataró; blood, 10 pools	(198)	95	BSOW	1.6	4.9		39.4		70.1	484	13.3

Table 25 (contd)

| Reference | Origin; sample description (and no.) | Coll. period | Anal. meth. | PCDD concentration (ng/kg fat) | | | | | | | I-TEQ PCDD/PCDF |
				TCDD 2378	PeCDD 12378	HxCDD 123478	123678	123789	HpCDD 1234678	OCDD	
Sweden											
Rappe (1984b)	Background; adipose (6)	82	CS[c]	1.5	12		11		73	240	
Nygren *et al.* (1986)	Adipose; Unexposed (18)	84	BSIW[c]	3 (2–6)	9 (4–18)		12 (3–18)	4 (3–5)	85 (12–176)	421 (98–679)	
	Cancer patients (17)			3 (2–9)	9 (4–24)		18	4 (3–13)	100 (12–380)	408 (90–620)	
	Non-cancer patients (14)			3 (2–6)	9 (3–18)		12 (8–18)	4 (3–5)	85 (20–168)	421 (182–763)	
Rappe (1992)	Blood; No fish consumption	90	BSIW[c]	1.8	5.7	2.8	35	5.7	56	357	17.5
	Normal fish consumption			2.5	7.6	3.0	43	6.0	80	458	25.8
	High fish consumption			8.0	16	3.9	48	6.5	71	473	63.5
Svensson *et al.* (1995a)	Blood pool[f] Sea of Bothnia Fishermen		BSI	27	35	6.2	66	12	84	551	154[f]
	Controls			6.1	12	4.2	38	6.6	67	574	40[f]
	Baltic proper Fishermen			6.9	20	4.6	44	ND	58	351	80[f]
	Controls			4.0	10	3.4	32	5.7	58	364	37[f]
	Baltic south Fishermen			17	33	8.8	75	ND	110	585	131[f]
	Controls			6.4	14	5.8	53	8.5	100	605	54[f]
	West coast Fishermen 100			5.7	11	4.9	36	6.0	54	367	42[f]
	Controls 88			4.0	13	ND	34	ND	85	553	39[f]
Hardell *et al.* (1995)	Blood Cancer patients (7)	>86	BSI	10.1 (<0.4–36)	24 (9–57)	1.2 (0.9–2.6)	45.3 (13–130)	6.3 (2.6–13)	118 (9–380)	510 (154–1600)	64.7[g] (19.9–187)
	Non-cancer patients (12)			2.8 (<0.4–6)	9.6 (<0.4–19)	<1	12.2 (8–18)	3.7 (3–5)	85 (32–168)	413 (247–672)	29.7[g] (12.9–53.4)

Table 25 (contd)

Reference	Origin; sample description (and no.)	Coll. period	Anal. meth.	PCDD concentration (ng/kg fat)							I-TEQ PCDD/PCDF
				TCDD 2378	PeCDD 12378	HxCDD 123478	123678	123789	HpCDD 1234678	OCDD	
Switzerland											
Wacker et al. (1990)	Background		CSO^c								
	Adipose (21)			–	24.1	15.3	144.3	–	195	1161	
	Liver (21)			–	1.1	1.1	10.5	–	81	491	
Taiwan											
Ryan et al. (1994)	Control children; serum	91	BSW	3.0	7.3		23		52	612	22.7
United Kingdom											
Duarte-Davidson et al. (1993)	Wales, 5 pools; adipose	90–91	CSO	<10	23 (21–24)	37 (29–47)	182 (160–210)	28 (22–210)	154 (120–230)	816 (590–1100)	57
United States											
Ryan et al. (1985c)	New York State: adipose (6)	83–84	CSOW	6.4 ± 1.6 (3.7–8.3)	9.7 ± 2.4 (7.5–13.8)	–	57.8 ± 6.5 (46.2–64.2)	–	95.2 ± 29.2 (39.4–119)	585 ± 98 (428–695)	
Ryan et al. (1986)	New York State;	<83	BSTW^c								
	Adipose (3) (mean LC, 67%)			5.4 (3.7–8.4)	7.4 (7.8–11)	–	73.7 (61–130)	–	95 (53–120)	528 (201–700)	
	Liver (3) (mean LC, 24%)			2.4 (ND–4.6)	2.3	–	36.8 (6.5–56)	–	34 (22–44)	250	
	Adrenal (2) (LC, 28.25%)			3.8–3.7	3.1–4.8	–	35–39	–	36–55	180–350 210–600	
	Bone marrow (1) (LC, 26%)			ND	12	–	30	–	48	540	
	Muscle (3) (mean LC, 11%)			<2.5 (ND–2.5)	1.3 (1.2–1.5)	–	11.6 (5.8–21)	–	11.7 (5–16)	122 (76–170)	
	Spleen (2) (LC, 1.8–1.7%)			(ND–1.3)	(1.1–11)	–	(1.5–1.9)	–	(4.7–13)	(20–46)	
	Kidney (2) (LC, 3.0–4.0%)			ND	ND	–	(2.5–4.0)	–	(5.2–13)	(31–39)	
	Lung (1) (LC, 2.2%)			ND	ND	–	1.4	–	2.9	21	
Gross et al. (1984)	Adipose	84	BNN								
	Controls (11)			5.6 (ND–14)	–	–	–	–	–	–	
	Air Force scientists (3)			5 (4–6)	–	–	–	–	–	–	

Table 25 (contd)

Reference	Origin; sample description (and no.)	Coll. period	Anal. meth.	PCDD concentration (ng/kg fat)							I-TEQ PCDD/PCDF
				TCDD 2378	PeCDD 12378	HxCDD 123478	123678	123789	HpCDD 1234678	OCDD	
United States (contd)											
Ryan (1986)	New York State; Adipose	85	BSIW^r								
	6 months(LC, 75%)			ND	–		4.5		–	130	
	22 y (LC, 83%)			2.2	–		74		–	920	
	Liver										
	6 months (LC, 4.0%)			ND	–		ND		–	22	
	22 y (LC, 4.4%)			ND	–		21		–	420	
Graham *et al.* (1985)	Background; adipose (8)	<84	CSI	5.4 (1.8–10)	10.3 (4–16)	–	–	–	–	–	
	(3)			7.7 (2–14)							
Schecter *et al.* (1986a)	Binghamton; adipose (1)	<84	CRO^s	8.3	13.8	–	46.2	7.4	95.8	534	
	(1)			7.2	10.3	–	54.5	7.5	39.4	593	
	(1)			6.0	8.2	–	60.3	7.4	119	695	
	(1)			3.7	7.5	–	60.4	6.8	93.1	586	
	L.C. 70.6% (46–88) (8)		BNW	7.2 (1.4–17.7)	11.1 (5.2–25.2)	–	95.9 (46.2–355)	–	164 (53–691)	707 (214–1931)	
Patterson *et al.* (1986a)	Georgia and Utah; adipose	<86	BSIW								
	Black women, 60.6 years old (7)			12.2	–	–	–	–	–	–	
	Black men, 55.9 years old (7)			10.4							
	White women, 52.2 years old (8)			10.9	–	–	–	–	–	–	
	White men, 54.8 years old (9)			8.8							
Stanley *et al.* (1986)	General population; adipose (46)	82	BSO	5.0 ± 2.8 (<1–10)	32 ± 38 (<1–180)	–	72 ± 70 (7.9–330)	–	87 ± 78 (<23–390)	560 ± 290 (64–1250)	
Patterson *et al.* (1986b)	Missouri; adipose (57)	86	BSIW	7.4 (1.4–20.2)	–	–	–	–	–	–	

Table 25 (contd)

Reference	Origin; sample description (and no.)	Coll. period	Anal. meth.	PCDD concentration (ng/kg fat)							I-TEQ PCDD/PCDF
				TCDD 2378	PeCDD 12378	HxCDD 123478	123678	123789	HpCDD 1234678	OCDD	
United States (contd)											
Centers for Disease Control Veterans Health Studies (1988)	Non-Viet Nam veterans; serum (97)	87	BSIW	4.1 ± 2.3 (ND–15)	–	–	–	–	–	–	–
Nygren et al. (1988)	Era control; serum (1)	<88	BSIW	1.5	9.0	<4	36	<4	59	84	
	(1)			7.3	15	11.6	191	<5	59	675	
	(1)			7.1	26	17.6	231	38	428	3246	
	(1)			2.4	16	3.6	47	4.0	188	468	
	(1)			2.2	6.9	4.7	36	6.0	65	1747	
	(1)			5.5	14	8.7	64	10.1	72	1052	
	(1)			6.0	13.5	13.2	69	15	105	566	
Andrews et al. (1989)	Missouri controls Adipose Men (51)	86	BSIW	6.8 ± 4.1 (ND–20)	–	–	–	–	–	–	
	Women (77)			7.2 ± 4.0 (1.4–20.2)	–	–	–	–	–	–	
Fingerhut et al. (1989)	Referents; serum (19)	<89	BSIW	8.2 (3.7–17.1)	–	–	–	–	–	–	
Schecter et al. (1989b)	One patient[c] Abdominal fat (LC, 75%) (1)	<89	N	5.7	7.8		64		110	680	
	Subcutaneous fat (LC, 75%) (1)			6.0	8.2		60		120	700	
	Adrenal fat (LC, 28%) (1)			3.8	3.1		35		55	600	
	Bone marrow (LC, 26%) (1)			ND	12		30		48	540	
	Liver (LC, 6%) (1)			ND	ND		6.5		22	220	
	Muscle (LC, 9%) (1)			ND	1.2		7.9		14	170	
	Spleen (LC, 1.8%) (1)			ND	11		1.9		13	46	
	Kidney (LC, 3.0%) (1)			ND	ND		2.5		5.2	31	
	Lung (LC, 2.2%) (1)			ND	ND		1.4		2.9	21	

Table 25 (contd)

Reference	Origin; sample description (and no.)	Coll. period	Anal. meth.	PCDD concentration (ng/kg fat)							I-TEQ PCDD/PCDF
				TCDD 2378	PeCDD 12378	HxCDD 123478	123678	123789	HpCDD 1234678	OCDD	
United States (contd)											
Wendling *et al.* (1990a)	Faeces; laboratory workers										
	Pool	<90	BSO	0.61 ± 0.09	—	—	—	—	—	—	
	Individual sample			0.74	—	—	—	—	—	—	
Schecter *et al.* (1990b; 1991a)	US veterans										
	Adipose (20)	<90	BSOW	6.9	7.7		59.3	6.3	82.5	429	24
	Plasma (20)			5.7	7.1		56.0	8.5	107.9	843	23
Kang *et al.* (1991)	Adipose	78	N								
	Viet Nam veterans (36)			13.4	20.6		170.4	19.4	276	1262	
	Non-Viet Nam veterans (79)			12.5	18.3		152.9	17.2	245	1109	
	Civilians (80)			15.8	18.3		165.1	17.9	300	1393	
Piacitelli *et al.* (1992)	Referents; serum (79)	87–88	BSIW	7 (2–20)	12 (3.5–51)	13 (3.2–58)	84 (17–183)	13 (3.6–33)	160 (39–460)	1010 (480–2300)	
Patterson *et al.* (1994)	Atlanta; adipose	84–86	BSIW								
	All data (28)			10.4 (1.6–38)							
	Men (14)			7.4 (1.6–19.4)							
	Women (14)			11.6 (3.1–24.3)							
	General population (4)			4.4 (1.6–8.3)	11.6 (8.5–16)	5.1 (3 pos.) (3.7–6.4)	94.2 (81–121)	16.9 (12.5–22)	56 (2 pos.) (48–63)	446 (2 pos.) (396–495)	
Schecter *et al.* (1994b)	Placenta, pooled (14)	<94	BSOW	2.4	4.0	2.4	15.9	3.2	36.2	282	10.1
	Placenta (1)			2.0	9.5	6.4	11.2	5.3	47.7	236	14.4
	Blood, pool (50)			3.8	9.3	9.8	72.1	11.9	118.6	793.9	27.0
Schecter *et al.* (1996b)	Fetal tissue, 8–14 weeks, pool (10)	94		1.4	2.0	2.3	8.9	1.7	22.9	98.8	5.3

Table 25 (contd)

Reference	Origin; sample description (and no.)	Coll. period	Anal. meth.	PCDD concentration (ng/kg fat)							I-TEQ PCDD/PCDF
				TCDD 2378	PeCDD 12378	HxCDD 123478	123678	123789	HpCDD 1234678	OCDD	
United States (contd)											
Schecter et al. (1996c)	Adipose (5)	96	BSNW	1.3	2.8	3.3	22.3	3.1	45.4	214	8.5
	Blood, before nursing (5)			1.7	3.2	4.0	19.9	4.2	57.9	374	9.9
	Placenta (5)			2.7	4.5	2.5	10.2	2.6	21.5	103	9.4
	Cord blood (5)			1.3	1.3	1.6	10.5	2.2	24.1	95.8	4.7
	Mother's milk (5)			1.4	2.5	3.0	20.1	3.5	34.0	104	8.1
	Blood after 4–8 weeks of nursing (5)			1.5	2.6	3.2	18.7	4.1	45.2	226	8.3
Schecter et al. (1996d)	Blood, pool (100)	96	BSTW	4.3	8.7	9.7	63.7	7.8	102	781	27.1
	Serum, pool (100)			4.2	9.8	10.6	67.9	10.7	117	878	27.6
Viet Nam											
Schecter et al. (1986b)	Adipose North Viet Nam; LC, 50% (7)	84	BSOW[c]	< 2	< 2	–	4.6	–	19.0	36.1	
	South Viet Nam; LC, 60% (13)			22.1 (10 pos.)	9.9	–	46.7	–	105	514	
Schecter et al. (1986c)	Adipose North Viet Nam; LC, 56% (9)	84	BSOW	< 2	3.8 (1 pos.)	–	11.4 (6 pos.) (ND–23.9)	–	28.8 (6 pos.) (ND–56.3)	104 (8 pos.) (ND–205)	
	South Viet Nam; LC, 62% (15)			27.9 (12 pos.) (ND–103)	15.4 (14 pos.) (ND–43.3)		99.8 (22.6–347)		178 (13.7–710)	1326 (141–3410)	
Schecter et al. (1989c)	Adipose North Viet Nam; pool (10)	84–88	BN	< 2	–	–	–	–	–	–	
	South Viet Nam (27)			19 (16 pos.) (ND–36)	–	–	–	–	–	–	
Nguyen et al. (1989)	Ho Chi Minh City; adipose; mean LC, 76% (9)	84–85	BSNW	23 (4–103)	12 (4.5–27)		89 (23–261)		272 (77–710)	2114 (25–4284)	
Hoang et al. (1989)	Adipose North Viet Nam (11)	< 89	N	1.3[a] (1 pos.)	–	–	–	–	–	–	
	South Viet Nam (44)			20.5 (40 pos.)	–	–	–	–	–	–	
Huteau et al. (1990b)	South Viet Nam; adipose (27)	< 90	BRO	16.2 (24 pos.) (1.5–129)	17.5 (4 pos.) (9.7–34.6)	11.7 (16 pos.) (4.5–23.5)	56.1 (23 pos.) (9.5–157)	12.7 (22 pos.) (2.4–48.5)	95.5 (23 pos.) (8.4–303)	569 (25 pos.) (35–2113)	

Table 25 (contd)

Reference	Origin; sample description (and no.)	Coll. period	Anal. meth.	PCDD concentration (ng/kg fat)							I-TEQ PCDD/PCDF
				TCDD 2378	PeCDD 12378	HxCDD 123478	123678	123789	HpCDD 1234678	OCDD	
Viet Nam (contd)											
Schecter *et al.* (1990c)	Adipose		BSO								
	North Viet Nam (10)	80s		1.4	2.5	1.4	6.0	·1.2	30.1	230	
	South Viet Nam (13)			6.7	6.4	5.0	27.6	6.1	69.2	470	
Schecter *et al.* (1990d)	Liver, stillborn infants		BSOW								
	(1)	<89		4.3	7.8	4.5	5.1	2.9	15	64	12
	(1)			3.5	8.3	3.8	6.1	2.3	11	65	12
	(1)			1.3	3.8	4.1	4.6	3.9	22	58	6.4
Schecter *et al.* (1992)	Whole blood; pool		BSOW								
	North Viet Nam (82)	<91		2.2	4.1	3.7	13.4	4.8	25.5	132	15
	South Viet Nam (383)			14.6	9.1	7.5	33.8	9.4	87.3	696	36
Schecter *et al.* (1995)	Blood		BSOW								
	South Viet Nam (433)	91–92		12.9	8.0	6.6	29.9	8.3	77.2	616	31.3
	Central Viet Nam (183)			13.2	16.3	13.0	46.2	13.4	78.1	751	50
	North Viet Nam (82)			2.2	4.1	3.7	13.4	4.8	25.5	132	15.3
Le *et al.* (1995)	Blood; pool		BSOW pool								
	North Viet Nam (133)	91		2.7	–	–	–	–	–	–	15.2
	Military region I (315)	91–92		12.8	–	–	–	–	–	–	56.4
	Military region II (176)	91–92		4.2	–	–	–	–	–	–	30.6
	Military region III (1443)	91–92		12.1	–	–	–	–	–	–	34.5
	Military region IV (569)	91–92		8.05	–	–	–	–	–	–	27.4

Data presented are arithmetic means and, if available, ± standard deviation, with range in parentheses, unless otherwise indicated. Levels of congeners not detected at a known detection limit (for example, 4.2 ng/kg) are presented as < 4.2 when detection limit is given.

Explanation for analytical methods: All analyses use high-resolution gas chromatography: B, high-resolution mass spectrometry; C, low-resolution mass spectrometry; I, isomer-specific; O, others; N, no information; S, sophisticated clean-up; R, reduced clean-up; W, WHO-accepted laboratory; –, not reported; ND, not detected; +, contains 50% of detection limit; LC, lipid content; pos., positive; S, south; N, north; C, control;
[ ] Calculated by the Working Group

[a] Overlap between these studies
[b] Detection limit, > 2–3 ng/kg
[c] WW, weight-based
[d] Contained also 22 ng/kg 1,2,3,4,6,7,9-HpCDD
[e] PCDD-I-TEQ only
[f] Nordic TEQ
[g] 50 fishermen and 150 controls for the 3 groups
[h] Mean level, ND are included at 1 ng/kg (half the detection limit)

Ryan *et al.* (1985c) analysed 46 and 10 adipose tissue samples originating from people who had died accidentally in 1976 and 1972, respectively, in Canada for various reasons, as well as 10 others from deceased hospital patients. Total PCDD levels were about an order of magnitude higher than total PCDFs. PCDD levels increased with increasing chlorination from 2,3,7,8-TCDD (average, 5–13 ng/kg) to OCDD (average, 528–1355 ng/kg). Only the penta-, hexa- and hepta-CDF congeners were detected at these levels (10–60 ng/kg); TCDF and OCDF were not detected.

Human adipose tissue samples obtained during autopsies in five Canadian municipalities within the Great Lakes basin (Cornwall, London, St Catherine's, Welland, Windsor) were analysed for PCDDs and PCDFs (LeBel *et al.*, 1990). The mean congener levels for male and female donors in each municipality were similar to those previously reported. The ages of the 40 men ranged from 29 to 83 years (mean, 63 years) and that of the 36 women from 12 to 88 years (mean, 69 years). No significant differences in congener levels between male and female donors or between municipalities were detected. However, in four cases, the values for women were 15–45% higher than the corresponding values for men. Additionally, a positive correlation with age was observed for the levels of several congeners as well as for the I-TEQ.

In connection with the forestry industry, there has been concern that by-products of pulp and paper production and chlorophenol fungicides used in sawmills may result in residents being environmentally or occupationally exposed to PCDDs/PCDFs. To examine this possibility, PCDD and PCDF levels were measured in the adipose tissue of 41 British Columbians selected to match the age and sex distribution of the exposed population. The group consisted of 18 men and 23 women. The mean age of the subjects was 45 years (range, 18–77 years) and the mean weight was 96 kg (range, 50–193 kg). The mean of the 41 samples was 29.1 ng I-TEQ/kg (range, 8.4–56.4). The highest 2,3,7,8-TCDD level measured was 9.2 ng/kg (lipid-based) (Teschke *et al.*, 1992).

Ryan (1986) examined the relationship between the PCDD/PCDF level and age (between 14 and 76 years) in 46 Canadian individuals.

(c)   *China*

Human adipose tissue from seven patients (four men, three women; mean age, 54 years) undergoing general surgery in Shanghai was analysed by Ryan *et al.* (1987). Compared with data from other countries, the values were low. At a detection limit of 2.0 ng/kg (based on wet weight), no 2,3,7,8-TCDD was found.

In connection with a study to examine the exposure of agricultural workers to PCP (for snail control) and PCDDs/PCDFs, Schecter (1994) reported data on two pooled age-matched control groups. For the two groups from the general population, very low blood concentrations of PCDDs/PCDFs were found at 4.8 ng I-TEQ/kg (age, 15–19 years) and 5.7 ng/kg (over 40 years), respectively. These are consistent with values found in mothers' milk (see Section 1.4(*b*)).

(d) Finland

In a study of pulp and paper mill workers in Finland (Rosenberg *et al.*, 1995), a comparison group with no known exposure was analysed. This control group consisted of 14 persons with a mean age of 41 years (range, 28–60 years). The mean total I-TEQ level in plasma was 49 ng/kg (range, 20–99 ng/kg) (see Section 1.3.1(*a*)(iv)).

(e) France

The levels of PCDDs and PCDFs in adipose tissue from eight persons living in Paris were reported by Huteau *et al.* (1990a). Most of the 2,3,7,8-substituted isomers were found, in some cases at unexpectedly high values (2,3,7,8-TCDF, 1,2,3,7,8-PeCDF and 2,3,4,7,8-PeCDF). Surprisingly, non-2,3,7,8-substituted isomers were also reported at relatively high values (TCDFs, TCDDs, HpCDFs). [Sample contamination cannot be excluded.]

(f) Germany

The first German data on background levels of PCDDs in human adipose tissue were reported by Beck *et al.* (1989b). Concentrations in 20 unexposed individuals (mean age, 50 years) were used for comparison in a study of 45 occupationally exposed employees at a chemical plant in Hamburg. The values for the comparison group ranged between 18 and 122 ng I-TEQ/kg (mean, 56 ng/kg).

No correlation was seen between adipose tissue or liver concentrations and age or sex in 28 subjects aged between 26 and 80 years (Thoma *et al.*, 1989, 1990). Large differences in the concentrations of PCDDs and PCDFs between adipose and liver tissues were demonstrated for most of the isomers (see **Table 26**). Thoma *et al.* (1990) also reported concentrations of PCDDs and PCDFs in adipose tissue from eight infants (age 2–12 months). The levels were lower than in adults for nearly all isomers.

Background data on PCDDs and PCDFs in human blood from Germany published by Päpke *et al.* (1989b) have been updated since 1991 by various authors (see **Table 27**). The results suggest a decrease in PCDD/PCDF blood levels in Germany over the past decade.

Age-related increases in blood levels of most of the PCDD congeners and the I-TEQ have been reported (Sagunski *et al.*, 1993; Schrey *et al.*, 1992; Päpke, 1996).

The Kieselrotstudie (Wittsiepe *et al.*, 1993) was designed to assess the degree of exposure to PCDDs and PCDFs in 56 persons living in the vicinity of a former copper smelter located in Marsberg (see monograph on PCDFs in this volume; Section 1.3.2(*c*)). The copper smelter was in operation until 1945. In 1991, high levels of PCDDs/PCDFs were found in materials from the slag dumps (10–100 μg I-TEQ/kg). The median I-TEQ values of the Marsberg group (43.2 ng/kg blood lipid) and the reference group from Steinfurt (43.0 ng/kg blood lipid) were similar, whereas the mean of the Marsberg group (52.7 ng/kg) was higher than that of the control group (44.4 ng/kg).

Near a metal reclamation plant in Baden-Württemberg, Rastatt, PCDD/PCDF contamination of soil, dust from homes, indoor air and vegetables was investigated in 1987. Blood samples from 22 volunteers living in the vicinity of the plant were analysed for

PCDDs and PCDFs. Levels of certain Pe-, Hx- and HpCDF isomers were increased, in a similar pattern to the contamination throughout the area. The increase in PCDD/PCDF levels was traced to occupational exposure in the case of workers and to food intake in the other cases. For children (four samples), soil and/or dust ingestion may be a pathway of special importance (Wuthe *et al.*, 1990).

Table 26. Concentrations of PCDD isomers in adipose and liver tissues of German adults and adipose tissue of infants

Compound	Adult; ratio liver : adipose	Adipose tissue; ratio infant : adult
TCDD	2.05	0.55
PeCDD	1.22	0.30
HxCDD	1.76	0.23
HpCDD	9.39	0.23
OCDD	11.83	0.19

From Thoma *et al.* (1989, 1990)

Table 27. Time trend in background data on concentrations of PCDDs/PCDFs in human blood

Reference	Collection year	No.	Mean I-TEQ ng/kg, lipid-based
Päpke *et al.* (1989b)	1988	10	[45.8]
Päpke *et al.* (1992)	1989–90	102	40.8
Kieselrotstudie (1991)	1991	56	44.4
Päpke *et al.* (1993b)	1992	44	26.0
Schrey *et al.* (1992)	1991	95[a]	42.7
Päpke *et al.* (1994b)	1993	70	21.7
Päpke *et al.* (1996)	1994	134	19.1
Päpke *et al.* (1996)	1996	139	16.1

[a] Contains 56 samples from Kieselrotstudie (1991)
[Calculated by the Working Group]

In Rheinfelden in southern Germany, soil concentrations of PCDDs/PCDFs of up to approximately 1000 ng German TEQ/kg were found. The source of contamination of the soils was identified as residues from a PCP production process. Locally produced food, such as eggs, chicken and vegetables, with high PCDD/PCDF levels were reported to be an important source of elevated human levels. Good agreement between human blood and milk concentrations was demonstrated in one woman (Wuthe *et al.*, 1993).

PCDD/PCDF levels were determined in the venous blood of 21 allotment gardeners from Duisburg (Ewers *et al.*, 1994). Soil analysis showed elevated levels of PCDDs/-PCDFs in garden soil (range, 16.4–77.6 ng I-TEQ/kg). Vegetable plants also had elevated levels (up to 65.6 ng I-TEQ/kg). The mean I-TEQ of 44.3 ng/kg (range, 29.2–81.1 ng/kg) in blood fat of the gardeners was within the range of a control group.

In seven breast cancer patients without known occupational exposure to PCDDs/PCDFs, the levels of PCDD/PCDF congeners in mammary carcinoma tissue were not elevated above the concentrations in tumour-free tissue (Körner *et al.*, 1994).

PCDD/PCDF levels in various organs from infants were measured by Beck *et al.* (1990, 1994). Adipose tissue, liver, spleen, thymus and brain from eight infants (age, 3–23 months) who had mostly died from sudden infant death syndrome were analysed. Five of the infants had been breast-fed exclusively for between 21 and 91 days. The lipid-based PCDD/PCDF levels in liver, thymus and spleen were higher than those in adipose tissue. Very often the concentrations were below the detection limits. The lowest levels were found in brain.

Elimination of PCDDs/PCDFs through the faeces was studied in a three-month-old breast-fed infant (Jödicke *et al.*, 1992). Little excretion of Cl_4–Cl_6 congeners was found. The data suggest that more than 90% had been absorbed by the infant. However, 1,2,3,4,6,7,8-HpCDD as well as OCDD were found to be highly concentrated in stool fat (by a factor of 5–12 over the concentration in milk fat).

(g) Guam

Schecter *et al.* (1992) reported a mean PCDD/PCDF level of 28 ng I-TEQ/kg in blood samples from 10 residents of the Pacific island of Guam. This was suggested to be due to consumption of food mainly imported from the United States and Japan. [A local source cannot be excluded.]

(h) Japan

In adipose tissue from six individuals 20–70 years old in Japan collected in 1984 (Ryan, 1986), the mean 2,3,7,8-TCDD concentration was 6.6 ng/kg and that of OCDD 1360 ng/kg.

Thirteen samples of human adipose tissue from cancer patients were analysed for Cl_4–Cl_8 PCDDs and PCDFs (Ono *et al.*, 1986). These compounds were identified in all of the analysed samples. 2,3,7,8-TCDD concentrations ranged from 6 to 18 ng/kg.

In a large study, more than 500 human milk and 17 adipose tissue samples were analysed for PCDDs (Ogaki *et al.*, 1987). Adipose tissues from inhabitants of a large city and its suburbs had higher levels of PCDDs that those of rural towns.

Muto *et al.* (1991) investigated the tissue distribution of 2,3,7,8-substituted PCDDs in humans who died of cancer. The values for OCDD were the highest in each organ and tissue. All data were wet weight-based, and no lipid concentrations for the tissues were reported.

(i) The Netherlands

Intake and faecal excretion of PCDDs/PCDFs in breast-fed infants at a range of ages were studied (Pluim *et al.*, 1993a). In three totally breast-fed infants, the amount of PCDDs/PCDFs consumed via breast milk and excreted in the stools was measured at the ages of four, eight and 12 weeks. Intake was high, especially at the age of four weeks (mean, 257 pg/kg bw). A strong decline was observed in the second month, mainly due to a reduction in PCDD/PCDF concentrations in whole breast milk as a result of reduced fat content. With the exception of OCDD, faecal excretion of the congeners was below 5% of their intake, indicating a bioavailability of more than 95% from breast milk. No influence of age on faecal excretion of PCDDs/PCDFs during the first three months of life was observed.

(j)   New Zealand

In a study to determine whether blood serum levels of 2,3,7,8-TCDD in a group of professional 2,4,5-T applicators in New Zealand were greater than those of a matched control group not involved in 2,4,5-T spraying, the mean level of 2,3,7,8-TCDD in the control group was 5.6 ng/kg ± 1.1 (standard error) (Smith *et al.*, 1992a) (see Section 1.3.1(*a*)(ii) and Table 17).

(k)   Norway

PCDDs/PCDFs have been analysed in human blood in relation to consumption of crabs from a contaminated fjord area in Norway (Johansen *et al.*, 1996). The analyses were performed in three different groups: reference, moderate crab intake and high crab intake (age between 40 and 54 years). A significant increase in blood levels of many PCDD and PCDF congeners was found in crab consumers; the differences were greatest for several of the PCDFs that are characteristic of the contamination of marine biota in the fjord caused by a magnesium-producing plant. Almost all subjects in the high-intake group exceeded the tolerable weekly intake of 35 pg 2,3,7,8-TCDD/kg bw per week proposed by the Nordic Expert Group (see Section 1.5).

(l)   Poland

Changes over time in PCDD/PCDF levels in the adipose tissue of a person with long-term exposure to PCP were studied (Górski *et al.*, 1984). The analyses, performed by GC-ECD, yielded half-lives of 1,2,3,6,7,8-HxCDD, 3.5 years; 1,2,3,4,6,7,8-HpCDD, 3.2 years; OCDD, 5.7 years; 1,2,3,4,6,7,8-HpCDF, < 1.7 years; OCDF, 1.8 years.

(m)   Russian Federation

Schecter *et al.* (1992) found PCDD/PCDF concentrations in pooled blood samples from Baikalsk (eastern Siberia) and St Petersburg to be 18 and 17 ng I-TEQ/kg, respectively. Levels of OCDD were very low (57 and 89 ng/kg, respectively).

(n)   Spain

Jiménez *et al.* (1995) measured the blood levels of PCDDs and PCDFs from 11 individuals (age, 19–55 years) living in Madrid. The mean total level of PCDDs was 515.3 ng/kg, of which 1.5 ng/kg was 2,3,7,8-TCDD.

(o)   Sweden

After Rappe *et al.* (1983) found elevated PCDD/PCDF levels in the blood of occupationally exposed workers (chlorophenol workers, textile workers), samples from the general population in Sweden were analysed. Levels of all higher chlorinated (Cl_4–Cl_8) PCDDs and PCDFs in adipose tissue were measured (Rappe, 1984b). The samples originated from patients undergoing cancer or gall bladder surgery. It was concluded that the low ng/kg levels for tetra- to octa-CDDs/CDFs represented typical contamination of the general population.

In a continuation of this study (Nygren *et al.*, 1986; Rappe *et al.*, 1986a), PCDD/-PCDF patterns in adipose tissue from a group of 17 cancer patients and a group of 14 controls were compared. No difference was seen in the pattern of congeners between the two groups.

In order to study the influence of diet on the body burden of PCDDs/PCDFs, blood from three different Swedish groups was analysed (Svensson *et al.*, 1991; Rappe, 1992): Group 1, with no fish consumption (persons suffering from an allergy); Group 2, with normal fish consumption (around 50 g/day); and Group 3, with high fish consumption (> 100 g/day). Group 3 had a body burden, calculated as TEQ, approximately three times higher than Group 2. Group 1, however, had only slightly lower blood levels of PCDDs/PCDFs than Group 2. The dominant congener among the tetra- and penta-chlorinated congeners was 2,3,4,7,8-PeCDF. The difference between the three groups was also highest for this particular congener, which is also the major congener in fish from the Baltic Sea (see Section 1.3.2(*d*)). The mean PCDD/PCDF values for Groups 1, 2 and 3 were 17.5, 25.8 and 63.5 ng I-TEQ/kg, respectively.

This study was extended to cover the main fishing areas in Sweden (Svensson *et al.*, 1995a) and assessed dietary habits and exposure to selenium, persistent organochlorine compounds, including PCDDs/PCDFs, methylmercury and methylamines among Swedish fishermen. The interview data showed that 250 fishermen ate almost twice as much fish as the 250 referents from the general population. Fishermen from the Baltic Coast ate more fatty fish than fishermen from the Atlantic Coast, and they also had higher blood levels of persistent organochlorine compounds such as PCDDs/PCDFs than both the Atlantic Coast fishermen and the referents.

Measurements of PCDD/PCDF concentrations in adipose tissue from seven patients with malignant lymphoproliferative diseases and 12 surgical patients without malignant disease showed significantly higher concentrations of 1,2,3,7,8-PeCDD, 1,2,3,6,7,8-HxCDD and 2,3,4,7,8-PeCDF in the cases with lymphoproliferative diseases than in the patients in the other group (Hardell *et al.*, 1995). Nordic TEQ values also were significantly higher in the first group (mean, 64.7 ng/kg; range, 19.9–187) than in the second group (mean, 29.7 ng/kg; range, 12.9–53.4).

(p)   Switzerland

Wacker *et al.* (1990) analysed liver and adipose tissue samples of 21 Swiss inhabitants (age, 15–85 years; mean, 47 years) for PCDDs/PCDFs. All values were reported on a wet weight basis. **Table 28** shows the concentration ratios between adipose tissue and liver. No correlation between age or weight and tissue levels was detected.

Table 28. Concentration ratios (wet weight-based) of PCDDs in adipose and liver tissue of Swiss inhabitants

Congener	Adipose : liver	SD
1,2,3,7,8-PeCDD	21.1	6.6
1,2,3,4,7,8-HxCDD	14.6	6.8
1,2,3,6,7,8-HxCDD	13.8	6.1
1,2,3,4,6,7,8-HpCDD	2.4	0.9
OCDD	2.4	0.8

From Wacker *et al.* (1990)

(q)   United Kingdom

PCDD/PCDF background levels were measured in pooled human adipose tissue samples from five areas in Wales (Duarte-Davidson *et al.*, 1993). With the exception of OCDF, which was found at unexpectedly high values in all pooled samples (36–62 ng/kg), the concentrations were similar to those in other industrialized countries. 2,3,7,8-TCDD and 2,3,7,8-TCDF were not detected at detection limits of 10 ng/kg.

(r)   United States

Six samples from both biopsy and autopsy fat taken in 1983–84 from New York State residents were analysed (Ryan *et al.*, 1985c). PCDDs and PCDFs were found in all samples with total (Cl_4–Cl_8) PCDD levels about an order of magnitude higher than total (Cl_5–Cl_7) PCDFs. PCDD levels increased with increasing chlorination from tetra- (mean, 6.4 ng/kg) to octa-CDD (mean, 585 ng/kg). Only the penta-, hexa- and hepta-PCDF congeners were detected, at levels that were of the same order of magnitude. TCDF and OCDF were absent.

The tissue distribution of PCDDs and PCDFs was studied in three autopsy subjects from the general population of New York State (Ryan *et al.*, 1986). These were the first reports to show that several 2,3,7,8-chlorine-substituted PCDDs/PCDFs are present not only in adipose tissues from the general population, but also in all other tissues assayed. The ratios of the PCDD/PCDF congeners to each other were similar in each tissue, with overall levels on a wet weight basis decreasing in the order fat, adrenal, bone marrow, liver, muscle, spleen, kidney and lung. If the levels are expressed on a lipid basis rather than on a wet weight basis, liver had the highest value and the variation between tissues showed only a two- to four-fold difference.

Schecter *et al.* (1986a) reported PCDD/PCDF levels in adipose tissue of eight control samples from Binghamton, NY. All values were based on wet weight. The 2,3,7,8-TCDD levels ranged between 1.4 and 17.7 ng/kg. HpCDDs and OCDD were found at mean values of 164 and 707 ng/kg, respectively, with maximum values of 691 and 1931 ng/kg, respectively.

Patterson *et al.* (1986a) reported 2,3,7,8-TCDD levels in 61 adipose tissue samples from 35 autopsy cases from Georgia and Utah. The geometric mean for these samples on a wet-weight basis for 2,3,7,8-TCDD was 7.1 ng/kg. The geometric mean of values for 2,3,7,8-TCDD in 31 of these samples on a lipid basis was 9.6 ng/kg. On the basis of the wet-weight adipose concentrations, the authors concluded that concentrations of 2,3,7,8-TCDD increased with age in both sexes. There was no significant difference in the concentration of 2,3,7,8-TCDD between blacks and whites, and women had a slightly higher (2 ng/kg) mean concentration than men.

Analysis for Cl_4–Cl_8 PCDDs/PCDFs was performed for 46 adipose tissue samples prepared from the United States Environmental Protection Agency National Human Adipose Tissue Survey (NHATS) as composites from over 900 specimens to represent the nine United States census divisions and three age groups (0–14, 15–44 and $\geq$ 45 years) (Stanley *et al.*, 1986). The results demonstrate that PCDDs/PCDFs are prevalent in the general United States population and that differences exist with age. Only means and ranges of all data were reported.

Stanley *et al.* (1990) also found a decrease in 2,3,7,8-TCDD with time in a subset of the NHATS adipose tissue samples (age group, 15–44 years) collected between 1971 and 1987 (see **Table 29**).

Table 29. Differences in 2,3,7,8-TCDD levels in adipose tissues by year of sample collection in the United States

2,3,7,8-TCDD (ng/kg lipid)	Collection year	Remark
~ 18	1971–73	Individual specimen
~ 14.5	1974–76	Individual specimen
~ 10.5	1977–79	Individual specimen
~ 9.5	1980–82	Individual specimen
~ 8	1982	Composite specimen
~ 4	1987	Composite specimen

Adapted by the Working Group from Stanley *et al.* (1990)

In an interim report, Patterson *et al.* (1986b) described high concentrations of 2,3,7,8-TCDD in adipose tissue from persons (mean age, 52.6 years) exposed recreationally, residentially and occupationally in a highly contaminated area in Missouri, compared with 57 controls. The geometric and arithmetic means were 6.4 and 7.4 ng/kg (wet weight-based), respectively, with a range of 1.4–20.2 ng/kg.

The Missouri study control group (Patterson *et al.*, 1986b) was expanded in 1989 by 128 persons with no known exposure (Andrews *et al.*, 1989): adipose 2,3,7,8-TCDD levels ranged from non-detectable to 20.2 ng/kg, with 95% of the levels at 16.6 ng/kg or below.

Patterson *et al.* (1994) analysed adipose samples originating from Atlanta, GA, in 1984–86. They found mean 2,3,7,8-TCDD concentrations for men and women of 7.4 ng/kg and 11.6 ng/kg, respectively. Further adipose tissue samples were analysed for all isomers.

Piacitelli *et al.* (1992) compared serum 2,3,7,8-TCDD levels in 280 chemical plant workers with the levels in 99 unexposed referents. The mean serum level for the control group was 7 ng/kg (lipid-based).

A comparison of PCDD/PCDF levels in whole blood, plasma and adipose tissue was performed by Schecter *et al.* (1990b) and Päpke *et al.* (1992). There were few differences in PCDD/PCDF levels between blood plasma and adipose and also between whole blood and adipose tissue when reported on lipid basis. The difference was most striking for OCDD between plasma and adipose tissue, with a ratio of 2 : 1. Total PCDDs/PCDFs appeared higher in plasma than in adipose tissue, if reported by actual measurement, because OCDD is usually the most abundant congener. Comparing whole blood with adipose tissue, the values were more similar. When TEQs were used, however, the values were almost identical in the two series. Wendling *et al.* (1990a) found 2,3,7,8-TCDD levels in samples of faeces from laboratory workers of between 0.61 and 0.74 ng/kg, dry weight-based. The fat content of the faeces was not measured. With some assumptions, a faecal fat 2,3,7,8-TCDD concentration of 3.7 ng/kg was estimated.

PCDDs and PCDFs in adipose tissue of United States Viet Nam veterans and controls were determined by Kang *et al.* (1991). The samples were collected in 1978. The geometric mean (± SD) 2,3,7,8-TCDD levels in adipose tissue for Viet Nam veterans, non-Viet Nam veterans and civilian controls were 11.7 (± 1.7), 10.9 (± 1.7) and 12.4 (± 1.9) ng/kg on a lipid weight basis, respectively. The mean levels for these groups were not significantly different from each other.

The effect of fasting on blood PCDD/PCDF levels was tested in 13 Viet Nam veterans (Hansson *et al.*, 1989). Although 2,3,7,8-TCDD levels increased slightly, for no congener including 2,3,7,8-TCDD was the change statistically significant.

In connection with analysis of blood samples from various geographical locations for PCDDs/PCDFs, Schecter *et al.* (1992) reported a total I-TEQ of 41 ng/kg (lipid-based) in a pooled blood sample ($n = 100$) from the United States. [The Working Group noted that the dates of collection of these samples were not given.]

In a study by Schecter *et al.* (1994b; 1996b), levels of PCDDs/PCDFs in placenta, blood and fetal tissue were measured. The highest semen levels, reported on wet weight, were found for OCDD, OCDF and HpCDF. The highest I-TEQ values (lipid-based) were found in blood, followed by placenta. The fetal tissue contained approximately one third of the I-TEQ of the adult values.

In a further study of partitioning of PCDDs/PCDFs in human maternal tissues, including blood, milk, adipose tissue and placenta, Schecter *et al.* (1996c) collected samples from five American women (mean age, 21.6 years; range, 21–34 years) residing in upstate New York and undergoing caesarean section deliveries between September

1995 and January 1996. Blood, placenta and fat were collected at the time of delivery. The milk and second blood were collected about four to eight weeks later. The lowest concentrations were found in the cord blood, at about one half of the maternal adipose and blood levels. A reduction in PCDD/PCDF levels was observed in the 'second' blood samples after a breast-feeding period of between four and eight weeks.

PCDD/PCDF levels in two pools of whole blood and serum ($n = 100$) collected in 1996 were compared with older blood data; a decrease was not clearly shown. The mean age of the blood donors was not specified (Schecter *et al.*, 1996d).

(s) Viet Nam

2,3,7,8-TCDD was not detected in seven adipose tissue samples from north Viet Nam (no exposure to Agent Orange) but was found in 10/13 samples from south Viet Nam (mean level, 34 (range, 9–103) ng/kg). Most of the other chlorinated PCDDs and PCDFs were found in samples from south Viet Nam (Schecter *et al.*, 1986b). A further 27 individual and 10 pooled human adipose tissue specimens, collected from persons in south and north Viet Nam, respectively, were analysed for 2,3,7,8-TCDD and 2,3,7,8-TCDF (Schecter *et al.*, 1989c). The mean values were 19 ng/kg 2,3,7,8-TCDD and 7 ng/kg 2,3,7,8-TCDF in the samples from persons in the south; no 2,3,7,8-TCDD or 2,3,7,8-TCDF was detected in samples from persons in the north. Differences in 2,3,7,8-TCDD body burden continued to be substantial between the populations of south and north Viet Nam.

In 1984–85, adipose tissues were taken from nine patients at a hospital in south Viet Nam (Nguyen *et al.*, 1989) and analysed for PCDDs/PCDFs. Eight patients had detectable levels of 2,3,7,8-TCDD ranging from 4 to 103 ng/kg, with a mean of 23 ng/kg.

Effects of geographical conditions and other variables on the distribution of 2,3,7,8-TCDD levels in adipose tissues from Viet Nam have been studied (Hoang *et al.*, 1989). No 2,3,7,8-TCDD was detected in 10/11 samples from the north (the positive sample contained 5 ng/kg). In the south, 2,3,7,8-TCDD was not detected in 4/44 samples and the mean level was 20.5 ng/kg in the four positive samples.

PCDD/PCDF levels in 27 adipose tissue samples from south Viet Nam were reported by Huteau *et al.* (1990b). Besides the usual 2,3,7,8-substituted isomers, they found non-2,3,7,8-substituted isomers in many samples. [Sample contamination cannot be excluded.]

In connection with analysis of blood samples from various geographical locations for PCDDs/PCDFs, Schecter *et al.* (1992) reported results for pooled samples from north Viet Nam (two analyses with a total of 82 persons) and south Viet Nam (nine analyses totalling 383 persons). The 2,3,7,8-TCDD level and I-TEQ value for samples from north and south Viet Nam were 2.2 and 14.6 ng/kg and 15 and 36 ng I-TEQ/kg, respectively.

PCDD levels in persons living at various localities in Viet Nam were summarized (Le *et al.*, 1995) using data from pooled blood samples. Each sample was obtained from 30–100 adults over 40 years old, who had been living for more than five years in a given area. As from 1992, some samples were taken from younger age groups between 18–40 years. The results of 43 analyses (containing blood of 2722 individuals) indicated that most of the samples from the south had higher levels of 2,3,7,8-TCDD as well as I-TEQ than the ones from the north.

In a study of the persistence of elevated PCDD levels in human tissues from Viet Nam, Schecter *et al.* (1995) performed 160 analyses on tissues from 3243 persons. 2,3,7,8-TCDD levels of up to 103 ng/kg were found in adipose tissue collected in the 1980s. Pooled blood collected from south Viet Nam in 1991–92 also showed 2,3,7,8-TCDD levels up to 33 ng/kg, whereas tissues from north Viet Nam had 2,3,7,8-TCDD levels at or below 2.9 ng/kg.

1.4.2   *Human milk*

There have been a large number of studies of PCDD concentrations in human milk. Many of the results are shown in **Table 30** and summarized in **Table 31**.

Only 2,3,7,8-substituted congeners have been found in human milk. The concentrations of the individual congeners present have been shown to be significantly correlated (Van den Berg *et al.*, 1986a; Beck *et al.*, 1987). Several studies have involved analysis of quite large numbers of individual samples without pooling, and these results show inter-individual variation of about a factor of 5 to 10 for most congeners (Beck *et al.*, 1989c; Frommberger, 1990; Dewailly *et al.*, 1991; Fürst *et al.*, 1992b; Hashimoto *et al.*, 1995b; Liem *et al.*, 1995).

Fürst *et al.* (1989, 1992b) and Beck *et al.* (1992) have both shown, by statistical analysis of their results, that the concentrations of PCDDs in human milk decrease as the period of breast-feeding increases, and decrease significantly for successive breast-fed children. Fürst *et al.* (1992b) found the summed I-TEQ concentration of PCDDs and PCDFs for the third breast-feeding period to be about 75% of that for the first, while Beck *et al.* (1992) reported a corresponding reduction to 57%. In Japan, Hirakawa *et al.* (1995) found that a small group of multipara donors had an average summed I-TEQ level about 10% lower than that for primipara donors.

Beck *et al.* (1992) found that mean PCDD and PCDF levels in six mothers on a vegetarian diet were slightly lower than the mean of a larger control group. Pluim *et al.* (1993b) concluded that there was a direct relationship between the amount of animal fat consumed and the PCDD/PCDF concentrations in breast milk. Short-term dietary measures to reduce PCDD/PCDF intake have been found, however, to have no effect on human milk concentrations (Pluim *et al.*, 1994a).

Many of the data included in **Table 30** were obtained in studies coordinated by the World Health Organization European Centre for Environment and Health and involved the following selection criteria (Yrjänheikki, 1989; WHO, 1996):

– donors should be primiparae;
– both mother and child should be apparently healthy, and the pregnancy should have been normal;
– the mother should be breast-feeding one child only (i.e., no twins);
– mothers who had resided outside the area for more than six months during the last five years should be excluded;
– only mothers who were exclusively breast-feeding should be included.

Table 30. Concentrations of PCDDs in human milk

Reference	Origin	No.	Coll. period	Concentration (ng/kg fat)							I-TEQ[a] PCDD/PCDF
				TCDD	PeCDD	HxCDD			HpCDD	OCDD	
				2378	12378	123478	123678	123789	1234678		
WHO (1996)	Albania, Librazhd; pool; unpolluted area (WHO criteria)	10	1992–93	0.4	1	0.6	4.1	1.1	6.3	21.6	3.8
WHO (1996)	Albania, Tirana; pool; polluted area (WHO criteria)	10	1993–93	0.6	1.3	0.6	4.8	1.1	7	23.6	4.8
WHO (1996)	Austria, Brixlegg; pool; industrial area (WHO criteria)	13	1992–93	2.2	4.5	2.5	12.3	2.3	14.1	82.3	14
Yrjänheikki (1989)	Austria, Tulln; pool (WHO criteria)	51	1986–88	2.7	5.2		17.2	6.1	72.9	141	[18.7]
WHO (1996)	Austria, Tulln; pool; rural area (WHO criteria)	21	1992–93	2	3.5	2.2	13.2	3	18.6	110	10.9
Yrjänheikki (1989)	Austria, Vienna; pool (WHO criteria)	54	1986–88	2.9	4.4		14	4	46.5	159	[17.2]
WHO (1996)	Austria, Vienna; pool; urban area (WHO criteria)	13	1992–93	1.3	3.4	2.1	14	2.7	27.4	150	10.7
Yrjänheikki (1989)	Belgium; pool; industrial area (WHO criteria)	–	1986–88	10.2	10.7	5.8	28	7.7	52	283	[40.2]
Yrjänheikki (1989)	Belgium; pool; rural area (WHO criteria)	–	1986–88	–	10.5	7.9	39	9.3	121	555	[33.7]
Yrjänheikki (1989)	Belgium; pool; urban area (WHO criteria)	–	1986–88	9.1	9.6	7	30	9.6	88	517	[38.7]
WHO (1996)	Belgium, Brabant Wallou; pool (WHO criteria)	8	1992–93	2.5	6.9	4.1	22.3	4.8	31.5	152	20.8
WHO (1996)	Belgium, Brussels; pool (WHO criteria)	6	1992–93	3.4	8	5.2	27.2	27.6	55.6	310	26.6
WHO (1996)	Belgium, Liege; pool (WHO criteria)	20	1992–93	3.1	9.1	5.6	31.2	5.5	30.3	191	27.1

Table 30 (contd)

Reference	Origin	No.	Coll. period	Concentration (ng/kg fat)								
				TCDD	PeCDD	HxCDD			HpCDD	OCDD	I-TEQ PCDD/PCDF
				2378	12378	123478	123678	123789	1234678		
Schecter et al. (1991b)	Cambodia, Phnom Penh	8	–	0.49	1.6	0.6	3.4	1.1	11	59	3.1
WHO (1996)	Canada (all provinces); pool	200	1981	3.4	8.9		84	18	94	361	28.6
WHO (1996)	Canada (all provinces); pool	100	1992	2.1	6.2		37	7.2	33	138	14.5
Yrjänheikki (1989)	Canada, British Columbia; pool	23	1986–88	3.4	10.2	6.3	63	3.1	82	160	[23.5]
Yrjänheikki (1989)	Canada, Maritimes; pool	19	1986–88	2.5	5.9	5.1	35	4.8	63	148	[15.7]
Yrjänheikki (1989)	Canada, Ontario N&E; pool	32	1986–88	2.2	6.5	5.2	46	6.6	68	143	[17]
Yrjänheikki (1989)	Canada, Ontario SW; pool	44	1986–88	2.2	7.4	6.9	42	5.7	69	137	[17.9]
Yrjänheikki (1989)	Canada, Prairies; pool	31	1986–88	2.7	8.1	7.6	54	8.7	75	143	19.4
Yrjänheikki (1989)	Canada, Québec; pool	34	1986–88	2.8	8.1	5.6	41	6.8	73	152	[18.2]
Dewailly et al. (1991)	Canada, Québec; pool; rural regions	16	1988–89	2.3	4.8		35	6.4	41	132	[13.4]
Yrjänheikki (1989)	Croatia, Krk; pool (WHO criteria)	14	1986–88	1.6	3		15.1	4.2	19.8	101	[12]
Yrjänheikki (1989)	Croatia, Zagreb; pool (WHO criteria)	41	1986–88	1.9	2.4		20.6	4.7	14.6	90	[11.7]
WHO (1996)	Croatia, Krk; pool (WHO criteria)	10	1992–93	1.2	2.4	1.9	8	2.3	17	84.3	8.4

Table 30 (contd)

Reference	Origin	No.	Coll. period	Concentration (ng/kg fat)							I-TEQ PCDD/PCDF
				TCDD 2378	PeCDD 12378	HxCDD 123478	123678	123789	HpCDD 1234678	OCDD	
WHO (1996)	Croatia, Zagreb; pool (WHO criteria)	13	1992–93	2	3.6	3.3	10.1	2.6	21.5	99.4	13.5
WHO (1996)	Czech R, Kladno; pool (WHO criteria)	11	1992–93	0.9	1.9	1.1	5.2	1.6	8.9	39.8	12.1
WHO (1996)	Czech R, Uherske Hradiste; pool (WHO criteria)	11	1992–93	1.3	3	1.5 .	7.3	2.1	11.3	40.3	18.4
Yrjänheikki (1989)	Denmark; pool (WHO criteria)	10	1986–88	2.3	5.5	–	34	4.9	51	157	[17.5]
Yrjänheikki (1989)	Denmark; pool (WHO criteria)	42	1986–88	2.1	6.2	–	40	4.7	47	210	[17.7]
WHO (1996)	Denmark; 7 cities; pool (WHO criteria)	48	1992–93	1.7	5.6	7.7	25.9	5.1	26	141	15.2
Mussalo-Rauhamaa & Lindström (1995)	Estonia, Tallinn (primipara)	6	1991	3.3	3	1.6	6.6	3.5	10	111	13.5
Mussalo-Rauhamaa & Lindström (1995)	Estonia, Tarto (primipara)	6	1991	4.1	5.6	2.2	7.9	4.3	13.5	147	21.4
Abraham et al. (1995b)	Faeroe Islands	1	1994~	0.9	3.7	4.5	13	1.9	9.8	45	9
Abraham et al. (1995b)	Faeroe Islands	1	1994~	1	4	4	17	2.1	19	114	10
Abraham et al. (1995b)	Faeroe Islands	1	1994~	<1	5.2	3.5	16	2	9.3	75	[10.2]
Abraham et al. (1995b)	Faeroe Islands	1	1994~	<3	5	3.2	12	<3	22	63	[11.7]

Table 30 (contd)

Reference	Origin	No.	Coll. period	Concentration (ng/kg fat)							I-TEQ PCDD/PCDF
				TCDD 2378	PeCDD 12378	HxCDD 123478	123678	123789	HpCDD 1234678	OCDD	
Abraham et al. (1995b)	Faeroe Islands; pool	9	1994~	0.8	2.9	3.3	11	1.4	9.2	64	6.7
Yrjänheikki (1989)	Finland, Helsinki; pool (WHO criteria)	38	1986–88	2	5.6	< 0.5	36	7	49	154	18
WHO (1996)	Finland, Helsinki; pool (WHO criteria)	10	1992–93	2.3	6.9	2.6	34.7	5.9	50.1	238	21.5
Yrjänheikki (1989)	Finland, Kuopio; pool (WHO criteria)	31	1986–88	1.8	5.6	< 0.5	22	5.8	28	113	[15.7]
WHO (1996)	Finland, Kuopio; pool (WHO criteria)	24	1992–93	1.2	3.9	1.4	24.5	3.7	29.2	131	12
González et al. (1996)	France, Paris	15	1990	2.4	6.6		25.9		56	290	20.1
Beck et al. (1992a)	Germany (primipara)	34	–	4.3	13	10	48	9.7	56	292	33
Beck et al. (1992a)	Germany (multipara)	23	–	3.1	10	9.6	39	7.9	44	252	25.6
Beck et al. (1992a)	Germany (multipara)	6	–	2.3	7.8	6.6	28	5.8	32	187	18.9
Frommberger (1990)	Germany, Baden-Württemberg	490	1988–89	4.2	10	9.2	32	6.6	61	503	[36.2]
Beck et al. (1987)	Germany, Berlin	30	–	3.4	15	12	59	11	61	530	[32.6]
Beck et al. (1989c)	Germany, Berlin	35	–	3.5	15	12	57	11	60	500	[33]
Yrjänheikki (1989)	Germany, Berlin; pool (WHO criteria)	40	1986–88	3.3	14	12	57	10	44	210	[32.1]

Table 30 (contd)

Reference	Origin	No.	Coll. period	Concentration (ng/kg fat)							
				TCDD	PeCDD	HxCDD			HpCDD	OCDD	I-TEQ PCDD/PCDF
				2378	12378	123478	123678	123789	1234678		
WHO (1996)	Germany, Berlin; pool (WHO criteria)	10	1992–93	2.2	7.1	6.3	21.6	5.1	23.4	164	16.5
Beck et al. (1989c)	Germany, Flensburg (Baltic coast)	6	–	4.1	12	7.3	46	8.3	41	200	[31.6]
Fürst et al. (1989)	Germany, North Rhine Westphalia	189	1985–88	2.9	9.9	7.6	31.2	6.6	44.7	195	[27.5]
Fürst et al. (1992b)	Germany, North Rhine Westphalia	526	1986–91	3.2	10.1	8.4	35.8	6.4	41.2	208	29.3
Yrjänheikki (1989)	Germany, North Rhine Westphalia; pool; primipara (WHO criteria)	79	1986–88	2.7	11.8	8.6	35.2	7.5	50.6	224	[31.8]
Yrjänheikki (1989)	Germany, Oldenburg; pool (WHO criteria)	35	1986–88	3.3	7.2	9.6	40	8.8	49.8	255	[35.4]
Beck et al. (1989c)	Germany, Recklinghausen (industrial area)	10	–	3.9	12	13	46	8.3	45	260	[30.6]
Yrjänheikki (1989)	Germany, Recklinghausen; pool (WHO criteria)	23	1986–88	3.8	14	9.7	45	7.6	42	170	32.8
Beck et al. (1989c)	Germany, Rheinfelden; pool; rural area/PCP manufacture	9	–	4.5	16	13	54	12	79	441	[36.9]
Beck et al. (1989c); Yrjänheikki (1989)	Germany, Weiden; rural area	14	1986–88	3.7	12	9.3	44	9.6	60	264	30.1
Wuthe et al. (1993)	Germany, one woman	1	1992	2.1	5.9		39.3		39.5	199	–

Table 30 (contd)

Reference	Origin	No.	Coll. period	Concentration (ng/kg fat)							I-TEQ PCDD/PCDF
				TCDD 2378	PeCDD 12378	HxCDD 123478	123678	123789	HpCDD 1234678	OCDD	
Yrjänheikki (1989)	Hungary, Budapest; (WHO criteria)	100	1986–88	3.4	1	3.2	8.2	1	60	210	[9.36]
WHO (1996)	Hungary, Budapest; pool (WHO criteria)	20	1992–93	1.7	2.8	4.3	8.3	2.1	25.6	129	8.5
Yrjänheikki (1989)	Hungary, Szentes; pool (WHO criteria)	50	1986–88	3.7	1.4	5.2	12.8	1.6	63	271	[11.7]
WHO (1996)	Hungary, Szentes; pool (WHO criteria)	10	1992–93	1.3	2.6	3.1	7.8	2	31.1	149	7.8
Yrjänheikki (1989)	Japan, Fukuoka; pool	6	1986	[2.1]	[4.6]	[4]	[30]	[5.6]	[62]	[975]	[24.3]
Hirakawa et al. (1995)	Japan, Fukuoka; multipara	8	1994	1.2	5	2.6	18.9	3.6	31.3	195	[11.8]
Hirakawa et al. (1995)	Japan, Fukuoka; primipara	7	1994	2	8.9	4.7	32.3	6.9	29.8	174	[18.6]
Hashimoto et al. (1995b)	Japan, various locations	26	1993–94	2.7	12	3.5	57	10	21	160	[37]
Alawi et al. (1996b)	Jordan, Amman; pool	4 to 6	1994	<3.2	<3.2	<3.2	<3.2	<3.2	3.2	64.6	[9.38]
Alawi et al. (1996b)	Jordan, Amman; pool	4 to 6	1994	<6.3	<6.3	<6.3	<6.3	<6.3	15.7	56.1	[18.3]
Alawi et al. (1996b)	Jordan, Aqaba; pool	4 to 6	1994	7.8	<4.5	<4.5	19	<4.5	14.5	46.9	[22]
Alawi et al. (1996b)	Jordan, Irbid; pool	4 to 6	1994	3.7	21.3	<3.7	56.5	<3.7	47.2	75.8	[98.5]

Table 30 (contd)

Reference	Origin	No.	Coll. period	Concentration (ng/kg fat)							
				TCDD 2378	PeCDD 12378	HxCDD 123478	123678	123789	HpCDD 1234678	OCDD	I-TEQ PCDD/PCDF
Alawi et al. (1996b)	Jordan, Madaba; pool	4 to 6	1994	<11	55	11	11	11	96	147	[110]
Alawi et al. (1996b)	Jordan, Zarka; pool	4 to 6	1994	<2.6	6.1	<2.6	9.6	<2.6	14	29	[11.4]
Petreas et al. (1996)	Kazakstan (WHO criteria)	40	<1996	13.6	4.45	1.15	4.01	1.14	10	112	20.1
WHO (1996)	Lithuania, Anykshchiai; pool; rural area (WHO criteria)	12	1992–93	5.5	3.6	3.6	3.8	1.2	5.7	32.7	14.4
WHO (1996)	Lithuania, Palanga; pool; coastal area (WHO criteria)	12	1992–93	4.8	3.4	1.9	4.5	1.4	5.1	21.3	16.6
WHO (1996)	Lithuania, Vilnius; pool; urban area (WHO criteria)	12	1992–93	5.4	2.8	1.8	4.7	1.5	7.2	39.5	13.3
Liem et al. (1995)	Netherlands (primipara)	103	1993	3.1	8.1	8.6	37.1	6.9	44.9	295	23.5
Yrjänheikki (1989)	Netherlands; pool; urban area (WHO criteria)	13	1986–88	5.2	18	10	75	11	112	627	39.6
Yrjänheikki (1989)	Netherlands; pool; rural area (WHO criteria)	13	1986–88	5.4	17	10	72	7.6	82	545	37.4
Pluim et al. (1992, 1993c, 1994)	Netherlands, Amsterdam			3.8	10.6	1.3	49.1	6.5	54.3	297.5	–
Koopman-Esseboom et al. (1994)	Netherlands, Rotterdam/Groningen			4.0	10.6	8.7	47.4	6.7	63.2	799.6	–
WHO (1996)	Netherlands; pool (WHO criteria)	17	1992–93	2.9	7.6	7.9	35.6	6.8	46.1	324	22.4

Table 30 (contd)

Reference	Origin	No.	Coll. period	Concentration (ng/kg fat)							
				TCDD	PeCDD	HxCDD			HpCDD	OCDD	I-TEQ PCDD/PCDF
				2378	12378	123478	123678	123789	1234678		
Tuinstra et al. (1995)	Netherlands, Groningen/Rotterdam; collected at 10 and 42th day after delivery	168	–	–	–	–	–	–	–	–	30
Yrjänheikki (1989)	Norway, Hamar; pool; rural area (WHO criteria)	10	1985–86	2.5	4.7		18.8	4.9	40.3	150	[14.8]
WHO (1996)	Norway, Hamar; pool; rural area (WHO criteria)	10	1992–93	1.8	2.8	1.6	9.2	2.4	17.4	116.7	9.3
Clench-Aas et al. (1992)	Norway, Skien-Porsgrunn; Mg production (WHO criteria)	10	1985–86	2.7	5.0		20.3	3.2	36.6	156	[19.2]
WHO (1996)	Norway, Skien-Porsgrunn; pool; industrial area (WHO criteria)	10	1992–93	2.1	3.8	1.9	10.7	3.5	19.1	112	12.5
Clench-Aas et al. (1992)	Norway, Tromsø; pool; coastal area (WHO criteria)	11	1985–86	2.9	4.7		19.2	4.7	36	155	15.9
WHO (1996)	Norway, Tromsø; pool; coastal area (WHO criteria)	10	1992–93	2.4	3.1	1.4	9.3	2.4	15.7	86.9	10.1
Buckland et al. (1990a)	New Zealand, Auckland (WHO criteria)	11	<1990	4.6	6		26	5.1	53	200	15
Buckland et al. (1990a)	New Zealand, Christchurch (WHO criteria)	9	<1990	5.7	8.2		34	6.3	51	240	19
Buckland et al. (1990a)	New Zealand, N. Canterbury (WHO criteria)	8	<1990	5.6	8.4		38	7.2	53	220	19
Buckland et al. (1990a)	New Zealand, Northland (WHO criteria)	9	<1990	4.7	6.8		39	5.5	51	180	17
Schecter et al. (1990e)	Pakistan; pool	7	–	3.3	5.2		15.3	4.8	40.7	180	12.6

Table 30 (contd)

Reference	Origin	No.	Coll. period	Concentration (ng/kg fat)							I-TEQ PCDD/PCDF
				TCDD 2378	PeCDD 12378	HxCDD 123478	123678	123789	HpCDD 1234678	OCDD	
Yrjänheikki (1989)	Poland; pool (WHO criteria)	5	1986–88	3.6	6	3	11	6.5	30.9	250	[21.1]
WHO (1996)	Russian Federation, Arkhangelsk; pool	1	1993	4.7	4	3.8	5.6	1.3	7.9	35.9	15.2
Schecter et al. (1990f)	Russian Federation, Baikalsk; pool	5	1988–89	2	2.7	0.9	4	0.7	5	30	10.4
Schecter et al. (1990f)	Russian Federation, Irkutsk; pool	4	1988–89	1.9	3.6	1.6	6.1	2	6.9	48	17.3
Schecter et al. (1990f)	Russian Federation, Kachug	4	1988–89	2.5	2.2	1	4.4	1.1	6	33	9.29
WHO (1996)	Russian Federation, Karhopol; pool	1	1992–93	1.9	1.6	0.7	1.9	0.5	1.5	9	5.9
Polder et al. (1996)	Russian Federation, Kola Peninsula	30	1992–93	–	–	–	–	–	–	–	15.8
Schecter et al. (1990f)	Russian Federation, Moscow	1	1988–89	8.7	6.3	4	14	1.8	16	88	20.6
Schecter et al. (1990f)	Russian Federation, Novosibirsk; pool	10	1988–89	3.4	3.9	2.2	6.6	1.2	11	68	11.9
WHO (1996)	Slovakia, Michalovce; pool (WHO criteria)	10	1992–93	1.3	2.4	1.5	5.5	1.3	7.2	30.2	15.1
WHO (1996)	Slovakia, Nitra; pool (WHO criteria)	10	1992–93	1.5	2.7	1.8	7.8	2	13.6	57.6	12.6
Schecter et al. (1990e)	South Africa; Black; pool	6	–	1.2	3.9		21.5	6.1	51.1	196	8.3

Table 30 (contd)

Reference	Origin	No.	Coll. period	Concentration (ng/kg fat)								
				TCDD	PeCDD	HxCDD			HpCDD	OCDD	I-TEQ PCDD/PCDF
				2378	12378	123478	123678	123789	1234678		
Schecter et al. (1990e)	South Africa; White; pool	18	–	1.7	5.8		26.5	6.9	60.7	254	12.6
WHO (1996)	Spain, Bizkaia; pool (WHO criteria)	19	1992–93	2	6	3.1	33.4	5.8	32.6	158	19.4
WHO (1996)	Spain, Gipuzkoa; pool (WHO criteria)	10	1992–93	2.3	7.7	4.2	53.5	9.3	59.6	164	25.5
González et al. (1996)	Spain, Madrid	13	1990	1.2	6.7		53.6		46	234	[14.3]
Yrjanheikki (1989); Clench-Aas et al. (1992)	Sweden, Borlänge; pool; rural area (WHO criteria)	10	1985–86	2.8	6.5		26.5	6.1	41.8	184	[20.1]
Yrjanheikki (1989)	Sweden, Gothenburg; pool; urban area (WHO criteria)	10	1985–86	3.2	7.5		39	6.2	67.3	237	22.8
Yrjanheikki (1989)	Sweden, Sundsvall; pool; industrial area (WHO criteria)	10	1985–86	3.3	7.8		28.1	7.1	52.2	209	22.6
Yrjanheikki (1989)	Sweden, Uppsala; pool; MSWI (WHO criteria)	10	1985–86	2.9	7.2		38.9	8.2	72.1	255	22.4
Schecter et al. (1991b)	Thailand, Bangkok	10	–	0.3	1.1	0.5	1.1	0.7	10	68	3
Wearne et al. (1996)	UK, Cambridge (WHO criteria)	20	1993–94	3.7	9.9	11	32	7.5	47	190	24
Startin et al. (1989)	UK, Glasgow (WHO criteria)	50	1987~	4.6	12		57	6.5	65	271	[29]

Table 30 (contd)

Reference	Origin	No.	Coll. period	Concentration (ng/kg fat)							I-TEQ PCDD/PCDF
				TCDD 2378	PeCDD 12378	HxCDD 123478	123678	123789	HpCDD 1234678	OCDD	
Wearne et al. (1996)	UK, Glasgow (WHO criteria)	20	1993–94	3.1	8.6	9.6	27	6.4	40	170	21
Startin et al. (1989)	UK, Sutton Coldfield (WHO criteria)	50	1987~	6.5	14		67	10	76	303	37
Wearne et al. (1996)	UK, Birmingham (WHO criteria)	20	1993	3.5	9	9.2	27	6.5	31	130	21
WHO (1996)	Ukraine, Kiev; pool (WHO criteria)	5	1992–93	2.8	2.4	1.9	3.9	1.4	6.6	40.2	11.0
WHO (1996)	Ukraine, Kiev; pool (WHO criteria)	5	1992–93	4.8	2.7	1.6	3.5	1.1	3.6	24.4	13.3
Schecter et al. (1989d)	USA	42	1988	3.3	6.7	4.95	30.5	6.2	42	233	[16.6]
Schecter et al. (1990e)	USA, Tennessee; pool	9	–	2.5	6.8		38.2	9.6	59.6	234	14.6
Schecter et al. (1990e)	Viet Nam, Binh Long; pool	4	NR	2.8	6.9		17	4.4	37.9	146	14.5
Schecter et al. (1991b)	Viet Nam, Da Nang	11	1985–90	5.6	15	5.1	22	11	55	292	34
Schecter et al. (1991b)	Viet Nam, Dong Nai	11	1985–90	10	7.2	2.1	10	4	28	119	26
Schecter et al. (1991b)	Viet Nam, Hanoi	30	1985–90	2.1	2.9	1.8	5.2	1.8	11.5	78.3	9
Schecter et al. (1989d)	Viet Nam, Ho Chi Minh	38	1985–90	7.1	6	2.9	15	4.2	36	231	18.5

Table 30 (contd)

Reference	Origin	No.	Coll. period	Concentration (ng/kg fat)							I-TEQ PCDD/PCDF
				TCDD 2378	PeCDD 12378	HxCDD 123478	123678	123789	HpCDD 1234678	OCDD	
Schecter et al. (1989d)	Viet Nam, Song Be	12	1985–90	17	8.2	6.6	18	6	36	185	31.7
Schecter et al. (1990e)	Viet Nam, Tay Ninh; pool	4	NR	5.7	14.1		43.8	10.9	88	415	[28.6]
Schecter et al. (1990e)	Viet Nam, Vung Tau; pool	5	NR	6.2	10.5		15.1	6	52.9	181	21.9
Schecter et al. (1995)	South Viet Nam; analytical method N	1	1970	1832	–	–	–	–	–	–	
		1	1970	1465	–	–	–	–	–	–	
		1	1970	732	–	–	–	–	–	–	
		1	1970	366	–	–	–	–	–	–	
		1	1970	333	–	–	–	–	–	–	
		1	1973	266	–	–	–	–	–	–	
		1	1973	280	–	–	–	–	–	–	
		1	1973	133	–	–	–	–	–	–	
		2	1985–88	5	–	–	–	–	–	–	
		2	1985–88	11	–	–	–	–	–	–	
		30	1985–88	2.1	–	–	–	–	–	–	

–, not reported; ND: not detected and limit of detection not reported

a Summed TEQ concentrations calculated by the Working Group [ ] where possible assuming congeners that were not detected were present at the full value of the limit of detection or as given by the authors when they correspond to the value calculated by the Working Group.

Table 31. Summary of concentrations (ng/kg fat) of PCDDs in human milk (as reported in Table 30)

	TCDD	PeCDD	HxCDD			HpCDD	OCDD	Total TEQ (PCDDs/ PCDFs)
	2378	12378	123478	123678	123789	1234678		
Mean	3.4	7.2	5.0	26	5.4	39	180	20
Minimum	0.3	1	0.5	1.1	0	1.5	9	3.1
5th percentile	1.03	1.71	0.83	3.9	1.1	6.17	30.11	8.16
25th percentile	2	3.68	1.9	10.25	2.3	15.93	89.5	12.35
Median	2.85	6.15	4	22.15	5.5	38.95	155	17.9
75th percentile	3.73	8.9	7.6	37.78	7.1	53.5	233.25	24.9
95th percentile	7.70	15	11.35	57	11	82	501.35	37.15
Maximum	17	55	13	84	27.6	121	975	110

By involving only primiparous women, these criteria may lead to slight over-estimation of average concentrations in milk, but the results provide a good basis for comparing different regions and variations over time. Laboratories generating data have also participated in an extended series of quality assurance intercomparisons (Rappe *et al.*, 1989c; Yrjänheikki, 1989; Stephens *et al.*, 1992; Carlé *et al.*, 1995).

Most of the regional comparisons within countries have shown no significant differences between donor cohorts from rural and industrial areas. Koopman-Esseboom *et al.* (1994a) reported significantly higher levels of a number of PCDDs and PCDFs in women living in industrialized areas of the Netherlands, compared with women living in rural areas. Rather larger differences were found by Alawi *et al.* (1996b) for different samples from Jordan, but variable detection limits and a high incidence of non-detection make interpretation uncertain. Pioneering work by Baughman, R. showed elevated 2,3,7,8-TCDD levels as high as 1450 ng/kg in milk lipid (Schecter, 1994) collected from south Viet Nam in 1970, while Agent Orange spraying was still occurring or had only just ceased. More recent samples from Viet Nam, analysed by Schecter *et al.* (1989d,e, 1990e,g, 1991b, 1995), have not shown any exceptional concentrations.

There is evidence of differences between certain parts of the world, and of a decrease over time. Samples taken in the second half of the 1980s from the industrialized countries of western Europe contribute most of the upper-quartile data in **Table 31**. Relatively low average levels have been found in samples from Albania, Cambodia, Croatia, the Faeroe Islands, Hungary, Pakistan and Thailand.

There is now clear evidence of a decrease in PCDD/PCDF levels in human milk over time in almost every region for which suitable data exist (Alder *et al.*, 1994; Liem *et al.*, 1995; WHO, 1996). The WHO (1996) study also shows that the highest rates of decrease, nearly 14% per annum, have been in the areas with the highest initial concentrations (**Figure 1**). These data imply that a substantial reduction in intake of PCDDs and PCDFs has occurred in recent years.

Figure 1. Annual percentage decrease of PCDD/PCDF levels in human milk for 11 countries as a function of the dioxin levels in 1988

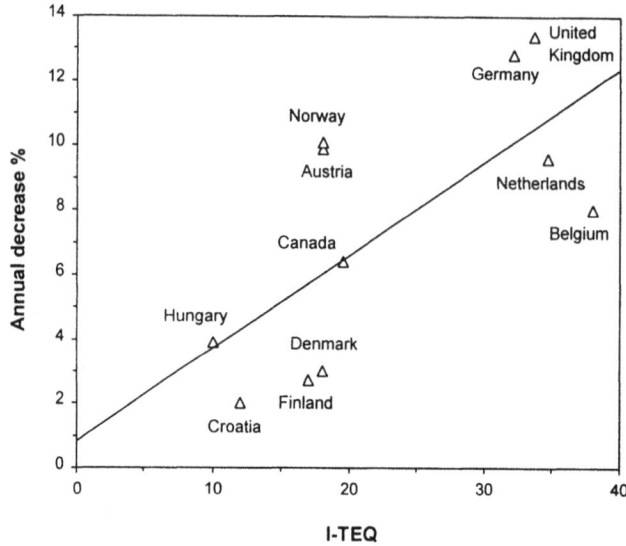

From WHO (1996)

1.5   Regulations and guidelines

In Germany, an occupational technical exposure limit (TRK) value of 50 pg I-TEQ/m^3 in air has been established for PCDDs and PCDFs. 2,3,7,8-TCDD is classified in Germany as a III A2 compound (shown to be clearly carcinogenic only in animal studies but under conditions indicative of carcinogenic potential at the workplace) (Deutsche Forschungsgemeinschaft, 1996).

The United States Occupational Safety and Health Administration (OSHA) has not set a permissible exposure level (PEL) for the PCDDs. The United States National Institute for Occupational Safety and Health (NIOSH) has not set a recommended exposure level (REL) for PCDDs, but states that 2,3,7,8-TCDD should be treated as a potential occupational carcinogen and occupational exposures should be limited to the lowest feasible concentration (United States National Institute for Occupational Safety and Health, 1994). The American Conference of Governmental Industrial Hygienists (1995) has not set a threshold limit value (TLV) for the PCDDs.

The United States Environmental Protection Agency (1996b) has established a final drinking water standard for 2,3,7,8-TCDD. The maximum contaminant level (MCL) (the maximum permissible level of a contaminant in water delivered to any user of a public water system) is set at 3×10^{-8} mg/L (30 pg/L).

The Canadian Government has proposed a tolerable daily intake (TDI) of 10 pg I-TEQ/kg bw per day for PCDDs and PCDFs (Government of Canada, 1993).

A Nordic tolerable weekly intake of 0–35 pg 2,3,7,8-TCDD/kg bw was proposed (Ahlborg et al., 1988). A TDI of 1 pg dioxin-like compounds/kg bw per day has been recommended in the Netherlands (Health Council for the Netherlands, 1996) and one of 5 pg/kg bw per day has been established in Sweden (Ahlborg *et al.*, 1988). A TDI of 10 pg PCDDs/PCDFs per kg bw per day from food has been recommended by WHO/EURO (WHO, 1991; Ahlborg *et al.*, 1992b) as well as by the Ministry of Health and Welfare of the Japanese Government (Kurokawa, 1997).

At present, the regulatory requirements for incinerator emissions vary widely among the countries of the European Union. The European Commission (1994) published a Council Directive on the incineration of hazardous waste which would require that 'the emission of PCDDs and PCDFs shall be minimized by the most progressive techniques' and which defines 0.1 ng/m^3 as a guide value which should not be exceeded by all average values measured over the sample period of 6 to 16 h.

Germany and the Netherlands have set daily average limit values of 0.1 ng I-TEQ/m^3 of exhaust gas for PCDDs/PCDFs from municipal waste incinerator emissions; in Sweden, the corresponding value is 0.1–0.5 ng Eadon TEQ/m^3. The United Kingdom has set a limit value of 1 ng I-TEQ/m^3 with a goal to reduce PCDD/PCDF emissions to 0.1 ng I-TEQ/m^3 for industrial and municipal waste incinerators (ECETOC, 1992; Liem & van Zorge, 1995).

In Japan, a limit of 0.5 ng I-TEQ/m^3 2,3,7,8-TCDD/TCDF is recommended for municipal waste incinerators (Liem & van Zorge, 1995).

In Germany, sewage sludge used as a fertilizer for farmland is not allowed to contain more than 100 ng I-TEQ/kg dry matter (Ordinance on Sewage Sludge, 1992; Liem & van Zorge, 1995).

The European Union has specified that 2,3,7,8-TCDD must not form part of the composition of cosmetic products (European Commission, 1992).

For milk and milk products, a maximal tolerable concentration for PCDDs/PCDFs of 17.5 ng I-TEQ/kg fat has been set in the United Kingdom. In Germany, PCDDs/PCDFs must not exceed 5 ng I-TEQ/kg milk fat and, in the Netherlands, their level must not exceed 6 ng I-TEQ/kg milk and milk product fat (Liem & van Zorge, 1995).

2. Studies of Cancer in Humans

2,3,7,8-TCDD is thought to be the most toxic PCDD congener, followed in presumed toxicity by the higher chlorinated PCDDs. Lower chlorinated PCDDs are thought to be much less toxic.

The focus of this review of human studies is on studies in which exposure to 2,3,7,8-TCDD or higher chlorinated PCDDs can be presumed or is documented. Typically this involves exposure to phenoxy herbicides contaminated by 2,3,7,8-TCDD (particularly 2,4,5-T) or to other contaminated chemicals used in manufacturing processes (e.g., TCP).

Studies involving only exposure to herbicides not contaminated by PCDDs (e.g., 4-chloro-2-methylphenoxyacetic acid (MCPA)) are not reviewed (e.g., Coggon *et al.*, 1986; Lynge, 1993). Studies involving only exposure to unspecified combinations of pesticides and herbicides are also not reviewed (e.g., Blair *et al.*, 1983) because the

extent of exposure to PCDD-containing herbicides (if any) is unknown. Studies involving only exposure to 2,4-D, that is not likely to have been contaminated by higher
chlorinated PCDDs, are also not discussed. Studies involving exposure to substances
contaminated with higher chlorinated PCDDs without 2,3,7,8-TCDD, e.g., PCP, are
discussed separately from studies involving exposure to 2,3,7,8-TCDD.

Blood concentrations reported are lipid-based, unless otherwise noted (see Section
1.4).

2.1   Industrial exposures and industrial accidents

The cohort study populations considered by various authors overlap in many
instances. However, different publications on overlapping study groups may have
different focuses, e.g., incidence/mortality, different follow-up periods, different exposure assessment and other characteristics. Therefore, **Table 32** presents the relationship
between different publications which are considered relevant for this monograph in terms
of study population size.

2.1.1   *Exposure to 2,3,7,8-TCDD and higher chlorinated PCDDs/PCDFs in chemical plants*

Cohort studies are summarized in **Table 33**.

Workers at chemical plants in the United States which produced chemicals contaminated with PCDDs/PCDFs (primarily TCP and/or 2,4,5-T) have been studied extensively. There has been a series of publications on two separate plants and a larger study
of 12 plants which included most United States workers manufacturing these products
who were exposed specifically to 2,3,7,8-TCDD. In the latter study, serum PCDD
measurements were available for some workers.

(a)   Two United States plants

Nitro plant

Workers at a Monsanto plant in Nitro, WV, have been studied by Zack and Suskind
(1980), Zack and Gaffey (1983) and Collins *et al.* (1993). Zack and Suskind (1980)
studied 121 male workers (one woman is not included in the mortality analysis) who
developed chloracne after an accident during production of TCP in 1949. These workers
were followed through 31 December 1978 with person–time at risk beginning at the
accident. United States referent rates were used. Thirty-two deaths were observed
(standardized mortality ratio (SMR), 0.7; $p < 0.05$), of which nine were cancer deaths
(SMR, 1.0). No significant excess was found for any specific cancer, although lung
cancer was elevated (5 observed; SMR, 1.8). One soft-tissue sarcoma was observed — a
fibrous histiocytoma (classified as a skin cancer (ICD-8, 172–173)), with 0.2 skin
cancers expected. Three deaths from lymphatic and haematopoietic cancers were
observed (SMR, 3.4).

Table 32. Relationship between industrial cohort study groups with exposure to 2,3,7,8-TCDD

Kogevinas *et al.* (1997)	> Fingerhut *et al.* (1991a,b) (USA, NIOSH, 12 plants)	> Bond *et al.* (1989a), Ott *et al.* (1987), Cook *et al.* (1986) (Dow, Midland, MI) > Zack & Gaffey (1983) (Monsanto, Nitro, WV) > Collins *et al.* (1993) (Monsanto, Nitro, WV)	> Ramlow *et al.* (1996) (Dow, Midland, MI)
	> Saracci *et al.* (1991)	> Bueno de Mesquita *et al.* (1993), Hooiveld *et al.* (1996a) (Netherlands) > Coggon *et al.* (1991) (United Kingdom)	
	> Becher *et al.* (1996) (Boehringer-Ingelheim, Bayer, BASF (not the accident))	> Flesch-Janys *et al.* (1995) (Boehringer-Ingelheim)	Manz *et al.* (1991) (Boehringer-Ingelheim)
Ott & Zober (1996), Zober *et al.* (1994), Zober *et al.* (1990) (accident, BASF)			

A > B denotes that the study population of B is a subset of A.
A, B denotes that the study populations A and B are almost identical.
All publications mentioned contain results considered to be relevant by the Working Group.
The study populations of Collins *et al.* (1993) and Zack & Gaffey (1983) overlap in part.
Specific female cohorts (Kogevinas *et al.*, 1993; Nagel *et al.*, 1994) are not included.

Zack and Gaffey (1983) studied 884 white male employees at the Nitro plant who were active on or after 1 January 1955 with one or more years of employment as hourly workers. This cohort included all workers at the plant, not just those exposed to PCDDs. Follow-up was through 31 December 1977 and United States referent rates were used. There were 163 deaths in this cohort (SMR, 1.0). Nine deaths from urinary bladder cancer were observed (SMR, 9.9). The excess of urinary bladder cancer was attributed to the use of 4-aminobiphenyl (see IARC, 1987f), a known urinary bladder carcinogen. Seven of these cancers had been detected earlier in a screening programme. Work history of decedents was examined to determine if the men had been assigned to 2,4,5-T production. For 58 men so identified, a proportionate mortality study was conducted. Nine cancers were observed (proportionate mortality ratio [PMR], 0.8). Six were lung cancers (PMR, 1.7). No haematopoietic cancer occurred in this group. One soft-tissue sarcoma (a liposarcoma) was observed; no expected number for soft-tissue sarcoma was given. [An unknown, but probably small, number of workers who worked with TCP but not with 2,4,5-T would have been omitted from this analysis].

Collins *et al.* (1993) studied 754 workers who had worked at the Nitro plant for one day or more between 8 March 1949 (the date of the above-mentioned accident) and

Table 33. Industrial cohort studies and populations exposed to industrial exposures and industrial accidents

Reference, country	Study subjects	Study type/ Period of follow-up	Exposure	Gender	Cancer site/cause of death	No. obs.	RR	95% CI	Comments
Fingerhut et al. (1991a), USA	5172 workers 12 plants	Mortality followed from first exposure to 31 December 1987	1987 serum levels of exposed (n = 253) averaged 233 ng/kg fat compared with 7 ng/kg for unexposed workers (n = 79)	Men	All cancers				Combined 2,3,7,8-TCDD-exposed production workers from 12 plants exposed during 1942–84, including Monsanto (Nitro, WV) and Dow (Midland, MI) workers
					≥ 20 years latency	265	1.2	1.0–1.3	
					≥ 1 year exposure	114	1.5	1.2–1.8	
					Digestive system				
					≥ 20 years latency	67	1.1	0.9–1.4	
					≥ 1 year exposure	28	1.4	0.9–2.0	
					Lung				
					≥ 20 years latency	89	1.1	0.9–1.4	
					≥ 1 year exposure	40	1.4	1.0–1.9	
					Haematopoietic (all)				
					≥ 20 years latency	24	1.1	0.7–1.6	
					≥ 1 year exposure	8	1.3	0.5–2.5	
					NHL				
					≥ 20 years latency	10	1.4	0.7–2.5	
					≥ 1 year exposure	2	0.9	0.1–3.4	
					Multiple myeloma				
					≥ 20 years latency	5	1.6	0.5–3.9	
					≥ 1 year exposure	3	2.6	0.5–7.7	
					Leukaemia				
					≥ 20 years latency	6	0.7	0.2–1.5	
					≥ 1 year exposure	2	0.8	0.1–2.8	
					Connective tissue/STS				
					≥ 20 years latency	4	3.4	0.9–8.7	
					≥ 1 year exposure	3	9.2	1.9–27.0	

Table 33 (contd)

Reference, country	Study subjects	Study type/ Period of follow-up	Exposure	Gender	Cancer site/cause of death	No. obs.	RR	95% CI	Comments
Ott & Zober (1996), (BASF) Germany	243 workers accidentally exposed to 2,3,7,8-TCDD in a TCP unit in a chemical plant	Mortality and incidence 1953–92	2,3,7,8-TCDD serum levels in 138 subjects in 1988–92. Model-based estimation for other workers	Men	All cancers				Mortality [p_{trend} = 0.07]; local reference
					< 0.1 µg/kg bw	8	0.8	0.4–1.6	
					0.1–0.99 µg/kg bw	8	1.2	0.5–2.3	
					1.0–1.99 µg/kg bw	8	1.4	0.6–2.7	
					≥ 2.0 µg/kg bw	7	2.0	0.8–4.0	
					All cancers	13	2.0	1.0–3.4	> 1 µg/kg bw, ≥ 20 years of latency
					Respiratory	6	3.1	1.1–6.7	
					All cancers	18	1.9	1.1–3.0	113 chloracne cases, latency > 20 years; mortality
					Digestive system	6	1.8	0.7–4.0	
					Respiratory tract	7	2.4	1.0–5.0	
					Respiratory tract	8	2.0	0.9–3.9	Incidence, > 1.0 µg/kg bw
					Digestive tract	11	1.5	1.1–1.9	Cox's regression; deaths
					Digestive tract	12	1.4	1.1–1.7	Cox's regression; incident cases; internal comparison controlling for known confounders
Manz et al. (1991), (Boehringer-Ingelheim) Germany	1184 men and 399 women employed in a herbicide plant; 496 high exposure; 901 medium exposure; 186 low exposure	Mortality 1952–89	TCP, 2,4,5-T and 2,3,7,8-TCDD; fat levels in 48 subjects in 1985 Median fat 2,3,7,8-TCDD, 137 ng/kg high exposure Median fat 2,3,7,8-TCDD medium + low, 60 ng/kg	Men	All cancers	29	1.8	1.2–2.6	Gas workers reference [p_{trend} = 0.24]
					High exposure	39	1.2	0.9–1.6	
					Medium exposure	7	1.5	0.6–3.0	
					Low exposure				
				Women	All cancers	NG	0.9	0.6–1.5	National reference
					Breast	9	2.2	1.0–4.1	

Table 33 (contd)

Reference, country	Study subjects	Study type/ Period of follow-up	Exposure	Gender	Cancer site/cause of death	No. obs.	RR	95% CI	Comments
Flesch-Janys et al. (1995); Flesch-Janys et al. (1996b) (Boehringer-Ingelheim) Germany	1189 workers employed in a herbicide plant contaminated with PCDDs/PCDFs	Mortality 1952–92	PCDD/PCDF-contaminated herbicides. 2,3,7,8-TCDD biological levels in 190 workers in 1992. Model-based estimation for other workers	Men	All cancers	NG	1.0	0.6–1.8	Blood TEQ 1.0–12.2 ng/kg
						NG	1.3	0.8–2.1	Blood TEQ 12.3–39.5 ng/kg
						NG	1.2	0.7–1.9	Blood TEQ 39.6–98.9 ng/kg
						NG	1.2	0.8–1.9	Blood TEQ 99.0–278.5 ng/kg
						NG	1.3	0.7–2.3	Blood TEQ 278.6–545 ng/kg
						NG	2.7	1.7–4.4	Blood TEQ 545.1–5362 ng/kg
						NG	2.0	1.1–3.8	$P_{trend} < 0.01$, Cox's regression 2,3,7,8-TCDD, 344.7–3890 ng/kg, internal comparison
						NG	2.3	1.1–4.6	Internal comparison; subjects exposed to dimethyl sulfate excluded
Becher et al. (1996); Kogevinas et al. (1997) Germany	2479 workers from four plants involved in production of phenoxy herbicides and chlorophenols	Mortality 1950s–89	Herbicides, PCDDs, PCDFs, 2,4,5-T, TCP, 2,3,7,8-TCDD, chlorophenols	Men	All cancers	138	1.2	1.0–1.4	National reference
					Buccal, pharynx	9	2.9	1.3–5.6	
					Lung	47	1.4	1.0–1.9	
					All haematopoietic	13	1.7	0.9–2.9	
					NHL	6	3.3	1.2–7.1	
			TCP, chlorophenols, 2,3,7,8-TCDD		All cancers	97	1.3	1.1–1.6	Plant I (Boehringer-Ingelheim). Blood 2,3,7,8-TCDD in 190 workers: 3–2252 ng/kg. Numerous cases of chloracne
					Lung	31	1.5	1.0–2.1	
					All haematopoietic	11	2.4	1.2–4.3	
					Multiple myeloma	4	3.8	1.0–9.6	
					NHL	3	5.4	1.1–15.9	Plant II (Bayer-Uerdingen). Blood 2,3,7,8-TCDD in 19 workers: 23–1935 ng/kg. Some cases of chloracne
			2,4,5-T, 2,3,7,8-TCDD		NHL	2	12.0	1.5–43.5	
Coggon et al. (1991), (Plant A) United Kingdom	1082 chemical workers producing or formulating phenoxy herbicides and chlorophenols in 1975–85. 2,4,5-T was produced during 1968–78	Mortality 1975–87	Phenoxy compounds including 2,4,5-T and chlorophenols	Men	All cancers	12	1.0	[0.7–1.4]	Workers in one (Factory A) out of four factories included in study
					Lung	6	1.3	[0.5–2.8]	
					NHL	0			

Table 33 (contd)

Reference, country	Study subjects	Study type/ Period of follow-up	Exposure	Gender	Cancer site/cause of death	No. obs.	RR	95% CI	Comments
Bueno de Mesquita *et al.* (1993), The Netherlands	Workers in synthesis and formulation of phenoxy herbicides and chlorophenols in two plants (963 exposed, 1111 unexposed); Factory A, accident in 1963; exposure to 2,3,7,8-TCDD	Mortality 1955–86	2,4,5-T, PCDDs, 2,3,7,8-TCDD	Men	All cancers	26	1.2	0.5–1.7	Factory A only, exposed workers versus national population
					Pancreas	3	2.9	0.6–8.4	
					Large intestine	3	2.4	0.5–7.0	
					Lung	9	1.0	0.5–1.9	
					Prostate	2	2.2	0.3–7.8	
					Lymphosarcoma	1	2.0	0.1–11.4	
					Myeloid leukaemia	1	2.9	0.1–15.9	
					All cancers	31	1.7	0.9–3.4	Both plants; exposed versus unexposed
					Respiratory tract	9	1.7	0.5–6.3	
			Accidental exposure in 1963		All cancers	10	1.4	0.7–2.5	Factory A; national reference
						Case/control	OR		
Kogevinas *et al.* (1995), international	11 STS cases and 55 healthy controls; 32 NHL cases and 158 healthy controls	Nested case–control study within the IARC cohort reported by Saracci *et al.* (1991)	Exposure to 21 chemicals including major phenoxy herbicides, PCDDs, raw materials and other process chemicals	Men and women	STS	10/30	10.3	1.2–90.6	Any phenoxy herbicide
						9/24	5.6	1.1–27.7	Any PCDD or PCDF
						5/13	5.2	0.9–31.9	2,3,7,8-TCDD
					NHL	19/85	1.3	0.5–2.9	Any phenoxy herbicide
						20/78	1.8	0.8–4.3	Any PCDD or PCDF
						11/39	1.9	0.7–5.1	2,3,7,8-TCDD

Table 33 (contd)

Reference, country	Study subjects	Study type/ Period of follow-up	Exposure	Gender	Cancer site/cause of death	No. obs.	RR	95% CI	Comments
Kogevinas et al. (1997), international	21 863 in 36 cohorts from 12 countries	Mortality	2,3,7,8-TCDD or higher chlorinated PCDDs versus not exposed to 2,3,7,8-TCDD or higher chlorinated PCDDs or no PCDD exposure	20851 men, 1012 women	All cancers				Combined PCDD-exposed workers (production and spraying) from 36 cohorts with varied follow-up from 1939 to 1992. Includes and updates IARC cohort (Saracci et al., 1991), adds NIOSH cohort (Fingerhut et al., 1991a,b) and adds four plants in Germany (Manz et al., 1991; Becher et al., 1996; Flesch-Janys et al., 1995). Largest combined cohort of PCDD-exposed workers.
					Exposed to 2,3,7,8-TCDD and higher	710	1.1	1.0–1.2	
					Exposed to lower or no PCDD	398	1.0	0.9–1.1	
					Digestive system				
					Exposed to 2,3,7,8-TCDD and higher	190	[1.0]	[0.9–1.2]	
					Exposed to lower or no PCDD	106	[0.9]	[0.7–1.1]	
					Lung				
					Exposed to 2,3,7,8-TCDD and higher	225	1.1	1.0–1.3	
					Exposed to lower or no PCDD	148	1.0	0.9–1.2	
					Haematopoietic (all)				
					Exposed to 2,3,7,8-TCDD and higher	57	1.1	[0.8–1.4]	
					Exposed to 2,3,7,8-lower or no PCDD	35	1.2	[0.8–1.6]	
					NHL				
					Exposed to 2,3,7,8-TCDD and higher	24	1.4	0.9–2.1	
					Exposed to lower or no PCDD	9	1.0	0.5–1.9	
					Multiple myeloma				
					Exposed to 2,3,7,8-TCDD and higher	9	1.2	0.6–2.3	
					Exposed to lower or no PCDD	8	1.6	0.7–3.1	

Table 33 (contd)

Reference, country	Study subjects	Study type/ Period of follow-up	Exposure	Gender	Cancer site/cause of death	No. obs.	RR	95% CI	Comments
Kogevinas et al. (1997), international (contd)					Leukaemia				
					Exposed to 2,3,7,8-TCDD and higher	16	0.7	0.4–1.2	
					Exposed to lower or no PCDD	17	1.4	0.8–2.3	
					Connective tissue/STS				
					Exposed to 2,3,7,8-TCDD and higher	6	2.0	0.8–4.4	
					Exposed to lower or no PCDD	2	1.4	0.2–4.9	
Bertazzi et al. (1993), Italy	Residents in contaminated zones after the Seveso accident: Zone A, 724; Zone B, 4824; Zone R, 31 647; age, 20–74 years	Incidence 1977–86	2,3,7,8-TCDD: Zone A; soil levels, 15.5–580 µg/m²; median blood levels in adults, 389 ng/kg (back-calculation)	Men	All cancers	7	0.7	0.3–1.5	Local reference. Median 2,3,7,8-TCDD level in the reference area (52 samples in 1992–93), 5.5 ng/kg blood (Landi et al., 1996)
					Digestive system	2	0.7	0.2–2.8	
					Lung	2	0.8	0.2–3.4	
				Women	All cancers	7	1.0	0.5–2.1	
					Digestive tract	3	1.7	0.6–5.4	
			Zone B; soil levels, <50 µg/m²; median blood levels in adults, 78 ng/kg (back-calculation)	Men	All cancers	76	1.1	0.9–1.4	Local reference
					Digestive system	18	0.9	0.6–1.5	
					Hepatobiliary	5	1.8	0.7–4.4	
					Liver	4	2.1	0.8–5.8	
					Lung	18	1.1	0.7–1.8	
					Haematopoietic	8	2.1	1.0–4.3	
					NHL	3	2.3	0.7–7.4	
					Lymphoreticulosarcoma	3	5.7	1.7–19.0	
					Multiple myeloma	2	3.2	0.8–13.3	
					Leukaemia	2	1.6	0.4–6.5	

Table 33 (contd)

Reference, country	Study subjects	Study type/ Period of follow-up	Exposure	Gender	Cancer site/cause of death	No. obs.	RR	95% CI	Comments
Bertazzi et al. (1993), Italy (contd)				Women	All cancers	36	0.8	0.6–1.1	Local reference
					Digestive system	12	1.1	0.6–1.9	
					Hepatobiliary	5	3.3	1.3–8.1	
					Gall-bladder	4	4.9	1.8–13.6	
					Breast	10	0.7	0.4–1.4	
					Haematopoietic	6	1.9	0.8–4.4	
					Multiple myeloma	2	5.3	1.2–22.6	
					Myeloid leukaemia	2	3.7	0.9–15.7	
			Zone R; soil levels, < 5 µg/m²	Men	All cancers	447	0.9	0.9–1.0	Local reference
					Digestive system	131	0.9	0.8–1.1	
					Lung	96	0.8	0.7–1.0	
					STS	6	2.8	1.0–7.3	
					Haematopoietic	25	1.0	0.6–1.5	
					NHL	12	1.3	0.7–2.5	
					Myeloid leukaemia	5	1.4	0.5–3.8	
				Women	All cancers	318	0.9	0.8–1.1	Local reference
					Digestive tract	75	0.9	0.7–1.1	
					Lung	16	1.5	0.8–2.5	
					STS	2	1.6	0.3–7.4	
					Breast	106	1.1	0.9–1.3	
					Haematopoietic	18	0.8	0.5–1.3	
					NHL	10	1.2	0.6–2.3	
					Lymphoreticulosarcoma	6	1.7	0.7–4.2	
Bertazzi et al. (1996), Italy	Residents in contaminated zones after the Seveso accident: Zone A, 750; Zone B, 5000; Zone R, 30 000; all ages	Mortality 1976–91	Zone A	Men	All cancers	6	0.4	0.2–1.0	Local reference. Median level in the reference area (52 samples in 1992–93), 5.5 ng/kg (Landi et al., 1996)
					Lung	4	1.0	0.4–2.6	
				Women	All cancers	10	1.2	0.6–2.2	
					Digestive system	5	1.5	0.6–3.6	
					Colon	2	2.6	0.6–10.5	

Table 33 (contd)

Reference, country	Study subjects	Study type/ Period of follow-up	Exposure	Gender	Cancer site/cause of death	No. obs.	RR	95% CI	Comments
Bertazzi et al. (1996), Italy (contd)			Zone B	Men	All cancers	104	1.1	0.9–1.3	Local reference
					Digestive system	33	0.9	0.7–1.3	
					Rectum	7	2.9	1.4–6.2	
					Lung	34	1.2	0.9–1.7	
					Haematopoietic	12	2.3	1.3–4.2	
					NHL	2	1.5	0.4–6.0	
					Hodgkin's disease	2	3.3	0.8–14.0	
					Leukaemia	7	3.1	1.4–6.7	
				Women	All cancers	48	0.9	0.7–1.2	
					Digestive system	18	0.8	0.5–1.3	
					Stomach	7	1.0	0.5–2.2	
					Hepatobiliary	4	1.1	0.4–3.1	
					Liver	3	1.3	0.4–4.0	
					Breast	9	0.8	0.4–1.5	
					Haematopoietic	7	1.8	0.8–3.8	
					Hodgkin's disease	2	6.5	1.5–30.0	
					Myeloma	4	6.6	2.3–18.5	
				Men and women	Thyroid	2	[3.9]	[0.4–14.1]	
			Zone R	Men	All cancers	607	0.9	0.8–1.0	Local reference
					Digestive system	226	0.9	0.8–1.0	
					Oesophagus	30	1.6	1.1–2.4	
					Lung	176	0.9	0.8–1.1	
					STS	4	2.1	0.7–6.5	
					Haematopoietic	27	0.8	0.5–1.2	
				Women	All cancers	401	0.9	0.8–1.0	Local reference
					Digestive system	158	0.9	0.8–1.0	
					Lung	29	1.0	0.7–1.6	
					Breast	67	0.8	0.6–1.0	
					Haematopoietic	29	0.9	0.6–1.4	

Abbreviations: NHL, non-Hodgkin lymphoma; STS, soft-tissue sarcoma; NG, not given

22 November 1949 (the date of the last reported case of chloracne resulting from the accident clean-up) (this study includes the 122 chloracne cases of Zack & Suskind, 1980). Person–time at risk began on 8 March 1949 or at date of hire, if hired between 8 March and 22 November 1949, and extended through 31 December 1987 (23 198 person–years). Follow-up was complete for 733 workers. United States referent rates were used. The cohort was further subdivided into four groups: (1) 461 workers without chloracne and judged not to have been exposed to 4-aminobiphenyl; (2) 171 workers without chloracne but with exposure to 4-aminobiphenyl; (3) 97 workers with chloracne and no exposure to 4-aminobiphenyl; and (4) 25 workers with chloracne and exposure to 4-aminobiphenyl. Three deaths from soft-tissue sarcoma occurred in the cohort: one in the group without chloracne but with exposure to 4-aminobiphenyl (upon review, this case was not a soft tissue sarcoma) and two in the group with chloracne and with exposure to 4-aminobiphenyl. Excesses of urinary bladder cancer occurred in all groups, but primarily in the group without chloracne but with exposure to 4-aminobiphenyl (10 observed; SMR, 22; 95% CI, 10.4–40.0). The authors considered that the deaths due to soft-tissue sarcoma may have been caused by 4-aminobiphenyl. [The Working Group considered that this argument is weakened by two points. First, the one case of soft-tissue sarcoma occurring in the group without chloracne but with exposure to 4-aminobiphenyl apparently may have been exposed to 2,3,7,8-TCDD, as suggested by additional data presented in the study. Second, there are no human data indicating that 4-aminobiphenyl or other aromatic amines cause soft-tissue sarcoma and hence no strong reason to believe it could act as a confounder for soft-tissue sarcoma occurrence due to PCDDs.] (All but one of the confirmed cases of soft-tissue sarcomas of the Fingerhut *et al.* (1991a) study are included in Collins *et al.* (1993)).

Midland plant

Workers at a Dow plant in Midland, MI, have been studied in a series of publications. Ott *et al.* (1980) studied 204 male workers exposed to 2,4,5-T from 1950 to 1971 (the period during which it was manufactured) (157 with less than one year's exposure). The method of worker selection may have missed some short-term workers, but all workers with at least one year of employment in the 2,4,5-T work area would have been included. Some workers with exposure to TCP (but no exposure to 2,4,5-T) may have been excluded from this analysis. No case of chloracne was identified in this group. Follow-up extended through 1976. United States referent rates were used. Only 11 deaths occurred in this cohort (20 expected) and only one cancer death (a respiratory cancer in a smoker) (3.6 expected).

Cook *et al.* (1980) studied 61 men at the same plant in Midland, MI, who worked in TCP production in 1964 (there was an incident in June 1964 in the plant and these employees have been exposed to 2,3,7,8-TCDD); 49 developed chloracne at that time. Follow-up extended through 1978 and 40 men were still working at the end of 1978. United States referent rates were used. Only four deaths were observed versus 7.8 expected; three were due to cancer versus 1.6 expected (one soft-tissue sarcoma (fibro-sarcoma) occurred).

A cohort of 2189 (later 2192) workers at the Midland, MI, plant exposed to higher chlorinated phenols (three or more chlorines) and related products (including 2,4,5-T) was studied by Cook *et al.* (1986), Ott *et al.* (1987) and Bond *et al.* (1989a). (Bond *et al.* (1989a) also included a sub-cohort analysis of the mortality of 323 men diagnosed with chloracne.) The cohort was defined on the basis of work in departments manufacturing TCP, PCP, 2,4,5-T and 2,4,5-T esters. Among these, only PCP did not contain 2,3,7,8-TCDD (Fingerhut *et al.*, 1991b), although it did contain hexa-, hepta- and octa-CDDs. Production of these chemicals began at various dates from 1937 to 1955, and ended between 1971 and 1982. Workers were ranked on a scale of 0 to 4 for intensity of exposure to 2,3,7,8-TCDD and from 0 to 2 for intensity of exposure to hexa-, hepta- and octa-CDDs, with each unit representing an increase on a logarithmic scale. Exposure data were available from wipe samples, process streams and intermediate products. 2,3,7,8-TCDD was present at 1818 mg/kg (mean of 28 samples) in TCP waste streams in the 1960s and 1970s and at much lower levels in other process streams and in the intermediate product (range, 0.1–116 mg/kg) (Ott *et al.*, 1987). Almost all of these workers were included in the United States NIOSH 12-plant cohort studied by Fingerhut *et al.* (1991a,b), which was restricted to workers with some exposure to 2,3,7,8-TCDD; the only workers in the Midland, MI, cohort of 2192 who were excluded from Fingerhut *et al.* (1991a,b) were approximately 100 workers with exposure to PCP only.

Cook *et al.* (1986) followed the cohort of 2189 men from 1940 through 1979 and found an SMR for all causes of death of 0.9 and for all cancers of 1.0. No specific cancer site showed an increase.

Ott *et al.* (1987) followed up the same cohort (2187 men) through 1982 with only 25 (1%) lost to follow-up; United States referent rates were used. Approximately 50% of the cohort had worked in exposed areas for less than one year and only 209 men had worked for 10 years or more; 823 were still employed at the end of follow-up. The overall SMR was 0.9 (95% confidence interval [CI], 0.8–1.0) based on 370 deaths. There were 102 cancer deaths (SMR, 1.0; 95% CI, 0.8–1.3) and the SMR for cancer with 20 or more years' latency was not significantly elevated (SMR, 1.3; 95% CI, 1.0–1.6). There was no significant elevation for cancer deaths, except for the category of other and unspecified neoplasms (12 observed; SMR, 2.6). Respiratory tract cancer mortality (23 deaths; SMR, 0.82) was not elevated. Elevations based on small numbers were observed for stomach cancer (6 observed, SMR, 1.6; 95% CI, 0.6–3.4) and lymphatic and haematopoietic cancers (12 observed; SMR, 1.5; 95% CI, 0.8–2.6), with the excess in the latter category accounted for mainly by non-Hodgkin lymphoma (5 observed; SMR, 1.9; 95% CI, 0.6–4.5) and multiple myeloma (2 observed; SMR, 2.0; 95% CI, 0.2–7.2). One death was initially classified as due to soft-tissue sarcoma (a fibrosarcoma); however, upon pathology review, this cancer was determined to be a renal clear-cell carcinoma. Analyses by cumulative exposure intensity scores showed no significant trend (at the $p = 0.05$ level) with increased exposure to 2,3,7,8-TCDD or to hexa-, hepta- or octa-CDDs for any specific cancer, although there was some increase in digestive tract cancers with increasing 2,3,7,8-TCDD exposure.

Bond *et al.* (1989a) increased by two years (through 1984) the follow-up of the cohort studied by Ott *et al.* (1987) (vital status was established for 2191 subjects). There was an increase in the number of deaths by 36, bringing the total to 406 (SMR, 0.9; [95% CI, 0.8–1.0]). Cancer deaths increased in number by 14 to make a total of 95 (SMR, 1.0; [95% CI, 0.8–1.3]). Two additional deaths from stomach cancer (8 observed [SMR, 2.0; [95% CI, 0.9–3.9]), one (additional) death from soft-tissue sarcoma (2 observed (one misclassified); [SMR, 5.0; 95% CI, 0.6–18.1]) and one additional death from non-Hodgkin lymphoma (6 observed; [SMR, 2.1; 95% CI, 0.8–4.5]) occurred. These elevations felt short of statistical significance. The two cases of soft-tissue sarcoma (one of which was actually misclassified) occurred in workers with chloracne. No other statistically significant trend with cumulative dose (of either 2,3,7,8-TCDD or hexa-, hepta- or octa-CDDs) occurred. Results from a sub-cohort of 323 male workers diagnosed with chloracne were presented, based on a review of 2072 (95% of the cohort) company medical records. Diagnoses of chloracne were included if they were considered 'probable' or 'definite'; person–time at risk began at the time of diagnosis. This sub-cohort had 4871 person–years of observation and 37 deaths (SMR, 0.8; 95% CI, 0.6–1.1) and only seven cancer deaths (SMR, 0.7; 95% CI, 0.3–1.4). The presence of chloracne was more prevalent in those who had the highest cumulative exposure to either 2,3,7,8-TCDD or hexa-, hepta- or octa-CDDs. Mortality in this sub-cohort was unremarkable except for soft-tissue sarcoma, for which two deaths (which included the misclassified case) were observed versus < 0.1 expected.

(b)   Comprehensive United States study

The largest study of United States production workers exposed to PCDDs was conducted by the United States National Institute for Occupational Safety and Health (NIOSH) and published by Fingerhut *et al.* (1991a). A more detailed technical report of this study is also available (Fingerhut *et al.*, 1991b). This 12-plant study included the Nitro, WV, plant of Monsanto and the Midland, MI, plant of Dow discussed above, which represented 9% and 40% of the cohort, respectively. In order to be included into the cohort, all workers had to have had presumed exposure to 2,3,7,8-TCDD. The cohort was constructed by NIOSH after a review of personnel records at 12 United States plants producing chemicals known to be contaminated with 2,3,7,8-TCDD (principally TCP and 2,4,5-T). The cohort included most workers in the United States likely to have been exposed to 2,3,7,8-TCDD in chemical manufacturing, comprising 5000 men with work records showing assignment to a production or maintenance job in a process involving 2,3,7,8-TCDD contamination, as well as an additional 172 men without work history records but known to have been exposed at the Nitro, WV, plant based upon inclusion in a prior cross-sectional medical study by Suskind & Hertzberg (1984). These latter 172 men and an additional 30 men in the NIOSH study lacked sufficient work history information for their inclusion in more detailed analyses by duration of exposure. Follow-up was conducted through 1987 and United States referent rates were used. Serum levels of 2,3,7,8-TCDD in 253 cohort members at two plants measured in 1987 averaged 233 ng/kg lipid, compared with 7 ng/kg lipid in a group of 79 unexposed workers. Levels increased to 418 ng/kg for 119 workers exposed for more than one year

(Fingerhut *et al.*, 1991a). Extrapolation to the date when these workers were employed, assuming a half life of 7.1 years, indicated a mean serum level at that time of 2000 ng/kg lipid (highest level, 32 000 ng/kg). Workers had last been exposed 15–37 years earlier. The correlation between serum 2,3,7,8-TCDD level and duration of exposure was 0.72 (Fingerhut *et al.*, 1991b). There were 1052 deaths in this cohort, with 116 748 person–years. The SMR for all causes was 1.0 (95% CI, 0.9–1.1). Mortality from all cancers (265 deaths) was slightly but significantly elevated (SMR, 1.2; 95% CI, 1.0–1.3). Soft-tissue sarcoma mortality was elevated based on four deaths (SMR, 3.4; 95% CI, 0.9–8.7). Two of the deaths from soft-tissue sarcoma, upon further review of medical records, were found to be misclassified (false positives), but three deaths from other causes, upon review, were found to be soft-tissue sarcomas (false negatives). Other causes of death of interest in this study were not remarkable. There were 10 deaths from non-Hodgkin lymphoma (SMR, 1.4; 95% CI, 0.7–2.5); stomach cancer mortality was not elevated (10 deaths observed; SMR, 1.0; 95% CI, 0.5–1.9); lung cancer showed a slight increase (89 observed; SMR, 1.1; 95% CI, 0.9–1.4). Sub-cohort analyses focused on those workers with more than one year's duration of 2,3,7,8-TCDD exposure and at least 20 years' potential latency (1520 workers, 29% of the cohort; mean duration of employment, 19 years; mean duration of exposure to 2,3,7,8-TCDD, 7 years). In this sub-cohort, mortality from all cancers combined was significantly elevated (114 observed; SMR, 1.5; 95% CI, 1.2–1.8). A wide variety of cancer sites showed some excess, but only soft-tissue sarcoma was significantly elevated (3 observed; SMR, 9.2; 95% CI, 1.9–27). The SMR for lung cancer was 1.4 (95% CI, 1.0–1.9) based on 40 deaths. Conversely, the SMR for non-Hodgkin lymphoma was not elevated in this sub-cohort with presumed higher exposure (2 deaths observed; SMR, 0.9; 95% CI, 0.1–3.4). Internal analyses comparing longer duration of exposure to 2,3,7,8-TCDD to a short duration (< 1 year) referent category found nonsignificant positive trends for all cancers and lung cancer ($p = 0.3$ and $p = 0.2$, respectively). Rate ratios also increased with latency (all cancer SMRs, 0.7, 1.1 and 1.3; lung cancer SMRs, 0.8, 1.0 and 1.2 with latency of < 10 years, 10–20 years and ≥ 20 years, respectively). The authors considered that smoking was not likely to be responsible for the excess of lung cancer for several reasons including that (*a*) there was no increase in non-malignant respiratory disease, which is strongly related to smoking; (*b*) an indirect adjustment for smoking based on known smoking habits for a sample of the cohort did not account for the observed increase; and (*c*) there was no increase in lung cancer among the group with 20 years' potential latency but short duration (< 1 year) of exposure to 2,3,7,8-TCDD (17 observed; SMR, 1.0). [The Working Group noted that these are indirect ways of controlling for confounding.]

(c)   German accident cohort

In the 1953 accident at the BASF TCP production unit at Ludwigshafen, Germany, the total number of employees identified as being involved directly or in the subsequent clean-up, repair or maintenance activities was 247 (243 men, 4 women). Analyses of adipose tissue and blood from groups of these workers are described in Section 1.3.1(*a*)(i). Part of the cohort was first studied by Thiess *et al.* (1982). It was completed by Zober *et al.* (1990) and further studied by Zober *et al.* (1994) and Ott and Zober

(1996). Out of the 247, 69 (1 woman) were identified by a company physician early after the accident as the most directly involved (cohort C1); 84 (2 women) were identified by August 1983 as probably involved (cohort C2); and 94 (1 woman) were recognized by the end of 1987 as possibly exposed during participation in demolition and toxicology investigations, or because they were members of the safety department and plant management at the time of the accident (cohort C3). Their mortality was investigated through 1987, with no loss to follow-up (Zober et al., 1990). Death certificates were obtained for 67 deceased subjects, and 11 additional deaths were ascertained through other means (information from physicians, autopsy reports). Expected deaths were calculated from national rates. All members of cohort C1 were affected by chloracne and their mortality from malignancies was moderately higher than expectation (9 deaths; SMR, 1.3; 95% CI, 0.7–2.3). Other nonsignificant increases were seen for stomach cancer (3 deaths; SMR, 3.0; 95% CI, 0.8–7.7), colon and rectum (2 deaths; SMR, 2.5; 95% CI, 0.4–7.8) and lung cancer (4 deaths; SMR, 2.0; 95% CI, 0.7–4.6). In cohort C2, 17 workers were affected by chloracne and four had other exposure-related skin lesions. Their mortality from all cancers combined after 20 years since first exposure was significantly increased (8 deaths; SMR, 2.4; 95% CI, 1.2–4.3), as was mortality from other and unspecified cancer sites (5 deaths; SMR, 3.2; 95% CI, 1.3–6.8) (whole cohort). A nonsignificant increase was noted for colorectal cancer (2 deaths; SMR, 2.7; 95% CI, 0.5–8.5) (whole cohort). Suicides were elevated in both cohorts C1 and C2. In cohort C3, where 28 persons had experienced mild forms of chloracne, no significant increase for deaths from any cause was seen, although one single leukaemia death represented a greater than five-fold elevated risk. Among all 127 workers affected by chloracne or other skin lesions (erythema), the mortality from all cancers combined was significantly elevated after 20 years since exposure (14 deaths; SMR, 2.0; 95% CI, 1.2–3.2). Nonsignificant increases were seen for cancer of the stomach (3 deaths; SMR, 1.8; 95% CI; 0.5–4.7), colon and rectum (3 deaths; SMR, 2.2; 95% CI, 0.6–5.8) and lung (6 deaths; SMR, 1.8; 95% CI, 0.8–3.6). In 1986, blood concentrations of 2,3,7,8-TCDD were measured in 28 workers. The median values were 24.5 ng/kg in cohort C1 (10 subjects), 9.5 ng/kg in C2 (7 subjects) and 8.4 ng/kg in C3 (11 subjects). The median value for workers with chloracne and other skin lesion was 15 ng/kg versus 5.8 ng/kg in those without skin manifestations. The small size of the study population precludes definitive conclusions.

The cancer incidence and the updated mortality, through 1992, have been reported (Ott & Zober, 1996). The study population comprised the 243 exposed men. One death from a motor vehicle accident had occurred among the four exposed women, and they were not further considered in the analysis. Incident cases were ascertained from available medical and necropsy data and from survey results (the area was not covered by a cancer registry). Death certificates were obtained for all but one of the deceased workers. Expected numbers of incident cases were calculated from the cancer statistics of the state of Saarland and expected deaths were calculated on the basis of national rates. At that time, serum measurements of 2,3,7,8-TCDD were available for 138 cohort members (Ott et al., 1993) (see Section 1.3.1(a)(i)). Model-based estimates of the cumulative dose of 2,3,7,8-TCDD (µg/kg bw) were calculated for each study subject.

Chloracne status was also adopted as an indicator of past exposure to 2,3,7,8-TCDD; 113 workers had a diagnosis of chloracne, and 55 were classified as severe. Standardized mortality and incidence ratios and their 95% CIs were estimated using standard techniques. Internal dose–response analyses were performed with the Cox's proportional hazard model, taking into account — among other variables — cigarette smoking and other potentially confounding exposures. Results of the models were reported in terms of conditional risk ratios (CRRs). The conditional risk represents the risk per unit increase (1 μg/kg bw) in 2,3,7,8-TCDD dose. In the mortality analysis, an increased cancer mortality with increasing dose was apparent: 2,3,7,8-TCDD level < 0.1 μg/kg bw, eight deaths (SMR, 0.8; 95% CI, 0.4–1.6); 0.1–0.99 μg/kg bw, eight deaths (SMR, 1.2; 95% CI, 0.5–2.3); 1.0–1.99 μg/kg bw, eight deaths (SMR, 1.4; 95% CI, 0.6–2.7); ≥ 2 μg/kg bw, seven deaths (SMR, 2.0; 95% CI, 0.8–4.0) [p for trend = 0.07]. Digestive system and respiratory tract cancers also tended to increase with increasing dose. In the 2,3,7,8-TCDD category > 1 μg/kg bw, after 20 or more years since initial exposure, all-cancer mortality (13 deaths; SMR, 2.0; 95% CI, 1.1–3.4) and respiratory cancer mortality (6 deaths; SMR, 3.1; 95% CI, 1.1–6.7) were significantly increased. In the sub-cohort with chloracne, 20 or more years after first exposure, 18 cancer deaths were observed (SMR, 1.9; 95% CI, 1.1–3.0). An increase was also seen for digestive tract cancer (6 deaths; SMR, 1.8; 95% CI, 0.7–4.0) and respiratory tract cancer (7 deaths; SMR, 2.4; 95% CI, 1.0–5.0). In the incidence analysis, a slight, nonsignificant increase in the risk for all cancers combined with increasing 2,3,7,8-TCDD dose was obtained. Respiratory tract cancer incidence was elevated in the high-dose group (8 cases; SMR, 2.0; 95% CI, 0.9–3.9). With the Cox's regression model, after controlling for other relevant variables, a significant association between 2,3,7,8-TCDD dose and increase in digestive system cancer was obtained, as both cause of death (CRR, 1.5; 95% CI, 1.1-1.9) and incident cases (CRR, 1.4; 95% CI, 1.1–1.7). Joint analysis of 2,3,7,8-TCDD dose and cigarette smoking showed a positive relationship between 2,3,7,8-TCDD dose and all cancers combined among current cigarette smokers (2,3,7,8-TCDD dose, SMR (95% CI) in current smokers: < 0.1, 1.2 (0.3–3.1); 0.1–0.99, 1.4 (0.3–4.2); 1.0–1.99, 3.0 (1.1–6.5); ≥ 2 μg/kg bw, 4.0 (1.5–8.6)) but not among nonsmokers.

(d) Other German plants

Several reports have considered workers from a chemical plant operated by Boehringer-Ingelheim, in Hamburg, Germany, that produced herbicides heavily contaminated with 2,3,7,8-TCDD and other PCDDs/PCDFs (Manz *et al.*, 1991; Nagel *et al.*, 1994; Flesch-Janys *et al.*, 1995; Becher *et al.*, 1996). In the latter study, workers from three other German plants were also considered.

Manz *et al.* (1991) reported the mortality experience of workers at the Hamburg plant since late 1951. An outbreak of chloracne in 1954 led to a halt in the production of TCP and 2,4,5-T. In 1957, production was resumed using a new process that reduced 2,3,7,8-TCDD formation. The vital status of all permanent employees at the plant for at least three months between 1 January 1952 and 31 December 1984 (1184 men, 399 women) was investigated through 1989. Causes of death were derived from medical records or, when not available, from death certificates. 2,3,7,8-TCDD concentrations were measured in workers from various production departments, mainly after the plant had closed in 1984. Workers were classified in exposure groups according to their work history: high (496 subjects), medium (901) and low (186). Mean concentrations of 2,3,7,8-TCDD in adipose tissue in 1985 from 48 volunteer surviving members of the cohort were 296 ng/kg (SD, 479; median, 137) in 37 workers in the high-exposure group and 83 ng/kg (SD, 73; median, 60) in 11 workers in the combined medium-/low-exposure groups. For comparison, national death rates and rates from a cohort of some 3500 workers at the Hamburg gas supply company were used. In the latter case, the follow-up period was restricted to 1985. SMRs and 95% CIs were estimated using standard techniques assuming a Poisson distribution. Follow-up was 97% successful. In men, mortality due to all cancers combined was increased in comparison with both the general population (93 deaths; SMR, 1.2; 95% CI, 1.0–1.5) and the gas workers (75 deaths; SMR, 1.4; 95% CI, 1.1–1.8). The increase was highest among those who entered the plant before 1954 (who had the highest exposure to 2,3,7,8-TCDD based on the history of the plant and subsequent serum measurement) and remained employed for 20 or more years. In men, in comparison with gas workers, deaths from all cancers combined were: high exposure, 29 deaths (SMR, 1.8; 95% CI, 1.2–2.6); medium exposure, 39 deaths (SMR, 1.2; 95% CI, 0.9–1.6); and low exposure, seven deaths (SMR, 1.5; 95% CI, 0.6–3.0) [p for trend = 0.24]. Among specific sites, significant increases were seen for lung cancer (26 deaths; SMR, 1.7; 95% CI, 1.1–2.4) and malignancies of the haematopoietic system (9 deaths; SMR, 2.7; 95% CI, 1.2–5.0). Smoking prevalence was similar in chemical (73%) and gas (76%) workers. Suicides were also significantly increased in comparison with both reference populations. Among women, mortality from all cancers combined was close to expectation; an increase was seen for breast cancer (9 deaths; SMR, 2.2; 95% CI, 1.0–4.1).

Mortality of the female workers in the cohort was further investigated by Nagel *et al.* (1994). Compared with the results of Manz *et al.* (1991), one additional breast cancer death was identified (10 cases; SMR, 2.4; 95% CI, 1.1–4.4). Cox's regression analysis yielded increasing breast cancer risk with duration of employment. 2,3,7,8-TCDD levels in blood or adipose tissue were measured for 26 women (22 for blood and 4 for adipose tissue), with an arithmetic mean of 109.7 ng/kg (median, 23 ng/kg; range, 7–1439 ng/kg).

The mortality experience of 1189 male workers employed for at least three months between 1952 and 1984 in the same plant in Hamburg was investigated through 1992 (Flesch-Janys *et al.*, 1995). A quantitative exposure index was constructed. Fourteen relevant production departments were identified and levels of PCDDs/PCDFs were determined in the buildings, products and wastes. A detailed work history for each worker ever employed in these departments was constructed. In a sample of 190 workers, concentrations of each PCDD/PCDF congener in adipose tissue or whole blood were determined, and their levels at the end of workers' exposure were calculated assuming a one-compartment first-order kinetic model; the contribution of working time in each production department to the end-of-exposure levels in these 190 workers was estimated. Based on this model, an estimated total end-of-exposure level was then calculated for each worker employed in these departments. The strongest association with 2,3,7,8-TCDD levels was found for duration of employment in 2,4,5-T (estimated yearly increase, 75.6 ng/kg blood) and TCP (estimated yearly increase < 1957, 292 ng/kg) production departments. For the entire cohort, the mean estimated 2,3,7,8-TCDD level was 141.4 ng/kg (median, 38.2 ng/kg). Blood measurements of PCDDs are presented in **Table 14**. Exposure to other carcinogens (e.g., dimethyl sulfate (see IARC, 1987g) and benzene (see IARC, 1987h) had occurred in some departments. As a reference, a cohort of 2528 workers from a gas supply company was adopted. Causes of death were ascertained from hospital and medical records whenever possible, or from death certificates, insurance data or next-of-kin interview. The validity of cause of death determination was successfully tested. Relative risks at seven exposure levels (reference, the first four quintiles and the ninth and tenth deciles of the estimated 2,3,7,8-TCDD levels) were estimated using Cox's regression techniques. An internal comparison group was also adopted composed of the chemical workers in the two lowest quintiles of the exposure levels distribution. Follow-up was 99% successful. Total mortality was elevated in all 2,3,7,8-TCDD exposure categories and showed a significant trend ($p = 0.01$) with increasing exposure level. Updated relative risks (RR) for total TEQ levels (not 2,3,7,8-TCDD levels) were published in an erratum (Flesch-Janys, 1996) and were as follows for all cancers combined (124 cases): 1.0–12.2 ng TEQ/kg, RR, 1.0 (95% CI, 0.6–1.8); 12.3–39.5 ng TEQ/kg, RR, 1.3 (95% CI, 0.8–2.1); 39.6–98.9 ng TEQ/kg, RR, 1.2 (95% CI, 0.7–1.9); 99.0–278.5 ng TEQ/kg, RR, 1.2 (95% CI, 0.8–1.9); 278.6–545.0 ng TEQ/kg, RR, 1.3 (95% CI, 0.7–2.3); 545.1–4362 ng TEQ/kg, RR, 2.7 (95% CI, 1.7–4.4). A significant pattern of increasing risk with increasing TEQ levels was also obtained for cardiovascular and ischaemic heart diseases, but not for other causes of death. The mortality pattern for all causes, all cancers, cardiovascular diseases and ischaemic heart diseases remained virtually unchanged when 2,3,7,8-TCDD exposure levels were used. When the internal comparison group of chemical workers was adopted, the relative risk estimates were lower and the confidence intervals wider. Nevertheless, total mortality (RR, 1.4; 95% CI, 1.0–2.1) and all-cancer mortality (RR, 2.0; 95% CI, 1.1–3.8) remained clearly elevated in the highest exposure category. When the 149 workers with exposure to one of the possible confounders (dimethyl sulfate) were excluded from analysis, the all-cancer mortality remained elevated, especially in the highest exposure category (RR, 2.3; 95% CI, 1.1–4.6) and the dose–response pattern was significant ($p < 0.01$). Smoking habits and socioeconomic status were similar in the chemical and gas worker cohorts. No data on specific cancer sites were reported.

Becher *et al.* (1996) reported the mortality of 2479 male workers employed in four German plants who were involved in the production of phenoxy herbicides and chlorophenols or who were likely to have been in contact with these substances and their contaminants, PCDDs (often including 2,3,7,8-TCDD) and PCDFs. Only workers with German nationality and at least one month of employment were included. The follow-up was performed through 1989 (1992 in one plant). Cause of death was recorded from death certificates or, in some cases, hospital or physician reports. Expected figures were calculated from national rates. Blood concentrations of 2,3,7,8-TCDD were measured in workers from three of the four plants (Kogevinas *et al.*, 1997). Workers in the Hamburg plant (plant I), including a group of females not considered here, had already been under investigation (see above; Manz *et al.*, 1991; Nagel *et al.*, 1994; Flesch-Janys *et al.*, 1995;

Flesch-Janys *et al.*, 1996b). In this plant (1144 male workers), concentrations of 2,3,7,8-TCDD in the order of 5–10 mg/kg were measured in 1957–70 in some products (chlorophenols and 2,4,5-T and its esters) and of 10–50 mg/kg in some process and waste streams. After the early 1970s, the concentrations were below 1 mg/kg. Numerous cases of chloracne occurred in 1954, at the early stage of development of herbicide manufacture. Measurements of blood concentrations from 190 workers in 1985–94 ranged between 3 and 2252 ng/kg (mean, 141 ng/kg). In plant II (135 workers), TCP was manufactured with 2,3,7,8-TCDD levels on average about 10 μg/kg. Eleven cases of chloracne were reported among maintenance workers in the early 1970s and measurements in 1989–92 from 20 workers ranged between 23 and 1935 ng/kg fat (mean, 401.7 ng.kg). In plant III (520 workers), a variety of phenoxy herbicides were produced. 2,3,7,8-TCDD levels in the products were reported to be in the 'sub-ppm range'. In plant IV (680 workers) (BASF, but the cohort is different from that of the accident study), phenoxy herbicides were synthesized in a large building where many other chemicals were also produced. Measurements in 1996 from 19 workers ranged between 1.3 and 6.49 ng/kg fat (mean, 3.2 ng/kg). In this plant, slightly elevated concentrations of higher chlorinated PCDDs were found in synthesis workers. No cases of chloracne were reported in plants III or IV. In the total cohort, mortality increases were seen for all cancers combined (138 deaths; SMR, 1.2; 95% CI, 1.0–1.4), cancer of the buccal cavity and pharynx (9 deaths; SMR, 3.0; 95% CI, 1.4–5.6), lung cancer (47 deaths; SMR, 1.4; 95% CI, 1.1–1.9), lymphatic and haematopoietic neoplasms (13 deaths; SMR, 1.7; 95% CI, 0.9–2.9) and non-Hodgkin lymphoma (6 deaths; SMR, 3.3; 95% CI, 1.2–7.1). Examination of trends with increasing time since first exposure showed: for all cancers combined (0–10 years: 15 deaths; SMR, 0.9; 95% CI, 0.5–1.5; 10–< 20 years: 46 deaths; SMR, 1.3; 95% CI, 0.9–1.7; ≥ 20 years: 77 deaths; SMR, 1.2; 95% CI, 1.0–1.5 [*p* for trend = 0.67]), for lymphatic and haematopoietic neoplasms (0–10 years: 2 deaths; SMR, 1.1; 95% CI, 0.1–4.0; 10–< 20 years: 4 deaths; SMR, 1.7; 95% CI, 0.5–4.4; ≥ 20 years: 7 deaths; SMR, 1.9; 95% CI, 0.8–4.0 [*p* for trend = 0.51]) and for non-Hodgkin lymphoma (0–10 years: 0 deaths; 10–< 20 years: 2 deaths; SMR, 3.6; 95% CI, 0.4–13.1; ≥ 20 years: 4 deaths; SMR, 4.3; 95% CI, 1.2–10.9; [*p* for trend = 0.24]). All-cause (345 deaths; SMR, 1.2; 95% CI, 1.0–1.3) and all-cancer mortality (97 deaths; SMR, 1.3; 95% CI, 1.1–1.6) was elevated only for plant I, where statistically significant increases were also seen for lung cancer (31 deaths; SMR, 1.5; 95% CI, 1.0–2.1), lymphatic and haematopoietic neoplasms (11 deaths; SMR, 2.4; 95% CI, 1.2–4.3), non-Hodgkin lymphoma (4 deaths; SMR, 3.8; 95% CI, 1.0–9.6) and multiple myeloma (3 deaths; SMR, 5.4; 95% CI, 1.1–15.9). Mortality from accidents and suicide was also increased. An increase in the incidence of non-Hodgkin lymphoma for plant II (2 deaths; SMR, 12.0; 95% CI, 1.5–43.5), and in that of cancer of the buccal cavity and pharynx for plant IV (6 deaths; SMR, 8.2; 95% CI, 3.0–17.9) were seen.

(e)   British plants

Four cohorts of workers employed between 1963 and 1985 in British factories producing or formulating — among other chemicals — phenoxy herbicides, including 2,4,5-T (Kauppinen *et al.*, 1993) and chlorophenols (some of which may have been contaminated by PCDDs) were investigated (Coggon *et al.*, 1991). In one of the plants (factory A), 2,4,5-T was synthesized between 1968 and 1978. In the other plants, 2,4,5-T was formulated only. The study was restricted to men. A total of 2239 subjects (employed during 1963–85) met the inclusion criteria. Job histories were used to classify workers according to potential exposure to phenoxy herbicides and chlorophenols. Approximately 50% of employees had directly worked with phenoxy herbicides. No environmental or personal monitoring had been carried out. Subjects were traced up to December 1987. Information was obtained on cause of death for deceased persons and on any cancers registered among living study subjects. Expected figures were obtained from rates for England and Wales, and in some analyses adjustment for local differences in mortality was applied. In the combined cohort, all-cause mortality was slightly higher than expected (152 deaths; SMR, 1.1; 95% CI, 0.9–1.3), and this was largely due to excesses of circulatory diseases and deaths from violent causes. Mortality from all-cancers combined was as expected (37 deaths; SMR, 1.0; 95% CI, 0.7–1.4). Statistically nonsignificant excesses were present for lung cancer (19 deaths; SMR, 1.3; 95% CI, 0.8–2.1) and non-Hodgkin lymphoma (2 deaths; SMR, 2.3; 95% CI, 0.3–8.3), even after local adjustment. When analysis was restricted to subjects with greater than background exposure to phenoxy compounds or chlorophenols, the SMR for lung cancer was 1.2 (14 observed deaths; [95% CI, 0.7–2.1]). Both non-Hodgkin lymphoma deaths occurred among these workers (SMR, 2.8; [95% CI, 0.3–10.2]). In factory A, 12 cancer deaths were observed (12.3 expected) and six were from lung cancer (SMR, 1.3 [95% CI, 0.5–2.8]).

(f) Dutch plants

The mortality of two cohorts of workers employed between 1955 and 1986 in the synthesis and formulation of phenoxy herbicides and chlorophenols in the Netherlands was examined (Bueno de Mesquita *et al.*, 1993). In one of the plants (A), where the main production was 2,4,5-T and derivatives, an accident in 1963 caused a release of PCDDs, including 2,3,7,8-TCDD. In factory B, production included MCPA, 4-chloro-2-methyl-phenoxypropionic acid (MCPP) and 2,4-D. The study enrolled 2074 manufacturing male workers from the two plants (963 exposed to phenoxy herbicides and 1111 not exposed). In addition, 145 workers probably exposed to 2,3,7,8-TCDD during the industrial accident and the clean-up operations were examined. Definition of individual exposure to phenoxy herbicides, chlorophenols or contaminants (PCDDs/PCDFs) was based on occupational history derived from job records and personal interviews, including periods of employment in different departments and positions held. Follow-up was 97% complete. The 190 female workers were excluded from the analysis. Of the accident workers, only 139 had sufficient data for analysis. Expected numbers of deaths were calculated from national rates. In addition, mortality rates of exposed and non-exposed workers were internally compared by Poisson regression analysis. Among subjects in factory A only, in comparison with the general population, all-cancer mortality was increased (26 deaths; SMR, 1.2; 95% CI, 0.8–1.7). Statistically nonsignificant increases were also seen for cancers of the pancreas (3 deaths; SMR, 2.9; 95% CI, 0.6–8.4), large intestine (3 deaths; SMR, 2.4; 95% CI, 0.5–7.0) and prostate (2 deaths; SMR, 2.2; 95%

CI, 0.3–7.8), lymphosarcoma (non-Hodgkin lymphoma) (1 death; SMR, 2.0; 95% CI, 0.1–11.4) and myeloid leukaemia (1 death; SMR, 2.9; 95% CI, 0.1–15.9). No death due to soft-tissue sarcoma was reported. In comparison with the non-exposed workers, exposed subjects in both plants exhibited increased mortality from all cancers combined (31 exposed deaths; rate ratio (RR), 1.7; 95% CI, 0.9–3.4) and respiratory tract cancer (9 deaths; RR, 1.7; 95% CI, 0.5–6.3). Six cancers of the urogenital organs were observed among the exposed and none among the non-exposed. A nonsignificant increase in deaths from lymphatic and haematopoietic neoplasms was also noted (4 deaths; RR, 2.6; 95% CI, 0.3–125). Increases in all cancers combined (RR, 2.0; 95% CI, 0.8–4.9) and lung cancer (RR, 3.9; 95% CI, 0.5–31.1) were confined to factory A, where the accident occurred and where the opportunity for exposure to 2,3,7,8-TCDD was highest. In the small group of accident-exposed workers, 10 cancer deaths were observed (SMR, 1.4; 95% CI, 0.7–2.5).

The study was later extended in time (1955–91) and enlarged in size (2298 subjects including 191 females) (Hooiveld et al., 1996a; Kogevinas et al., 1997). More accurate and elaborate proxies of exposure were used in the analysis, based on modelled 2,3,7,8-TCDD levels in serum, measured in 1993 in a subset of 31 surviving exposed (mean concentration, 53 ng/kg; range, 1.9–194) and 16 unexposed (mean concentration, 8 ng/kg) cohort members. Fourteen subjects exposed during the accident in factory A in 1963 had the highest levels (mean concentration, 96 ng/kg; range, 15.8–194). In this factory, both all-cause (139 observed; SMR, 1.3; 95% CI, 1.1–1.5) and all-cancer mortality (51 observed; SMR, 1.5; 95% CI, 1.1–1.9) were significantly increased. Excesses at specific sites were seen for urinary bladder (4 observed; SMR, 3.7; 95% CI, 1.0–9.5), kidney cancer (4 observed; SMR, 4.1; 95% CI, 1.1–10.4) and non-Hodgkin lymphoma (3 observed; SMR, 3.8; 95% CI, 0.8–11.0). Non-Hodgkin lymphoma was also increased in factory B (1 case only). Age- and time-adjusted relative risks comparing exposed and unexposed workers in factory A showed significant increases in mortality from all causes (139 observed; RR, 1.8; 95% CI, 1.2–2.5) and all cancers (51 observed; RR, 3.9; 95% CI, 1.8–8.8). Lung and urinary tract cancers showed numerically higher, but statistically nonsignificant increases. Three non-Hodgkin lymphomas were seen among the exposed and one among the unexposed (a nonsignificant increase). When workers were subdivided into three categories (low, medium and high exposure) according to model-predicted serum levels of 2,3,7,8-TCDD, relative risks for all causes, all cancers and lung cancer were significantly elevated in both middle and high categories, and were highest in the highest exposure group.

(g) IARC multi-country study

An international cohort of workers exposed to phenoxy herbicides and chlorophenols was set up by the International Agency for Research on Cancer in association with the United States National Institute of Environmental Health Sciences (Saracci et al., 1991). The cohort included 16 863 men and 1527 women employed in production or spraying, distributed among 20 cohorts from 10 countries, including the British and Dutch cohorts described above. Their mortality from 1955 onwards was examined, and follow-up was successful for 95% of the cohort members. National mortality rates were used for reference. Exposure assessment was based on work histories collected in each factory through questionnaires with the assistance of industrial hygienists, workers and factory personnel. A total of 13 482 workers were classified as 'exposed' to phenoxy herbicides, 416 were classified as 'possibly exposed', 541 had 'unknown' exposure and 3951 were classified as 'non-exposed'. In the entire cohort, all-cause mortality was lower than expected (SMR, 0.95; 95% CI, 0.9–1.0). Among men exposed to phenoxy herbicides or chlorophenols, mortality from all cancers combined was close to expectation (499 observed; SMR, 1.0; 95% CI, 0.9–1.1). Significant increases were seen for thyroid cancer (4 observed; SMR, 3.7; 95% CI, 1.0–9.4) and benign and unspecified neoplasms (12 observed; SMR, 2.0; 95% CI, 1.0–3.5); significant deficits were observed for skin (3 observed; SMR, 0.3; 95% CI, 0.1–0.9) and brain cancer (6 observed; SMR, 0.4; 95% CI, 0.1–0.8). Elevated risks were also seen for cancers of the nose and nasal cavities (3 observed; SMR, 2.9; 95% CI, 0.6–8.5), testis (7 observed; SMR, 2.3; 95% CI, 0.9–4.6) and other endocrine glands (3 observed; SMR, 4.6; 95% CI, 1.0–13.5) and for soft-tissue sarcomas (4 observed; SMR, 2.0; 95% CI, 0.6–5.2). In the probably exposed category, lung cancer mortality was significantly increased (11 observed; SMR, 2.2; 95% CI, 1.1–4.0). Significant increases were also seen among non-exposed workers, for unspecified digestive organs and for benign and unspecified neoplasms. The increase in soft-tissue sarcoma concerned workers after 10–19 years since first exposure (4 observed; SMR, 6.1; 95% CI, 1.7–15.5); no differentiation in risk was noted in relation to duration of exposure or probable 2,3,7,8-TCDD exposure. The SMR estimates for testicular and thyroid cancer were highest among workers probably exposed to 2,3,7,8-TCDD (SMR, 3.0 and 4.3, respectively) compared with those probably not exposed (SMR, 1.6 and 3.1, respectively).

Two nested case–control studies of soft-tissue sarcoma (11 incident cases, 55 controls) and non-Hodgkin lymphoma (32 incident cases, 158 controls) were conducted by Kogevinas *et al.* (1995) within the IARC cohort studied by Saracci *et al.* (1991). Exposures to 21 chemicals or mixtures were estimated by a panel of three industrial hygienists. Levels of exposure were evaluated using a relative scale, since few actual measurements of past exposure were available. A cumulative exposure score was calculated for each subject and chemical, on the basis of estimated level of exposure and duration of exposure (in years). The model that was used as the conceptual framework in deriving levels of exposure included variables related to department/job, emission of chemicals, contact with chemicals, personal protection, and other relevant determinants of exposure. Excess risk for soft-tissue sarcoma was associated with exposure to any phenoxy herbicide (odds ratio, 10.3; 95% CI, 1.2–91.0) and to each of the three major classes of phenoxy herbicides (2,4-D, 2,4,5-T and MCPA). Soft-tissue sarcoma was also associated with exposure to any PCDD/PCDF (odds ratio, 5.6; 95% CI, 1.1–28.0) and with exposure to 2,3,7,8-TCDD (odds ratio, 5.2; 95% CI, 0.9–32.0). Associations between non-Hodgkin lymphoma and phenoxy herbicides were generally weaker. The odds ratio between non-Hodgkin lymphoma and 2,3,7,8-TCDD exposure was 1.9 (95% CI, 0.7–5.1). A monotonic increase in risk was observed for cumulative exposure (categorized in four categories, non-exposed, low, medium, high exposure) to 2,4-D (odds ratio for highest category, 13.7; 95% CI, 0.9–309; *p*-value for trend = 0.01), 2,4,5-T (odds ratio for highest category, 7.7; 95% CI, 0.5–477; *p*-value for trend = 0.07), any PCDD/PCDF (odds ratio for highest category, 19.0; 95% CI, 1.3–1236; *p*-value for trend = 0.008) and 2,3,7,8-TCDD (odds ratio for highest category, 10.6; 95% CI, 0.6–671; *p*-value for trend = 0.04). [The Working Group noted that analysis for specific exposures was complicated by the exposure of most workers to a multitude of herbicides.]

While Saracci *et al.* (1991) studied the men in the IARC cohort, 701 women were studied by Kogevinas *et al.* (1993) for both cancer incidence and mortality. Among 169 women probably exposed to 2,3,7,8-TCDD, excess incidence was observed for all cancers combined (9 cases; standardized incidence ratio (SIR), 2.2; 95% CI, 1.0–4.2). There was one case of breast cancer (SIR, 0.9; 95% CI, 0.0–4.8). For 532 women probably not exposed to 2,3,7,8-TCDD, the rate ratio for incidence of all cancers combined was 0.8 (20 cases; 95% CI, 0.5–1.2). Cause-specific analyses were based on small numbers. Mortality results paralleled those for incidence.

The international cohort studied by Saracci *et al.* (1991) was updated and expanded with the data of Fingerhut *et al.* (1991a,b) and Becher *et al.* (1996) (Kogevinas *et al.*, 1997). Follow-up differed by plant, but most European plants were followed through 1991–92, while the United States plants were followed through 1987. Each of the 21 863 male and female workers exposed to phenoxy herbicides or chlorophenols was placed in one of three categories: (1) those exposed to 2,3,7,8-TCDD or higher chlorinated PCDDs (*n* = 13 831); (2) those not exposed to 2,3,7,8-TCDD or higher chlorinated PCDDs (*n* = 7553); and (3) those of unknown exposure to 2,3,7,8-TCDD or higher chlorinated PCDDs (*n* = 479). The latter category included all workers in one British cohort for which production history, particularly for 2,4,5-T, was incomplete. Three criteria were used to classify workers as exposed to 2,3,7,8-TCDD or higher chlorinated PCDDs: (i) employment during the period of production, formulation or spraying of 2,4,5-T, 2,4,5-trichlorophenoxypropionic acid, TCP, hexachlorophene, Erbon, Ronnel, PCP or 2,3,4,6-tetrachlorophenol; and (ii) employment in plants with documented (through serum, adipose tissue or environmental measurements) exposure to 2,3,7,8-TCDD or higher chlorinated PCDDs at levels above background; or (iii) in the absence of PCDD measurements, employment in plants or companies with documented large-scale production, formulation or spraying of the above-mentioned phenoxy herbicides and chlorophenols. An average production of these chemicals of 10 tonnes per year was chosen *a priori*, below which it was considered that the probability of contamination and significant exposure to 2,3,7,8-TCDD and higher chlorinated PCDDs would be minimal for most workers in a cohort. Current mean levels of 2,3,7,8-TCDD, measured in 574 workers from 10 companies in 7 countries, ranged from 3 to 389 ng/kg lipid. Among workers exposed to 2,3,7,8-TCDD or higher chlorinated PCDDs, mortality was elevated for soft-tissue sarcoma (6 deaths; SMR, 2.0; 95% CI, 0.8–4.4). Mortality from all cancers combined (710 deaths; SMR, 1.1; 95% CI, 1.0–1.2), non-Hodgkin lymphoma (24 deaths; SMR, 1.3; 0.9–2.1) and lung cancer (225 deaths; SMR, 1.1; 95% CI, 1.0–1.3) was slightly elevated. Risks for all cancers combined and for soft-tissue sarcomas and lymphomas increased with time since first exposure. Workers not exposed to 2,3,7,8-TCDD or higher chlorinated PCDDs had SMRs of 1.0 for all cancers, for non-Hodgkin lymphoma and for lung cancer; soft-tissue sarcoma was slightly elevated, based on two deaths (SMR, 1.4; 95% CI, 0.2–4.9). In a direct comparison between those exposed to higher chlorinated PCDDs versus lower ones or none, a rate ratio of 1.3 (95% CI, 1.0–1.8) for all cancers combined was found. This study represents the largest overall cohort of 2,3,7,8-TCDD-exposed workers.

2.1.2 *Population exposure due to industrial accident*

The mortality and cancer incidence among the population of Seveso exposed in the industrial accident described in Section 1.3.1 were investigated. The contaminated area was subdivided into three exposure zones (zone A, zone B and zone R), according to the average levels of 2,3,7,8-TCDD measured in soil samples. The most contaminated, Zone A, extended for 87 hectares and average soil levels between 15.5 μg/m^2 and 580 μg/m^2 were found. In Zone B (270 hectares), soil levels did not exceed, on average, 50 μg/m^2. In Zone R (1430 hectares), soil levels were generally below 5 μg/m^2. All persons residing in these zones at the time of the accident, as well as all newborn infants and new residents in the subsequent 10-year period, were considered to have been exposed. Measurements of blood levels of 2,3,7,8-TCDD in members of the exposed population are described in Section 1.3.1. Three exposure categories were formed, corresponding to the zone of residence of the subjects at the time of the accident or later entry into the area. As a reference, the population of 11 municipalities surrounding the contaminated area was adopted. Ethnic, social, cultural and occupational characteristics were closely comparable. The exposed and referent populations were followed up as if they were a unique cohort, blindly to the exposure status of the subjects. The follow-up after 15 years was > 99% successful (Bertazzi *et al.*, 1993). Causes of death were derived from death certificates. In the period 1976–91, there were 750 subjects in Zone A and 16 cancer deaths, 5000 subjects in Zone B and 152 cancer deaths, and 30 000 subjects in Zone R and 1008 cancer deaths. The reference population comprised over 200 000 subjects (Bertazzi *et al.*, 1996).

The cause-, age-, gender- and calendar time-specific mortality rates in the exposed and reference populations were compared using Poisson regression methods (Bertazzi *et al.*, 1996). All-cause and all-cancer mortality did not differ significantly from those expected in any of the contaminated zones. Mortality from gastrointestinal cancer was increased. Women had a relative risk for all digestive system cancers combined of 1.5 (5 deaths; 95% CI, 0.6–3.6) in Zone A and liver cancer (3 deaths; RR, 1.3; 95% CI, 0.4–4.0) in Zone B. Among men, increases were seen for rectal cancer (7 deaths; RR, 2.9; 95% CI, 1.4–6.2) in Zone B and for cancer of the oesophagus (30 deaths; RR, 1.6; 95% CI, 1.1–2.4) in Zone R. Neoplasms of the lymphatic and haematopoietic tissues were clearly elevated in Zone B. The highest risks were seen for leukaemia in men (7 deaths; RR, 3.1; 95% CI, 1.4–6.7), multiple myeloma in women (4 deaths; RR, 6.6; 95% CI, 2.3–18.5) and Hodgkin's disease in both men and women (men: 2 deaths; RR, 3.3; 95% CI, 0.8–14.0; women: 2 deaths; RR, 6.5; 95% CI, 1.5–30.0). Two cases of thyroid cancer in Zone B, one each in men and women, represented a notable, although nonsignificant increase [RR, 3.9; 95% CI, 0.4–14.1]. Four cases of soft-tissue sarcoma were seen in

Zone R among men (RR, 2.1; 95% CI, 0.7–6.5). Breast cancer was below expectation in all zones.

Cancer incidence data are available for the period 1977–86 (Bertazzi et al., 1993) for the population aged 20–74 years and residing in the area at the date of the accident. Cancer diagnoses were obtained from the regional registration system of hospital admissions and discharges. Of the 41 801 relevant medical records, 41 778 were successfully reviewed. The proportion of non-detected cases ranged from 2.6% to 6.8% across hospitals, and the overall histological confirmation rate was 72%. Quality and completeness of cancer case ascertainment did not vary appreciably across zones or with the referent population. In Zone A, no significant differences from expectation were seen (14 cancer cases in total). In Zone B, hepatobiliary cancer was increased among both women (5 cases; RR, 3.3; 95% CI, 1.3–8.1) and men (5 cases; RR, 1.8; 95% CI, 0.7–4.4). Haematopoietic system neoplasms were significantly increased. Among women, increases were seen for multiple myeloma (2 cases; RR, 5.3; 95% CI, 1.2–22.6) and myeloid leukaemia (2 cases; RR, 3.7; 95% CI, 0.9–15.7) and, among men, increases were seen for lymphoreticulosarcoma (3 cases; RR, 5.7; 95% CI, 1.7–19.0) and multiple myeloma (2 cases; RR, 3.2; 95% CI, 0.8–13.3). In Zone R, soft-tissue sarcoma incidence was increased in both women (2 cases; RR, 1.6; 95% CI, 0.3–7.4) and men (6 cases; RR, 2.8; 95% CI, 1.0–7.3). Breast and endometrial cancers were below expectation. The cancer incidence among subjects aged 0–19 years was analysed separately (Pesatori et al., 1993). Given the small number of events, the three contaminated zones and both genders were grouped together. Seventeen cancer cases were observed (RR, 1.2; 95% CI, 0.7–2.1). Two ovarian cancer cases were observed versus none expected. Two thyroid gland cancers among girls gave a relative risk of 4.6 (95% CI, 0.6–32.7). Lymphatic and haematopoietic neoplasms were increased (9 cases; RR, 1.6; 95% CI, 0.7–3.4), particularly Hodgkin's lymphoma (3 cases; RR, 2.0; 95% CI, 0.5–7.6) and myeloid leukaemia (3 cases; RR, 2.7; 95% CI, 0.7–11.4). [The Working Group noted that the size of the most exposed population is small and that the latency of 15 years may be short for certain health effects to manifest themselves. Measurements of blood levels of 2,3,7,8-TCDD (see Section 1.3.1) are available for only small samples of the exposed populations.]

2.1.3 *Industrial exposure to higher chlorinated PCDDs*

Two United States studies have focused on cohorts exposed to PCP or chlorophenates (penta and tetra); these chemicals contain predominantly higher chlorinated PCDDs (Cl_6–Cl_8) but not 2,3,7,8-TCDD (United States Environmental Protection Agency, 1994). Many workers in one of these studies also had exposure to 2,3,7,8-TCDD.

In another study of pentachlorophenate-exposed industrial workers, Hertzman et al. (1997) studied 23 829 workers from 11 Canadian sawmills in British Columbia which used chlorophenates from the 1940s to the 1970s. Another 2658 unexposed workers from three sawmills not using chlorophenates were also studied. Cohort members had to have worked for at least one year between 1 January 1950 and 31 December 1985. Follow-up was through 1990. Jobs were rated according to level of chlorophenate exposure and a quantitative exposure score was developed. Most exposure was dermal, although some inhalation exposure could occur. In the 1960s and 1970s, sawmills switched from using predominantly pentachlorophenates, which would be expected to have contained higher chlorinated PCDDs and PCP, to tetrachlorophenates (less contaminated with higher chlorinated PCDDs). Exposure to chlorophenates was widespread in the industry. Wood was dipped in chlorophenates and then planed; exposures occurred during both processes. Urine samples taken in the 1980s showed significant levels of chlorophenates (median, 180 µg/L) (Hertzman *et al.*, 1988). Mortality and cancer incidence rates were compared with the population of British Columbia; cases were identified from either cancer registry data or death certificates. There were 583 190 person–years in chlorophenate mills and 41 280 in non-chlorophenate mills, with 70 119 potential person–years lost to follow-up (11.2%); analyses were conducted either assuming that lost-to-follow-up workers were alive until the end of 1990 (method 1) or assuming that person–time ended when a worker was lost to follow-up (method 2). There were 4710 deaths in the cohort (1950–89) (4539 in exposed mill workers and 171 in non-exposed mill workers) and 1547 incident cancer cases (1969–89) (1498 in exposed mill workers and 49 in non-exposed mill workers). The SMR for all causes of death among workers at chlorophenate mills was 0.81 (95% CI, 0.79–0.83) by method 1 of treating loss to follow-up and 0.96 (95% CI, 0.94–0.99) by method 2; the SMR for non-chlorophenate mills was 0.89 (95% CI, 0.78–1.01) with method 2. In the chlorophenate mill workers, there were six deaths from soft-tissue sarcoma (SMR using method 1 for loss to follow-up, 1.2; 95% CI, 0.5–2.3; SMR using method 2, 1.4; 95% CI, 0.6–2.8). There were 11 incident cases of soft-tissue sarcoma (SIR using method 1, 1.0; 95% CI, 0.6–1.7; and using method 2, 1.2; 95% CI, 0.7–1.9). There were 36 deaths from non-Hodgkin lymphoma (SMR using method 1, 0.9; 95% CI, 0.7–1.2 or SMR using method 2, 1.1; 95% CI, 0.8–1.4) and 23 deaths from lymphosarcoma (SMR using method 1, 1.3; 95% CI, 0.9–1.8 or SMR using method 2, 1.5; 95% CI, 1.0–2.1). There were 63 incident cases of non-Hodgkin lymphoma during the study period (SMR using method 1, 1.0; 95% CI, 0.8–1.2 or SMR using method 2, 1.2; 95% CI, 1.0–1.5). While no trend was observed for mortality from non-Hodgkin lymphoma with cumulative exposure, a significant positive trend of SIR for non-Hodgkin lymphoma was seen with increasing cumulative exposure to chlorophenate ($p = 0.02$). The SIR for the group with the highest cumulative exposure and 20 or more years' exposure was 1.5 ($p = 0.04$).

Ramlow *et al.* (1996) studied 770 workers from the occupational cohort in Midland, MI, studied by Ott *et al.* (1987) and Bond *et al.* (1989a) (see Section 2.1.1), but restricted to those cohort members with some exposure to PCP. Although the authors provide no details, most of these workers (approximately 85%) were also exposed to 2,3,7,8-TCDD based on detailed data from the United States NIOSH cohort (Fingerhut *et al.*, 1991b). Follow-up was from 1940 through 1989; both the United States population and another group of unexposed male workers from the same company were used as referent groups. Exposure scores for PCP were developed, in addition to the exposure scores for 2,3,7,8-TCDD and hexa-, hepta- or octa-CDDs used previously by Ott *et al.* (1987). The average length of follow-up was 26.1 years and there were 20 107 person–years in the study. There were 229 deaths from all causes in the whole cohort (SMR, 0.9; 95% CI, 0.8–1.1) and 50 cancer deaths (SMR, 1.0; 95% CI, 0.7–1.3). The SMR for a category of non-Hodgkin lymphoma and myeloma combined was 2.0 (5 deaths; 95% CI, 0.7–4.7); the authors noted that two of these cancers were myeloma (versus approximately 0.8 expected), while three were non-Hodgkin lymphomas [approximately 1.7 expected]. Stomach cancer mortality was slightly elevated (4 deaths; SMR, 1.7; 95% CI, 0.5–4.3), as was kidney cancer mortality (3 deaths; SMR, 2.3; 95% CI, 0.5–6.7). No deaths from liver cancer were observed (1.1 expected) nor from thyroid cancer (0.1 expected), cancers *a priori* of interest from animal studies. Results of analyses for ≥ 15 years' potential latency were also presented, which differed little from those of the overall analysis. Analyses by cumulative exposure to PCP were conducted for 'low PCP' and 'high PCP' groups compared with unexposed workers using a variety of lag periods. A significant positive trend was noted for kidney cancer with increasing exposure when a 15-year lag was used (p = 0.03) and a nearly significant positive trend was noted for the combined category of non-Hodgkin lymphoma and myeloma (p = 0.08). Similar trends were seen for these two cancer categories when the data were stratified by level of exposure to 2,3,7,8-TCDD or hexa-, hepta or octa-CDDs.

In three cohorts included in the IARC international cohort, 842 workers were evaluated to have been exposed to higher chlorinated PCDDs but not to 2,3,7,8-TCDD. The workers had been producing PCP in a plant in England, 2,3,4,6-tetrachlorophenol in a plant in Finland and a variety of phenoxy herbicides in a plant in Germany. In the latter group of workers, serum levels of 2,3,7,8-TCDD were around background, while an elevation was seen for higher chlorinated PCDDs, especially among synthesis workers (Messerer *et al.*, 1996). Mortality from all neoplasms was around that expected from national mortality rates (41 deaths; SMR, 1.0; 95% CI, 0.7–1.4). No deaths from soft-tissue sarcoma (0.2 expected) or non-Hodgkin lymphoma (0.7 expected) were registered in these three cohorts, while mortality from lung cancer was higher (19 deaths; SMR, 1.5; 95% CI, 0.9–2.3) than in 2,3,7,8-TCDD-exposed workers (Kogevinas *et al.*, 1997).

2.2 Herbicide exposures

Introduction

Studies of herbicide exposure among farmers, pesticide applicators and other non-industrial populations were included in this review either if there was explicit evidence that exposure included 2,4,5-T (known to be contaminated with 2,3,7,8-TCDD), or if data on individual exposure to phenoxy herbicides as a class was available and it was known that 2,4,5-T was used in the area. Several studies of applicators without adequate documentation of exposure to 2,4,5-T or other phenoxy herbicides were not considered informative, such as those of Barthel (1981), Corrao *et al.* (1989) and Eriksson *et al.* (1992). In addition, studies with exposure to phenoxy herbicides limited to 2,4-D, MCPA or other compounds typically not found to be contaminated with higher chlorinated PCDDs were excluded, such as those of Wigle *et al.* (1990) and Morrison *et al.* (1993, 1994). Similarly, studies of paper and pulp mill workers were not considered, because measurements of PCDDs in biological tissues of workers have not shown that their levels were elevated (Rosenberg *et al.*, 1994, 1995; Mouradian *et al.*, 1995; see Section 1.3.1).

In these studies, direct evidence of exposure to 2,3,7,8-TCDD is often lacking. The limited data available indicate that exposure to 2,3,7,8-TCDD is likely to be substantially lower than exposure in industrial cohorts (see Section 1.3.1). For example, in the most heavily exposed applicators of 2,4,5-T in New Zealand, who applied 2,4,5-T for at least 180 months, the estimated mean serum level of 2,3,7,8-TCDD at the time of blood drawing was 53 ng/kg (Smith *et al.*, 1992a). Back extrapolation of this level to the period when 2,4,5-T was likely to be most contaminated with 2,3,7,8-TCDD gave a value of around 300 ng/kg. Among United States Air Force personnel (Ranch Hand) who applied Agent Orange from 1962 to 1971, generally for relatively short periods, the median serum 2,3,7,8-TCDD level in 1987 was 13 ng/kg, which when back-extrapolated would be about 50 ng/kg (Roegner *et al.*, 1991). These levels are about one order of magnitude lower than the back-extrapolated 2,3,7,8-TCDD levels estimated for many industrial cohorts. In data from Australia (Johnson *et al.*, 1992a), the range of serum 2,3,7,8-TCDD levels at time of blood drawing in 1990 in 33 applicators randomly selected from a group of 654 men who had applied 2,4,5-T and 2,4-D for at least 12 months was 2–34 ng/kg. Back-extrapolation to the time exposure ceased, using a half life of 7.1 years, revealed that those who sprayed after 1974 (the period when 2,3,7,8-TCDD contamination of 2,4,5-T was markedly reduced) had a significantly lower mean exposure rate (0.06 ng/kg per month) compared with workers who sprayed before 1965 (2.7 ng/kg per month) or during 1965–74 (2.3 ng/kg per month). For those workers who sprayed during 1965–74, the estimated serum TCDD concentrations at termination of employment ranged from 13 to 329 ng/kg.

In Sweden, no difference in 2,3,7,8-TCDD levels in adipose tissue was found between 13 exposed (mean 2,3,7,8-TCDD, 2 ng/kg) and 18 non-exposed subjects (mean 2,3,7,8-TCDD, 3 ng/kg) (Nygren *et al.*, 1986; see Section 1.3.1(*a*)(ii)). Exposure was defined as in the Swedish case–control studies on soft-tissue sarcoma and non-Hodgkin lymphoma (e.g., Hardell *et al.*, 1981) (see Section 2.2.2). The 13 exposed subjects sampled were not a representative sample of phenoxy herbicide applicators in Sweden, and these results may not be generalizable.

Applicators of phenoxy herbicides in most of the epidemiological studies applied these herbicides for only a short time. Analyses restricted to 'long duration' often included only a few subjects exposed for more than a year. In light of the above data, it is to be expected that 2,3,7,8-TCDD levels in herbicide applicators would be very low.

2.2.1   *Applicator cohorts* (**Table 34**)

(*a*)   *Commercial*

A cohort study of 348 male railroad workers in Sweden exposed to herbicides during the period 1957–72 was initially followed through 1972 (Axelson & Sundell, 1974) and subsequently through 1978 (Axelson *et al.*, 1980). The workers had been exposed to amitrole (see IARC, 1987i) and to phenoxy herbicides, particularly 2,4-D and 2,4,5-T. Only workers with a minimum of 45 days of exposure, not necessarily continuous, were included in the cohort. Workers were classified into three sub-cohorts depending on the type of herbicide used: those with exposure to amitrole, those with exposure to

Table 34. Cohort studies of cancer in relation to herbicide application

Reference, country	Study subjects	Study type/ Period of follow-up	Exposure	Gender	Cancer site/ cause of death	No obs.	RR	95% CI	Comments
Axelson et al. (1980), Sweden	348 railroad herbicide sprayers	Mortality 1957–78. Latency ≥ 10 years	2,4-D, 2,4,5-T, amitrole and combinations, others	Men	All cancers	13	2.4	[1.3–4.1]	Exposed in 1957–61
					Stomach	3	5.3	[1.1–15.5]	Exposed in 1957–61
					All cancers	3	1.5	[0.3–4.4]	Exposed to amitrole
						6	1.9	[0.7–4.1]	Exposed to phenoxy herbicides
					All cancers	6	3.4	[1.2–7.4]	Exposed to both
					Stomach	6	2.3	[0.8–5.0]	Follow-up 1972–78
						2	7.7	[0.9–27.8]	Exposed to phenoxy herbicides
Riihimäki et al. (1982), Finland	1926 herbicide applicators during 1955–71	Mortality, 1972–80	2,4-D, 2,4,5-T, ≥ 2 weeks per year	Men	All cancers				
					No latency	26	[0.7]	[0.5–1.0]	
					≥ 10 years latency	20	[0.8]	[0.5–1.3]	
					≥ 15 years latency	5	[0.4]	[0.1–1.0]	
					Lung				
					≥ 10 years latency	12	[1.1]	[0.6–1.9]	
					≥ 15 years latency	4	[0.9]	[0.2–2.2]	
					Prostate				
					≥ 10 years latency	2	[1.8]	[0.2–6.6]	
					Multiple myeloma				
					≥ 10 years latency	1	[5.0]	[0.1–28]	
			Most heavily exposed ≥ 8 weeks per year or during 5 years		All cancers				
					≥ 10 years latency	5	[0.5]	[0.2–1.2]	
					≥ 15 years latency	1	[0.2]	[0.0–1.1]	

Table 34 (contd)

Reference, country	Study subjects	Study type/ Period of follow-up	Exposure	Gender	Cancer site/ cause of death	No obs.	RR	95% CI	Comments
Hansen et al. (1992), Denmark	4015 gardeners, 1975–84	Incidence, 1975–84	Greenhouse workers (10–20%): fungicides, insecticides; outdoor gardeners (80–90%): 2,4-D, 2,4,5-T, MCPA, amitrole, other herbicides	Men	All cancers	184	1.1	0.9–1.2	
					Respiratory tract	41	1.0	0.7–1.3	
					STS	3	5.3	1.1–15	
					Haematopoietic (all)	15	1.4	0.8–2.4	
					NHL	6	1.7	0.6–3.8	
					CLL	6	2.8	1.0–6.0	
					Other leukaemia	3	1.4	0.3–4.2	
				Women	All cancers	33	0.9	0.6–1.3	
					Respiratory tract	2	0.7	0.1–2.6	
					Breast	10	1.1	0.5–2.1	
					STS	0	0	0–41	
					Haematopoietic (all)	2	1.4	0.2–5.0	
					NHL	2	3.6	0.4–13	
					CLL	0	0	0–17	
					Other leukaemias	0	0	0–11	
Hogstedt & Westerlund (1980), Sweden	145 forestry workers, 251 unexposed foresters	Mortality 1954–78, incidence 1958–78	2,4-D, 2,4,5-T ≥ 5 days	Men	All cancers (mortality)	2	[0.4]	[0.0–1.3]	Exposed
						3	[3.0]	[0.6–8.8]	Foremen
						5	[0.8]	[0.3–1.8]	Unexposed
					All cancers (incidence)	3	[0.4]	[0.1–1.0]	Exposed
						5	[3.6]	[1.2–8.3]	Foremen

Table 34 (contd)

Reference, country	Study subjects	Study type/ Period of follow-up	Exposure	Gender	Cancer site/ cause of death	No obs.	RR	95% CI	Comments
Wiklund et al. (1987, 1988, 1989), Sweden	20 245 pesticide applicators, licensed 1965–76	Incidence, 1965–82	Herbicides (20–70%): MCPA, dinoseb, 2,4-D, 2,4,5-T; insecticides (15–50%): DDT, fenitrothion; fungicides (10–30%): maneb, triadimefon	Men (99%); Women (1%)	All cancers				
					No latency	558	0.9	0.8–0.9	
					≥ 10 years latency	281	0.9	[0.8–1.0]	
					Lung				
					No latency	38	0.5	0.4–0.7	
					≥ 10 years latency	23	0.6	[0.4–0.8]	
					NHL				
					No latency	21	1.0	0.6–1.5	
					≥ 10 years latency	12	1.2	0.6–2.0	
					Hodgkin's disease				
					No latency	11	1.2	0.6–2.2	
					≥ 10 years latency	4	1.5	0.4–3.7	
					STS				
					No latency	7	0.9	0.4–1.9	
					≥ 10 years latency	4	1.0	0.3–2.7	
Ketchum & Akhtar (1996), USA	1261 Ranch Hand veterans (Viet Nam)	Mortality through 1993	Agent Orange median serum 2,3,7,8-TCDD 12 ng/kg in 1987 (comparison 4 ng/kg)	Men	All cancers	30	0.9	0.6–1.3	US Air Force Viet Nam veterans who applied Agent Orange, compared to 19 101 Air Force Viet Nam veterans who did not apply Agent Orange
					Lung	3	[0.9	0.5–1.6]	
					All haematopoietic	12	[0.9	0.2–2.5]	
					NHL	1	[1.4	0.0–7.7]	
					STS	1	[2.4	0.1–13.6]	
					Digestive system	5	[0.7	0.2–1.5]	

Abbreviations: NHL, non-Hodgkin lymphoma; STS, soft-tissue sarcoma; CLL, chronic lymphocytic leukaemia phenoxyherbicides and those with exposure to both. Workers had also been exposed to some less commonly used herbicides such as monuron, diuron, or atrazine (see IARC, 1991). None of the 348 individuals was lost to follow-up. Underlying cause of death was recorded on the basis of information from death certificates as classified by the National Central Bureau of Statistics. Expected numbers of deaths were calculated using cause-, calendar period- and age-specific national mortality rates. Mortality rates for 1975 were used for the period 1975–78 since national rates were not available at the time of the study for the last three years. In the total cohort, all-cause mortality was approximately that expected (45 deaths; SMR, 0.9, [95% CI, 0.7–1.2]) and mortality from all cancers combined was slightly elevated (17 deaths; SMR, 1.4 [95% CI, 0.8–2.3]). The SMRs for all cancers in the sub-cohort exposed to phenoxy herbicides was 1.1 (6 deaths [95% CI, 0.4–2.3]), with an excess observed for stomach cancer (2 deaths; SMR, 3.1 [95% CI, 0.4–11.1]). The SMR for all cancers combined in the sub-cohort exposed to both phenoxy herbicides and amitrole was 2.1 (6 deaths [95% CI, 0.8–4.5]) with an excess for stomach cancer based on only one death (0.3 expected) and lung cancer (one death; 0.5 expected). When a 10-year latency period was applied, the SMR for all cancers combined for the phenoxy herbicides sub-cohort was 1.9 (6 deaths [95% CI, 0.7–4.2]) and that for the sub-cohort exposed to both phenoxy herbicides and amitrole was 3.4 (6 deaths [95% CI, 1.2–7.3]).

A follow-up study was conducted among forestry workers in Sweden (Hogstedt & Westerlund, 1980). One hundred and forty-five male forestry workers registered as having worked with phenoxy herbicides (2,4-D and 2,4,5-T) for at least five days, 16 foremen (claimed to be highly exposed) and 251 unexposed foresters were identified from pay lists of a timber company in Hälsingland between 1954 and 1967. Persons who worked for more than five days with other herbicides were not included. Vital status and cause of death were assessed for the period 1954–78 from national health registers, except for three exposed and seven unexposed foresters. Incident cancer cases between 1958 and 1978 were identified through cancer registries. National statistics were used as a reference. The average duration of exposure was 30 days (range, 6–114) among forest workers and 176 days (range, 16–317) among foremen. In the exposed cohort, 29 deaths occurred versus 28.0 expected; 47 deaths were observed in the unexposed versus 64.4 expected. Tumour deaths were three (versus 1.0 expected) among foremen, two (versus 5.4 expected) among exposed workers and five (versus 6.4 expected) among unexposed workers. Incident cancer cases were in excess among foremen (5 versus 1.4 expected; $p < 0.02$) and less than expected in the other exposed workers (3 versus 8.4 expected). No specific cancer site was remarkable (stomach (1), pancreas (2), lung (1), skin (1), prostate (2), urinary bladder (1)).

A cohort of male phenoxy herbicide applicators in Finland was followed prospectively from 1972 to 1980 (Riihimäki *et al.*, 1982). The herbicides 2,4-D and 2,4,5-T had been used in Finland since the mid-1950s, with the peak consumption (about 50–70 tonnes of active ingredient per year) occurring in the late 1960s. Analysis of some old herbicide preparations used in Finland in 1962–67 suggested that the 2,3,7,8-TCDD content ranged between 0.1 and 0.9 mg/kg. After 1972, the use of these chemicals declined. The cohort of herbicide applicators was identified in 1972 from the personnel records of the four main Finnish employers involved in chemical control of brushwood. The cohort included 1971 men exposed to 2,4-D and 2,4,5-T for at least two weeks during 1955–71. The data were collected by office personnel in the companies from various sources such as payrolls. In some cases, supplementary information was sought through interviews with foremen and clerks. About a quarter of the population had been exposed for more than eight weeks, as of 1971. During 1955–71, 45 individuals died, leaving 1926 subjects alive followed during 1972–80; fifteen subjects were not located in the population data register and were excluded from the cohort. The underlying cause of death for all deceased subjects was retrieved from death certificates registered at the Central Statistical Office. National age- and sex-specific mortality rates for 1975 were used to calculate expected numbers of deaths. Mortality from all cancers during the period 1972–80 was lower than expected from national rates (26 deaths [SMR, 0.7; 95% CI, 0.5–1.0]), with a slightly higher rate observed during the last years of follow-up, (1977–80; 17 deaths [SMR, 0.9; 95% CI, 0.5–1.5]). Similar results were obtained when allowing for a 10-year or a 15-year latency period, or when the analysis was restricted to subjects with the longest duration of exposure. The SMR for lung cancer, allowing for a 10-year latency period, was 1.1 (12 deaths [95% CI, 0.6–1.9]). There were no deaths registered from malignant lymphomas or soft-tissue sarcoma.

Cancer incidence was studied in a cohort of 20 245 licensed pesticide applicators in Sweden (Wiklund et al., 1987, 1988, 1989). Since 1965, a licence has been mandatory for using the most acutely toxic pesticides. The workers in the study had been issued a licence between 1965 and 1976 and were followed up for cancer incidence to 31 December 1982. A survey of a random sample of 273 workers showed that 72% had been exposed to phenoxy herbicides for one day or more during the 1950s, 1960s and 1970s. Phenoxy herbicides had been used in Sweden since the late 1940s. The main compound used in agriculture was MCPA and, since the mid-1960s, MCPP and dichlorprop (2-(2,4-dichlorophenoxy)propionic acid). 2,4-D and 2,4,5-T were used to a lesser extent. Cancer incidence rates for the Swedish population were used for comparison. A total of 558 cancer cases were observed in the cohort (SIR, 0.86; 95% CI, 0.79–0.93). Excess risks were observed for lip cancer (14 observed; SIR, 1.8; 95% CI, 1.0–2.9), testicular cancer (18 observed; SIR, 1.6; 95% CI, 0.9–2.5) and Hodgkin's disease (11 observed; SIR, 1.2; 95% CI, 0.6–2.2) but not for lung cancer (38 observed; SIR, 0.5; 95% CI, 0.4–0.7), non-Hodgkin lymphoma (21 observed; SIR, 1.0; 95% CI, 0.6–1.5) or cancer at any other site. The SIR for testicular cancer increased with time since licence (0–4 years, 0.9; 5–9 years, 1.4; ≥ 10 years, 2.5; based on four, six and eight cases, respectively). The SIR for lung cancer increased with years since first employment from 0.3 (0–4 years) to 0.5 (5–9 years) to 0.6 (≥ 10 years). The authors provided data showing that smoking was less prevalent among pesticide applicators than among other occupational categories in Sweden, strongly suggesting that the observed deficit of lung cancer was due to lower cigarette consumption. A follow-up from the date of licence until 31 December 1984 indicated no excess risk for soft-tissue sarcoma (7 cases observed; SIR, 0.9; 95% CI, 0.4–1.9) (Wiklund et al., 1988).

A historical cohort study was conducted among Danish gardeners heavily exposed to pesticides (Hansen et al., 1992). The cohort comprised 859 women and 3156 men and included all employed persons who, in May 1975, were members of one of the 10 local trade unions of gardeners associated with the Danish Union of General Workers. Subjects were followed from 1 May 1975 to 1 January 1985 through the records of the Danish Central Population Register, with 100% of the subjects being traced. Cancer incidence was recorded through the Danish Cancer Registry. The analysis was limited to subjects 30–79 years of age. The gardeners constituted three fairly separate groups, namely workers in greenhouses (nearly all female), a small group of nursery gardeners and gardeners in public parks, gardens and cemeteries (the majority of workers). Gardeners working outdoors had been exposed to phenoxy herbicides (2,4-D, MCPA, 2,4,5-T) and amitrole. This exposure took place regularly throughout the growing season. Data on individual job histories were not obtained, except for a limited subset of cancer cases. A total of 219 cancer cases were identified in the study, 217 among subjects aged 30–79 years. There was no elevation in incidence of all cancers combined (SIR, 1.0; 95% CI, 0.9–1.2) or of most common neoplasms. An increased risk was seen for soft-tissue sarcoma (code 197 in ICD 7th revision), with an SIR of 4.6 (3 cases; 95% CI, 0.9–13.3) which was statistically significant among men (3 cases; SIR, 5.3; 95% CI, 1.1–15.4). Elevated risks were seen for non-Hodgkin lymphoma (8 cases; SIR, 2.0; 95% CI, 0.9–3.9) and for chronic lymphatic leukaemia (6 cases; SIR, 2.5; 95% CI, 0.9–5.5). Two individuals with soft-tissue sarcoma, six with non-Hodgkin lymphoma and three with chronic lymphatic leukaemia had worked as gardeners for more than 10 years. No additional soft-tissue sarcoma cases were identified in this cohort when the records of the cancer registry were searched for sarcomas which might have occurred in parenchymal organs and consequently not been included in the ICD code (code 197, 7th rev.) used for the main analysis.

(b) Military

United States Viet Nam veterans as a group, with the exception of those known to have directly handled Agent Orange, show no evidence of exposure to PCDDs or PCDFs above that of other veterans who did not serve in Viet Nam (i.e., beyond background levels), on the basis of serum measurements. However, veterans actually involved in spraying, as members of the Air Force Operation Ranch Hand or of the Army Chemical Corps, have shown elevated serum levels of 2,3,7,8-TCDD (see Section 1.3.1(*a*)(ii)).

The mortality of 1261 Ranch Hand veterans has been compared with that of 19 101 other Air Force Viet Nam veterans who were not exposed to Agent Orange (Michalek *et al.*, 1990). Person–time at risk began when the tour of duty in Viet Nam began. The most recent mortality report extends follow-up through 1993 (Ketchum & Akhtar, 1996), with 31 394 person–years among Ranch Hand personnel and 490 792 person–years among the comparison group. The SMR for all causes of death was 1.0 (95% CI, 0.8–1.2), based on 118 deaths. There were 30 cancer deaths (SMR, 0.9; 95% CI, 0.6–1.3) and 12 lung cancer deaths (13.0 expected). There was one death from soft-tissue sarcoma (a fibroma; ICD 171.3) versus 0.4 expected for the category cancer of the connective tissue (ICD 171.0–171.9), and one from non-Hodgkin lymphoma (0.7 expected). No case of chloracne has been reported among Ranch Hand veterans.

The mortality of 894 members of the Army Chemical Corps was studied by Thomas and Kang (1990). Follow-up extended through 1987, and the United States population was used as the referent. Person–time at risk was taken to begin when service ended in Viet Nam. There were 53 deaths (SMR, 1.1) in this cohort, with about 16 000 person–years and an average follow-up of 18 years. There were six cancer deaths (SMR, 0.9): two lung cancer deaths versus 1.8 expected, two leukaemias versus 0.5 expected and two brain cancers versus 0.4 expected. Review of medical records found two incident cases of Hodgkin's disease, with approximately 0.7 expected.

2.2.2   *Community-based case–control studies*

Although many case–control studies may include one or more questions concerning exposure to herbicides, the Working Group considered only those in which exposure to PCDD-containing herbicides was a major hypothesis being tested, and where such exposure was evaluated in detail.

Studies of soft-tissue sarcoma and haematopoietic tumours have been systematically reviewed. For other sites (Section 2.2.2(*d*)), studies in which phenoxy herbicides were not a main focus of interest have not been examined.

(*a*)   *Soft-tissue sarcoma* (see **Table 35**)

A series of studies on soft-tissue sarcoma were conducted in Sweden applying similar methodology (Hardell & Sändstrom, 1979; Eriksson *et al.*, 1981; Hardell & Eriksson, 1988; Eriksson *et al.*, 1990). Relevant exposure measurements are presented in **Tables 16 and 17**.

The first case–control study associating phenoxy herbicides and chlorophenols with soft-tissue sarcoma was conducted in 1978 in the population of the region of Umeå, in northern Sweden (Hardell & Sändstrom, 1979). The study was initiated following a case report of three soft-tissue sarcoma patients who had been exposed to phenoxy herbicides (Hardell, 1977). The study included 21 living and 31 deceased pathologically verified soft-tissue sarcoma male cases, diagnosed in one hospital during 1970–77. Four population controls matched for age, sex, place of residence and vital status were selected per case. Living controls were selected from the national population registry and deceased controls from the national registry of causes of death. The response rate was 100% for cases and 99% for the controls. A self-administered questionnaire was sent to living subjects and to the next-of-kin of deceased subjects (approximately 60% of all questionnaires). Information was requested about a variety of exposures and the questionnaire was supplemented by telephone interviews of selected subjects. Any subject exposed for more than one day was characterized as exposed. Exposure to phenoxy herbicides and/or chlorophenols was associated with a six-fold increased risk. In the matched analysis, the odds ratio was 6.2 [confidence intervals not provided]. In an unmatched analysis, the odds ratio was 5.7 (95% CI, 2.9–11.3). The odds ratio among living subjects was 9.9 and that among deceased subjects was 3.8. The odds ratio for exposure only to phenoxy herbicides was 5.3 (95% CI, 2.4–11.5). After excluding the three index cases [but not

Table 35. Case–control studies on soft-tissue sarcoma containing information on exposure to phenoxy herbicides, chlorophenols or PCDDs

Reference, country	No. of cases/ controls	Gender	Exposure	Relative risk (95% CI)	Comments
Hardell & Sandström (1979), Sweden	52/208	Men	Exposure to phenoxy herbicides or chlorophenols for more than one day	5.7 (2.9–11.3)	Odds ratios for living subjects were higher than those for deceased subjects
			Exposure to phenoxy herbicides only	5.3 (2.4–11.5)	
Eriksson *et al.* (1981), Sweden	110/220	Men	Exposure to phenoxy herbicides or chlorophenols for more than one day	5.1 (2.5–10.4)	Odds ratio from matched analysis
			Exposure for more than one day to phenoxy herbicides contaminated with 2,3,7,8-TCDD	17.0 (NR)	
			Exposure for more than one day to phenoxy herbicides not contaminated with 2,3,7,8-TCDD	4.2 (NR)	
			Exposure to chlorophenols for one week continuously or one month discontinuously	3.3 (1.3–8.1)	
Hardell & Eriksson (1988), Sweden	54/490 (311 population controls, 179 cancer controls)	Men	Exposure to phenoxy herbicides for more than one day (comparison with population controls)	3.3 (1.4–8.1)	Odds ratio from matched analysis. Odds ratio was slightly lower (2.2; 95% CI, 0.9–5.3) when comparing with cancer controls.
Eriksson *et al.* (1990), Sweden	218/212	Men	Exposure to phenoxy herbicides for more than one day	1.3 (0.7–2.6)	Odds ratio from matched analysis. Risk for exposure to 2,4,5-T before 1950 was higher (odds ratio, 2.9; 95% CI, 1.1–8.0)
			Exposure to 2,4,5-T	1.8 (0.9–3.9)	
			Exposure to PCP for one week continuously or one month discontinuously	3.9 (1.2–12.9)	

Table 35 (contd)

Reference, country	No. of cases/ controls	Gender	Exposure	Relative risk (95% CI)	Comments
Hardell *et al.* (1991), Sweden	352/865	Men	*2,3,7,8-TCDD exposure*		Odds ratios (90% CI) Referent group non-exposed to phenoxy herbicides or chlorophenols. Pooled analysis of the four above-mentioned studies by Hardell, Eriksson and colleagues
			Non-exposed	1.0	
			Less than one year to phenoxy herbicides contaminated with 2,3,7,8-TCDD	3.0 (2.0–4.5)	
			More than one year to phenoxy herbicides contaminated with 2,3,7,8-TCDD	7.2 (2.6–20)	
			Exposure to other PCDDs		
			Non-exposed	1.0	
			Less than one year to phenoxy herbicides contaminated with other PCDDs	1.7 (1.0–2.9)	
			More than one year to phenoxy herbicides contaminated with other PCDDs	6.2 (2.9–13)	
Smith *et al.* (1984b), New Zealand	82/92	Men	*Phenoxy herbicides*		Odds ratios (90% CI)
			Potentially exposed > 1 day not in 5 years before cancer registration	1.3 (0.6–2.5)	
			Probably or definitely exposed for > 5 days not in 10 years before cancer registration	1.3 (0.6–2.9)	
			Chlorophenols		
			Potentially exposed > 1 day not in 5 years before cancer registration	1.5 (0.5–4.5)	
			Probably or definitely exposed for > 5 days not in 10 years before cancer registration	1.6 (0.5–5.2)	
Smith & Pearce (1986), New Zealand	51/315 (new study)	Men	*Phenoxy herbicides*		Odds ratios (90% CI)
			Potentially exposed for > 1 day not in 5 years before cancer registration	0.7 (0.3–1.5)	
	133/407 (combined)			1.1 (0.7–1.8)	

Table 35 (contd)

Reference, country	No. of cases/ controls	Gender	Exposure	Relative risk (95% CI)	Comments
Woods *et al.* (1987), USA	128/694	Men	All occupations with potential exposure to phenoxy herbicides or chlorophenols	0.8 (0.5–1.2)	Risk for soft-tissue sarcoma was not associated with exposure to phenoxy herbicides or chlorophenols and no incresed risk with increasing length of exposure
			Estimated intensity of exposure to phenoxy herbicides:		
			Low	0.6 (0.3–1.1)	
			Medium	1.0 (0.6–1.7)	
			High	0.9 (0.4–1.9)	
			Estimated intensity of exposure to chlorophenols:		
			Low	0.9 (0.5–1.6)	
			Medium	0.9 (0.6–1.5)	
			High	0.9 (0.5–1.8)	
Vineis *et al.* (1986), Italy	37/85	Men	Living men whose exposure could not be ruled out	0.9 (0.2–3.9)	Age-adjusted estimates. 90% CI. Risk higher in women exposed during 1950–55 when highest exposures occurred. No excess risk in men. No excess risk for deceased cases and controls
	31/73	Women	Living women 'definitely' exposed to phenoxy herbicides	2.7 (0.6–12.4)	
Smith & Christophers (1992), Australia	30/30/30 cancer and population controls	Men	At least one day of exposure to phenoxy herbicides or chlorophenols	1.0 (0.3–3.1)	Exposure to phenoxy herbicides and chlorophenols coded as 'none', 'possible' and 'definite/probable' by expert assessment. Matched analysis on age, gender and residence
			At least one day only to phenoxy herbicides	1.3 (0.4–4.1)	
			More than 30 days of exposure to phenoxy herbicides or chlorophenols	2.0 (0.5–8.0)	

NR, not reported

four additional cases included in a pilot study], this odds ratio became 4.7 (95% CI, 2.0–10.7). Tobacco smoking, exposure to DDT, exhaust fumes and emulsion agents did not appear to be associated with risk for soft-tissue sarcoma.

Responding to criticisms that selection and information bias could have affected the results of the previous study (Hardell & Sändstrom, 1979) and of a study on malignant lymphomas (Hardell *et al.*, 1981), Hardell (1981) conducted a further analysis using colon cancer patients as controls. The study is fully described in Section 2.2.4(*d*). Results obtained when using colon cancer patients as controls were very similar to the original results obtained when using population controls.

A case–control study of the association between soft-tissue sarcoma and phenoxy herbicides and chlorophenols was conducted among the population of the five southern-most counties of Sweden (Eriksson *et al.*, 1981). The study included 110 pathologically verified soft-tissue sarcoma cases (including 38 deceased cases) reported to the cancer registry during 1974–78. Two population controls matched for age, place of residence and vital status were selected per case. Living controls were selected from the national population registry and deceased controls from the national registry of causes of death. A self-administered questionnaire was sent to living subjects and to the next-of-kin (approximately 35% of all questionnaires) of deceased subjects. Information was requested about a variety of exposures. The questionnaire was supplemented by tele-phone interviews for subjects with incomplete or obscure replies to questions on expo-sure to solvents or pesticides, and also for all subjects reporting work in agriculture, forestry or horticulture. Any subject exposed to phenoxy herbicides for more than one day was characterized as exposed. The predominant exposure in this area was to MCPA, considered to be free of 2,3,7,8-TCDD contamination, to 2,4-D and the analogous phenoxypropionic acids, MCPP and dichlorprop, possibly contaminated by PCDDs other than 2,3,7,8-TCDD. A high level of exposure to chlorophenols used as wood preser-vatives was defined as one week of continuous or one month of discontinuous exposure. The odds ratio for exposure to phenoxy herbicides and/or chlorophenols was 5.1 in the matched analysis (95% CI, 2.5–10.4). The odds ratio for exposure to any phenoxy herbicide was 6.8 (95% CI, 2.6–17.3). A higher relative risk was observed for exposure to phenoxy herbicides considered to be contaminated with 2,3,7,8-TCDD (odds ratio, 17.0) compared with herbicides uncontaminated with 2,3,7,8-TCDD (odds ratio, 4.2). Longer duration of exposure to phenoxy herbicides (more or less than 30 days) was not associated with an increased risk. High-level exposure to chlorophenols was associated with an increased risk (odds ratio, 3.3; 95% CI, 1.3–8.1), while low-level exposure was not associated with an increased risk. Tobacco smoking or exposure to organic solvents, various pesticides or other chemical agents did not appear to be associated with risk for soft-tissue sarcoma.

A case–control study on soft-tissue sarcoma was conducted in the population of three northern counties of Sweden (Hardell & Eriksson, 1988). The study included 55 male histopathologically confirmed soft-tissue sarcoma cases (18 alive, 37 deceased) aged 25–80 years. Cases were diagnosed during 1978–83 and were identified through the regional cancer registry in Umeå. In eight cases, the tumour was classified as probable soft-tissue sarcoma but another malignancy could not be excluded. Three groups of controls were selected. A first group of 220 living population controls was matched with cases by age and residence at the time of diagnosis. The second group consisted of 110 dead controls. The third group consisted of 190 cancer cases (112 alive) (except for malignant lymphomas and nasopharyngeal cancer) drawn at random from the population cancer registry. A self-administered postal questionnaire was used and information was requested on lifetime occupational history, exposure to specific agents at work or leisure and lifestyle factors. The questionnaire was supplemented by telephone interviews for subjects with incomplete or obscure replies, and also for all subjects reporting work in agriculture, forestry, horticulture, carpentry and sawmills. The participation rate among both cases and controls was about 95%. The odds ratios for at least one day of exposure to phenoxy herbicides were 3.3 (95% CI, 1.4–8.1) when the two combined population control groups were used and 2.2 when cancer controls were used (95% CI, 0.9–5.3). Exclusion of the eight soft-tissue sarcoma cases with uncertain diagnosis gave a higher estimate of the risk (odds ratio, 3.7 (95% CI, 1.5–9.1) for population controls and 2.4 (95% CI, 1.0–5.9) for cancer controls). No association with exposure to chlorophenols was found. Exposure to 2,3,7,8-TCDD gave a crude rate ratio of 3.5 when population-based referents were used and 3.1 with cancer referents. A higher risk associated with exposure to DDT was present only among subjects with concomitant exposure to phenoxy herbicides. No statistically significant results were observed for other occupational exposures or for smoking.

A case–control study on soft-tissue sarcoma was conducted among the population of seven counties of central Sweden covered by the population cancer registry of Uppsala (Eriksson *et al.*, 1990). The study included 218 male histopathologically confirmed soft-tissue sarcoma cases (78 alive, 140 deceased) aged 25–80 years. Cases were diagnosed during 1978–86 and were identified through the regional cancer registry. One group of population controls was selected, matched for age, gender, county of residence and vital status. A self-administered postal questionnaire was used and information was requested on lifetime occupational history (including details of 16 specific occupations), exposure to specific agents at work or leisure and lifestyle factors. The questionnaire was supplemented by telephone interviews for subjects with incomplete or obscure replies, and also for all subjects reporting work in agriculture, forestry, horticulture, carpentry and sawmills. The participation rate for the cases was 92% (218/237 originally identified cases) and that for controls was 89% (212/237 originally identified controls). The odds ratio for exposure (at least one day) to phenoxy herbicides was 1.3 (95% CI, 0.7–2.6). The risk associated with use of 2,4,5-T was higher (odds ratio, 1.8; 95% CI, 0.9–3.9), especially for use before the 1950s (odds ratio, 2.9; 95% CI, 1.1–8.0) when contamination with PCDDs could be expected to be highest. A high risk was associated with exposure to chlorophenols (odds ratio, 5.3; 95% CI, 1.7–16.3), particularly PCP (odds ratio, 3.9; 95% CI, 1.2–12.9) among subjects characterized as having a high level of exposure (continuous exposure for more than one week or discontinuous exposure for more than one month). No clear dose–response relationship was observed for exposure to phenoxy herbicides. Exposure to phenoxy herbicides not contaminated with 2,3,7,8-TCDD was not associated with an increased risk. No statistically significant associations were observed for other occupational exposures or for smoking.

The data from the four Swedish case–control studies on soft-tissue sarcoma were aggregated (for a total of 434 cases and 948 controls) and re-analysed according to duration of exposure, latency and type of PCDD exposure, reported in a letter to the editor (Hardell *et al.*, 1991). For exposure to PCDDs of any type, less than one year of exposure gave an odds ratio of 2.4 (58 exposed cases; 90% CI, 1.7–3.4), and more than one year gave an odds ratio of 6.4 (24 exposed cases; 90% CI, 3.5–12). Forty-six cases were exposed to 2,4,5-T, presumed to be contaminated with 2,3,7,8-TCDD, yielding odds ratios of 3.0 (40 exposed cases; 90% CI, 2.0–4.5) for less than one year of exposure and 7.2 (6 exposed cases; 90% CI, 2.6–20) for more than one year of exposure. However, even exposure to other PCDDs was associated with an increased risk for soft-tissue sarcoma (< 1 year: 18 exposed cases; odds ratio, 1.7; 90% CI, 1.0–2.9; > 1 year: 18 exposed cases; odds ratio, 6.2; 90% CI, 2.9–13). It was concluded that PCDDs other than 2,3,7,8-TCDD might have contributed to the noted effect.

A case–control study evaluating the association between exposure to phenoxy herbicides and chlorophenols with the occurrence of soft-tissue sarcoma was carried out in New Zealand (Smith *et al.*, 1984b). Preliminary results had been reported earlier (Smith *et al.*, 1982a, 1983). The study included 82 living or deceased male cases with histopathologically verified soft-tissue sarcoma reported to the national cancer registry between 1976 and 1980. One control per case was selected randomly from other cancer patients in the national cancer registry matched for age, gender and year of registration. The participation rate was 84% among cases (82/98 eligible) and 83% among controls (92/111 eligible). Interviews were conducted with the subjects or the next-of-kin (43% of cases, 34% of controls). Subjects were interviewed by telephone concerning work in particular occupations with potential exposure to phenoxy herbicides or chlorophenols. Exposure to phenoxy herbicides and chlorophenols was ascertained through a combination of information on occupation, industry, type of cultivation sprayed and self-reported exposure to specific agents. In a separate study, PCDD levels were determined in serum of nine workers first employed before 1960 and having sprayed 2,4,5-T for a minimum of 180 months (Smith *et al.*, 1992a). The mean value of 2,3,7,8-TCDD was 53.3 ng/kg (range, 3–131 ng/kg) (see Table 17). Any potential exposure to a phenoxy herbicide was associated with a small non-statistically significant excess risk (odds ratio, 1.3; 90% CI, 0.7–2.5). A slightly higher risk was observed in subjects with more than one day of probable or definite exposure, after excluding the last five years of exposure before registration (odds ratio, 1.6; 90% CI, 0.7–3.3). Potential exposure to chlorophenols was associated with a small increased risk (odds ratio, 1.3; 90% CI, 0.5–3.6), particularly for those subjects who were potentially exposed for more than five days (odds ratio, 1.6; 90% CI, 0.5–5.2). However, a review of the working histories of those subjects through additional interviews and contacts with their employers indicated that only two cases, out of the seven characterized as potentially exposed, actually had potential for exposure to TCP.

An update was conducted by Smith and Pearce (1986) combining new data, including a general population control group, with the study population of Smith *et al.* (1984b). New cases diagnosed from 1980 to 1982 (n = 51) were compared with population controls (n = 315). The odds ratio estimate was 0.7 (90% CI, 0.3–1.5) for probable or definite exposure to phenoxy herbicides for more than one day not in the five years before cancer registration. The odds ratio estimate for the combined studies was 1.1 (90% CI, 0.7–1.8). There was no evidence in either study of an increase in risk with longer duration of exposure or longer latency since first exposure.

A population-based case–control study was conducted in three provinces of northern Italy where rice growing is the predominant agricultural activity and phenoxy herbicides have been used since 1950 (Vineis *et al.*, 1986). During 1950–55, rice weeding was still done manually, mostly by a seasonal work force of women, who were presumed to have had the highest exposure to phenoxy herbicides, predominantly 2,4,5-T. Incident cases of soft-tissue sarcoma aged 20 years or older, with a proven or suspected histological diagnosis in 1981–83 were identified through all the pathology departments of the three provinces, and six pathology departments of the city of Turin and the National Cancer Institute in Milan. Out of 135 cases initially identified, 37 were excluded because the diagnosis was not confirmed or because the cases were prevalent or were visceral sarcomas. Of the remaining 98 eligible cases, interviews were obtained from 68 patients or next-of-kin (44 living, 24 deceased). The participation rate was 69%. A random sample of living controls was drawn from electoral registers. Deceased controls (any cause of death apart from suicide) matched by age, sex, year of death and municipality were selected through demographic offices of the relevant municipalities. Interviews were obtained from 122/168 eligible controls (participation rate 73%) and 36/40 relatives of deceased subjects (participation rate 90%). Direct interviews were carried out with subjects, who were asked for information on lifetime occupational history, and additional information on jobs with titles indicating potential exposure to phenoxy herbicides or chlorophenols. In addition, supplementary questionnaires were administered to subjects working in agriculture, particularly cultivation of rice and other crops. Two experts assessed exposure to phenoxy herbicides and classified subjects into three categories: (1) those not exposed to phenoxy herbicides; (2) those for whom exposure could not be ruled out; and (3) those 'definitely' exposed, based on occupational histories primarily as rice weeders. Among living subjects, no men were 'definitely' exposed. Among living women, four cases and five controls were 'definitely' exposed (odds ratio, 2.7; 90% CI, 0.6–12.4). The odds ratio for the combined categories 2 and 3 was 2.4 (5 exposed cases; 90% CI, 0.6–10.3). Among living women continuously exposed during 1950–55, the crude odds ratio was [9.9] (3 exposed cases, 1 exposed control). No excess risk was observed when analyses were limited to deceased subjects. [The Working Group noted that no distinction was made between herbicides likely to be contaminated with PCDDs and others.]

A population-based case–control study was conducted in western Washington State, United States, to evaluate the relationship between occupational exposure to phenoxy herbicides and chlorophenols and risk for soft-tissue sarcoma and non-Hodgkin lymphoma (Woods *et al.*, 1987). Living and deceased cases, aged 20–79 years and diagnosed during 1981–84, were identified from the population-based tumour registry that covers 13 counties of the state. Enrolled in the study were 128 pathologically reviewed soft-tissue sarcoma cases (97 alive, 31 dead). Population controls were selected using random digit dialling or from social security records (for older cases) or non-cancer death certificates (for deceased cases). Controls were matched for age and vital status with a parallel series of non-Hodgkin lymphoma cases. The participation rate was 62% for soft-tissue sarcoma cases (128/206) and 76% for controls. Subjects were interviewed in person and information was requested on occupational exposures to phenoxy herbicides and chlorophenols and to other potential risk factors. Additional information was requested for specific occupations and job activities involving potential exposure to the chemicals of interest. The risk for soft-tissue sarcoma associated with all occupations involving potential exposure to phenoxy herbicides was 0.8 (95% CI, 0.5–1.2). Exposure to phenoxy herbicides or chlorophenols was not associated with increased risk for soft-tissue sarcoma. No association was seen with estimated intensity of exposure to either phenoxy herbicides or chlorophenols. [The Working Group noted that no information was provided on use of specific herbicides.]

A case–control study on patients with soft-tissue sarcoma was undertaken in Victoria, Australia, during 1982–88 (Smith & Christophers, 1992). The study included 30 male cases with soft-tissue sarcoma registered in the Victoria Cancer Registry. Cases were first diagnosed between 1976 and 1987. For each case, one cancer control was selected from the cancer registry, matched for age, sex and residence. A second set of population controls was selected from the electoral register using the same matching criteria. The response rates were 70% for cases, 56% for cancer controls and 70% for population controls. Cases were interviewed mostly before 1986, while both series of controls were mostly interviewed after 1986. A comprehensive occupational history was obtained through a personal interview. Exposures to phenoxy herbicides and to chlorophenols were coded by expert assessment as none, possible or definite/probable. Exposures within the five-year period before the year of diagnosis of a case were ignored, for both cases and their matched controls. The main chlorinated herbicides used in Victoria were 2,4-D, 2,4,5-T and MCPA. There were no significant differences between population and cancer controls with respect to definite exposure and these two groups were combined for the analysis. For soft-tissue sarcoma, the odds ratio was 1.0 (95% CI, 0.3–3.1) for at least one day's exposure to phenoxy herbicides or chlorophenols and 1.3 (95% CI, 0.4–4.1) for exposure only to phenoxy herbicides. The odds ratio for more than 30 days of exposure to phenoxy herbicides or chlorophenols was 2.0 (95% CI, 0.5–8.0). [The Working Group noted that no distinction was made between herbicides likely to be contaminated with PCDDs and others.]

(b)   Malignant lymphomas (see **Table 36**)

A case–control study followed the report in Sweden of 17 cases of histiocytic malignant lymphoma, 11 of whom had been exposed to phenoxy herbicides or chlorophenols (Hardell, 1979). All men aged 25–85 years admitted between 1974 and 1978 to the oncology department of the University Hospital in Umeå, Sweden, with histologically verified malignant lymphoma were included in the study (Hardell et al., 1981). For every living

Table 36. Case–control studies on malignant lymphoma containing information on exposure to phenoxy herbicides, chlorophenols or dioxins

Reference, country	No. of cases/ controls	Gender	Exposure	Relative risk (95% CI)	Comments
Hardell *et al.* (1981), Sweden	109 cases with NHL and 60 with Hodgkin's disease/338 controls	Men	Exposure to phenoxy herbicides or chlorophenols for more than one day	6.0 (3.7–9.7)	Odds ratios from matched analysis
			Exposure to phenoxy herbicides for more than one day	4.8 (2.9–8.1)	
			Exposure to chlorophenols for one week continuously or one month discontinuously	8.4 (4.2–16.9)	
Hoar *et al.* (1986), USA	170 with NHL/948	Men	Phenoxy herbicide use	2.2 (1.2–4.1)	Phenoxy herbicide used was almost exclusively 2,4-D. Significant but inconsistent increases in risk were observed in relation to duration, frequency and latency. The increased risk persisted after adjusting for use of other pesticides.
Woods *et al.* (1987), USA	576 with NHL /694	Men	Estimated intensity of exposure to phenoxy herbicides: None Low Medium High	1.0 0.9 (0.6–1.3) 1.0 (0.7–1.3) 1.2 (0.8–1.9)	Higher risks observed for specific occupational groups
			Estimated intensity of exposure to chlorophenols: None Low Medium High	1.0 1.0 (0.7–1.3) 0.9 (0.7–1.2) 0.9 (0.9–1.4)	

Table 36 (contd)

Reference, country	No. of cases/ controls	Gender	Exposure	Relative risk (95% CI)	Comments
Olsson & Brandt (1988), Sweden	167 with NHL/130	Men	One day handling phenoxy herbicides One day handling chlorophenols 'Skin lymphoma' exposed to phenoxy herbicides	1.3 (0.8–2.1) 1.2 (0.7–2.0) 10.0 (2.7–31.1)	Age-adjusted odds ratios. No interactions between exposures. Risk not associated with length of exposure

Woods & Polissar (1989), USA	576 with NHL/694
	
	181/196
		Men	Used more than once or twice per year:
			All subjects
			  'Phenoxy *per se*'
			  2,4,5-T
			Farmers
			  'Phenoxy *per se*'
			  2,4,5-T
				
				0.9 (0.5–1.5)
				1.0 (0.4–2.0)
				
				0.7 (0.3–1.5)
				0.7 (0.3–2.1)
					Mantel-Haenszel estimates

Pearce *et al.* (1987), New Zealand	183 with malignant lymphoma/ 338 cancer controls	Men	Ever potentially exposed to 2,4,5-T Ever potentially exposed to chlorophenols	1.0 (0.7–1.5) 1.4 (0.8–2.3)	No association of the risk with any specific herbicide or with duration or frequency of herbicide use
Cantor *et al.* (1992), USA	622 with NHL/1245	Men	Use of one or more herbicides Ever handling, mixing or applying 2,4-D Ever handling, mixing or applying 2,4,5-T Prior to 1965	1.3 (1.0–1.6) 1.2 (0.9–1.6) 1.2 (0.7–1.9) 1.7 (0.8–3.6)	Odds ratios and CI adjusted for many potential confounding factors. Risk for 2,4,5-T was slightly higher in farmers not using protective equipment
Smith & Christophers (1992), Australia	30 with malignant lymphoma/ 30/30 cancer and population controls	Men	At least one day of exposure to phenoxy herbicides or chlorophenols At least one day only to phenoxy herbicides At least one day only to chlorophenols More than 30 days of exposure to phenoxy herbicides or chlorophenols	1.5 (0.6–3.7) 1.1 (0.4–3.0) 1.4 (0.3–6.1) 2.7 (0.7–9.6)	Exposure to phenoxy herbicides and chlorophenols coded as 'none', 'possible' and 'definite/probable' by expert assessment. Matched analysis on age, gender and residence.

NHL, Non-Hodgkin lymphoma

case (in total 107), eight controls matched for sex, age and place of residence were extracted from the national population registry and the two closest in age were used in the analysis. For the 62 deceased cases, 10 controls per case were selected from the national registry of causes of death among those who had died from causes other than malignant tumour, matched for sex, age, municipality and year of death. The two deceased controls closest in age to the cases were used in the analysis. Exposures were reconstructed by means of a self-administered questionnaire. The data concerning deceased subjects were obtained by contact with next-of-kin. For exposure to phenoxy herbicides or chlorophenols, an odds ratio of 6.0 (95% CI, 3.7–9.7) was obtained. For phenoxy herbicides alone (41 exposed cases), the odds ratios were 4.8 (95% CI, 2.9–8.1) and 7.0 for those exposed for more than 90 days. Five cases and no controls were exposed only to MCPA; 7 cases and 1 control only to 2,4-D. These herbicides were not likely to be contaminated with PCDDs or PCDFs. Fifty cases were exposed to chloro-phenols, giving an odds ratio of 2.9 (95% CI, 1.6–5.2) for those with low-level exposure and 8.4 (95% CI, 4.2–16.9) for high-level exposure. High-level exposure to organic solvents was also associated with a significantly increased risk. Combined exposure to solvents and phenoxy herbicides or chlorophenols further increased the odds ratio estimate. Separate analysis for Hodgkin's disease (60 cases) and non-Hodgkin lymphoma (109 cases) yielded similarly increased risks. [The Working Group noted that no distinction was made between herbicides likely to be contaminated with PCDDs and others.]

A population-based case–control study on lymphoma was conducted in Kansas, a major wheat-producing state in the United States (Hoar *et al.*, 1986). All newly diagnosed cases of Hodgkin's disease and non-Hodgkin lymphoma among white male residents in Kansas aged 21 years or older, diagnosed from 1976 through 1982, were identified through the population-based cancer registry covering the state of Kansas. All cases included in the study were histologically confirmed. Interviews were conducted with 121 cases with Hodgkin's disease and 170 with non-Hodgkin lymphoma (96% participation rate). One-half of the patients with non-Hodgkin lymphoma and one-third of those with Hodgkin's disease had died before the study began. Controls were 948 white men resident in Kansas matched to cases for age and vital status. The response rate for controls was 94%. Subjects were interviewed by telephone and detailed information was obtained concerning farming practices, including years lived or worked in farms, crops grown or livestock raised, herbicides and insecticides used, numbers of years and acres of treatment and protective equipment used. Corroborative evidence was sought for a sample of 130 subjects by contacting their suppliers. Farm herbicide use was associated with an increased risk for non-Hodgkin lymphoma (odds ratio, 1.6; 95% CI, 0.9–2.6). The relative risk for non-Hodgkin lymphoma increased significantly with the number of days of herbicide exposure per year and with latency. Men exposed to herbicides for more than 20 days per year had a six-fold increased risk for non-Hodgkin lymphoma (odds ratio, 6.0; 95% CI, 1.9–19.5). Frequent users (> 20 years per year) who mixed or applied the herbicides themselves had an odds ratio of 8.0 (95% CI, 2.3–27.9). Use of phenoxy herbicides (odds ratio, 2.2; 95% CI, 1.2–4.1) essentially indicated use of 2,4-D, since only three cases and 18 controls had used 2,4,5-T, and all but two of these controls had also used 2,4-D. Farm herbicide use was not associated with risk for Hodgkin's disease (odds ratio, 0.9; 95% CI, 0.5–1.5). For this neoplasm, no consistent pattern of excess risk was observed either with duration or frequency of exposure. The authors noted that the observed excess risk for non-Hodgkin lymphoma was associated with exposure to phenoxy herbicides (2,4-D) which were not contaminated with 2,3,7,8-TCDD, although they might be contaminated with other PCDD congeners.

A population-based case–control study from western Washington State (Woods *et al.*, 1987), described above, included 576 non-Hodgkin lymphoma cases (402 alive, 174 dead). Population controls were selected using random digit dialling or from social security records (for older cases) or non-cancer death certificates (for deceased cases). Controls were frequency matched for age and vital status with the non-Hodgkin lymphoma cases. The participation rate was 77% for non-Hodgkin lymphoma cases and 76% for controls. The risk for non-Hodgkin lymphoma associated with all occupations involving potential exposure to phenoxy herbicides was 1.1 (95% CI, 0.8–1.4). Exposure to phenoxy herbicides or chlorophenols was not associated with increased risk for non-Hodgkin lymphoma. No association was seen with estimated intensity of exposure to either phenoxy herbicides or chlorophenols. A statistically significant excess risk for non-Hodgkin lymphoma was observed for specific occupational groups, including farmers (odds ratio, 1.3; 95% CI, 1.0–1.7) and subjects spraying forests with herbicides (odds ratio, 4.8; 95% CI, 1.2–19.4). All forestry sprayers reported combined use of 2,4-D and 2,4,5-T. [The Working Group noted that no information was provided on use of specific herbicides.]

Following the same methodology, a population-based case–control study was conducted in western Washington State on non-Hodgkin lymphoma and phenoxy herbicide exposure in farmers (Woods & Polissar, 1989). Cases of non-Hodgkin lymphoma occurring between 1983 and 1985 were identified from the cancer surveillance system. A total of 694 control men without cancer selected randomly from the same geographical area were matched with the 576 cases by five-year age group and vital status. Among them, 181 non-Hodgkin lymphoma cases and 196 controls reported having worked as farmers. Information on exposure to phenoxy herbicides was obtained through personal interviews. Regular use was defined as 'more than just once or twice per year'. Mantel–Haenszel odds ratios were calculated for farmers, for all subjects for 2,4,5-T and for 'phenoxy *per se*' exposures, among others. No excess risks were observed in all subjects nor in the group of farmers for the above exposures: for 2,4,5-T, the odds ratios were 0.7 (95% CI, 0.3–2.1) in farmers and 1.0 (95% CI, 0.4–2.0) for all subjects; for 'phenoxy *per se*', the odds ratios were 0.7 (95% CI, 0.3–1.5) and 0.9 (95% CI, 0.5–1.5), respectively.

Pearce *et al.* (1987) expanded a previously reported case–control study on malignant lymphomas and farming in New Zealand (Pearce *et al.*, 1986). The study included male public hospital patients registered under ICD codes 200 or 202 during the period 1977–81, who were under the age of 70 years. All cases were pathologically verified. Out of a total of 215 eligible cases, 183 cases were enrolled in the study (participation rate 85%). For each of the cases, two cancer controls were randomly selected from the cancer registry files, matched for age and year of cancer registration. In total, 338 controls were enrolled (81% participation rate). Interviews were conducted by telephone with the patients or their next-of-kin [no information was given on the proportion of interviews with next-of-kin]. Information was requested concerning work in particular occupations with potential exposure to phenoxy herbicides or chlorophenols. If the response to a stem question was affirmative, then a series of subsidiary questions were asked to clarify the work done and the actual potential for exposure to specific chemicals. Exposure to phenoxy herbicides and chlorophenols was ascertained through a combination of information on occupation, industry, type of cultivation sprayed and self-reported exposure to specific agents. The proportions of cases and controls who had worked in the occupations examined in this study were very similar. The odds ratio for any potential exposure to phenoxy herbicides was 1.0 (95% CI, 0.7–1.5) and none of the odds ratios relating to specific phenoxy herbicides was elevated. The odds ratio for any potential exposure to chlorophenols was slightly elevated (odds ratio, 1.4; 95% CI, 0.8–2.3), largely due to the results for meat workers, which included workers potentially exposed to 2,4,6-TCP in pelt departments. In a re-analysis of the data (Pearce, 1989), little evidence was found of an association of non-Hodgkin lymphoma either with duration or with frequency of phenoxy herbicide use. Findings were similar in the earlier publication using general population controls (Pearce *et al.*, 1986). [The Working Group noted that no distinction was made between herbicides likely to be contaminated with PCDDs and others.]

Olsson and Brandt (1988) examined the lifetime work history of 167 incident cases of non-Hodgkin lymphoma diagnosed at a hospital in Lund (Sweden) between 1978 and 1981 in adult men and in 130 age-matched population controls, 50 from the same geographical area as the cases and 80 from different parts of Sweden. Exposure to organic solvents, phenoxy herbicides and chlorophenols was given special attention. Interviewers were not blind to subject status (case or control). One day of handling was taken to constitute exposure to phenoxy acids or chlorophenols. Odds ratios were estimated using logistic models, adjusting for age. The roles of different exposures, of their interaction and of length of exposure were examined using logistic regression analysis. In the multivariate analysis, the odds ratio for exposure to phenoxy herbicides was 1.3 (95% CI, 0.8–2.1) and that for chlorophenols was 1.2 (95% CI, 0.7–2.0). Separate analysis for localized 'skin lymphoma' yielded a significantly increased risk (odds ratio, 10.0; 95% CI, 2.7–37.1) for exposure to phenoxy herbicides. No interaction between exposures was detected. Risk for non-Hodgkin lymphoma was significantly associated with length of exposure to solvents but not to phenoxy herbicides and chlorophenols. [The Working Group noted that no distinction was made between herbicides likely to be contaminated with PCDDs and others.]

Concurrent population-based case–control interview studies of leukaemia, non-Hodgkin lymphoma and multiple myeloma in Iowa, United States, and leukaemia and non-Hodgkin lymphoma in Minnesota, United States, were conducted during 1981–84. The studies used the same questionnaire and the same controls. Results from the case–control study on non-Hodgkin lymphoma were reported by Cantor *et al.* (1992). Results for the studies on leukaemia (Morris Brown *et al.*, 1990) and multiple myeloma (Morris

Brown *et al.*, 1993) are described in Section 2.2.2(*c*). All male cases of non-Hodgkin lymphoma aged 30 years or older and newly diagnosed during 1980–82 were ascertained from Iowa State Health Registry records and a special surveillance of Minnesota hospitals and pathology laboratory records. Residents of Iowa and of selected areas of Minnesota were eligible. A review panel of four pathologists confirmed diagnoses. Out of 780 reported non-Hodgkin lymphoma cases, 622 (438 living, 184 deceased) were confirmed as non-Hodgkin lymphoma and interviewed. The participation rate was slightly above 80% [exact proportion not estimable]. A population control group of 1245 white men without haematopoietic or lymphatic cancer was randomly selected and frequency matched with the non-Hodgkin lymphoma and leukaemia cases by five-year age group, vital status at time of interview and state of residence. Random digit dialling was used to select controls for living cases under 65 years of age. A 1% random listing of Medicare files was used for the selection of controls for living cases over 65 years of age. State death certificates were used for deceased cases. The participation rate was around 77% in all three groups of controls. Direct structured interviews were conducted during 1981–84. Detailed information on farming and pesticide use was requested for all subjects who had worked on a farm for at least six months since the age of 18 years. The information recorded included years of farming activity, total acreage, crops grown and detailed history of pesticide use. There was a small increase in risk (odds ratio, 1.2; 95% CI, 1.0–1.5) associated with ever living or working on a farm. The odds ratio for use of one or more herbicides was 1.3 (95% CI, 1.0–1.6), but no single family of herbicides was significantly associated with risk for non-Hodgkin lymphoma. No significant risk elevations were observed for ever handling, mixing or applying specific phenoxy herbicides. The odds ratio for 2,4-D was 1.2 (95%, 0.9–1.6) and that for 2,4,5-T was 1.2 (95% CI, 0.7–1.9). The risk for 2,4,5-T was slightly higher among farmers who did not use protective gear (odds ratio, 1.4; 95% CI, 0.7–2.5). The odds ratios for handling these herbicides before 1965 (assuming a latency of about 15 years) were 1.3 (95% CI, 0.9–1.8) for 2,4-D and 1.7 (95% CI, 0.8–3.6) for 2,4,5-T. The authors stated that there was minimal confounding of results for any single pesticide by exposure to pesticides belonging to other chemical families.

The case–control study conducted in Victoria, Australia, described in Section 2.2.2(*a*) (Smith & Christophers, 1992), also included 52 male cases with malignant lymphoma. The odds ratios for malignant lymphoma were 1.5 (95% CI, 0.6–3.7) for at least one day's exposure to phenoxy herbicides or chlorophenols, 1.1 (95% CI, 0.4–3.0) for exposure only to phenoxy herbicides and 1.4 (95% CI, 0.3–6.1) for exposure only to chlorophenols. The odds ratio for more than 30 days of exposure to phenoxy herbicides or chlorophenols was 2.7 (95% CI, 0.7–9.6). [The Working Group noted that no distinction was made between herbicides likely to be contaminated with PCDDs and others.]

(*c*)   *Other haematopoietic malignancies* (see **Table 37**)

A case–control study on leukaemia was conducted in Iowa and Minnesota, United States (Morris Brown *et al.*, 1990) using the same methodology and same control group as that described in Section 2.2.2(*b*) (Cantor *et al.*, 1992). All newly diagnosed cases of

Table 37. Case–control studies on other tumour sites containing information on exposure to phenoxy herbicides, chlorophenols or dioxins

Reference, country	No. of cases/ controls	Gender	Exposure	Relative risk (95% CI)	Comments
Leukaemia					
Morris-Brown et al. (1990), USA	578/1245	Men	Use of one or more herbicides	1.2 (0.9–1.6)	Cases (340 living/238 deceased). Adjusted for vital status, age, state, tobacco, family history, high-risk occupations and exposures. No consistent dose–response pattern by days per year handled for any herbicide used
			Use of phenoxy herbicides	1.2 (0.9–1.6)	
			Exposure to 2,4,5-T (20 years before interview)	1.8 (0.8–4.0)	
			Mixed, handled or applied 2,4,5-T		
			Acute non-lymphocytic leukaemia	2.1 (0.9–4.9)	
			Chronic lymphocytic leukaemia	1.6 (0.7–3.4)	
			Mixed, handled or applied 2,4,5-T at least 20 years before interview		
			Chronic lymphocytic leukaemia	3.3 (1.2–8.9)	
Multiple myeloma					
Morris-Brown et al. (1993), USA	173/650	Men	Mixed, handled or applied 2,4,5-T	0.9 (0.4–2.1)	Adjusted for vital status and age by logistic regression
Liver					
Hardell et al. (1984), Sweden	103/206	Men	Exposure to phenoxy herbicides and chlorophenols	1.8 (0.9–4.0)	Analysis restricted to 98 hepatocellular and cholangiocellular carcinomas and 200 controls with exposure data. Mantel–Haenszel estimates adjusted by alcohol consumption
			Exposure to phenoxy herbicides only	1.7 (0.7–4.4)	
			Exposure to chlorophenols only for one week continuously or one month discontinuously	2.2 (0.7–7.3)	
Cordier et al. (1993), Viet Nam	152/241	Men	Exposure to Agent Orange during military service in south Viet Nam		Cases were hepatocellular carcinoma. Risks adjusted for matching variables, hepatitis virus status and alcohol
			Any service	1.3 (0.8–2.1)	
			10 years or more	8.8 (1.9–41)	

Table 37 (contd)

Reference, country	No. of cases/ controls	Gender	Exposure	Relative risk (95% CI)	Comments
Colon					

Hardell (1981), Sweden	157/451	Men	More than one day of exposure to:
			  Phenoxy herbicides
			  Chlorophenols
				1.3 (0.6–2.8)
				1.8 (0.6–5.3)
					Mantel-Haenszel estimates adjusted by age, vital status and place of residence

Nasopharynx + nasal					
Hardell *et al.* (1982), Sweden	71/541	Men	Exposure to phenoxy herbicides for more than one day Exposure to chlorophenols for one week continuously or one month discontinuously	2.1 (0.9–4.7) 6.7 (2.8–16.2)	Mantel-Haenszel estimates adjusted by age and vital status

leukaemia among white men aged 30 years or older were ascertained from tumour registry or hospital records retrospectively (one year before the start of the study) or prospectively (two years after the start of the study). Interviews were completed with 86% of the cases (or next-of-kin). The final study population consisted of 578 cases (340 living, 238 deceased) and 1245 population controls. Apart from the main interview (described above), a supplementary interview was conducted including 92 cases and 211 controls (or their next-of-kin) from Iowa who had reported agricultural use of pesticides in their initial interview. There was a small risk for all leukaemias among persons who had lived or worked on a farm as an adult (odds ratio, 1.2; 95% CI, 1.0–1.5). A similar risk was seen for farmers reporting ever having used herbicides (odds ratio, 1.2; 95% CI, 0.9–1.6) or phenoxy herbicides (odds ratio, 1.2; 95% CI, 0.9–1.6). Risks for all leukaemias were not significantly increased among subjects who personally mixed, handled or applied specific herbicides. When analyses were restricted to persons first exposed to specific herbicides more than 20 years before interview, increased risks were observed for exposure to MCPA (odds ratio, 2.4; 95% CI, 0.7–8.2) and 2,4,5-T (odds ratio, 1.8; 95% CI, 0.8–4.0). Among specific cell types, the highest risk for those who handled 2,4-D was seen for chronic myelogenous leukaemia (odds ratio, 1.9; 95% CI, 0.9–3.9). The odds ratios for those who handled 2,4,5-T were 2.1 (95% CI, 0.9–4.9) for acute non-lymphocytic leukaemia and 1.6 (95% CI, 0.7–3.4) for chronic lymphocytic leukaemia. The risk for those who handled 2,4,5-T at least 20 years before interview was significantly elevated for chronic lymphocytic leukaemia (odds ratio, 3.3; 95% CI, 1.2–8.9). No consistent dose–response pattern in terms of days of handling per year was seen for any of the herbicides used.

A case–control study on multiple myeloma was conducted in Iowa, United States (Morris-Brown *et al.*, 1993), using the same methodology and same control group as that described above in Section 2.2.2(*b*) (Cantor *et al.*, 1992). All cases of multiple myeloma among adult white men aged 30 years or older and diagnosed during 1981–84 were identified from the Iowa State Health Registry. Pathological material and laboratory reports were reviewed by an expert pathologist. Included the study were 173 cases (101 alive, 72 deceased) and 650 controls (452 alive, 198 deceased). Interviews were completed for 84% of multiple myeloma cases and 78% of controls. Some farming activity was reported by 64% of the cases and 58% of the controls (odds ratio, 1.2; 95% CI, 0.8–1.7). Risks were not elevated for subjects who handled the phenoxy herbicides 2,4-D (odds ratio, 1.0; 95% CI, 0.6–1.6) or 2,4,5-T (odds ratio, 0.9; 95% CI, 0.4–2.1).

(*d*)   *Other solid tumours* (**Table 37**)

Hardell (1981) conducted a case–control study on colon cancer patients following the same methodology as that described earlier (see Section 2.2.2(*a*); Hardell & Sändstrom, 1979; Eriksson *et al.*, 1981; Hardell *et al.*, 1981). Cases were 157 men with colon cancer (response rate, 98.1%) aged 25–85 years who were residents of the region of Umeå, Sweden, and who had been reported to the Swedish Cancer Registry in 1978–79. All had a histopathological diagnosis of adenocarcinoma. Sixty-five cases (41%) were deceased. The 541 controls were derived from two earlier studies (Hardell & Sändstrom, 1979; Hardell *et al.*, 1981). A low excess risk was observed for exposure to phenoxy herbicides (odds ratio, 1.3; 95% CI, 0.6–2.8) and for exposure to chlorophenols (odds ratio, 1.8; 95% CI, 0.6–5.3). [The Working Group noted that no distinction was made between herbicides likely to be contaminated with PCDDs and others.]

In a case–control study on nasal and nasopharyngeal cancer in the region of Umeå, Sweden, Hardell et al. (1982) followed the same methodology as that described above (Hardell & Sändstrom, 1979; Hardell et al., 1981). The cases comprised all male patients aged 25–85 years with histopathologically confirmed nasopharyngeal cancer (n = 27) and cancer of the nose and nasal sinuses (n = 44). All cases had been reported to the Swedish Cancer Registry in 1970–79 and were residents in the three most northern counties of Sweden. The 541 controls were derived from two earlier studies in the same region (Hardell & Sändstrom, 1979; Hardell et al., 1981). Fifty (70.4%) of the cases were deceased, compared with 245 (45.3%) of the controls. [No information was provided on response rates.] Exposure to phenoxy herbicides was associated with a two-fold risk for the combination of nasopharyngeal and nasal cavity cancer (odds ratio, 2.1; 95% CI, 0.9–4.7). A high risk was found for high-level exposure to chlorophenol, defined as a cumulative exposure of one week of continuous or one month of discontinuous exposure (odds ratio, 6.7; 95% CI, 2.8–16.2). No obvious difference was reported between cases and controls for low-level exposure to chlorophenols. The risk associated with use of chlorophenol exposure was higher among wood workers (odds ratio, 8.4) than in other occupations (odds ratio, 2.7) but, in a stratified analysis, it was shown that occupation as a wood worker was not a confounding factor for exposure to chlorophenols. [The Working Group noted that no distinction was made between herbicides likely to be contaminated with PCDDs and others.]

Men aged 25–80 who had been diagnosed with liver cancer between 1974 and 1981 and reported to the Department of Oncology, Umeå, Sweden, were included in another case–control study (Hardell et al., 1984). Microscope slides were reviewed for the 166 assembled cases, and 103 cases of primary liver cancer were retained for the study; 206 population-based controls were matched with cases for age and residence. Information on exposure was obtained as in previous studies (see Hardell & Sandström, 1979); responses were obtained for 102 cases and 200 controls. The analyses were restricted to the 98 cases of hepatocellular and cholangiocellular carcinoma. Odds ratios, without controlling for other agricultural exposures, were 1.8 (95% CI, 0.9–4.0) for exposure to phenoxy herbicides and chlorophenols, 1.7 (95% CI, 0.7–4.4) for exposure to phenoxy herbicides only and 2.2 (95% CI, 0.7–7.3) for high-level exposure to chlorophenols only. [The Working Group noted that no distinction was made between herbicides likely to be contaminated with PCDDs and others.]

A case–control study conducted in two hospitals in Hanoi (Viet Nam) between 1989 and 1992 included 152 male cases of hepatocellular carcinoma and 241 hospital controls, admitted mainly in abdominal surgery departments, matched for age, sex and area of residence at the time of admission (Cordier et al., 1993). Exposure to Agent Orange may have occurred during stays in the south of Viet Nam after 1960 (date of the beginning of spraying missions) especially for military purposes. Duration of military service in the south, for North Vietnamese soldiers, was considered as a proxy for exposure to Agent

Orange. This is justified by the fact that sprayings were principally aimed at uncovering trails used by the Vietnamese combatants, who stayed one or two years on average in these areas and consumed locally grown (and contaminated) foodstuffs. The overall odds ratio associated with military service in the south was 1.3 (95% CI, 0.8–2.1). The risk rose with increasing duration of stay in the south, reaching 8.8 (95% CI, 1.9–41) after 10 years. Odds ratios were adjusted for matching variables (hospital, age, area of residence), hepatitis B virus surface antigen, anti-hepatitis C virus status and alcohol consumption.

2.3 Combined evidence from high-exposure human populations

Causal inference about the effects of chemicals can best be drawn from studies with well documented exposures. It is important to focus on human studies in which it is clear that exposure to the chemical in question actually occurred. The ideal is to have biological markers of such exposure. In the case of 2,3,7,8-TCDD, the long half-life in humans means that recent biological measurements allow assessment of past human exposure. In addition, chloracne may be an indication of exposure for some studies, although its absence does not rule out exposure.

The most informative studies for causal inference are those with the highest exposures, which if they are causal will produce the highest cancer risks. For these reasons, the Working Group abstracted from published studies data concerning the most highly exposed populations studied in the world. Evidence for their exposure being high is given in Section 1.3.1 (see **Table 22**). The Working Group focused on the most exposed sub-cohorts within cohorts, and also confined its attention to findings with adequate latency when available. The reasons for doing this are that if associations are truly causal, they will become more apparent at the highest exposures with adequate latency. Such studies are identified in **Table 38**. The first line gives the results from the large international cohort study conducted by IARC. The next lines give data from four separate cohorts of industrial production workers, three of which were included within this large cohort. These have been selected because of known high exposure to 2,3,7,8-TCDD, whereas the total combined IARC cohort also included sub-cohorts with much lower exposure. Data from the community exposures resulting from the Seveso accident, although high exposures, are not included because of inadequate duration of follow-up since the accident.

The focus of attention within each of the published studies has been on all cancers combined, and on particular sites of interest, namely cancers of the lung and gastrointestinal tract, non-Hodgkin lymphoma and soft-tissue sarcoma. Observed numbers, SMRs and 95% CIs are given for each of these sites for each study. Below the presentation of the high-exposure industrial cohorts are summary estimates by the Working Group obtained by adding the observed and expected numbers for all cancers combined and each cancer site.

There is an overall increase in mortality from all cancers combined in the high-exposure industrial cohorts in several studies. The overall SMR for all cancers combined calculated by the Working Group was 1.4 (95% CI, 1.2–1.6). Although this overall SMR is low, these findings concerning all cancers are most unlikely to be due to chance, and

Table 38. Summary of the combined international cohort and selected industrial cohort studies with high exposure levels

Reference	All cancers			Lung cancer			Non-Hodgkin lymphoma			Soft-tissue sarcoma			Gastrointestinal cancer		
	Obs.	SMR	95% CI	Obs.	SMR	95% CI	Obs.	SMR	95% CI	Obs.	SMR	95% CI	Obs.	SMR	95% CI
International cohort															
Kogevinas et al. (1997)[a]	394	1.2	1.1–1.3	127	1.2	1.0–1.4	14	1.6	0.9–2.7	3	2.3	0.5–6.6	190	1.0	0.9–1.2
Industrial populations (high-exposure subcohorts)															
Fingerhut et al. (1991a)[b] (USA)	114	1.5	1.2–1.8	40	1.4	1.0–1.9	2	0.9	0.1–3.4	3	9.2	1.9–27.0	28	1.4	0.9–2.0
Becher et al. (1996)[c] (Germany)	105	[1.3]	[1.0–1.5]	33	[1.4]	[1.0–2.0]	6	[4.6]	[1.7–10.0]	0	0.0	–	27	[0.9]	[0.6–1.4]
Hooiveld et al. (1996a)[d] (Netherlands)	51	1.5	1.1–1.9	14	1.0	0.5–1.7	3	3.8	0.8–11.0	0	0.00	–	NR		
Ott & Zober (1996)[e] (BASF, accident)	18	1.9	1.1–3.0	7	2.4	1.0–5.0	NR			NR			6	1.8	0.7–4.0
Total	[288]	[1.4]	[1.2–1.6]	[94]	[1.4]	[1.1–1.7]	[11]	[2.6]	[1.3–4.7]	[3]	[4.7]		[61]	[1.2]	[0.9–1.5]
p value		*< 0.001*			*< 0.01*			*< 0.01*						*0.23*	

NR, not reported

[a] Kogevinas et al. (1997): men and women > 20 years since first exposure, except for digestive cancer for which no latency data were available. These data include the cohorts of Fingerhut et al. (1991a,b), Becher et al. (1996), Hooiveld et al. (1996a), the original IARC cohort (Saracci et al., 1991) and other cohorts.

[b] Fingerhut et al. (1991a): Men ≥ 20 years latency and > 1 year exposure

[c] Becher et al. (1996): Men, Cohort I and II, summed (Boehringer-Ingelheim, Bayer-Uerdingen cohorts)

[d] Hooiveld et al. (1996a): Men and women, Factory A

[e] Ott & Zober (1996): Men, chloracne subgroup, ≥ 20 years latency. Data presented for lung cancer are all respiratory tract cancers combined. No data were available for soft-tissue sarcoma and non-Hodgkin lymphoma.

are consistent across the studies with the highest exposure. Increases in all cancers combined of this magnitude have rarely been found in occupational cohorts.

The combined SMR for lung cancer was calculated to be 1.4 (95% CI, 1.1–1.7). The findings are unlikely to be due to chance. It is the view of the Working Group that these lung cancer results are not the result of confounding by cigarette smoking. As with all cancers combined, the strength of association is again low .

The overall estimate for non-Hodgkin lymphoma was significantly elevated [SMR, 2.6; 95% CI, 1.3–4.7], but there was no increased risk in the large NIOSH cohort. The SMR for gastrointestinal cancer was 1.2 (95% CI, 0.9–1.5). For soft-tissue sarcoma, the overall SMR was approximately 4.7 [calculated by the Working Group, estimating expected values of 0.20 and 0.12 for Becher *et al.* (1996) and Hooiveld *et al.* (1996a) respectively].

The available dose–response data are presented in **Table 39**. Two studies give dose–response relationship data for all cancers combined based on evidence for 2,3,7,8-TCDD exposure. In the Boehringer-Ingelheim cohort (cohort I in Becher *et al.*), the relative risks are given for seven levels of toxic equivalents for 2,3,7,8-TCDD (Flesch-Janys *et al.*, 1995). The rate ratios fluctuate, but there is a clear elevation for the highest exposure group, which involves workers with markedly higher blood and fat 2,3,7,8-TCDD levels than for the other categories (RR, 2.7; 95% CI, 1.7–4.4). The overall test for trend resulted in a *p* value less than 0.01, but this is largely the result of the high RR for the highest exposure group.

The second study giving dose–response data for all cancers involves the BASF accident cohort, based on the entire cohort (*n* = 243). Workers were divided into four categories of measured and estimated 2,3,7,8-TCDD levels. There was a trend for increasing SMR with measured exposure up to a relative risk of 2.0 (95% CI, 0.8–4.0). The test for trend using cumulative dose as a continuous variable in Cox's regression analysis yielded confidence intervals indicating a *p* value of 0.05. Thus this study and the Boehringer-Ingelheim cohort together provide dose–response evidence supporting a causal relationship between 2,3,7,8-TCDD exposure and mortality from all cancers combined. Further subdivision of the data indicates that the positive dose–response was restricted to smokers.

Concerning specific cancer sites, dose–response information from highly exposed populations is available in one publication only involving two cancer sites, non-Hodgkin lymphoma and soft-tissue sarcoma. For each site, there are trends of increasing risks with increasing exposures classified as low, medium and high. While confidence limits are broad, the test for trend gave *p* values of 0.1 for non-Hodgkin lymphoma and 0.04 for soft-tissue sarcoma.

In summary, the epidemiological evidence from the most highly 2,3,7,8-TCDD-exposed populations studied produces strong evidence of increased risks for all cancers combined, along with less strong evidence of increased risks for cancers of particular sites. This situation appears to be unique, compared with established human carcinogens. The overall findings are unlikely to be due to chance. There is no obvious basis to infer

Table 39. Cohort or nested case–control studies of industrial workers presenting dose–response data

Boehringer-Ingelheim cohort, Germany (Flesch-Janys, 1996), all cancers

PCDD/PCDF TEQ (ng/blood fat)[a]	Rate ratio	(95% CI)
0	1.0	
1.0–12.2	1.0	(0.6–1.8)
12.3–39.5	1.3	(0.8–2.1)
39.6–98.9	1.2	(0.7–1.9)
99.0–278.5	1.2	(0.8–1.9)
278.6–545.0	1.3	(0.7–2.3)
545.1–4 361.9	2.7	(1.7–4.4)
Test for linear trend $p < 0.01$		

BASF accident cohort, Germany (Ott & Zober, 1996), all cancers

2,3,7,8-TCDD (µg/kg bw)	No. of subjects	No. of deaths	SMR	(95% CI)
< 0.1	108	8	0.8	(0.4–1.6)
0.1–0.99	66	8	1.2	(0.5–2.3)
1.0–1.99	47	8	1.4	(0.6–2.7)
≥ 2.0	22	7	2.0	(0.8–4.0)
	[$p = 0.05$]			

IARC nested case–control study (Kogevinas et al., 1995)

2,3,7,8-TCDD exposure	Number of cases/controls	Odds ratio	(95% CI)
Non-Hodgkin lymphoma			
Non-exposed	21/119	1.0	
Low	4/18	1.4	(0.4–4.6)
Medium	3/8	3.6	(0.7–18.7)
High	4/13	3.6	(0.6–19.2)
Test for linear trend $p = 0.1$			
Soft-tissue sarcoma			
Non-exposed	6/42	1.0	
Low	1/4	2.8	(0.1–54.8)
Medium	1/4	6.6	(0.1–540)
High	3/5	10.6	(0.6–671)
Test for linear trend $p = 0.04$			

[a] Estimated German PCDD/PCDF TEQ levels at the end of exposure above German median background

that the findings are due to confounding with smoking, nor with occupational exposures to other chemicals, but such confounding cannot be ruled out. There is evidence in some studies of dose–response relationships, although dose–response data are not available for some of the largest studies. The relative risk estimates for all cancers, lung cancer and gastrointestinal cancer involve relatively low strengths of association. Higher relative risk estimates are present in some studies concerning non-Hodgkin lymphoma and soft-tissue sarcoma, but the total numbers of cancers are small, in particular for soft-tissue sarcoma.

3.   Studies of Cancer in Experimental Animals

2,3,7,8-Tetrachlorodibenzo-*para*-dioxin (2,3,7,8-TCDD)

Long-term carcinogenicity studies of 2,3,7,8-TCDD in experimental animals are summarized in **Table 40**.

3.1   Oral administration

3.1.1   *Mouse*

Groups of 45 male outbred Swiss/H/Riop mice, 10 weeks of age, were given gastric instillations of 0.007, 0.7 or 7.0 µg/kg bw 2,3,7,8-TCDD [purity unspecified] dissolved in sunflower oil once a week for one year. A control group received vehicle only. Animals were followed for the rest of their life span. Survival was significantly decreased in the high-dose animals (average life span, 424 days compared with 588 days in controls). It was reported that all organs [unspecified] were examined histologically. Treatment with 2,3,7,8-TCDD caused severe chronic, ulcerous skin lesions, followed by generalized lethal amyloidosis and was associated with an increased incidence of liver tumours (hepatocellular adenomas and carcinomas combined) [the two histological types were not reported separately]: control, 7/38; low-dose, 13/44; mid-dose, 21/44 ($p < 0.01$, χ^2 test) and high-dose, 13/43. No statistically significant increase in the incidence of lung tumours or lymphomas was observed (Toth *et al.*, 1979). [The Working Group noted that mortality-adjusted analysis was not performed and, therefore, the tumour incidence in the high-dose group may be underestimated.]

Groups of 50 male and 50 female B6C3F1 mice, six weeks of age, were given gastric instillations of 0.01, 0.05 or 0.5 µg/kg bw (males) and 0.04, 0.2 or 2.0 µg/kg bw (females) 2,3,7,8-TCDD (purity, 99.4%) in a vehicle of 9 : 1 corn oil–acetone twice a week for 104 weeks. One control group of 75 males and 75 females received vehicle alone and another group of 50 males and 50 females was untreated. Mean body weights of the treated groups were comparable with those of the vehicle-control group. Treatment did not affect survival: 30/50 untreated control, 38/74 vehicle-control, 30/50 low-dose, 31/50 mid-dose and 31/50 high-dose males were still alive at 105–107 weeks and 34/50 untreated control, 58/75 vehicle-control, 37/50 low-dose, 36/50 mid-dose and 32/50 high-dose females were still alive at 106–107 weeks. Treatment-related increases in

Table 40. Summary of long-term carcinogenicity studies on 2,3,7,8-TCDD in experimental animals

Species	Sex	Dose and route	Target organ	Tumour type	Lowest effective dose for significant increase in tumours	Reference
Mouse	M	0.007, 0.7, 7.0 µg/kg bw orally once a week for 1 year and observed for lifetime	Liver	Hepatocellular adenoma and carcinoma	0.7 µg/kg/bw	Toth *et al.* (1979)
	M	0.01, 0.05, 0.5 µg/kg bw orally twice a week, 104 weeks	Liver Lung	Hepatocellular carcinoma Alveolar/bronchiolar adenomas or carcinoma	Dose-related trend Dose-related trend	United States National Toxicology Program (1982a)
	F	0.04, 0.2, 2.0 µg/kg bw orally twice a week, 104 weeks	Liver Thyroid Haematopoietic system Skin	Hepatocellular carcinoma Follicle-cell adenoma Lymphoma Subcutaneous fibrosarcoma	Dose-related trend Dose-related trend Dose-related trend Dose-related trend	
	F	0.005 µg/animal, skin, 3 times per week for 104 weeks	Integumentary system	Fibrosarcoma	0.001 µg/animal	United States National Toxicology Program (1982b)
	M	2.5, 5.0 µg/kg bw orally once a week for 52 weeks, followed until 104 weeks of age	Liver	Hepatocellular carcinoma	2.5 µg/kg bw	Della Porta *et al.* (1987)
	F	2.5, 5.0 µg/kg bw orally once a week for 52 weeks, followed until 104 weeks of age	Liver	Hepatocellular carcinoma	2.5 µg/kg bw	

Table 40 (contd)

Species	Sex	Dose and route	Target organ	Tumour type	Lowest effective dose for significant increase in tumours	Reference
Mouse (immature)	M	1, 30, 60 μg/kg bw i.p. once a week for 5 weeks and observed until 78 weeks of age	Thymus Liver	Lymphoma Hepatocellular adenoma and carcinoma	Dose-related trend Dose-related trend	Della Porta *et al.* (1987) (contd)
	F	1, 30, 60 μg/kg bw i.p. once a week for 5 weeks and observed until 78 weeks of age	Thymus Liver	Lymphoma Hepatocellular adenoma and carcinoma	Dose-related trend Dose-related trend	
Rat	M	22, 210, 2200 ppt in diet, for 2 yrs (equiv. to 0.001, 0.01, 0.1 μg/kg bw)	Hard palate Nasal turbinates Tongue	Squamous-cell carcinoma Squamous-cell carcinoma Squamous-cell carcinoma	0.1 μg/kg bw 0.1 μg/kg bw 0.1 μg/kg bw	Kociba *et al.* (1978)
	F	22, 210, 2200 ppt in diet, for 2 yrs (equiv. to 0.001, 0.01, 0.1 μg/kg bw)	Liver Liver Hard palate Nasal turbinates Lung Tongue	Hyperplastic nodule Hepatocellular carcinoma Squamous-cell carcinoma Squamous-cell carcinoma Squamous-cell carcinoma Squamous-cell carcinoma	0.01 μg/kg bw 0.1 μg/kg bw 0.1 μg/kg bw 0.1 μg/kg bw 0.1 μg/kg bw 0.1 μg/kg bw	
	M	0.01, 0.05, 0.5 μg/kg bw orally, twice a week, 104 weeks	Thyroid Liver	Follicular-cell adenoma Neoplastic nodule	Dose-related trend Dose-related trend	United States National Toxicology Program (1982a)
	F	0.01, 0.05, 0.5 μg/kg bw orally, twice a week, 104 weeks	Thyroid Liver	Follicular-cell adenomas Neoplastic nodules	0.5 μg/kg bw 0.5 μg/kg bw	
Hamster	M	50, 100 μg/kg bw i.p. or s.c. 6 times at 4 wk intervals and observed for 1 year	Skin	Squamous-cell carcinomas	100 μg/kg bw	Rao *et al.* (1988)

i.p., intraperitoneally; s.c., subcutaneously

hepatotoxicity were found in high-dose animals of both sexes. The incidences of hepato-cellular carcinoma were dose-related, with significantly higher incidence in the high-dose groups (males, $p = 0.002$; females, $p = 0.014$, Fisher's exact test) than in the vehicle-control groups (males: vehicle-control, 8/73; low-dose, 9/49; mid-dose, 8/49; and high-dose, 17/50; females: vehicle-control, 1/73; low-dose, 2/50; mid-dose, 2/48; and high-dose, 6/47; males, $p = 0.002$; females, $p = 0.008$ Cochran–Armitage test for trend). Dose-related increases in the incidence of follicular-cell adenomas of the thyroid were observed in female mice, with significantly higher incidence ($p = 0.009$) in the high-dose group than in the vehicle-control group (vehicle-control, 0/69; low-dose, 3/50; mid-dose, 1/47; and high-dose, 5/46; $p = 0.016$ for trend). In female mice, there was a significant increase in the incidence of lymphomas at the high dose (18/74 controls, 11/50 low-dose, 13/48 mid-dose and 20/47 high-dose; $p = 0.029$). There was also a significant increase in the incidence of subcutaneous fibrosarcomas in high-dose females (1/74 controls, 1/50 low-dose, 1/48 mid-dose and 5/47 high-dose; $p = 0.032$). A dose-related increase ($p = 0.04$, Cochran–Armitage test for trend) in lung tumours (alveolar/bronchiolar ade-nomas or carcinomas) was observed in male mice (10/71 controls, 2/48 low-dose, 4/48 mid-dose and 13/50 high-dose) (United States National Toxicology Program, 1982a).

Groups of 45–55 male and female (C57BL/6J × C3Hf)F1 mice, six weeks of age, were given gastric instillations of 0, 2.5 or 5.0 µg/kg bw 2,3,7,8-TCDD [laboratory grade; purity unspecified] in 0.01 mL/kg bw corn oil vehicle (containing 1.2% acetone) once a week for 52 weeks. At 31–39 weeks of age, 41 males and 32 females in the 2.5-µg/kg bw group were erroneously treated once with a dose of 25 µg/kg bw 2,3,7,8-TCDD. The treatment of these mice was interrupted for five weeks and then continued until week 57, as for the other treated mice. At the end of treatment, all groups were kept under observation until 110 weeks of age, when all survivors were killed. Histopatho-logical examination was carried out on Harderian glands, pituitary, thyroid, tongue, oeso-phagus, trachea, lungs, liver, pancreas, mesenteric lymph nodes, small intestine, spleen, kidney, adrenal glands, testis or ovaries, uterus, urinary bladder and all other organs with apparent or suspected pathological alterations. Treatment with 2,3,7,8-TCDD at both dose levels caused a marked depression in mean body weight in both males and females. Survival was significantly reduced in male and female 2,3,7,8-TCDD-treated mice ($p < 0.001$). Long-term administration of 2,3,7,8-TCDD increased the incidence of some non-neoplastic lesions, including liver necrosis, amyloidosis of multiple tissues and nephrosclerosis. Dermatitis developed in most 2,3,7,8-TCDD-treated mice and regressed after cessation of treatment. Tumour incidence was evaluated statistically adjusting for intercurrent mortality. [The authors report that, due to the toxicity of the treatment, it was not possible to distinguish between fatal and incidental tumours and both statistical methods were used.] Hepatocellular adenomas occurred in 10/45 control, 11/51 low-dose and 10/50 high-dose males ($p > 0.05$, incidental tumour test). However, when fatal tumours were considered, there was a significant increase ($p < 0.001$, fatal tumour test). In females, the incidence of hepatocellular adenomas was 2/49 control, 4/42 low-dose and 11/48 high-dose animals ($p < 0.01$, fatal tumour test; $p < 0.001$, incidental tumour test). The incidences of hepatocellular carcinomas were: 5/43 control, 15/51 low-dose and 33/50 high-dose males ($p < 0.001$ for both fatal and incidental tumour tests); and

1/49 control, 12/42 low-dose and 9/48 high-dose females ($p < 0.01$, fatal tumour test; $p < 0.05$, incidental tumour test). The incidence of any other tumour type was not associated with treatment (Della Porta *et al.*, 1987).

3.1.2   *Rat*

Groups of 10 male Sprague-Dawley rats, weighing approximately 60 g, were fed diets containing 1, 5, 50, 500 ng/kg diet (parts per trillion; ppt), 1, 5, 50, 500 or 1000 μg/kg diet (parts per billion; ppb) 2,3,7,8-TCDD [purity unspecified]. One control group was maintained on basal diet. Animals were maintained on the diets for 78 weeks, at which time the treated animals were changed to the basal diet. At 65 weeks of the experiment, laparotomies were performed on all surviving animals and at 95 weeks all surviving animals were killed. All animals treated with the three highest doses (50, 500 and 1000 ppb) died between the second and fourth week of the experiment. At the end of the experiment, four, eight, six, six and five, zero and zero animals were alive in the control, 1-, 5-, 50- and 500-ppt and 1- and 5-ppb groups, respectively. Various types of neoplasm were observed in the treated rats and none in the control rats. The numbers of animals with neoplasms were zero, zero, five, three, four, four and seven in the control, 1-, 5-, 50- and 500-ppt and 1- and 5-ppb groups, respectively. In the 5-ppb group, four squamous-cell tumours of the lung, four neoplastic nodules of the liver and two cholangio-carcinomas of the liver were observed. One cholangiocarcinoma was observed in the 1-ppb group (Van Miller *et al.*, 1977). [The Working Group noted the small number of animals per group, but that cholangiocarcinomas are relatively rare in rats and may be related to treatment.]

Groups of 50 male and 50 female Sprague-Dawley rats, six to seven weeks of age, were fed 22, 210 or 2200 ppt (ng/kg) 2,3,7,8-TCDD (purity, > 99%) in the diet, corresponding to 0.001, 0.01 or 0.1 μg/kg bw daily for two years. Control groups of 86 male and 86 female rats received a basal diet containing the vehicle (acetone) only. Terminal necropsy was performed at 105 weeks. Representative portions of most organs and any additional gross lesions were preserved in formalin fixative. Histological examination was conducted on an extensive list of tissues from control and high-dose rats. All rats in the low- and mid-dose groups were subjected to histological examination of tissues identified as possible target organs and all gross lesions. Reduced survival was observed in high-dose females and in mid- and high-dose males. Mean body weights of high-dose males and mid- and high-dose females were below those of the control animals throughout the major portion of the study [details not reported]. Non-neoplastic, treatment-related pathological changes were reported, especially in the liver. High- and mid-dose rats had multiple hepatocellular necrosis and inflammatory changes. In males, the incidences of hepatocellular hyperplastic nodules (6/85 controls, 0/50 low-dose, 3/50 mid-dose and 2/50 high-dose) and hepatocellular carcinomas (2/85 controls, 0/50 low-dose, 0/50 mid-dose and 1/50 high-dose) were not increased. In female rats, the incidence of hepatocellular hyperplastic nodules was 8/86 control, 3/50 low-dose, 18/50 mid-dose and 23/49 high-dose animals ($p < 0.05$, Fisher's exact test) and that of hepatocellular carcinomas was 1/86 control, 0/50 low-dose, 2/50 mid-dose and 11/49 high-dose animals

($p < 0.05$). The lipid concentrations of 2,3,7,8-TCDD in the low-, mid- and high-dose rats were 540, 1700 and 8100 ng/kg. Squamous-cell carcinomas of the hard palate or nasal turbinates occurred in 4/49 ($p < 0.05$) high-dose and 1/50 mid-dose females, squamous-cell carcinomas of the lung were observed in 7/49 ($p < 0.05$) high-dose females and squamous-cell carcinomas of the tongue occurred in 2/49 high-dose females; tumours at these sites were not observed in the other groups. In high-dose males, 4/50 rats developed squamous-cell carcinomas of the hard palate or nasal turbinates ($p < 0.05$), one developed a squamous-cell carcinoma of the lung and three squamous-cell carcinomas of the tongue ($p < 0.05$). In comparison with the high incidence of endocrine-related tumours (pituitary adenomas, phaeochromocytomas and pancreatic islet-cell tumours) in controls, reduced incidences were observed in the high-dose group (Kociba *et al.*, 1978).

A re-evaluation of the slides of liver specimens from the female animals studied by Kociba *et al.* (1978) was performed by a panel of pathologists (Keenan *et al.*, 1991). In contrast to the original findings, they found about two-thirds fewer tumours present in the livers of female Sprague-Dawley rats. On the basis of their results, they established a no-observed-adverse-effect level for hepatocellular carcinomas of 0.01 μg/kg bw per day 2,3,7,8-TCDD. [The Working Group noted that the results of this re-evaluation do not change substantially the positive findings of Kociba *et al.* (1978) on the liver carcinogenicity of 2,3,7,8-TCDD in female rats.]

Liver slides from the study by Kociba *et al.* (1978) were further reviewed by a pathology working group with the aim of evaluating proliferative lesions in the livers of female rats. The results of the working group substantially confirmed the previous results on dose-related increased tumour incidence (hepatocellular adenomas: 2/81 control, 1/50 low-dose, 9/50 mide-dose and 14/45 high-dose; hepatocellular carcinomas: 0/86, 0/50, 0/50 and 4/45). There was a dose-related increase in the incidence of hepatic eosinophilic foci (31/86 control, 23/50 low-dose, 37/50 mid-dose and 40/45 high-dose) (Goodman & Sauer, 1992).

Groups of 50 male and 50 female Osborne-Mendel rats, six weeks of age, were given gastric instillations of 0.01, 0.05 or 0.5 μg/kg bw 2,3,7,8-TCDD (purity, > 99.4%) in a vehicle of 9 : 1 corn oil–acetone twice a week for 104 weeks. One control group of 75 male and 75 female rats received vehicle alone and another control group of 50 males and 50 females was untreated. Mean body weights of the high-dose groups were lower than those of the corresponding controls after week 55 in males and after week 45 in females. Treatment did not affect survival: 23/50 untreated control, 29/75 vehicle-control, 17/50 low-dose, 20/50 mid-dose and 19/50 high-dose males were alive at the end of the experiment at 105–108 weeks; 29/50 untreated control, 39/75 vehicle-treated control, 29/50 low-dose, 34/50 mid-dose and 32/50 high-dose females were alive at the end of the experiment at 105–107 weeks. Treatment-related increased hepatotoxicity was observed in high-dose males and females. Treatment-related increased incidences of follicular-cell adenomas of the thyroid were seen in males and were significantly higher ($p = 0.001$; Fisher's exact test) in the high-dose group than in the vehicle controls (1/69 vehicle-control, 5/48 low-dose, 6/50 mid-dose and 10/50 high-dose; $p = 0.006$, Cochran–

Armitage test for trend) and in high-dose female rats (3/73 vehicle-control, 2/45 low-dose, 1/49 mid-dose and 6/47 high-dose; $p = 0.022$, Cochran–Armitage test for trend). The incidence of neoplastic nodules of the liver was significantly higher ($p = 0.006$) in high-dose females than in vehicle-control females (5/75 vehicle-control, 1/49 low-dose, 3/50 mid-dose and 12/49 high-dose). In males, a dose-related positive trend ($p = 0.005$) was seen (0/74, 0/50, 0/50 and 3/50, respectively) (United States National Toxicology Program, 1982a).

3.2   Administration to immature animals

Mouse: Groups of 89–186 male and female (C57BL/6J × C3Hf)F1 (B6C3) and (C57BL/6J × BALB/c)F1 (B6C) mice, 10 days old, were given five weekly intraperitoneal injections of 0, 1, 30 or 60 µg/kg bw 2,3,7,8-TCDD [laboratory grade; purity unspecified] in 0.01 mL/g bw corn oil vehicle (containing 1.2% acetone). Treatment-related mortality was high, especially with the mid and high doses. In both hybrids, 2–6% of vehicle-control and low-dose mice died between the end of treatment and week 13 of age, compared with 12–20% of mid-dose and 26–30% of high-dose mice. A mean body weight depression of 5% was observed throughout the experiment in mid- and high-dose B6C3 and B6C males compared with the control groups. Animals received no further treatment until 78 weeks of age, when all survivors (73–100% of males and 81–100% of females) were killed. Gross examination was performed on all animals that died or were killed. Histopathological examination was carried out on the liver, kidney and any other organ with apparent or suspected pathological alterations. The incidences of thymic lymphomas were: 0/45 control, 0/55 low-dose, 1/52 mid-dose and 2/43 high-dose B6C3 males; 0/42 control, 0/57 low-dose, 0/48 mid-dose and 5/57 high-dose B6C3 females; 0/32 control, 0/54 low-dose, 2/27 mid-dose and 2/30 high-dose B6C males; and 0/48 control, 0/57 low-dose, 1/39 mid-dose and 2/38 high-dose B6C females. Thymic lymphomas developed between 16 and 41 weeks of age and most of them (11/15) were seen within 26 weeks of age. The χ^2 test for trend was significant ($p < 0.05$) in all four groups (male and female B6C3 and B6C mice). The authors considered the development of thymic lymphomas to be treatment-related due to the rarity of this tumour type in untreated groups of B6C3 and B6C mice. The incidences of hepatocellular adenomas were: 6/45 control, 5/55 low-dose, 5/52 mid-dose and 11/43 high-dose B6C3 males ($p = 0.043$, χ^2 test for trend); and 0/42 control, 1/57 low-dose, 1/48 mid-dose and 5/57 high-dose B6C3 females ($p = 0.014$, χ^2 test for trend). The incidences of hepatocellular carcinomas were: 3/45 control, 1/55 low-dose, 9/52 mid-dose and 14/43 high-dose B6C3 males ($p < 0.001$, χ^2 test for trend; $p = 0.002$, Fisher's exact test, high-dose compared with control); and in 0/42 control, 0/57 low-dose, 1/48 mid-dose and 1/57 high-dose B6C3 females. Hepatocellular carcinomas were not observed in B6C mice of either sex (Della Porta *et al.*, 1987).

3.3   Intraperitoneal or subcutaneous administration

Hamster: Groups of 10–24 male Syrian golden hamsters, weighing 65–80 g [age unspecified] received six intraperitoneal or subcutaneous injections of 50 or 100 µg/kg bw 2,3,7,8-TCDD [purity unspecified] in dioxane or dioxane alone at four-week intervals. A further group received only two intraperitoneal injections of 100 µg/kg bw 2,3,7,8-TCDD. Animals were observed until 12–13 months after the beginning of treatment. Complete necropsies were performed on all animals, and tissues were fixed in formalin and examined microscopically. Toxicity and early mortality were observed in the high-dose groups. Squamous-cell carcinomas of the facial skin developed in 4/18 intraperitoneally high-dosed animals and 3/14 subcutaneously high-dosed animals. No animal in the control groups, the low-dose groups or the groups receiving two intra-peritoneal injections of the high dose developed tumours at any site (Rao *et al.*, 1988). [The Working Group noted the small number of animals per group.]

3.4   Skin application

Mouse: Groups of 30 male and 30 female Swiss-Webster mice (six weeks old) received 2,3,7,8-TCDD (purity, 99.4%) on the clipped back at doses of 0.001 µg/animal (males) and 0.005 µg/animal (females), suspended in 0.1 mL acetone, on three days per week for 99 (males) or 104 weeks (females). As vehicle controls, 45 mice of each sex received 0.1 mL acetone three times per week. Thirty animals of each sex served as untreated controls. Mean body weights were similar in the 2,3,7,8-TCDD- and vehicle-treated groups, but untreated controls of both sexes had slightly higher body weights. Survival in both sexes was decreased by 2,3,7,8-TCDD treatment ($p = 0.005$ and $p = 0.031$ in males and females, respectively, Cox's test). Among males, 27/30, 33/45 and 27/30 untreated control, vehicle-control and 2,3,7,8-TCDD-treated mice, respec-tively, were alive at week 52 of the study; 28/30, 43/45 and 29/30 untreated control, vehicle-control and 2,3,7,8-TCDD-treated females, respectively, were alive at week 52 of the study. In males, the incidence of fibrosarcomas of the integumentary system was 3/42 and 6/28 in the vehicle-control and 2,3,7,8-TCDD-treated mice, respectively (not a statistically significant difference). In female mice, the incidence of fibrosarcomas of the integumentary system was significantly higher in animals treated with 2,3,7,8-TCDD (8/27) compared with vehicle-controls (2/41; $p = 0.007$, Fisher's exact test) (United States National Toxicology Program, 1982b).

3.5   Exposure by immersion in water

Fish: Preliminary results of a study in progress reported in an abstract indicate that exposure of medaka fish [*Oryzias latipes*] to 2,3,7,8-TCDD producing a body concen-tration of 2 µg/kg was associated with tumours at several sites — gills, thyroid and swim bladder (Johnson *et al.*, 1992b).

3.6   Administration with known carcinogens and modifying factors

For an overview of studies on administration of 2,3,7,8-TCDD and related PCDDs with known carcinogens, see **Table 41**. [The Working Group noted that the experimental approach used in these studies is frequently termed a tumour promotion protocol. This terminology is used in Section 4.6.2 of the present monograph.]

Table 41. Studies on 2,3,7,8-TCDD and related PCDDs administered with known carcinogens and modifying factors

Tumour type Strain/species (sex)	Known carcinogen	Route of administration	Interval	Dose and frequency of PCDD (times per week/number of weeks)	Route of administration	Enhancement[a]	Reference
Skin							
CD1 mice (F)	200 nmol DMBA	Skin	1 week	0.1 µg 2,3,7,8-TCDD/2 per wk/30 wk	Skin	−	Berry et al. (1978)
HRS/J haired mice (hr/+) (F)	200 nmol DMBA	Skin	None	20 ng 2,3,7,8-TCDD/2 per wk/8 wk then 50 ng/17 wk	Skin	−	Poland et al. (1982)
HRS/J hairless mice (hr/hr) (F)	200 nmol DMBA	Skin	None	20 ng 2,3,7,8-TCDD/2 per wk/8 wk then 50 ng/17 wk	Skin	+	
HRS/J hairless mice (hr/hr) (F)	5 µmol MNNG	Skin	None	3.75 ng 2,3,7,8-TCDD/2 per wk/20 wk	Skin	+	
	5 µmol MNNG	Skin	None	7.5 ng 2,3,7,8-TCDD/2 per wk/20 wk	Skin	+	
	5 µmol MNNG	Skin	None	15 ng 2,3,7,8-TCDD/2 per wk/20 wk	Skin	+	
	5 µmol MNNG	Skin	None	30 ng 2,3,7,8-TCDD/2 per wk/20 wk	Skin	+	
	5 µmol MNNG	Skin	None	50 ng 2,3,7,8-TCDD/5 wk/ then 20 ng/15 wk	Skin	+	
	5 µmol MNNG	Skin	None	20 µmol 2,7-DCDD/2 per wk/20 wk	Skin	−	
HRS/J hairless mice (hr/hr) (F)	5 µmol MNNG	Skin	7 days	2.5 ng 2,3,7,8-TCDD/2 per wk/20 wk	Skin	+	Hébert et al. (1990a)
	5 µmol MNNG	Skin	7 days	5 ng 2,3,7,8-TCDD/2 per wk/20 wk	Skin	+	
	5 µmol MNNG	Skin	7 days	10 ng 2,3,7,8-TCDD/2 per wk/20 wk	Skin	+	
Lung							
Swiss mice (M)	25 mg/kg bw NDMA	i.p.	3 weeks	1 × 1.6 µg/kg bw 2,3,7,8-TCDD	i.p.	+	Beebe et al. (1995a)
	25 mg/kg bw NDMA	i.p.	3 weeks	1 × 16 or 48 µg/kg bw 2,3,7,8-TCDD	i.p.	− (toxic)	
	25 mg/kg bw NDMA	i.p.	3 weeks	20 × 0.05 µg/kg bw 2,3,7,8-TCDD	i.p.	−	
C57BL/6 mice (M)	90 mg/kg bw NDEA	i.p.	3 weeks	0.05 µg/kg bw 2,3,7,8-TCDD/weekly/20 wk	i.p.	−	Beebe et al. (1995b)
B6D2F1 mice (M)	90 mg/kg bw NDEA	i.p.	3 weeks	0.05 µg/kg bw 2,3,7,8-TCDD/weekly/20 wk	i.p.	−	
DBA/2 mice (M)	90 mg/kg bw NDEA	i.p.	3 weeks	0.05 µg/kg bw 2,3,7,8-TCDD/weekly/20 wk	i.p.	−	
SD rats (F)	200 mg/kg bw NDEA	i.p.	10 days	1.4 µg/kg bw 2,3,7,8-TCDD/biweekly/60 wks	Oral	−	Clark et al. (1991)
SD rats (F) (ovariectomized)	200 mg/kg bw NDEA	i.p.	10 days	1.4 µg/kg bw 2,3,7,8-TCDD/biweekly/60 wks	Oral	+	

Table 41 (contd)

Strain/species (sex)	Known carcinogen	Route of administration	Interval	Dose and frequency of PCDD	Route of administration	Enhancement[a]	Reference
Liver							
C57BL/6 mouse	90 mg/kg bw NDEA	i.p.	3 weeks	0.05 µg/kg bw 2,3,7,8-TCDD/weekly/20 wk	i.p.	–	Beebe et al. (1995b)
B6D2F1 mouse	90 mg/kg bw NDEA	i.p.	3 weeks	0.05 µg/kg bw 2,3,7,8-TCDD/weekly/20 wk	i.p.	+	
DBA/2 mouse	90 mg/kg bw NDEA	i.p.	3 weeks	0.05 µg/kg bw 2,3,7,8-TCDD/weekly/20 wk	i.p.	–	
SD rats (F)	PH/10 mg/kg bw NDEA	oral	7 days	0.14 µg/kg bw 2,3,7,8-TCDD/biweekly/7 mo	i.m.	–	Pitot et al. (1980)
	PH/10 mg/kg bw NDEA	oral	7 days	1.4 µg/kg bw 2,3,7,8-TCDD/biweekly/7 mo	i.m.	+	
Fischer 344 rats (F)	PH/ 10 mg/kg bw NDEA	oral	14 days	0.0014 mg/kg bw 2,3,7,8-TCDD/biwekkly/6 mo	i.m.	–	Pitot et al. (1987)
	PH/ 10 mg/kg bw NDEA	oral	14 days	0.014 µg/kg bw 2,3,7,8-TCDD/biweekly/6 mo	i.m.	–	
	PH/ 10 mg/kg bw NDEA	oral	14 days	0.14 µg/kg bw 2,3,7,8-TCDD/biweekly/6 mo	i.m.	–	
	PH/ 10 mg/kg bw NDEA	oral	14 days	1.4 µg/kg bw 2,3,7,8-TCDD/biweekly/6 mo	i.m.	+	
SD rats (F)	PH/30 mg/kg bw NDEA	i.p.	7 days	0.7 µg/kg bw 2,3,7,8-TCDD/weekly/14 wk	s.c.	–	Flodström & Ahlborg (1989); Flodström et al. (1991)
	PH/30 mg/kg bw NDEA	i.p.	7 days	0.7 µg/kg bw 2,3,7,8-TCDD/weekly/26 wk	s.c.	+	
	PH/30 mg/kg bw NDEA	i.p.	35 days	3.5 then 0.7 µg/kg bw 2,3,7,8-TCDD/weekly/9 wk	s.c.	+	
	PH/30 mg/kg bw NDEA	i.p.	35 days	3.5 then 0.7 µg/kg bw 2,3,7,8-TCDD/weekly/21 wk	s.c.	+	
	PH/30 mg/kg bw NDEA	i.p.	35 days	0.35 then 0.07 µg/kg bw 2,3,7,8-TCDD/weekly/15 wk (normal vitamin A)	s.c.	–	
		i.p.	35 days	0.35 then 0.07 µg/kg bw 2,3,7,8-TCDD/weekly/15 wk (marginal or low vitamin A)	s.c.	+	
		i.p.	35 days	3.5 then 0.7 µg/kg bw 2,3,7,8-TCDD/weekly/15 wk (normal, marginal, low vitamin A)	s.c.	+	
Fischer 344 rats (F)	PH/10 mg/kg bw NDEA	oral	2 weeks	0.14 µg/kg bw 2,3,7,8-TCDD/biweekly/6 mo	s.c.	+	Dragan et al. (1991)
SD rats (F)	PH/30 mg/kg bw NDEA	i.p.	35 days	0.44 then 0.088 µg/kg bw 1,2,3,7,8-PeCDD/weekly/20 wk	s.c.	+	Waern et al. (1991)
	PH/30 mg/kg bw NDEA	i.p.	35 days	1.75 then 0.35 µg/kg bw 1,2,3,7,8-PeCDD/weekly/20 wk	s.c.	+	(1991)
	PH/30 mg/kg bw NDEA	i.p.	35 days	7 then 1.4 µg/kg bw 1,2,3,7,8-PeCDD/weekly/20 wk	s.c.	+	
	PH/30 mg/kg bw NDEA	i.p.	35 days	0.22 then 0.044 µg/kg bw 2,3,7,8-TCDD/weekly/20 wk	s.c.	+	
	PH/30 mg/kg bw NDEA	i.p.	35 days	0.88 then 0.175 µg/kg bw 2,3,7,8-TCDD/weekly/20 wk	s.c.	+	
	PH/30 mg/kg bw NDEA	i.p.	35 days	3.5 then 0.7 µg/kg bw 2,3,7,8-TCDD/weekly/20 wk	s.c.	+	

Table 41 (contd)

Strain/species (sex)	Known carcinogen	Route of administration	Interval	Dose and frequency of PCDD	Route of administration	Enhancement[a]	Reference
Liver (contd)							
SD rats (F)	200 mg/kg bw NDEA	i.p.	7 days	1.4 µg/kg bw 2,3,7,8-TCDD/biweekly/30 wk	Oral	+	Lucier et al. (1991)
SD rats (F) (ovariectomized)	200 mg/kg bw NDEA	i.p.	7 days	1.4 µg/kg bw 2,3,7,8-TCDD/biweekly/30 wk	Oral	+	
SD rats (F)	PH/10 mg/kg bw NDEA	oral	7 days	0.14 µg/kg bw 2,3,7,8-TCDD/biweekly/1 mo	i.p.	+	Dragan et al. (1992)
	PH/10 mg/kg bw NDEA	oral	7 days	0.14 µg/kg bw 2,3,7,8-TCDD/biweekly/3 mo	i.p.	+	
	PH/10 mg/kg bw NDEA	oral	7 days	0.14 µg/kg bw 2,3,7,8-TCDD/biweekly/5 mo	i.p.	+	
SD rats (F)	175 mg/kg bw NDEA	i.p.	14 days	3.5 ng/kg bw 2,3,7,8-TCDD/biweekly/30 wk	Oral	−	Maronpot et al. (1993)
	175 mg/kg bw NDEA	i.p.	14 days	10.7 ng/kg bw 2,3,7,8-TCDD/biweekly/30 wk	Oral	−	
	175 mg/kg bw NDEA	i.p.	14 days	35.7 ng/kg bw 2,3,7,8-TCDD/biweekly/30 wk	Oral	−	
	175 mg/kg bw NDEA	i.p.	14 days	125 ng/kg bw 2,3,7,8-TCDD/biweekly/30 wk	Oral	+	
Wistar rats (F)	5 × 10 mg/kg bw NDEA	oral	14 days	1.4 µg/kg bw 2,3,7,8-TCDD/biweekly/9 wk	s.c.	+	Buchmann et al. (1994)
	5 × 10 mg/kg bw NDEA	oral	14 days	1.4 µg/kg bw 2,3,7,8-TCDD/biweekly/13 wk	s.c.	+	
	5 × 10 mg/kg bw NDEA	oral	14 days	1.4 µg/kg bw 2,3,7,8-TCDD/biweekly/17 wk	s.c.	+	
	5 × 10 mg/kg bw NDEA	oral	14 days	70 µg/kg bw HpCDD/biweekly/9 wk	s.c.	+	
	5 × 10 mg/kg bw NDEA	oral	14 days	70 µg/kg bw HpCDD/biweekly/13 wk	s.c.	+	
	5 × 10 mg/kg bw NDEA	oral	14 days	70 µg/kg bw HpCDD/biweekly/17 wk	s.c.	+	
Wistar rats (F)	80 mg/L *N*-nitroso-morpholine in drinking-water for 25 days	oral	14 days	2 ng/kg bw 2,3,7,8-TCDD/daily/13 wk	s.c.	+	Schrenk et al. (1994a)
		oral	14 days	20 ng/kg bw 2,3,7,8-TCDD/daily/13 wk	s.c.	+	
		oral	14 days	200 ng/kg bw 2,3,7,8-TCDD/daily/13 wk	s.c.	+	
		oral	14 days	100 ng/kg bw HpCDD/daily/13 wk	s.c.	−	
		oral	14 days	1000 ng/kg bw HpCDD/daily/13 wk	s.c.	+	
		oral	14 days	10 000 ng/kg bw HpCDD/daily/13 wk	s.c.	+	
		oral	14 days	200 ng/kg bw PCDD mixture/daily/13 wk	s.c.	+	
		oral	14 days	2000 ng/kg bw PCDD mixture/daily/13 wk	s.c.	+	
		oral	14 days	20 000 ng/kg bw PCDD mixture/daily/13 wk	s.c.	+	
SD rats (F)	10 mg/kg bw NDEA	i.p.	30 days	0.007 µg/kg bw 2,3,7,8-TCDD/day (150 ppt in diet) until day 450	Oral	+	Sills et al. (1994)
	10 mg/kg bw NDEA	i.p.	170 days	0.007 µg/kg bw 2,3,7,8-TCDD/day (150 ppt in diet) until day 450	Oral	+	
	10 mg/kg bw NDEA	i.p.	240 days	0.007 µg/kg bw 2,3,7,8-TCDD/day (150 ppt in diet) until day 450	Oral	+	

Table 41 (contd)

Strain/species (sex)	Known carcinogen	Route of administration	Interval	Dose and frequency of PCDD	Route of administration	Enhancement[a]	Reference
Liver (contd)							
SD rats (F)	PH/30 mg/kg bw NDEA	i.p.	35 days	0.5 then 0.1 µg/kg bw 2,3,7,8-TCDD/weekly/20 wk	s.c.	−	Hemming et al. (1995)
	PH/30 mg/kg bw NDEA	i.p.	35 days	1.58 then 0.316 µg/kg bw 2,3,7,8-TCDD/weekly/20 wk	s.c.	−	
	PH/30 mg/kg bw NDEA	i.p.	35 days	5 then 1 µg/kg bw 2,3,7,8-TCDD/weekly/20 wk	s.c.	+	
Wistar rats (F)	10 × 10 mg/kg bw NDEA	oral	56 days	1.4 µg/kg bw 2,3,7,8-TCDD once	s.c.	−	Stinchcombe et al. (1995)
	10 × 10 mg/kg bw NDEA	oral	56 days	1.4 µg/kg bw 2,3,7,8-TCDD/biweekly/16 wk	s.c.	+	
SD rats (F)	175 mg/kg bw NDEA	i.p.	14 days	1.75 µg/kg bw 2,3,7,8-TCDD/biweekly/30 wk	Oral	+	Tritscher et al. (1995)

DMBA, 7,12-dimethylbenz[a]anthracene; MNNG, N-methyl-N -nitro-N -nitrosoguanidine; NDMA, N-nitrosodimethylamine; NDEA, N-nitrosodiethylamine; SD, Sprague-Dawley; PH, partial hepatectomy; F, female; M, male; i.p., intraperitoneal injection; s.c., subcutaneous injection; i.m., intamuscular injection
[a]Enhancement corresponds to promotion as used in Section 4.6.2.

3.6.1 *Skin*

Mouse: Groups of 30 female CD1 mice, seven to nine weeks of age, received skin applications of 2 µg 2,3,7,8-TCDD or 2.56 µg 7,12-dimethylbenz[*a*]anthracene (DMBA) per animal or both chemicals together in 0.2 mL acetone solvent. Starting one week later, the mice received thrice weekly applications of 12-*O*-tetradecanoylphorbol-13-acetate (TPA) (5 µg/animal) in 0.2 mL acetone for 32 weeks. The 2,3,7,8-TCDD/TPA-treated mice had 0.1 papillomas/mouse (14% incidence), the 2,3,7,8-TCDD + DMBA/TPA-treated mice had 2.2 papillomas/mouse (63% incidence) and the DMBA/TPA-treated mice had approximately 1.8 papillomas/mouse (40% incidence) (DiGiovanni *et al.*, 1977). [The Working Group noted that adequate control groups were not available, precluding an evaluation.]

Three groups of 30 female CD1 mice, six to eight weeks of age, received single skin applications of 0.2 µmol/animal (60 µg) DMBA in 0.2 mL acetone or solvent alone. Starting one week later, mice were treated with an acetone solution of 0.1 µg 2,3,7,8-TCDD or 2 µg TPA per animal (positive control) or acetone solvent alone twice weekly for 30 weeks, at which time the experiment was terminated. The percentages of mice with skin papillomas were DMBA/2,3,7,8-TCDD, 0%; DMBA/TPA, 92% and acetone/-TPA, 0% (Berry *et al.*, 1978).

In groups of female HRS/J haired (*hr*/+) mice given single skin applications of DMBA (0.2 µmol in acetone) followed by twice weekly applications of 20 ng/animal 2,3,7,8-TCDD for eight weeks then 50 ng/animal for 17 weeks, no skin tumours were found. In contrast, in HRS/J hairless (*hr*/*hr*) mice treated with 0.2 µmol/animal DMBA and the same regimen of 2,3,7,8-TCDD (25 weeks), 15/19 surviving mice developed skin tumours (1.4 tumours per mouse). In hairless animals treated with DMBA alone, one skin papilloma was found and, in the absence of DMBA, 2,3,7,8-TCDD produced no skin tumour (Poland *et al.*, 1982).

In a further experiment, groups of 20 female HRS/J hairless (*hr*/*hr*) mice, seven weeks of age, were given single skin applications of 5 µmol (0.75 mg)/animal *N*-methyl-*N*'-nitro-*N*-nitrosoguanidine (MNNG) in 50 µL acetone followed by twice weekly doses of 0 or 3.75–30 ng/animal 2,3,7,8-TCDD or 1 µg or 3 µg/animal TPA as positive controls. The numbers of mice with skin tumours at 20 weeks are shown in **Table 42** (Poland *et al.*, 1982).

Groups of 26 female HRS/J hairless (*hr*/*hr*) mice, eight weeks of age, were given single skin applications of 0 or 5 µmol/animal MNNG in 50 µL acetone followed by 50 ng/animal 2,3,7,8-TCDD for five weeks then 20 ng/animal for 15 weeks, both in 50 µL acetone twice weekly during the 20-week period. Skin tumours developed in 16/19 (1.6 tumours per mouse) mice treated with MNNG plus 2,3,7,8-TCDD compared with 0/18 in mice treated with 2,3,7,8-TCDD alone (Poland *et al.*, 1982).

Three groups of 20 female HRS/J hairless (*hr*/*hr*) mice, five to eight weeks of age, were given single skin applications of 5 µmol/animal MNNG in 50 µL acetone. Seven days later, the mice were treated with 2.5, 5 or 10 ng/animal 2,3,7,8-TCDD in 25 µL acetone twice weekly for 20 weeks. A control group of 20 mice received acetone

followed by 10 ng/animal 2,3,7,8-TCDD. The numbers of surviving mice with papillomas, carcinomas or hyperproliferative nodules of the skin were 8/20, 8/19 and 7/18
after treatment with MNNG and 2.5, 5 or 10 ng/animal 2,3,7,8-TCDD compared with
0/18 mice treated with 2,3,7,8-TCDD alone (Hébert *et al.*, 1990a).

**Table 42. Induction of skin tumours in female HRS/J hairless
mice**

Initiation	Promotion		Tumour incidence (surviving mice with tumours/ surviving mice)	Tumour multiplicity (average no. of papillomas/ surviving mice)
MNNG	Acetone		1/19	0.05
MNNG	TCDD	3.75 ng	11/20	0.7
MNNG	TCDD	7.5 ng	13/17	1.5
MNNG	TCDD	15 ng	10/10	4.0
MNNG	TCDD	30 ng	15/19	1.6
Acetone	TCDD	30 ng	0/19	0
MNNG	TPA	1 µg	5/19	0.4
MNNG	TPA	3 µg	13/18	1.6

From Poland *et al.* (1982)

In two experiments with female Sencar mice, it was shown that prior skin application
of 2,3,7,8-TCDD reduced tumorigenesis of DMBA (or monofluoro derivatives of
DMBA) and benzo[*a*]pyrene (Cohen *et al.*, 1979; DiGiovanni *et al.*, 1983).

3.6.2   *Lung*

(a)   *Mouse*

Groups of male Swiss mice [initial numbers unspecified], five weeks of age, were
given a single intraperitoneal injection of 25 mg/kg bw *N*-nitrosodimethylamine
(NDMA) in saline. Three weeks later, the mice were given either single intraperitoneal
injections of 1.6, 16 or 48 µg/kg bw 2,3,7,8-TCDD in olive oil, weekly doses of
0.05 µg/kg bw 2,3,7,8-TCDD weekly for 20 weeks or olive oil alone. All mice were
killed after 52 weeks. Alveolar-cell adenomas and carcinomas were found in 100% of
mice in all treatment groups (NDMA/olive oil, 24/24; NDMA/2,3,7,8-TCDD (repeated
0.05 µg/kg bw/week), 30/30; NDMA/2,3,7,8-TCDD (1.6 µg/kg bw), 15/15; NDMA/-
2,3,7,8-TCDD (16 µg/kg bw), 19/19; NDMA/2,3,7,8-TCDD (48 µg/kg bw), 11/11).
However, tumour multiplicity was significantly increased in mice receiving weekly
injections of 0.05 µg/kg bw 2,3,7,8-TCDD (18 ± 1.7 versus 12 ± 1.5; $p = 0.031$) and in
mice given a single dose of 1.6 µg/kg bw 2,3,7,8-TCDD (20 ± 2.6 versus 12 ± 1.5;
$p = 0.016$) compared with those given NDMA only (Beebe *et al.*, 1995a).

In another experiment with male C57BL/6, DBA/2 and B6D2F1 mice, lung tumour
incidence following a single intraperitoneal injection of 90 mg/kg bw *N*-nitrosodiethyl-
amine (NDEA) was not increased by weekly intraperitoneal injections of 0.05 µg/kg bw

2,3,7,8-TCDD given three weeks later for 20 weeks followed by observation up to 52 weeks (C57BL/6: NDEA alone, 20/26; NDEA + 2,3,7,8-TCDD, 25/31; DBA/2: NDEA alone, 24/28; NDEA + 2,3,7,8-TCDD, 22/26; B6D2F1: NDEA alone, 33/34; NDEA + 2,3,7,8-TCDD, 33/33) (Beebe *et al.*, 1995b). [The Working Group noted that the high incidence of lung tumours induced by NDEA alone precluded the detection of an effect of 2,3,7,8-TCDD.]

(b) Rat

Groups of 45 female Sprague-Dawley rats were ovariectomized or sham-operated at 56 days of age. At 70 days of age, they were given a single intraperitoneal injection of 200 mg/kg bw NDEA in saline followed 10 days later by oral administration of 0 or 1.4 μg/kg bw 2,3,7,8-TCDD in olive oil every two weeks for 60 weeks. Lung carcinomas were found in 0/37 sham-operated and 4/39 (3 adenocarcinomas and 1 squamous-cell carcinoma) ovariectomized rats treated with NDEA and 2,3,7,8-TCDD (Clark *et al.*, 1991a). [The Working Group noted that no information was reported on whether NDEA alone caused lung tumours in sham-operated or ovariectomized rats.]

3.6.3 Liver

(a) Mouse

Groups of 18–30 male C57BL/6, DBA/2 and B6D2F1 mice were given a single intra-peritoneal injection of 90 mg/kg bw NDEA or the solvent tricaprilyn at five weeks of age. Starting three weeks later, 0.05 μg/kg bw 2,3,7,8-TCDD was given weekly for 20 weeks, and animals were observed until the terminal killing at 52 weeks. No significant increase was observed in liver tumours (all types) due to co-administration of NDEA and 2,3,7,8-TCDD in C57BL/6 (NDEA alone, 4/28; NDEA + 2,3,7,8-TCDD, 6/32) or DBA/2 (NDEA alone, 6/28; NDEA + 2,3,7,8-TCDD, 10/39) mice. However, 2,3,7,8-TCDD did increase the incidence of liver tumours (all types) as compared to NDEA alone in B6D2F1 mice (NDEA alone, 7/33; NDEA + 2,3,7,8-TCDD, 17/33). This increase was particularly due to an increase in hepatoblastomas (NDEA alone, 1/33; NDEA + 2,3,7,8-TCDD, 8/33) (Beebe *et al.*, 1995b). [The Working Group noted that only one dose level of 2,3,7,8-TCDD was used in this study.]

(b) Rat

Groups of 4–7 female Sprague-Dawley rats, weighing 200–250 g, were subjected to 70% partial hepatectomy and 24 h later treated once with saline or 10 mg/kg bw NDEA in saline by gastric instillation. Starting seven days later, the rats were given 0, 0.14 or 1.4 μg/kg bw 2,3,7,8-TCDD by subcutaneous injection every two weeks for 28 weeks at which time all surviving rats were killed. There was an increase in the number and size of focal and nodular hepatic lesions with 2,3,7,8-TCDD in the low- and high-dose groups. Focal and nodular hepatic lesions were identified by γ-glutamyl transpeptidase (GGT), canalicular adenosine triphosphatase (ATPase) and glucose-6-phosphatase (G6Pase). The number of focal lesions was 309 ± 98 (NDEA alone), 34 ± 17 (low-dose 2,3,7,8-TCDD), 25 ± 7 (high-dose 2,3,7,8-TCDD), 1068 ± 166 (NDEA followed by low-dose 2,3,7,8-TCDD) and 871 ± 66 (NDEA followed by high-dose 2,3,7,8-TCDD). The corresponding volume fractions of liver occupied by these lesions were 0.7, 0.2, 0.1, 9.0 and 43.0% (Pitot *et al.*, 1980).

Female Fischer 344 rats (150–220 g) [number not stated] were subjected to a 70% partial hepatectomy and given 10 mg/kg bw NDEA orally 24 h after the surgery. Starting two weeks after surgery, the rats were given intramuscular injections of 0, 0.0014, 0.014, 0.14 or 1.4 µg/kg bw 2,3,7,8-TCDD in corn oil every two weeks for six months. Treatment with 2,3,7,8-TCDD alone had virtually no effect on the number or volume fraction of altered hepatic foci. No effect on the number or volume fraction of focal hepatic lesions was observed at the three lowest doses. Only the highest dose (0.1 µg/kg bw per day) significantly increased the number and volume fraction of hepatic foci (detected by GGT, ATPase and G6Pase) (approximately 10 000 foci/liver with NDEA + 2,3,7,8-TCDD compared with 4000 foci/liver with NDEA alone; volume fraction approximately 2.8% with NDEA + 2,3,7,8-TCDD compared with 0.8% with NDEA alone) (Pitot *et al.*, 1987).

Groups of 10 female Sprague-Dawley rats (140–160 g) were subjected to a 70% partial hepatectomy and 24 h later were given a single intraperitoneal injection of 30 mg/kg bw NDEA. Starting one week later, the rats were given weekly subcutaneous injections of the corn oil solvent or 2,3,7,8-TCDD (0.7 µg/kg bw) for 14 or 26 weeks. Alternatively, some groups of rats were given a single loading dose (3.5 µg/kg bw) of 2,3,7,8-TCDD at five weeks after NDEA treatment or solvent in order to attain the same total dose. These latter groups were then given a weekly maintenance dose of 0.7 µg/kg bw 2,3,7,8-TCDD for nine or 21 weeks until killing. Focal hepatic lesions (detected by GGT) were significantly increased with weekly administration of 0.7 µg/kg bw 2,3,7,8-TCDD for 26 weeks. In the group receiving a loading dose of 2,3,7,8-TCDD, the percentage of liver occupied by hepatic foci was even greater than in the group treated with the same cumulative dose (Flodström & Ahlborg, 1989). Using the same experimental design, the influence of vitamin A deficiency upon the 2,3,7,8-TCDD response was investigated. Vitamin A deficiency increased the mean volume fraction of foci following NDEA + 2,3,7,8-TCDD treatment (Flodström *et al.*, 1991).

Female Fischer 344 rats (130–220 g) were subjected to a 70% partial hepatectomy and 24 h later were given a single gastric instillation of 10 mg/kg bw NDEA. Starting two weeks later, nine rats were administered oil and four rats were given 0.14 µg/kg bw 2,3,7,8-TCDD by subcutaneous injection every two weeks for six months. The number and volume fraction of the liver occupied by focal hepatic lesions (detected by gluta-thione *S*-transferase P (GSTP), GGT, ATPase, G6Pase) in the 2,3,7,8-TCDD-treated group was significantly increased compared with controls. The numbers of focal hepatic lesions per liver were 90 ± 30 (NDEA alone) and 14 220 ± 1340 (NDEA followed by 2,3,7,8-TCDD), while the volume fractions of liver were 0.14 ± 0.05% (NDEA alone) and 1.23 ± 0.11% (NDEA followed by 2,3,7,8-TCDD) (Dragan *et al.*, 1991).

Groups of 10–20 female Sprague-Dawley rats were subjected to a 70% partial hepa-tectomy followed by a single intraperitoneal injection of 30 mg/kg bw NDEA. Starting five weeks later, rats were given a loading dose of 0.22, 0.88 or 3.5 µg/kg bw 2,3,7,8-

TCDD by subcutaneous injection followed by a weekly maintenance dose of one fifth of the loading dose of 2,3,7,8-TCDD. One group received no 2,3,7,8-TCDD. The rats were killed after 20 weeks of treatment. A significant increase in the percentage of liver occupied by GGT-positive focal hepatic lesions was observed for all doses compared with NDEA controls (approximately 0.15% in controls, 0.6% in the low-dose, 0.59% in the mid-dose and 1.15% in the high-dose rats). A significant increase was seen in the number of foci at all doses (approximately: low-dose, 5000; mid-dose, 4250, high-dose, 7500) as compared to NDEA alone (2000) (Waern *et al.*, 1991).

Groups of nine female Sprague-Dawley rats, 70 days of age, were ovariectomized or sham-operated and were given an intraperitoneal injection of saline or 200 mg/kg bw NDEA. One week later, the rats were administered 2,3,7,8-TCDD in corn oil by intragastric instillation biweekly to provide a daily dose of approximately 100 ng/kg bw per day. The rats were killed after 30 weeks of 2,3,7,8-TCDD administration and GSTP- and GGT-positive foci were examined. For the GGT-positive foci, the percentages of the liver occupied by foci were 0.01 ± 0.01 (control), 0.01 ± 0.01 (2,3,7,8-TCDD alone), 0.3 ± 0.1 (NDEA alone) and 0.87 ± 0.06 (NDEA followed by 2,3,7,8-TCDD) in the intact animals. In the ovariectomized animals, the corresponding GGT-positive volume fractions were 0, 0, 0.03 ± 0.01 and 0.08 ± 0.04. The percentages of liver occupied by GSTP-positive foci were 0.04 ± 0.02 (control), 0.02 ± 0.01 (2,3,7,8-TCDD alone), 0.35 ± 0.11 (NDEA alone) and 1.17 ± 0.26 (NDEA followed by 2,3,7,8-TCDD) in the intact animals and 0.01 ± 0.01, 0.03 ± 0.01, 0.16 ± 0.05 and 0.57 ± 0.1 in the corresponding groups of ovariectomized animals. There was a reduction in the volume fraction of liver occupied by GSTP lesions in ovariectomized rats treated with NDEA alone and NDEA followed by 2,3,7,8-TCDD (Lucier *et al.*, 1991).

Groups of 5–10 female Sprague-Dawley rats were subjected to a 70% partial hepatectomy and administered oil vehicle or 10 mg/kg bw NDEA 24 h later by gastric instillation. Starting one week after the surgery, the rats were given biweekly subcutaneous injections of 0.14 µg/kg bw 2,3,7,8-TCDD for one, three or five months and either killed or maintained for a further six months before killing. The percentages of liver occupied by focal hepatic lesions (as identified by GSTP, GGT, ATPase and G6Pase) were 0.17 ± 0.03 (NDEA alone) and 1.47 ± 0.19 (NDEA and 2,3,7,8-TCDD) at the end of the first five months. The corresponding values in the group observed for an additional six months were 2.00 ± 0.27 (NDEA followed by 2,3,7,8-TCDD) and 1.35 ± 0.16 (NDEA alone, killed at the 11-month time point) (Dragan *et al.*, 1992).

Groups of 8–10 female Sprague-Dawley rats (70 days of age) were given a single intraperitoneal dose of saline or 175 mg/kg bw NDEA. Starting two weeks later, these rats were then administered an average of 0, 3.5, 10.7, 35.7 and 125 ng/kg bw 2,3,7,8-TCDD biweekly in corn oil by gastric instillation for 30 weeks and the number and volume fraction of GSTP-positive foci were determined. Dose-related increases in the number of foci per liver and the volume percentage of liver occupied by foci (as identified by GSTP) were found (see **Table 43**) (Maronpot *et al.*, 1993).

Groups of 20 female Wistar rats (100 g) were administered doses of 10 mg/kg bw NDEA in water by gastric instillation on five consecutive days. Starting two weeks after

NDEA administration, rats were treated with either corn oil or 1.4 µg/kg bw 2,3,7,8-TCDD biweekly by subcutaneous injection. Focal hepatic lesions (detected by ATPase deficiency) were quantitated at 9, 13 and 17 weeks for 4–8 rats per treatment group. In the control rats, the percentage of the liver occupied by foci was zero at all time points. In the group treated with NDEA alone, the percentages of liver occupied by foci were 0.025 ± 0.007 (at 9 weeks), 0.045 ± 0.017 (at 13 weeks) and 0.048 ± 0.018 (at 17 weeks). In the rats treated with 2,3,7,8-TCDD alone, the percentages of the liver occupied by ATPase-deficient hepatic foci were 0.030 ± 0.021 (at 9 weeks), 0.020 ± 0.011 (at 13 weeks) and 0.283 ± 0.211 (at 17 weeks). In the NDEA/2,3,7,8-TCDD-treated rats, the percentages of liver occupied by foci were 0.043 ± 0.02 (at 9 weeks), 0.211 ± 0.065 (at 13 weeks) and 0.313 ± 0.215 (at 17 weeks) (Buchmann *et al.*, 1994).

Table 43. Induction of focal hepatic lesions in rats treated with 2,3,7,8-TCDD and/or NDEA

2,3,7,8-TCDD dose (ng/kg bw)	2,3,7,8-TCDD only		+ NDEA (175 mg/kg bw)	
	No. of foci	Vol. %	No. of foci	Vol. %
0	327 ± 418	0.01 ± 0.01	$5748 \pm 3\,923$	0.57 ± 0.44
3.5	$457 \pm 1\,122$	0.02 ± 0.05	$10\,552 \pm 7\,941$	0.87 ± 0.40
10.7	447 ± 614	0.02 ± 0.03	$11\,482 \pm 8\,879$	1.00 ± 0.16
35.7	$1\,533 \pm 1\,794$	0.06 ± 0.11	$7\,157 \pm 3952$	0.93 ± 0.56
125	693 ± 921	0.04 ± 0.07	$11\,989 \pm 6\,798$	2.23 ± 1.47

From Maronpot *et al.* (1993)

Groups of five female Wistar rats (190–210 g) were given *N*-nitrosomorpholine (80 mg/L) in the drinking-water for 25 days. Starting two weeks later, the rats were given biweekly subcutaneous injections of corn oil or 2,3,7,8-TCDD for 13 weeks. The calculated average daily dose was 2, 20 or 200 ng/kg bw. The number and volume fraction of hepatic focal lesions (ATPase-deficient) were increased following 13 weeks of 2,3,7,8-TCDD administration at all doses. The numbers of hepatic focal lesions were approximately $125/cm^3$ (control), $250/cm^3$ (low-dose 2,3,7,8-TCDD), $250/cm^3$ (mid-dose 2,3,7,8-TCDD) and $500/cm^3$ (high-dose 2,3,7,8-TCDD), while the corresponding volume fractions were approximately 0.125% (control), 0.10% (low-dose 2,3,7,8-TCDD), 0.125% (mid-dose 2,3,7,8-TCDD) and 0.6% (high-dose 2,3,7,8-TCDD) (Schrenk *et al.*, 1994a).

Groups of 6–15 female Sprague-Dawley rats, 21 days of age, were treated with 10 mg/kg bw NDEA by intraperitoneal injection. After 30 days, rats were given either a basal diet or the basal diet supplemented with 2,3,7,8-TCDD (150 ppt [ng/kg diet], equivalent to a daily dose of about 0.007 µg/kg bw). Hepatic lesions were scored as ATPase-deficient foci. A time-dependent increase was noted in the volume fraction of hepatic foci in NDEA + 2,3,7,8-TCDD-treated rats (170 days after NDEA, 2%; 240 days, 4%;

450 days, 17%) as compared to NDEA alone (170 days, 0.6%; 240 days, 1.0%; 450 days, 4.0%). No hepatotoxicity was detected in any of the groups. Other rats were treated with NDEA (as above) followed by phenobarbital (PB) in the diet (500 ppm) for 30–170 days, at which time the rats were either returned to the basal diet or exposed to dietary 2,3,7,8-TCDD (150 ppt; 0.007 µg/kg bw per day). There was a time-dependent increase in the volume fraction of focal hepatic lesions, which was enhanced in the NDEA + PB + 2,3,7,8-TCDD group (240 days, 2%; 450 days, 13%) as compared to NDEA + PB (240 days, 1%; 450 days, 4%). However, when comparing the groups given NDEA + PB + 2,3,7,8-TCDD and NDEA + 2,3,7,8-TCDD (240 days, 4%; 450 days, 17%), no difference was seen. This suggests that phenobarbital does not enhance the ATPase-negative foci caused by NDEA + 2,3,7,8-TCDD. [The Working Group noted that loss of ATPase does not identify all possible preneoplastic lesions.] Hepatic tumours were examined at 450 days after NDEA treatment. They were primarily eosinophilic and expressed *ras*. The number of combined hepatocellular adenomas and carcinomas was 1/12 in the NDEA group, 5/15 in the NDEA + 2,3,7,8-TCDD group, 5/15 in the NDEA + PB group and 6/15 in the NDEA + PB + 2,3,7,8-TCDD group (Sills *et al.*, 1994).

The single and combined effects of 2,3,7,8-TCDD and 3,4,5,3′,4′-pentachlorobiphenyl (PCB 126) were examined in groups of 10–15 female Sprague-Dawley rats. Female rats (120–140 g) were subjected to a 70% partial hepatectomy and 24 h later received an intraperitoneal injection of corn oil or 30 mg/kg bw NDEA. Five weeks later, the rats were administered either PCB 126, 2,3,7,8-TCDD or a combination of the two, as an initial loading dose (equivalent to five single doses) followed by weekly injections for 19 weeks, at which time the rats were killed. Weekly doses of PCB 126 were 0, 0.316, 1, 3.16 or 10 µg/kg bw, while those of 2,3,7,8-TCDD were 0.1, 0.316 or 1 µg/kg bw. The doses of the combinations were 1 µg/kg bw PCB 126 plus 0.1 µg/kg bw 2,3,7,8-TCDD, 3.16 µg/kg bw PCB 126 plus 0.316 µg/kg bw 2,3,7,8-TCDD and 10 µg/kg bw PCB 126 plus 1 µg/kg bw 2,3,7,8-TCDD. The number and volume fraction of the liver occupied by altered hepatic foci expressing GGT were increased with the highest dose of PCB 126 (10 µg/kg bw per week), with the highest dose of 2,3,7,8-TCDD (1 µg/kg bw per week), and with two of the combinations of PCB 126 with 2,3,7,8-TCDD (3.16 + 0.316 and 10 + 1 µg/kg bw per week of PCB 126 and 2,3,7,8-TCDD, respectively) (Hemming *et al.*, 1995).

Groups of four female Wistar rats (120 g) were given gastric instillations of 10 mg/kg bw NDEA in water daily for 10 days and were then allowed to recover for eight weeks. One group of rats was given a single subcutaneous injection of 1.4 µg/kg bw 2,3,7,8-TCDD ('acute'), while a second group received biweekly subcutaneous injections of 1.4 µg/kg bw 2,3,7,8-TCDD for 115 days ('chronic'). All rats were killed 26 weeks after the start of NDEA treatment. The volume fraction of altered hepatic foci, identified as GSTP-positive, was significantly increased in the 'chronic' 2,3,7,8-TCDD + NDEA group (3.4%) as compared to NDEA alone (1.2%). There was no difference between the 'acute' 2,3,7,8-TCDD + NDEA group (1.7%) and the NDEA-alone group (1.2%) (Stinchcombe *et al.*, 1995).

Groups of 7–11 female Sprague-Dawley rats given 0 or 175 mg/kg bw NDEA in saline by intraperitoneal injection followed by biweekly treatment with 1.75 µg/kg bw 2,3,7,8-TCDD in corn oil by gastric instillation for 30 weeks. The percentages of the liver occupied by focal hepatic lesions (detected by GSTP) were 0.01 ± 0.01 (non-NDEA-treated controls at 30 weeks), 2.23 ± 1.47 (NDEA followed by 2,3,7,8-TCDD at 30 weeks), 0.32 ± 0.97 (non-NDEA-treated controls at 62 weeks) and 6.05 ± 4.3 (NDEA followed by 2,3,7,8-TCDD for 30 weeks and a 32-week observation period). [The Working Group noted that this study did not compare the NDEA/2,3,7,8-TCDD group to an NDEA group not given 2,3,7,8-TCDD.] The incidence of liver neoplasms was increased in the NDEA/2,3,7,8-TCDD group relative to the controls (5/7 and 0/11) (Tritscher et al., 1995).

Dibenzo-*para*-dioxin

Oral administration

Mouse

Groups of 50 male and 50 female B6C3F1 mice, five weeks of age, were administered 0 (control), 5000 (low-dose) or 10 000 (high-dose) mg/kg of diet (ppm) dibenzo-*para*-dioxin (purity, 99.5%) for 87 (high-dose males) or 90 (low-dose males and females, high-dose females) weeks. All surviving male mice were killed at 92–97 weeks, and all surviving female mice at 91–93 weeks. Mean body weights of the treated male and female mice were slightly lower than those of the corresponding controls. Survival of high-dose females was lower than that of the control and low-dose groups ($p < 0.001$, Tarone test). At week 90 of the study, 48/50 (96%), 50/50 (100%) and 46/50 (92%) control, low-dose and high-dose males, respectively, were still alive; and 44/50 (88%), 44/50 (88%) and 27/50 (54%) control, low-dose and high-dose females, respectively, were still alive. Tumours were not induced in mice of either sex at significantly higher incidence in the treated groups than in the corresponding control groups (United States National Toxicology Program, 1979a).

Rat

Groups of 35 male and 35 female Osborne-Mendel rats, five weeks of age, were administered 0 (control), 5000 (low-dose) or 10 000 (high-dose) mg/kg of diet (ppm) dibenzo-*para*-dioxin (purity 99.5%) in the diet for 110 weeks. Mean body weights of the treated male and female rats were lower that those of the corresponding controls. In male rats, survival in the control group was lower than in the treated groups ($p = 0.011$, Tarone test). Survival of high-dose female rats was lower than that of the control and low-dose groups ($p = 0.007$, Tarone test). At week 90 of the study, 24/35 control and 29/35 rats in each treated group of males were still alive, and 32/35, 31/35 and 20/35 control, low-dose and high-dose female rats, respectively, were still alive. Tumours were not induced in rats of either sex at significantly higher incidence in the treated groups than in the corresponding control groups (United States National Toxicology Program, 1979a).

2,7-Dichlorodibenzo-*para*-dioxin (2,7-DCDD)

3.1 Oral administration

3.1.1 *Mouse*

Groups of 50 male and 50 female B6C3F1 mice, five weeks of age, were given 0 (control), 5000 (low-dose) or 10 000 (high-dose) mg/kg of diet (ppm) 2,7-DCDD for 90 weeks. Three impurities with peak areas 3–6% of the major peak were detected by gas chromatography. One was identified as trichlorodibenzo-*para*-dioxin. No 2,3,7,8-TCDD was detected. All surviving male mice were killed at 92–101 weeks and all surviving female mice at 91–98 weeks. Mean body weights of the male mice were unaffected by administration of the test chemical, whereas those of female treated mice were slightly lower than those of the corresponding controls. Survival in male mice was unaffected by treatment. Survival in high-dose female mice was significantly lower than that in control and low-dose groups ($p < 0.001$, Tarone test). At the end of the study, 48/50, 36/50 and 38/50 control, low-dose and high-dose males, respectively, were still alive; and 45/50, 46/50 and 28/50 control, low-dose and high-dose females, respectively, were still alive. Treated male and female mice showed an increased incidence of focal necrosis of the liver. The incidence of hepatocellular carcinomas in male mice was unaffected by treatment: 4/49, 5/50 and 5/42 control, low-dose and high-dose mice, respectively. However, the incidence of hepatocellular adenomas was 4/49, 15/50 and 12/42 in control, low-dose and high-dose males, respectively. The incidence of hepatocellular adenomas and carcinomas combined (8/49, 20/50 and 17/42) was significantly higher in the treated groups than in the control group ($p = 0.008$, Cochran–Armitage test for trend). The incidences in the low- and high-dose groups were both significantly higher than that in the control group ($p = 0.008$ and $p = 0.010$, respectively, Fisher's exact test). In male mice, the incidence of lymphoma or leukaemia was higher in the low-dose (6/50) than in the control group (0/50) ($p = 0.006$, Fisher's exact test). However, the incidence in the high-dose group (3/50) was not statistically different from that of controls. In the female mice, no tumours were observed at significantly higher incidence in the dosed groups than in the corresponding controls (United States National Toxicology Program, 1979b). [The Working Group noted that the presence of three impurities makes it impossible to ascribe the observed carcinogenic effect specifically to the 2,7-dichloro congener.]

3.1.2 *Rat*

Groups of 35 male and 35 female Osborne-Mendel rats, five weeks of age, were given 0 (control), 5000 (low-dose) or 10 000 (high-dose) ppm 2,7-DCDD in the diet for 110 weeks. Three impurities with peak areas 3–6% of the major peak were detected by gas chromatography. All surviving male rats were killed at 110–112 weeks, and all surviving female rats at 110–117 weeks. Mean body weights of the dosed groups were lower that those in the corresponding controls. Survival was not significantly affected by administration of 2,7-DCDD. At week 78 of the study, 30/35, 26/35 and 29/35 control, low-dose and high-dose males, respectively, were still alive; and 33/35, 30/35 and 28/35 control, low-dose and high-dose females, respectively, were still alive. Toxic hepatic lesions characterized by centrilobular fatty metamorphosis (33–48%) and/or necrosis (6–20%) were observed in both low- and high-dose rats. Tumours were not induced in rats of either sex at significantly higher incidence in the dosed groups than in the corresponding control groups (United States National Toxicology Program, 1979b)

3.2   Administration with known carcinogens

Skin

Mouse: Groups of 20 female HRS/J hairless (*hr/hr*) mice, five to eight weeks of age, were treated with single skin applications of 0 or 5 µmol (0.75 mg) per animal MNNG in 50 µL acetone followed by 20 µg/animal 2,7-DCDD in 50 µL acetone twice weekly for 20 weeks. A control group of 20 mice was given acetone followed by 10 ng/animal 2,3,7,8-TCDD. Skin tumours developed in 0/19 mice treated with MNNG plus 2,7-DCDD and in 0/20 mice treated with 2,7-DCDD alone (Poland *et al.*, 1982).

1,2,3,6,7,8-Hexachlorodibenzo-*para*-dioxin and 1,2,3,7,8,9-hexachlorodibenzo-*para*-dioxin (mixture) (HxCDD)

3.1   Oral administration

3.1.1   *Mouse*

Groups of 50 male and 50 female B6C3F1 mice, six weeks of age, were administered HxCDD (purity, 98.6%; 31% 1,2,3,6,7,8-HxCDD and 67% 1,2,3,7,8,9-HxCDD of the total HxCDD content), suspended in a vehicle of 9 : 1 corn oil–acetone, by gastric instillation twice a week for 104 weeks at doses of 1.25 (low), 2.5 (mid) or 5 (high) µg/kg per week for male mice and 2.5 (low), 5 (mid) or 10 (high) µg/kg per week for female mice. Groups of 75 mice of each sex served as vehicle controls and 50 mice of each sex as untreated controls. All surviving animals were killed at 105–108 weeks. The mean body weights and survival in the treated groups were similar to those of the vehicle-control groups. At the end of the study, 32/50, 38/75, 29/50, 26/50 and 23/50 untreated control, vehicle-control, low-, mid- and high-dose male mice, respectively, were still alive; for females, the corresponding numbers were 36/50, 58/75, 31/50, 33/50 and 36/50 animals. In males, hepatocellular adenomas occurred at increased incidence in the high-dose group (7/73, 5/50, 9/49 and 15/48 vehicle-control, low-, mid- and high-dose mice, respectively; $p = 0.003$, Fisher's exact test). There was no significant increase in the incidence of hepatocellular carcinomas (8/73, 9/50, 5/49 and 9/48). In females, hepatocellular adenomas occurred at incidences that were dose-related (2/73, 4/48, 4/47 and 9/47 in the vehicle-control, low-, mid- and high-dose mice, respectively; $p = 0.002$, Cochran–Armitage test for trend); the incidence in the high-dose group was significantly higher ($p = 0.003$, Fisher's exact test) than that in the corresponding vehicle-control group. Hepatocellular carcinomas were found in 1/73, 0/48, 2/47 and 2/47 females, respectively (United States National Toxicology Program, 1980a). [The Working Group noted that it is unlikely that the impurities consisting of various polyhalogenated dibenzo-*para*-dioxins were responsible for the observed carcinogenic effects.]

3.1.2   *Rat*

Groups of 50 male and 50 female Osborne-Mendel rats, six weeks of age, were administered HxCDD (purity, 98.6%; 31% 1,2,3,6,7,8-HxCDD and 67% 1,2,3,7,8,9-HxCDD of the total HxCDD content), suspended in a vehicle of 9 : 1 corn oil–acetone, by gastric instillation twice a week for 104 weeks at doses of 1.25 (low), 2.5 (mid) or 5 (high) μg/kg per week. Groups of 75 rats of each sex served as vehicle controls and 50 rats of each sex as untreated controls. All surviving animals were killed at 105–108 weeks. A dose-related depression in mean body weight was seen in both sexes. At the end of the study, 24/50, 29/75, 18/50, 19/50 and 19/50 untreated control, vehicle control, low-, mid- and high-dose rats, respectively, were still alive; for females, the corresponding numbers were 33/50, 39/75, 36/50, 36/50 and 37/50 animals. In male rats, hepatic neoplastic nodules occurred at incidences that were dose-related (0/74, 0/49, 1/50 and 4/48 in the vehicle-control, low-, mid- and high-dose groups, respectively ($p = 0.003$, Cochran–Armitage test for trend). No hepatocellular carcinomas occurred in males. In female rats, hepatic neoplastic nodules occurred at incidences that were dose-related (5/75, 10/50, 12/50 and 30/50 in the vehicle-control, low-, mid- and high-dose groups, respectively; $p < 0.001$, Cochran–Armitage trend test); the incidences in the mid- and high-dose groups were significantly higher ($p = 0.006$ and $p < 0.001$, respectively, Fisher's exact test) than that in the corresponding vehicle-control group. In addition, four high-dose females had hepatocellular carcinomas (United States National Toxicology Program, 1980a). [The Working Group noted that it is unlikely that the impurities consisting of various polyhalogenated dibenzo-*para*-dioxins were responsible for the observed carcinogenic effects.]

3.2   Skin application

Mouse: Groups of 30 male and 30 female Swiss-Webster mice, six weeks of age, received skin applications on the clipped back of 0.01 μg/animal HxCDD (purity, 98.6%; 31% 1,2,3,6,7,8-HxCDD and 67% 1,2,3,7,8,9-HxCDD of the total HxCDD content) suspended in 0.1 mL acetone on three days per week for 104 weeks. During the first 16 weeks, doses were 0.005 μg/animal per application. As vehicle controls, 45 mice of each sex received 0.1 mL of acetone three times per week. Thirty animals of each sex served as untreated controls. HxCDD treatment did not affect mean body weights or survival in either sex. At week 60 of the study, 23/30, 30/45 and 25/30 untreated control, vehicle-control and HxCDD-treated males, respectively, were still alive; and 28/30, 43/45 and 24/30 untreated control, vehicle-control and HxCDD-treated females, respectively, were still alive. In male mice, the incidence of alveolar/bronchiolar carcinomas in the group administered only HxCDD was significantly higher (5/30; $p = 0.045$, Fisher's exact test) than that in the vehicle controls (1/41), but similar to that in untreated controls (4/28). In male mice, the incidence of lymphomas or leukaemias was significantly lower (0/30; $p = 0.011$) than that in untreated controls (6/29). In female mice, the incidence of fibro-sarcomas of the integumentary system was significantly higher in animals administered HxCDD (4/27; $p = 0.044$, Fisher's exact test) than that in untreated controls (0/30).

However, the incidences were not significantly elevated compared with those of the vehicle controls (2/41) (United States National Toxicology Program, 1980b).

1,2,3,7,8-Pentachlorodibenzo-*para*-dioxin (1,2,3,7,8-PeCDD)

Administration with known carcinogens

Liver

Rat: Waern *et al.* (1991) analysed the GGT-positive foci in groups of 10–20 female Sprague-Dawley rats subjected to a 70% partial hepatectomy followed by single intraperitoneal injection of 30 mg/kg bw NDEA and 1,2,3,7,8-PeCDD. Five weeks after NDEA administration, a loading dose of 1,2,3,7,8-PeCDD consisting of five times the weekly maintenance dose in each treatment group was given by subcutaneous injection. Weekly maintenance doses of 0.088, 0.35 and 1.4 µg/kg bw 1,2,3,7,8-PeCDD per week were then given for 20 weeks. The rats were killed at the end of the treatment. A significant increase in the percentage of liver occupied by GGT-positive focal hepatic lesions was observed for all doses of 1,2,3,7,8-PeCDD (approximately: low-dose, 0.35%; middose, 0.7%; high-dose, 1.6%) compared with NDEA alone (0.15%). A significant increase in the number of foci per liver was also seen in the two highest-dose groups (approximately: low-dose, 2750; mid-dose, 5000; high-dose, 10 250) compared with NDEA alone (2000).

1,2,3,4,6,7,8-Heptachlorodibenzo-*para*-dioxin (1,2,3,4,6,7,8-HpCDD)

Administration with known carcinogens

Liver

Rat: Groups of 4–8 female Wistar rats (100 g) were given five doses of 10 mg/kg bw NDEA in water by gastric instillation. Starting two weeks later, rats were treated with either corn oil solvent or 70 µg/kg bw 1,2,3,4,6,7,8-HpCDD biweekly by subcutaneous injection. The development of focal hepatic lesions was determined at 9, 13 and 17 weeks. ATPase-deficient lesions were quantitated and the GSTP-positive focal population was used to determine focal proliferation rates from pulse labelling with bromodeoxyuridine (BrdU) before sacrifice. The numbers of ATPase-deficient lesions were 619 ± 113 (at 9 weeks), 551 ± 158 (at 13 weeks) and 1691 ± 652 (at 17 weeks) per cm^3 in the NDEA-treated rats given 1,2,3,4,6,7,8-HpCDD. The corresponding numbers in the groups given 1,2,3,4,6,7,8-HpCDD but no NDEA were 63 ± 35 (at 9 weeks), 87 ± 16 (at 13 weeks) and 120 ± 30 (at 17 weeks) per cm^3. The percentage volume fractions of ATPase-deficient lesions were 0.093 ± 0.38 (at 9 weeks), 0.091 ± 0.037 (at 13 weeks) and 0.76 ± 0.40 (at 17 weeks) (Buchmann *et al.*, 1994).

Groups of five female Wistar rats (190–210 g) were given *N*-nitrosomorpholine (80 mg/L) in the drinking-water for 25 days. Starting two weeks later, the rats were given biweekly subcutaneous injections of corn oil or 1,2,3,4,6,7,8-HpCDD for 13 weeks. The calculated average daily doses were 100, 1000 or 10 000 ng/kg bw. The number and volume fraction of ATPase deficient lesions were assessed following 13 weeks of administration. The numbers of ATPase-deficient hepatic foci were approximately 125/cm³ (controls), 450/cm³ (low-dose), 250/cm³ (mid-dose) and 500/cm³ (high-dose), while the corresponding percentage volume fractions were approximately 0.125 (control), 0.25 (low-dose), 0.125 (mid-dose) and 0.9 (high-dose) (Schrenk *et al.*, 1994a).

Defined mixture of 49 polychlorinated dibenzo-*para*-dioxins (PCDDs)

Administration with known carcinogens

Liver

Rat: Groups of five female Wistar rats (190–210 g) were given *N*-nitrosomorpholine (80 mg/L) in the drinking-water for 25 days. Starting two weeks later, the rats were given biweekly subcutaneous injections of corn oil or a defined mixture of 49 PCDDs for 13 weeks at 200 ng, 2000 ng or 20 000 ng PCDD/kg. The number and volume fraction of ATPase-deficient lesions were assessed following 13 weeks of administration. The numbers of ATPase-deficient hepatic foci were approximately 125/cm³ (controls), 125/cm³ (200 ng/kg), 300/cm³ (2000 ng/kg) and 800/cm³ (20 000 ng/kg), while the corresponding percentage volume fractions were 0.125 (control), 0.2 (200 ng/kg), 0.25 (2000 ng/kg) and 0.75 (20 000 ng/kg) (Schrenk *et al.*, 1994a).

4. Other Data Relevant to an Evaluation of Carcinogenicity and its Mechanisms

4.1 Absorption, distribution, metabolism and excretion

4.1.1 *Humans*

The kinetic data on PCDDs have been reviewed (Olson, 1994).

In all vertebrate species studied so far, the 2,3,7,8-substituted PCDDs are almost exclusively retained in all tissue types, particularly fat and liver (Van den Berg *et al.*, 1994).

The penetration of 2,3,7,8-TCDD into human skin *in vitro* has been studied (Weber *et al.*, 1991a). At a dose level of 6.5 ng/cm² and using acetone as the vehicle, the absorption rate was about 5 pg/cm² per hour. When mineral oil was used as the vehicle, the absorption rate was about 1 pg/cm². These values represent a low rate of skin penetration. The stratum corneum appears to act as a reservoir.

The absorption and elimination kinetics of 2,3,7,8-TCDD were investigated in a 42-year-old male volunteer weighing 92 kg who ingested 105 ng [1,6-³H]2,3,7,8-TCDD (13.0 µCi) (Poiger & Schlatter, 1986); > 87% was absorbed and 11.5% of the dose was excreted in the faeces within three days, representing non-absorbed 2,3,7,8-TCDD. Thereafter, the daily faecal excretion amounted to 0.03% of the dose. Based on analytical results in adipose tissue obtained by biopsy and faecal samples from up to 125 days after dosing, an elimination half-life of 5.8 years was calculated. The data were compatible with first-order elimination kinetics. The maximal excretion of unmetabolized 2,3,7,8-TCDD in the faeces was 50% (Wendling et al., 1990b). In a follow-up of this experiment up to five years after dosage, an elimination half-life of 9.7 years was determined (Schlatter, 1991).

In a study of 36 Viet Nam veterans of Operation Ranch Hand (see Section 1.3.1(a)(i), (a)(ii)), the decline in serum levels of 2,3,7,8-TCDD indicated a half-life of 7.1 years (Pirkle et al., 1989). In a follow-up examination of 337 Ranch Hand veterans in 1994, a half-life of 11.3 years was found (Wolfe et al., 1994). In a 10-year follow-up study of these Ranch Hand veterans, a half-life estimate of 8.7 years with a 95% CI of 8.0–9.5 years was determined. Half-life increased significantly with increasing body fat, but not with age or relative changes in the percentage of body fat (Michalek et al., 1996).

In a group of 48 workers who were exposed to various PCDDs and PCDFs in a herbi-cide-producing plant, Boehringer Ingelheim, AG, in Hamburg, Germany (see Section 1.3.1(a)(i)), a median half-life of 7.2 years was calculated for 2,3,7,8-TCDD (Flesch-Janys et al., 1996).

In another study with 243 workers exposed to 2,3,7,8-TCDD in a reactor accident in a plant of BASF, AG, Ludwigshafen, Germany, estimated half-lives of 5.1 and 8.9 years were determined for individuals with 20% or 30% body fat, respectively (Ott & Zober, 1996).

In infants, less than 10% of ingested 2,3,7,8-TCDD is excreted in the faeces (Körner et al., 1993; Abraham et al., 1994; Dahl et al., 1995).

When expressed on a total tissue lipid basis, 2,3,7,8-TCDD is distributed equally in the liver and adipose tissue or in the blood and adipose tissue (Leung et al., 1990).

Mammalian (including human) data have been used to formulate kinetic models that have a broad applicability for any pattern of exposure from background to highly toxic levels. Relationships between 2,3,7,8-PCDD congener concentrations in adipose tissue and variations in the proportion of such tissue were established that indicate a need for caution in clearance rate measurements based solely on tissue lipids (Carrier et al., 1995a,b; Van der Molen et al., 1996).

There is a paucity of data on other PCDD congeners. Preliminary kinetic data, based on questionable analytical methods applied to fat samples from one individual exposed to technical pentachlorophenol, were derived for hexa-, hepta- and octa-CDDs (Górski et al., 1984). Half-lives of 3.2–5.7 years were calculated. Flesch-Janys et al. (1996) reported median half-lives for six PCDD congeners from 3.7 years (1,2,3,4,6,7,8-HpCDD) to 15.7 years (1,2,3,7,8-PeCDD) in a group of 48 occupationally exposed indi-viduals (see above). Comparison of daily intakes and body burdens of individual con-geners with the corresponding data for 2,3,7,8-TCDD yielded estimated elimination half-lives of about five years for 1,2,3,7,8-PeCCD, 15 years for 1,2,3,4,7,8-HxCDD, 25 years for 1,2,3,4,6,7,8-HpCDD and 50 years for OCDD (Schlatter, 1991).

4.1.2   *Experimental systems*

(a)   *Absorption*

Absorption across the gastrointestinal mucosa depends on the vehicle and on the molecular size and solubility of the congener. These factors seem to be most significant for the hepta- and octa-CDDs. There appear to be only minor differences in absorption between rodent species (Van den Berg *et al.*, 1994). Single-dose exposure studies with 2,3,7,8-TCDD showed 70–90% absorption from the gastrointestinal tract in rats, hamsters and guinea-pigs (Piper *et al.*, 1973; Allen *et al.*, 1975; Rose *et al.*, 1976; Olson *et al.*, 1985; Decad *et al.*, 1990), whereas less than 50% gastrointestinal absorption was found in female C57BL/6J and male ICR/Ha Swiss mouse strains (Koshakji *et al.*, 1984; Curtis *et al.*, 1990). When 2,3,7,8-TCDD was administered in the diet to rats for up to six weeks, absorption was only 50–60% (Fries & Marrow, 1975) compared with 70% following a single dose in corn oil (Piper *et al.*, 1973). No significant influence of age was found for gastrointestinal absorption of 2,3,7,8-TCDD in rats (Hébert & Birnbaum, 1987). Absorption of 1,2,3,7,8-PeCDD is in the same range as that of 2,3,7,8-TCDD (Yoshimura *et al.*, 1986; Brewster & Birnbaum, 1987). The only other PCDD congener of which the gastrointestinal absorption has been studied in some detail is OCDD; only 2–15% of a single oral dose was taken up by rats (Birnbaum & Couture, 1988). For metabolites of 2,3,7,8-TCDD, it has been shown that enterohepatic circulation is not significant in the rat (Ramsey *et al.*, 1982).

The uptake of PCDDs by dermal permeation and pulmonary absorption is much more limited than uptake after oral ingestion (Nessel *et al.*, 1992; Diliberto *et al.*, 1996). For 2,3,7,8-TCDD, dermal permeation is strongly dose-dependent in rats (Banks *et al.*, 1990). Uptake from the application site is slow but also depends on the vehicle used and shows a good inverse correlation with the octanol–water partition coefficient (Brewster *et al.*, 1989; Banks & Birnbaum, 1991; Jackson *et al.*, 1993). The bioavailability after dermal exposure is probably less than 1% for all congeners (Van den Berg *et al.*, 1994).

The adsorption of PCDDs on various environmental matrices can lead to a significant reduction in bioavailability, which depends strongly on the properties of the particles (Nessel *et al.*, 1992; Van den Berg *et al.*, 1994). On the basis of a number of studies with rodents, a bioavailability for PCDDs from soil of 25–50% was suggested for the Cl_4–Cl_6 congeners, while 10% was proposed for the Cl_7 and Cl_8 congeners. For combustion particles (fly ash), a bioavailability of 5–20% was proposed as a realistic estimate for PCDDs, this being high for the hepta- and octa-chlorinated PCDDs (Van den Berg *et al.*, 1994).

(b)   *Body distribution*

In all rodent species, the liver and adipose tissue are the major storage sites for PCDDs. However, in certain species, the skin can also act as an important storage site and high concentrations can be found in adrenals. Most detailed information is available for 2,3,7,8-TCDD, but reasonable quantities of data are available to support this primary tissue distribution in rodents for the higher chlorinated congeners. Long retention in tissues is caused primarily by the steric hindrance towards cytochrome P450 activity caused by chlorine atoms on the 2,3,7,8 positions, resulting in limited metabolism (Van den Berg *et al.*, 1994). Some tissue retention has been observed for certain non-2,3,7,8-substituted PCDDs in rodents and monkeys (Abraham *et al.*, 1989; Neubert *et al.*, 1990a), but the levels should not be considered as toxicologically relevant. Transport in the blood occurs through binding to plasma lipids and lipoproteins, with increasing affinity found for the higher chlorinated congeners in the plasma proteins (Patterson *et al.*, 1989; Schecter *et al.*, 1990h). The majority of 2,3,7,8-TCDD is bound to very low-density lipoprotein, followed by low-density lipoprotein and high-density lipoprotein (Marinovich *et al.*, 1983).

Depending on the experimental conditions, 25–70% of the administered dose of 2,3,7,8-TCDD is stored in the liver of rats, mice, hamsters and guinea-pigs approximately one day after exposure. Studies with mixtures of PCDDs showed that in rodents the Cl_5 and Cl_6 congeners have higher hepatic retention than 2,3,7,8-TCDD (Van den Berg *et al.*, 1994). As a result, the liver to adipose tissue concentration ratio strongly increases with increasing chlorination. Measurement of tritiated 2,3,7,8-TCDD administered in corn oil by gastric instillation to adult female rhesus monkeys, infant male rhesus monkeys and young adult male Sprague-Dawley rats indicated that liver retention of the dose was > 40% in rats, but < 10% in the rhesus monkeys. A large percentage of the dose was located in monkey tissues with a high lipid content, especially the skin, muscle and adipose tissue. In the rats, these tissues had much lower levels of 2,3,7,8-TCDD (Van Miller *et al.*, 1976). Differences in liver to adipose tissue ratio between rats and marmosets (*Callithrix jacchus*) have been observed (see **Figure 2**) (Olson, 1994).

Figure 2. The liver-to-adipose tissue ratios for 2,3,7,8-substituted PCDDs and PCDFs in marmosets and rats

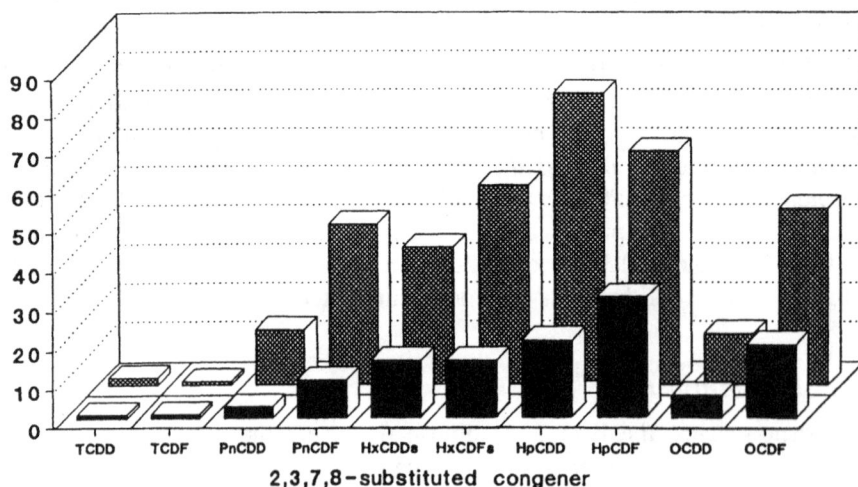

From Olson (1994)
Grey bars: rat; black bars: marmoset

Hepatic disposition of 2,3,7,8-TCDD is dose-dependent (Kociba *et al.*, 1978; Abraham *et al.*, 1988); this has been suggested to be caused by the presence in the liver of inducible protein binding sites, at least in mice (Poland *et al.*, 1989). As a possible mechanism, binding to CYP1A2 in the liver has been proposed (Voorman & Aust, 1987; Poland *et al.*, 1989; Voorman & Aust, 1989). In rats, 2,3,7,8-TCDD was equally distributed between hepatic P9 (mitochondrial, lysosomal, nuclear) and S9 (cytosol and microsomal) fractions, localization in the S9 being in microsomes. In extrahepatic tissues (lung/kidneys), 2,3,7,8-TCDD was concentrated in the P9 fraction, while in the S9 fraction localization was in the cytosol. Use of CYP1A1 and CYP1A2 immunoreactive proteins and measurement of marker enzyme activities, ethoxyresorufin *O*-deethylase and methoxyresorufin *O*-demethylase, respectively, showed that CYP1A1 was induced in microsomes of all three organs, while CYP1A2 was induced only in liver (Santostefano *et al.*, 1996). However, the role of other dioxin (inducible) hepatic binding proteins cannot be excluded (Landers *et al.*, 1990; Buckley-Kedderis *et al.*, 1992; Tritscher *et al.*, 1992; Van den Berg *et al.*, 1994).

Pre- and postnatal transfer of PCDDs has been studied in rats and mice. Lactational transfer was found to be one or two orders a magnitude higher than placental transfer in these rodents (Nau & Bass, 1981; Weber & Birnbaum, 1985; Nau *et al.*, 1986; Van den Berg *et al.*, 1987; Li *et al.*, 1995a). The level of placental transfer depends on the molecular size, with the highest fetal retention observed for 2,3,7,8-TCDD (Van den Berg *et al.*, 1987). In the mouse embryo, the liver is the major storage site, with two to five times higher concentrations than those found in other tissues (Nau & Bass, 1981; Krowke & Neubert, 1990). In contrast, there is no evidence for hepatic concentration in the fetal rat liver. From a quantitative point of view, lactational transfer in marmosets and rhesus monkeys is also more important than placental transport, but placental transport in marmosets can result in significant accumulation in fetal tissues (Hagenmaier *et al.*, 1990b; Krowke *et al.*, 1990). On the basis of studies with complex mixtures of PCDDs and PCDFs, it appears that these compounds are mobilized primarily from adipose tissue and not from the liver in rats (Van den Berg *et al.*, 1987). In marmosets, lactational transfer can lead to concentrations in the tissues of offspring that are equal to or higher than those found in maternal tissues. In both rats and marmosets, lactational transfer decreases with increasing number of chlorine atoms in the PCDD molecule (Van den Berg *et al.*, 1987; Krowke *et al.*, 1990).

(c) Metabolism

The metabolism of PCDDs has been studied primarily in rodents. In rats, oxidation by P450 occurs preferentially at the lateral, 2, 3, 7 and 8 positions, yielding primarily mono- and dihydroxylated metabolites. Furthermore, sulfur-containing metabolites have been identified, which probably arose through glutathione conjugation (Tulp & Hutzinger, 1978). Studies with 2,3,7,8-TCDF in rats suggest that CYP1A1 is directly involved in phase I metabolism of these compounds and not CYP1A2 (Tai *et al.*, 1993). If all of the 2, 3, 7 and 8-positions are substituted with chlorine atoms, metabolic conversion of the molecule is strongly hindered. Recent quantum-mechanical calculations determining highest occupied molecular orbital (HOMO) energy levels for the dibenzo-*para*-dioxin molecule have confirmed the higher susceptibility for epoxidation of the 2–3 or 7–8 positions in the molecule (Weber *et al.*, 1996). Although 2,3,7,8-TCDD is highly resistant towards biotransformation, small amounts of metabolites have been identified in rats and dogs. Metabolic transformation included oxidative and reductive dechlorination, including NIH shifts (shift of a chlorine substituent). In addition, oxygen bridge cleavage was found to be another important pathway (Poiger & Schlatter, 1979; Ramsey *et al.*, 1982; Poiger & Buser, 1984; Huwe *et al.*, 1996). Conjugation appears to be important for the elimination of PCDDs from the body, as many 2,3,7,8-TCDD metabolites were present as glucuronide conjugates in the bile of the rat (Poiger & Buser, 1984; Wroblewski & Olson, 1985; Huwe *et al.*, 1996). From a qualitative point of view, metabolic pathways are fairly similar among rodent species, but large quantitative differences can be observed (Van den Berg *et al.*, 1994; Larsen *et al.*, 1996). Guinea-pigs show a lower metabolic capacity than rats, Syrian hamsters and mice (Wroblewski & Olson, 1985). Limited information is available about the metabolic conversion of higher chlorinated 2,3,7,8-substituted PCDDs, but it can be expected that pathways will be similar to those for 2,3,7,8-TCDD, provided that susceptible positions are not sterically hindered by additional chlorines. In **Figure 3**, a generalized scheme of metabolic pathways for PCDDs is given (Van den Berg *et al.*, 1994).

(*d*) *Excretion*

The elimination of PCDDs has been studied in several laboratory species under a variety of experimental conditions (Van den Berg *et al.*, 1994). After exposure, the compounds are usually more rapidly eliminated from blood and muscle tissue than from liver and adipose tissue. In some species, such as primates, elimination from the skin is similar to that from the adipose tissue (Birnbaum *et al.*, 1980; Brewster & Birnbaum, 1987; Brewster *et al.*, 1988, 1989). For most body compartments, the elimination of 2,3,7,8-substituted PCDDs can be described by a one-compartment open model (Hiles & Bruce, 1976; Rose *et al.*, 1976), but models with two- or three-phase elimination have also been applied. In view of the non-linear distribution of PCDDs in many experimental systems, the use of physiologically based pharmacokinetic models has been successfully applied (Carrier *et al.*, 1995a,b). In almost all laboratory species which have been studied, elimination takes place through bile and faeces in the form of hydroxylated or conjugated metabolites that are rapidly eliminated from the body (Van den Berg *et al.*, 1994). Guinea-pigs seem to be an exception among rodents, as this species eliminates 2,3,7,8-TCDD more than its polar metabolites (Olson, 1986).

For 2,3,7,8-TCDD, whole body half-lives in the rat have been reported to range between 17 and 31 days, depending on the strain and experimental conditions used. Most studies with rodents have found similar elimination rates from the liver and adipose tissue for 2,3,7,8-TCDD (Piper *et al.*, 1973; Allen *et al.*, 1975; Fries & Marrow, 1975; Rose *et al.*, 1976; Abraham *et al.*, 1988, 1989; Pohjanvirta *et al.*, 1990a). In rats, lactation is a very effective route of elimination of 2,3,7,8-TCDD, leading to a 50% reduction of the half-life from the liver (Abraham *et al.*, 1988; Korte *et al.*, 1990). The half-life of 1,2,3,7,8-PeCDD elimination in the rat is approximately 30 days, which is

Figure 3. A generalized scheme of pathways for the biotransformation of PCDDs based on the information from mammalian studies *in vivo*

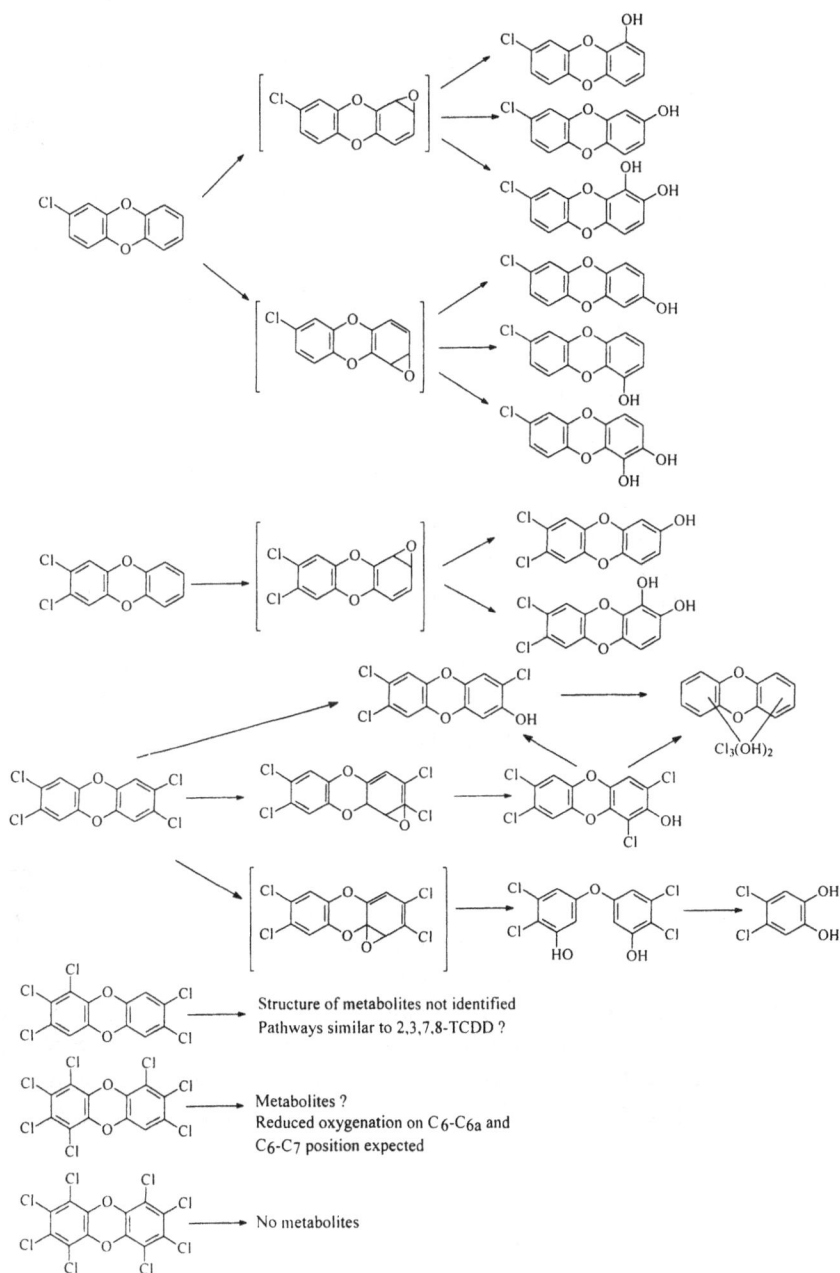

Structure of metabolites not identified
Pathways similar to 2,3,7,8-TCDD ?

Metabolites ?
Reduced oxygenation on C_6-C_{6a} and
C_6-C_7 position expected

No metabolites

From Van den Berg *et al.* (1994)

similar to that of 2,3,7,8-TCDD (Wacker *et al.*, 1986). However, with more chlorine atoms present in a 2,3,7,8-substituted PCDD, elimination is much slower. For the Cl_6–Cl_8 congeners, half-lives between 75 days and seven years have been calculated for the rat (Birnbaum & Couture,1988; Van den Berg *et al.*, 1989a, 1994). In the mouse, half-lives for 2,3,7,8-TCDD are in the same range as those in the rat, but there are distinct strain differences (Gasiewicz *et al.*, 1983; Birnbaum, 1986). Thus, the half-life of 2,3,7,8-TCDD in the non-responsive DBA strain is approximately twice as long as that in the responsive C57BL strain (Gasiewicz *et al.*, 1983). In the Syrian hamster, the half-life of 2,3,7,8-TCDD is two- to three-fold lower than in the rat (Olson *et al.*, 1980). Although this faster elimination of 2,3,7,8-TCDD in the Syrian hamster might contribute to the relative insensitivity of this species towards acute toxicity, it can be assumed that the 100-fold difference in sensitivity between Syrian hamsters and other rodents is dominated more by genetic background than kinetics (Van den Berg *et al.*, 1994). The half-life of 2,3,7,8-TCDD elimination in guinea-pigs has been estimated as 30 days (i.e., the same as in rats) (Gasiewicz & Neal, 1979) and 94 days (Olson, 1986). No clear reason for the discrepancy was discovered.

The half-life of 2,3,7,8-TCDD is much longer in primate species than in rodent species. In seven adult female rhesus monkeys, an average half-life of about 391 days was determined after four years of dietary exposure to 25 ng/kg diet (0.67 ng/kg bw/day). Lactation during four months resulted in a 21% decrease of the maternal body burden. During the first year after birth, the half-life of 2,3,7,8-TCDD in breast-fed rhesus monkeys was approximately 181 days, which was significantly lower than that observed in the mothers (Bowman *et al.*, 1989). In marmosets, longer half-lives for the 2,3,7,8-substituted PCDDs than in rodents were also observed. In liver and adipose tissue, half-lives from eight weeks up to several years were measured (Neubert *et al.*, 1990a).

During pregnancy, elimination from the dam is approximately twice as fast as in the non-pregnant female (Weber & Birnbaum, 1985).

(e)   Kinetics and toxicity

Kinetics to some extent influence the toxicity of individual PCDD and PCDF congeners. This was illustrated in experiments with B6C3F1 mice dosed with 2,3,7,8-TCDD or 2,3,7,8-TCDF, in which CYP1A1 activity was found to depend on the time period to acquire a steady-state situation (DeVito & Birnbaum, 1995). In addition, total body fat content in various species and strains of laboratory animals may contribute to some of the observed differences in species sensitivity for 2,3,7,8-TCDD (Geyer *et al.*, 1990). However, the available data seem to imply that kinetics are not a governing factor influencing the toxicity of these compounds, but genetic factors seem to predominate (Van den Berg *et al.*, 1994).

4.2 Toxic effects

4.2.1 *Humans*

Human exposure to 2,3,7,8-TCDD has been associated with many toxic effects other than cancer. The majority of these effects has been reported among occupationally exposed groups, such as chemical production workers, pesticide users and individuals who handled or were exposed to materials treated with 2,3,7,8-TCDD-contaminated pesticides, and among residents of areas contaminated with tainted waste oil and industrial effluent. These effects represent a complex network of responses ranging from changes in hepatic enzyme levels to observable alterations in the character and physiology of the sebaceous gland, as in chloracne. The Working Group noted that populations are exposed to a variety of chemicals and for some outcomes, it is difficult to separate the effects of the combined exposures. More comprehensive descriptions of studies cited in this section are included in other sections of this monograph (Taylor, 1979; Calvert *et al.*, 1992).

(a) Chloracne and other effects on the skin

Chloracne is a persistent acneiform condition characterized by comedones, keratin cysts and inflamed papules with hyperpigmentation and an anatomical distribution frequently involving the skin under the eyes and behind the ears. It occurs after acute or chronic exposure to a variety of chlorinated aromatic compounds by skin contact, ingestion or inhalation (Crow, 1978; Moses & Prioleau, 1985). This acne-like condition is reported to have occurred with or without other effects in at least a few workers after all reported accidents at TCP production facilities (Ashe & Suskind, 1950; Goldman, 1972; May, 1973; Zober *et al.*, 1990), among individuals involved in daily production of 2,3,7,8-TCDD-contaminated products (Bleiberg *et al.*, 1964; Poland *et al.*, 1971; Pazderova-Vejlupkova *et al.*, 1981; Moses *et al.*, 1984; Suskind & Hertzberg, 1984; Moses & Prioleau, 1985; Bond *et al.*, 1989b), among three laboratory workers exposed to pure 2,3,7,8-TCDD (Oliver, 1975) and among at least 193 (0.6%) Seveso residents, mostly children (at least 20% among children aged 0–14 years from Zone A) (Reggiani, 1978; Caramaschi *et al.*, 1981; Ideo *et al.*, 1985; Mocarelli *et al.*, 1986; Assennato *et al.*, 1989). Chloracne was not found among Missouri residents (Hoffman *et al.*, 1986; Webb *et al.*, 1989) examined 10 years after exposure or among Ranch Hand personnel (Roegner *et al.*, 1991). In United States Army Viet Nam veterans, chloracne-like skin lesions were rarely observed on examination (0.9% in Viet Nam veterans versus 0.8% in non-Viet Nam veterans; odds ratio, 1.4; 95% CI, 0.7–2.9) (Centers for Disease Control Vietnam Experience Study, 1988a).

Chloracne appears shortly after exposure to 2,3,7,8-TCDD-contaminated chemicals. In Seveso, the eruption of comedones, usually accompanied by cysts, was observed between two weeks and two months after the reactor release (Reggiani, 1980), and within six months of the explosion, 34 cases of chloracne were identified among children (Caramaschi *et al.*, 1981). In chemical workers involved in the TCP reactor release at the BASF plant in Ludwigshafen, Germany, most cases of chloracne developed within two days after first exposure (Zober *et al.*, 1990; Ott *et al.*, 1994). One case of chloracne developed only two years after the accident, but the authors suggest that the etiology of this case is unclear.

Among Seveso residents, despite high serum 2,3,7,8-TCDD levels, the chloracne resolved in all but one person by 1983 (Assennato *et al.*, 1989; Mocarelli *et al.*, 1991). However, for TCP workers at the Nitro, WV, USA, plant, Moses *et al.* (1984) reported that the mean duration of chloracne was 26.1 ± 5.9 years.

Positive associations between serum and adipose tissue levels of 2,3,7,8-TCDD and other PCDDs and the risk of chloracne among chemical production workers have been reported (Ott *et al.*, 1987; Beck *et al.*, 1989b; Bond *et al.*, 1989b); the risk was also shown to be greater for subjects of young age at exposure, long exposure duration and a history of employment in production areas of high potential exposure.

Mocarelli *et al.* (1991) described chloracne in people from Seveso Zone A who had 2,3,7,8-TCDD levels in serum lipids ranging from 828 to 56 000 ng/kg (sampled within one year of the reactor release) (see **Table 21**). The study also included other individuals from Zone A, but without chloracne, who had serum 2,3,7,8-TCDD levels that ranged from 1770 to 10 400 ng/kg. With the exception of one person with chloracne who was 16 years old at the time of the accident, all of the cases were in children under the age of 11 years. This contrasts with higher serum levels measured in some adult chloracne subjects among German production workers (**Table 44**). Cases had estimated adipose levels of greater than 200 ng/kg 2,3,7,8-TCDD and over 2000 ng/kg lipid HxCDD at the time of diagnosis. However, a threshold level above which chloracne occurs has not been established.

Other dermatological alterations, including hypertrichosis and hyperpigmentation, have been reported among workers exposed to 2,3,7,8-TCDD in the United States (West Virginia and New Jersey) (Ashe & Suskind, 1950; Bleiberg *et al.*, 1964; Poland *et al.*, 1971), Germany (Bauer *et al.*, 1961; Goldman, 1972) and Czechoslovakia (Jirasek *et al.*, 1974). Increased prevalence of actinic or solar elastosis was observed only in West Virginia TCP workers (59.1% exposed versus 30.1% unexposed; $p < 0.01$). In the same exposed population, three cases of Peyronie's disease (a rare progressive scarring of the penile membrane) were identified (Suskind & Hertzberg, 1984).

(b)   Hepatic effects

γ-Glutamyltransferase

The studies of Seveso children demonstrate an increase in γ-glutamyltransferase (GGT) levels that occured shortly after the explosion and then a gradual decline to near normal levels within five years (Caramaschi *et al.*, 1981; Mocarelli *et al.*, 1986).

Levels of GGT were also found to be elevated among some TCP production workers in the United Kingdom and the USA (West Virginia, Missouri and New Jersey) up to 30 years after last exposure to 2,3,7,8-TCDD-contaminated chemicals (May, 1982; Martin, 1984; Moses *et al.*, 1984; Calvert *et al.*, 1992). However, compared with controls, GGT was not elevated in another study of West Virginia workers (Suskind & Hertzberg, 1984).

Table 44. Chloracne and adipose tissue levels of 2,3,7,8-TCDD and HxCDD in German chemical workers

Population	2,3,7,8-TCDD level (ng/kg)[a]	HxCDD level (ng/kg)[a]	Year of chloracne diagnosis	Half-life extrapolated 2,3,7,8-TCDD[b] (ng/kg)	Half-life extrapolated HxCDD[b] (ng/kg)
Chemical	174	247	1955	7 050	10 000
workers[c]	99	166	1955	4 010	6 720
	147	5 101	1963	2 350	81 620
	61	172	[1955]	2 470	6 970
	50	517	1969	380	3 940
	16	58	1955	650	2 360
	1 280	1 019	1978	3 380	2 690
	49	3 442	[1974]	210	14 760
	50	9 613	[1972]	260	50 740
	2 252	3 087	1984	2 850	3 910
	158	1 191	[1977]	460	3 490
	6	283	1970	40	1 970

From Beck *et al.* (1989b)

Data on serum 2,3,7,8-TCDD levels in Seveso residents with or without chloracne are presented in Table 21.

[a] ng/kg lipid

[b] Half-life extrapolation calculated by authors (Beck *et al.*, 1989b) using the formula $C_0 = C_t \times 2^n$ where C_0 = original concentration of 2,3,7,8-TCDD or HxCDD, C_t = concentration at time t, n = number of half-life periods, and t = half-life of 5.8 years. Exposures occurred between 1949 and 1986.

[c] Measured in 1986

In a study of TCP production by Calvert *et al.* (1992), the increases in GGT were limited to workers with high serum 2,3,7,8-TCDD levels (> 100 ng/kg) and those with lifetime alcohol consumption of more than 30 alcohol–years (alcohol–year = 1 alcoholic beverage per day for one year). Contributions of other potentially confounding exposures were not explored.

Both the Viet Nam Experience Study and the United States Air Force Ranch Hand Study found statistically significant elevations in GGT levels among veterans (Centers for Disease Control Vietnam Experience Study, 1988a; Roegner *et al.*, 1991).

Aspartate aminotransferase and alanine aminotransferase

Reports on the Seveso children and on TCP production workers have found elevations in serum levels of aspartate aminotransferase (AST) and alanine aminotransferase (ALT) that appear to be transient effects of acute exposure to 2,3,7,8-TCDD (May, 1973; Jirasek *et al.*, 1974; Caramaschi *et al.*, 1981; Mocarelli *et al.*, 1986). Epidemiological studies conducted 10–30 years after last exposure found no effects in exposed workers, Viet Nam veterans and Missouri residents compared with unexposed control groups (May, 1982; Bond *et al.*, 1983; Martin, 1984; Suskind & Hertzberg, 1984; Hoffman *et al.*,

1986; Centers for Disease Control Vietnam Experience Study, 1988a; Webb *et al.*, 1989; Roegner *et al.*, 1991; Calvert *et al.*, 1992; Ott *et al.*, 1994; Grubbs *et al.*, 1995) or in workers with or without chloracne (Moses *et al.*, 1984).

ALT was increased in five of 14 TCP workers from the United Kingdom who were inside a manufacturing building at the time of a TCP reactor explosion in 1968, but no elevation in AST or ALT was found when workers from the same facility were re-evaluated later (May, 1982).

In Seveso children, levels of ALT were elevated in those with chloracne (Caramaschi *et al.*, 1981).

D-Glucaric acid

D-Glucaric acid (DGA) excretion is an indirect but valid indicator of hepatic microsomal activity.

Ideo *et al.* (1985) reported that DGA excretion was significantly elevated in adults residing in Seveso, Italy, at the time of the reactor explosion compared with residents of unexposed communities (Seveso, 27.1 μmol/g creatinine versus unexposed, 19.8 μmol/g creatinine; $p < 0.05$). In 1976, DGA excretion was significantly higher in children from Zone A with chloracne (39 μmol/g creatinine) compared with those without chloracne (20.5 μmol/g creatinine). However, by 1981, levels were within the normal range.

A significantly higher DGA : creatinine ratio was also observed in exposed TCP workers tested within one year after exposure to 2,3,7,8-TCDD ceased and 10 years after a TCP reactor explosion (Martin, 1984).

Other studies did not find increased DGA excretion in exposed populations 10–37 years after last exposure to 2,3,7,8-TCDD-contaminated chemicals (Roegner *et al.*, 1991; Calvert *et al.*, 1992).

[In summary, none of the studies reporting elevations in ALT, AST or DGA identified clinical evidence of liver disease in the study populations. Therefore, it is possible that the increases in ALT and AST levels and DGA excretion are related to high-level, acute exposure to 2,3,7,8-TCDD-contaminated chemicals and that, barring additional exposure, the levels decrease with time.]

Porphyrin metabolism

Whether 2,3,7,8-TCDD is associated with porphyrin changes in humans, particularly porphyria cutanea tarda (PCT), is a subject of some debate. PCT is a form of acquired or inherited porphyria caused by a deficiency of the enzyme uroporphyrinogen decarboxylase and the resulting overproduction and excretion of uroporphyrin (Sweeney, 1986). The predominant characteristics of PCT include skin fragility, blistering upon sun exposure, dark pigmentation, excess hair growth, hepatomegaly, reddish-coloured urine, and urinary excretion of uro- and heptacarboxyporphyrins (Strik, 1979).

In 1964, increased uroporphyrins, urinary coproporphyrins and urobilinogen were found in 11 of 29 TCP production workers in New Jersey (Bleiberg *et al.*, 1964). In the NIOSH study (which included the same cohort as reported by Bleiberg *et al.*, 1964)

(Calvert *et al.*, 1994), no difference was found between workers and an unexposed control group in the prevalence of PCT (odds ratio, 0.9; 95% CI, 0.2–4.5) and there were no differences in the risk between workers and the control group for an out-of-range uroporphyrin concentration or an out-of-range coproporphyrin concentration. Because this study was conducted at least 15 years after last occupational exposure to 2,3,7,8-TCDD, it was not possible to determine whether porphyrinuria occurred during the earlier years after exposure. Changes in porphyrin levels were measured in only one other study of workers exposed to 2,3,7,8-TCDD, the study of West Virginia TCP workers, in which no evidence of porphyrinuria was observed (Moses *et al.*, 1984).

Sixty Seveso residents were tested for elevated porphyrins in 1977 and again in 1980. None developed PCT. However, 13 (22%) exhibited secondary coproporphyrinuria, five of whom showed a slight increase of urocarboxyporphyrins, heptacarboxyporphyrins and coproporphyrins classified as a 'transition constellation to chronic hepatic porphyria type A'. In 1980, porphyrin levels had returned to normal in 12 individuals (Doss *et al.*, 1984).

Lipid levels

A number of case reports and epidemiological studies have described increases in levels of serum lipid fractions, particularly total cholesterol and triglycerides, in TCP production workers, laboratory workers, Seveso and Missouri residents and Viet Nam veterans. Others report no differences between subject and reference levels. A summary of the reported levels is presented in **Tables 45 and 46**.

Total cholesterol

The majority of epidemiological studies of workers and community residents have reported no significant increases in total cholesterol levels among exposed populations compared with controls (Moses *et al.*, 1984; Suskind & Hertzberg, 1984; Hoffman *et al.*, 1986; Mocarelli *et al.*, 1986; Assennato *et al.*, 1989; Webb *et al.*, 1989; Ott *et al.*, 1994; Calvert *et al.*, 1996). However, in one study of British TCP production workers, one year after exposure to 2,3,7,8-TCDD had ceased, total cholesterol levels in exposed workers with chloracne (6.02 mmol/L) and without chloracne (6.14 mmol/L) were significantly elevated compared with those of unexposed controls (5.6 mmol/L) (Martin, 1984) **(Table 45)**.

Similarly, a comparison of workers with persistent chloracne, no chloracne, or a history of chloracne revealed a significant association ($p < 0.05$) between the proportion of out-of-range low-density lipoprotein cholesterol values and persistent chloracne (Suskind & Hertzberg, 1984).

Among United States Army veterans, there was no difference in total cholesterol levels between groups who served in Viet Nam or in other countries (Centers for Disease Control Vietnam Experience Study, 1988a). In the United States Air Force Ranch Hand 1987 study, there was a statistically significant positive relationship between serum 2,3,7,8-TCDD levels above 33.3 ng/kg and total cholesterol levels (Roegner *et al.*, 1991). In the 1992 analysis, the difference was not observed (Grubbs *et al.*, 1995).

Table 45. Mean total cholesterol levels among Seveso and Missouri residents, TCP production workers, BASF accident cohort and Viet Nam veterans

Reference	Population	Exposed		Unexposed	
		No.	Mean level (mmol/L)	No.	Mean level (mmol/L)
Mocarelli et al. (1986)	Seveso children				
	1977	16[a]	4.62 (95% CI, 3.26–5.98)	28[a]	4.45 (95% CI, 3.12–5.77)
	1982	182[a]	4.48 (95% CI, 2.97–5.99)	250[a]	4.41 (95% CI, 2.99–5.83)
Caramaschi et al. (1981)	Seveso children	138	15.2[b,c]	120	12.5[b,d]
Assennato et al. (1989)	Seveso residents				
	1976	193[c]	4.78 ± 0.99	–	–
	1982–1983	152[c]	4.06 ± 0.80	123[d]	4.14 ± 0.77
	1983–1984	142[c]	4.09 ± 0.88	196[d]	4.12 ± 0.86
	1985	141[c]	4.14 ± 0.91	167[d]	4.13 ± 0.78
May (1982)	TCP production workers in the United Kingdom	41[c]	5.97	31	6.6
Martin (1984)	TCP production workers in the United Kingdom	39[c]	6.02[e]	126	5.6
Poland et al. (1971)	TCP production workers in New Jersey	71	6.12 ± 1.14	–	–
Moses et al. (1984)	TCP production workers in West Virginia	105[c]	5.38 ± 0.88	101[d]	5.37 ± 0.85

Table 45 (contd)

Reference	Population	Exposed		Unexposed	
		No.	Mean level (mmol/L)	No.	Mean level (mmol/L)
Suskind & Hertzberg (1984)	TCP production workers in West Virginia	200	5.46 ± 0.07	163	5.28 ± 0.08
	TCP production workers: chloracne versus never chloracne	105[c]	5.44 ± 0.08	28[d]	5.30 ± 0.18
Ott et al. (1994)	BASF accident cohort	135	6.14[f] ± 1.01	6 581	6.37[f] ± 1.17
Calvert et al. (1996)	TCP and 2,4,5-T production workers in Missouri and New Jersey	273	5.7[g,i]	259	5.6[g,i]
Hoffman et al. (1986)	Missouri residents in mobile home park	142	4.97[e] ± 0.96	148	5.2 ± 1.09
Webb et al. (1989)	Missouri residents				
	< 20 ng/kg[h]	16	5.88 ± 1.10	–	–
	20–60 ng/kg[h]	12	6.60 ± 0.93	–	–
	> 60 ng/kg[h]	12	6.76 ± 0.97	–	–
CDC Viet Nam Experience Study (1988a)	United States Army Viet Nam veterans	2 490	5.43[i,j]	1 972	5.36[i,j]
Roegner et al. (1991)	Ranch Hand personnel				
	Unknown ≤ 10 ng/kg[k]	338[l]	5.53	777	5.51
	Low 15–≤ 33.3 ng/kg[k]	191	5.55	–	–
	High > 33.3 ng/kg[k]	182	5.68[e]	–	–

Table 45 (contd)

Reference	Population	Exposed		Unexposed	
		No.	Mean level (mmol/L)	No.	Mean level (mmol/L)
Grubbs *et al.* (1995)	Ranch Hand personnel			1 025	5.69
	Background[a]	362	5.71[m]		
	Low[n]	251	5.68[m]		
	High[n]	251	5.76[m]		

Data are means ± SD unless otherwise specified
[a] Number of samples
[b] % abnormal
[c] Chloracne
[d] No chloracne
[e] $p < 0.05$
[f] Adjusted for age, body mass index, smoking history
[g] Adjusted for age, smoking, current diabetes
[h] Adipose tissue levels of 2,3,7,8-TCDD in ng/kg of lipid
[i] Geometric mean
[j] % abnormal: Viet Nam veterans, 5.1; non-Viet Nam veterans, 4.7; odds ratio, 1.1; 95% CI, 0.8–1.5
[k] Serum 2,3,7,8-TCDD levels in ng/kg of lipid
[l] Contrasted to unexposed comparisons
[m] Adjusted mean
[n] Serum 2,3,7,8-TCDD levels in ng/kg of lipid; background: current level ≤10 ng/kg of lipid; low: current level > 10 ng/kg of lipid, 10 ng/kg < initial level ≤ 143 ng/kg of lipid; high: current level > 10 ng/kg of lipid, 10 ng/kg < initial level > 143 ng/kg of lipid

Table 46. Mean triglyceride levels among Seveso children and Missouri residents, TCP production workers, BASF accident cohort and Viet Nam veterans

Reference	Population	Exposed		Unexposed	
		No.	Mean level (mmol/L)	No.	Mean level (mmol/L)
Mocarelli et al. (1986)	Seveso children				
	1977	38[a]	0.97 (95% CI, 0.60–1.50)	36[a]	0.95 (95% CI, 0.63–1.51)
	1982	207[a]	0.91 (95% CI, 0.52–1.60)	257[a]	0.86 (95% CI, 0.86–1.56)
Assennato et al. (1989)	Seveso residents				
	1976	193[b]	0.99 ± 0.43	–	–
	1982–1983	152[b]	0.87 ± 0.40	123[c]	0.85 ± 0.37
	1983–1984	142[b]	0.94 ± 0.59	196[c]	0.88 ± 0.46
	1985	141[b]	0.84 ± 0.44	167[c]	0.87 ± 0.55
May (1982)	TCP production workers, United Kingdom	41[b]	2.03	31[c]	1.83
Martin (1984)	TCP production workers, United Kingdom	39[b]	1.97[d] (95% CI, 0.4–4.0)	126[c]	1.41 (95% CI, 0.3–3.2)
Moses et al. (1984)	TCP production workers, West Virginia	93[b]	1.69[e] ± 1.26	93[c]	1.46 ± 0.73
Suskind & Hertzberg (1984)	TCP production workers, West Virginia	200	1.65 ± 0.08	163	1.76 ± 0.08
Ott et al. (1994)	BASF accident cohort	135	1.91[f] ± 1.19	4471	1.97[f] ± 1.65

Table 46 (contd)

Reference	Population	Exposed		Unexposed	
		No.	Mean level (mmol/L)	No.	Mean level (mmol/L)
Calvert et al. (1996)	TCP and 2,4,5-T production workers, Missouri and New Jersey	273	1.20[g,j]	259	1.15[g,j]
Hoffman et al. (1986)	Missouri residents in mobile home park	141	1.07 ± 0.73	146	1.19 ± 1.07
Webb et al. (1989)	Missouri residents				
	< 20 ng/kg[h]	16	2.17 ± 2.08	–	–
	20–60 ng/kg[h]	12	1.81 ± 1.19	–	–
	> 60 ng/kg[h]	12	2.69 ± 1.06	–	–
CDC Vietnam Experience Study (1988a)	United States Army Viet Nam veterans	2 490	1.06[i,j]	1 972	1.05[i,j]
Roegner et al. (1991)	Ranch Hand personnel			777	1.16
	Unknown ≤ 10 ng/kg[k]	338	1.02[d,l]		
	Low 15–≤ 33.3 ng/kg[k]	191	1.37[d,l]		
	High > 33.3 ng/kg[k]	182	1.35[d,l]		

Table 46 (contd)

Reference	Population	Exposed		Unexposed	
		No.	Mean level (mmol/L)	No.	Mean level (mmol/L)
Grubbs *et al.* (1995)	Ranch Hand personnel			1 025	1.47
	Background	362	1.43[l]		
	Low[m]	191	1.49[l]		
	High[m]	182	1.35[l]		

Data are means ± SD unless otherwise indicated
[a] Number of samples
[b] Chloracne
[c] No chloracne
[d] $p < 0.01$
[e] $p = 0.056$
[f] Adjusted for age, body mass index, smoking history
[g] Adjusted for body mass index, smoking, gender, race, current diabetes, use of β-blocker
[h] Adipose tissue levels of 2,3,7,8-TCDD in ng/kg of lipid
[i] % abnormal: Viet Nam veterans, 4.7; non–Viet Nam veterans, 5.3; odds ratio, 0.9; 95% CI, 0.7–1.2
[j] Geometric mean
[k] Serum 2,3,7,8-TCDD levels in ng/kg of lipid
[l] Contrasted to unexposed comparisons
[m] Serum 2,3,7,8-TCDD levels in ng/kg of lipid; background: current level ≤ 10 ng/kg of lipid; low: current level > 10 ng/kg of lipid, 10 ng/kg < initial level ≤ 143 ng/kg of lipid; high: current level > 10 ng/kg of lipid, 10 ng/kg < initial level > 143 ng/kg of lipid

Triglycerides

Elevated triglyceride levels were reported among British TCP workers with chloracne (Martin, 1984) and, in the United States Air Force Ranch Hand study, among subjects with serum 2,3,7,8-TCDD levels above 15 ng/kg lipid in 1987 (Roegner *et al.*, 1991) and only if above 33 ng/kg lipid in 1992 (Grubbs *et al.*, 1995). Among TCP production workers, there was a small rise in triglyceride levels with increasing serum 2,3,7,8-TCDD level, but this was found to be dependent on host factors (including sex and body mass index) in a multivariate regression analysis (Calvert *et al.*, 1996).

Triglyceride levels were not elevated in the BASF Ludwigshafen accident cohort (Ott *et al.*, 1994), in Missouri residents (Hoffman *et al.*, 1986; Webb *et al.*, 1989), in Seveso residents (Mocarelli *et al.*, 1986; Assennato *et al.*, 1989) or in United States Army Viet Nam veterans (Centers for Disease Control Vietnam Experience Study, 1988a) **(Table 46)**.

(c)   *Other gastrointestinal effects*

A variety of gastrointestinal disorders other than liver conditions have been reported following heavy, acute or chronic exposure of chemical workers (Ashe & Suskind, 1950; Baader & Bauer, 1951; Bauer *et al.*, 1961; Jirasek *et al.*, 1974). The most consistently reported symptoms were transient episodes of right upper quadrant pain, loss of appetite and nausea. None of the reports suggest an etiology for these symptoms and the symptoms were not reported in later follow-up studies of any cohort (Pazderova-Vejlupkova *et al.*, 1981; Moses *et al.*, 1984; Suskind & Hertzberg, 1984).

Three investigations of TCP production workers reported an increased prevalence of a history of upper gastrointestinal tract ulcer across all age strata of West Virginia workers (exposed, 20.7% versus unexposed, 5.5%) (Suskind & Hertzberg, 1984) and all digestive system diseases [not specified] among workers employed in a plant in Midland, MI (prevalence: exposed, 1.5% versus unexposed, 0.5%) (Bond *et al.*, 1983). The factors contributing to these conditions have not been examined fully. Neither the Ranch Hand study (Roegner *et al.*, 1991; Grubbs *et al.*, 1995) nor the NIOSH study (Calvert *et al.*, 1992) found an increased risk of upper gastrointestinal tract ulcers with increasing serum 2,3,7,8-TCDD level.

(d)   *Thyroid function*

Effects in adults

Little or no information has been reported on the effects of 2,3,7,8-TCDD specifically on thyroid function in production workers or Seveso residents, two groups with documented high serum 2,3,7,8-TCDD levels.

No difference was found between West Virginia TCP production workers and controls for thyroxine (T4) and thyroxine-binding globulin (TBG), although quantitative results were not presented (Suskind & Hertzberg, 1984). Thyroid-stimulating hormone (TSH), T4 and TBG levels were within the normal range in workers exposed in the BASF Ludwigshafen (Germany) accident (Ott *et al.*, 1994). The 1987 Ranch Hand study indicated a nonsignificant reduction in the percentage of triiodothyronine (T3) uptake

(Roegner *et al.*, 1991). A slight increase in the mean level of TSH with increasing serum 2,3,7,8-TCDD level was noted in both 1987 and 1991, but did not reach statistical significance (Roegner *et al.*, 1991; Grubb *et al.*, 1995). Among Army Viet Nam veterans, mean TSH levels, but not mean free thyroxine index (FTI) (biologically active) levels, were statistically significantly higher than among non-Viet Nam veterans, after adjustment for the six entry characteristics of age and year of enlistment, race, enlistment status, general technical test score and primary military occupation (**Table 47**) (Centers for Disease Control Vietnam Experience Study, 1988a).

Table 47. Levels of triidothyronine percentage (T3%) uptake and free thyroxine index in Viet Nam veterans

Reference	Population	Exposed		Adjusted RR (95% CI)	Unexposed	
		No.	Mean level		No.	Mean level
T3% uptake						
Roegner *et al.* (1991)	Ranch Hand personnel				772	30.7
	Unknown $\leq 10^a$	338	30.7	1.1 (0.6–2.1)		
	Low 15–$\leq 33.3^a$	194	30.4	0.9 (0.4–2.2)		
	High > 33.3^a	181^b	30.0	0.5 (0.1–1.5)		
	All Ranch Hand versus all comparisons	937	30.6	1.14 (0.7–1.8)	1 198	30.6
Free thyroxine index						
CDC Vietnam Experience Study (1988a)	United States Army Viet Nam veterans	2 490	2.2^c	1.2^d (0.9–1.5)	1 972	2.2^c

[a] Serum 2,3,7,8-TCDD in ng/kg lipid
[b] $p < 0.05$ comparison of veterans at background level with ≥ 33.3 ng/kg 2,3,7,8-TCDD
[c] Geometric mean
[d] Adjusted odds ratio

Effects in infants

Two studies in the Netherlands examined thyroid function in infants and related this to PCDD, PCDF and/or PCB levels in breast milk, cord blood or third trimester maternal serum samples.

Pluim *et al.* (1992, 1993c) examined thyroid function among 38 full-term breast-fed infants in relation to the total I-TEQ per kg of breast milk fat of seven PCDDs (see **Table 30**) and 10 PCDFs. Total T4, TBG and TSH levels were measured sequentially in cord blood and in the blood of infants at one week of age and at 11 weeks of age (**Table 48**). Total T3 was measured in plasma at 11 weeks. Infants were classified as 'high' or 'low' with respect to the median of the range of total I-TEQ. At one week and 11 weeks postnatally, mean total T4 and total T4 : TBG ratios were significantly higher

Table 48. Levels of thyroxine-binding globulin (TBG), thyroxine (T4), free thyroxine (FT4), T4/TBG ratio and thyroid-stimulating hormone (TSH) in nursing infants and workers of the BASF accident cohort

Measurement	Reference	Population	Exposed[a]		Unexposed[b]	
			No.	Mean ± SD	No.	Mean ± SD
Nursing infants						
Total T4 (nmol/L)	Pluim et al. (1992, 1993c)	Neonates; Amsterdam, The Netherlands				
		At birth/cord blood	15	134.3 ± 4.8[d]	18	122.5 ± 4.1[d]
		1 week postnatal	19	178.7 ± 5.5	19	154.5 ± 6.3
		11 weeks postnatal	16	122.2[c] ± 3.0	18	111.1 ± 4.0
	Koopman-Esseboom et al. (1994b)	Neonates; Rotterdam, The Netherlands				
		2nd week postnatal	39	159.9[c] ± 31.6	39	177.5 ± 39.2
Free T4 (nmol/L)	Koopman-Esseboom et al. (1994b)	Neonates; Rotterdam, The Netherlands				
		2nd week postnatal	39	23.0[c] ± 3.3	39	24.6 ± 3.5
TBG (nmol/L)	Pluim et al. (1992, 1993c)	Neonates; Amsterdam, The Netherlands				
		At birth/cord blood	15	589.5 ± 30.5[d]	18	520.1 ± 27.2[d]
		1 week postnatal	19	546.2 ± 19.1	19	532.6 ± 16.3
		11 weeks postnatal	16	500.7 ± 13.0	18	519.0 ± 29.4
T4/TBG	Pluim et al. (1992, 1993c)	Neonates; Amsterdam, The Netherlands				
		At birth/cord blood	15	0.232 ± 0.008[d]	18	0.240 ± 0.007[d]
		1 week postnatal	19	0.332[c] ± 0.011	19	0.291 ± 0.009
		11 weeks postnatal	16	0.247[c] ± 0.009	18	0.220 ± 0.008
TSH (IU/ml)	Pluim et al. (1992, 1993c)	Neonates; Amsterdam, the Netherlands				
		At birth/cord blood	11	11.9 ± 1.9[d]	14	10.4 ± 1.3[d]
		1 week postnatal	11	2.56 ± 0.41	15	2.93 ± 0.41
		11 weeks postnatal	12	2.50 ± 0.26	18	1.81 ± 0.19
	Koopman-Esseboom et al. (1994b)	Neonates; Rotterdam, the Netherlands				
		At birth/cord blood		11.6[c] ± 8.0		8.5 ± 6.0
		2nd week postnatal	39	2.6[c] ± 1.5	39	1.9 ± 0.8
		3 months	39	2.3[c] ± 1.0	39	1.6 ± 0.6

Table 48 (contd)

Measurement	Reference	Population	Exposed[a]		Unexposed[b]	
			No.	Mean ± SD	No.	Mean ± SD
Ludwigshafen accident cohort						
TBG (mg/L)	Ott et al. (1994)	BASF chemical workers	131	12.7 ± 3.2	141	12.7 ± 2.9
T4 (μg/dL)	Ott et al. (1994)	BASF chemical workers	131	7.8 ± 1.9	141	8.3 ± 1.5
T4/TBG	Ott et al.(1994)	BASF chemical workers	131	6.3 ± 1.3	141	6.7 ± 1.6
TSH (IU/mL)	Ott et al. (1993, 1994)	BASF chemical workers	130	1.19 ± 0.90	—[f]	—

[a] High exposure group: 29.2–62.7 ng toxic equivalents/kg (I-TEQ/kg milk fat) (Pluim et al., 1992, 1993c) or > 30.75–76.43 ng I-TEQ/kg fat (Koopman-Esseboom et al., 1994b)

[b] Low exposure group: 8.7–28.0 ng I-TEQ/kg (Pluim et al., 1992, 1993c) or 12.44–30.75 ng I-TEQ/kg fat (Koopman-Esseboom et al., 1994b)

[c] $p < 0.05$ compared to the unexposed group

[d] Standard error of the mean

[e] Total for both high and low = 75

[f] No referent values

among infants in the 'high' group. At 11 weeks, TSH was also significantly higher in the 'high' group. Total T3 was unchanged.

Koopman-Esseboom *et al.* (1994b) examined thyroid function in 78 mother–infant pairs in relation to the I-TEQ levels for PCDDs, planar PCBs, non-planar PCBs and total PCBs–PCDDs in breast milk collected in the first and second weeks after delivery. Total T4, total T3, free T4 and TSH levels were measured in the mother during the last month of pregnancy and 9–14 days after delivery, in cord blood and in the blood of infants at 9–14 days and three months after birth (**Table 48**). All the I-TEQs (PCDDs, co-planar PCBs, non-planar PCBs and total PCDDs/PCBs) were significantly correlated with infant plasma levels of TSH at the second week and third month, and inversely correlated with total T3 pre-delivery, and with total T3 and total T4 post-delivery for the mothers. The non-planar PCB TEQ was not significantly correlated with the mothers' total T4 after delivery and the infants' third month TSH. The measurements in infants with higher PCDD TEQ (based on median TEQ) during their second week of life showed a significant increase in TSH and significant decreases for total T4 and free T4.

These two studies of nursing infants suggest that ingestion of breast milk with elevated levels of PCDDs may alter thyroid function. Both studies covered a short observation period which limits the examination of persistent or long-term changes in thyroid status and the analyses did not control for other factors which might affect thyroid status.

(e)   Diabetes

Cross-sectional studies of workers from Nitro, West Virginia, found no difference in glucose levels between the exposed and control populations, although no quantitative values were presented in either report (Moses *et al.*, 1984; Suskind & Hertzberg, 1984). Similarly, the adjusted odds ratio for out-of-range fasting glucose levels comparing Viet Nam veterans with non-Viet Nam veterans was not statistically significant (odds ratio, 1.0; 95% CI, 0.4–2.2) (Centers for Disease Control Vietnam Experience Study, 1988a). Mean fasting glucose levels in the workers exposed in the BASF Ludwigshafen (Germany) accident were elevated compared with the control population and were associated with current levels of 2,3,7,8-TCDD ($p = 0.062$) but not with the levels back-extrapolated to the time of exposure (Ott *et al.*, 1994).

In the Ranch Hand study, diabetic status was assessed by measuring fasting serum glucose and 2-h postprandial glucose and by using a case definition of diabetes. Diabetes was defined as having a verified history of diabetes or an oral glucose tolerance test of ≥ 11.1 mmol/L (200 mg/dL) (Roegner *et al.*, 1991). The analyses of all three parameters suggested a consistent association between serum 2,3,7,8-TCDD levels above 33.3 ng/kg and an increased risk of diabetes. Adjusted relative risks in Ranch Hand veterans with serum 2,3,7,8-TCDD above 33.3 ng/kg compared with an unexposed group were statistically significantly elevated for fasting serum glucose levels and diabetes (glucose RR, 3.0; $p < 0.001$; diabetes RR, 2.5; $p < 0.001$) (**Table 49**) and for the 2-h postprandial glucose test (RR, 2.4; $p = 0.035$). In addition, Ranch Hand personnel meeting the case definition for diabetes were also more likely to have earlier onset of diabetes than the unexposed group (Wolfe *et al.*, 1992).

Table 49. Adjusted relative risk (RR) for fasting serum glucose levels, cases of diabetes and mean 2-h postprandial glucose levels by category of lipid-adjusted serum 2,3,7,8-TCDD level in Ranch Hand veterans

Serum 2,3,7,8-TCDD (ng/kg)	Fasting serum glucose (RR)	Diabetes (RR)[a]	2-H postprandial glucose level (RR)[b]
Unknown: ≤ 10 ng/kg lipid	0.66	0.82	0.88
Low: 15–≤ 33.3 ng/kg lipid	1.18	1.01	0.60
High: > 33.3 ng/kg lipid	2.95[d]	2.51[d]	2.35[c]

From Roegner *et al.* (1991)

[a] Defined as having a verified history of diabetes or 2-h postprandial glucose level of ≥ 11.1 mmol/L (200 mg/dL)

[b] Comparison of diabetics and normals

[c] $p = 0.035$

[d] $p < 0.001$

(*f*)   *Immunological effects* (**Tables 50–57**)

Nine epidemiological studies and one case report have assessed immunological function in populations exposed to 2,3,7,8-TCDD (Reggiani, 1978; Hoffman *et al.*, 1986; Centers for Disease Control Vietnam Experience Study, 1988a; Evans *et al.*, 1988; Jennings *et al.*, 1988; Webb *et al.*, 1989; Roegner *et al.*, 1991; Ott *et al.*, 1994; Tonn *et al.*, 1996). With the exception of the Tonn *et al.* (1996) study, none has found a clear relationship between exposure and impaired immunological status. Among the Seveso children resident in the area of highest 2,3,7,8-TCDD contamination, immunoglobulins, complement levels, lymphocyte subpopulations and lymphocyte activity analyses were within the normal range, with no differences from those of unexposed controls (Reggiani, 1978).

In Missouri residents with potential exposure to 2,3,7,8-TCDD-contaminated soil (see Section 1.3.2(*c*)), depression in cell-mediated immunity (delayed hypersensitivity) was reported by Hoffman *et al.* (1986). However, a follow-up study did not confirm the presence of anergy (Evans *et al.*, 1988). In a later study of a different cohort of Missouri residents, Webb *et al.* (1989) found no clinical evidence of immunosuppression in 40 individuals whose adipose 2,3,7,8-TCDD levels ranged from below 20 ng/kg to over 430 ng/kg [top of range not given].

The effect of past occupational exposure on parameters of the immune system was examined in 18 British workers who were evaluated 17 years after accidental industrial exposure to chemicals contaminated with 2,3,7,8-TCDD (Jennings *et al.*, 1988). There were no significant differences in the levels of immunoglobulins, T and B lymphocytes, responsiveness to phytohaemagglutinin A or the CD4 and CD8 counts. Three measurements were different in workers compared with controls: antinuclear antibodies (8 workers versus 0 controls, $p < 0.01$), immune complexes (11 workers versus 3 controls, $p < 0.05$) and natural killer cells (workers, 0.40×10^6/L versus controls, 0.19×10^6/L; $p < 0.002$).

Table 50. CD4/CD8 ratios in Missouri residents, Viet Nam veterans and BASF accident cohort

Reference	Population	Exposed			Unexposed	
		No.	Mean ratio (SD)		No.	Mean ratio (SD)
Roegner et al. (1991)	Ranch Hand personnel					
	Unknown: ≤ 10 ng/kg[a]	126	1.72		301	1.89
	Low: 15–≤ 3.3 ng/kg[a]	72	1.91			
	High: > 33.3 ng/kg[a]	72	1.99			
Grubbs et al. (1995)	Ranch Hand personnel					
	Background[b]	139	1.50		399	1.48
	Low[b]	94	1.58			
	High[b]	106	1.57			
CDC Vietnam Experience Study (1988a)	United States Army Viet Nam veterans	2 490	1.8[c]	Odds ratio < reference range, 0.9 Odds ratio > reference range, 1.1	1 972	1.8[c]
Hoffman et al. (1986)	Missouri residents in mobile home park	135	1.9 (0.8)	% abnormal, 8.2	142	1.9 (0.6) % abnormal, 6.3
Webb et al. (1989)	Missouri residents					
	< 20 ng/kg[d]	16	2.0 (0.7)		–	–
	20–60 ng/kg[d]	12	2.1 (1.0)			
	> 60 ng/kg[d]	12	1.4 (0.7)			
Ott et al. (1994)	BASF accident cohort	132	1.6 (0.9)		42[e]	1.5 (0.6)

[a] Serum 2,3,7,8-TCDD level in ng/kg of lipid
[b] Comparison: current dioxin ≤ 10 ng/kg of lipid; background: current dioxin > 10 ng/kg of lipid; low: current dioxin > 10 ng/kg, 10 ng/kg < initial dioxin ≤ 143 ng/kg; high: current dioxin> 10 ng/kg, 10 ng/kg < initial dioxin > 143 ng/kg
[c] Geometric mean
[d] Adipose tissue 2,3,7,8-TCDD level in ng/kg of lipid
[e] From Zober et al. (1992)

Table 51. Total lymphocytes in 2,4,5-T production workers, Missouri residents, Viet Nam veterans and BASF accident cohort

Reference	Population	Exposed			Unexposed		
		No.	Mean level[a]	SD	No.	Mean level[a]	SD
Roegner *et al.* (1991)	Ranch Hand personnel						
	Unknown: ≤ 10 ng/kg[b]	127	1954	–	301	1972	–
	Low: 15 ≤ 33.3 ng/kg[b]	73	2011	–			
	High: > 33.3 ng/kg[b]	74	2032	–			
Grubbs *et al.* (1995)	Ranch Hand personnel						
	Background[c]	141	2067[d]		400	2022	
	Low[c]	95	1989				
	High[c]	108	2034				
CDC Vietnam Experience Study (1988a)	United States Army Viet Nam veterans	2490	1973	1.0/1.2[f]	1972	1936	–
Hoffman *et al.* (1986)	Missouri residents in mobile home park	135	2465	724	142	2311	634
Webb *et al.* (1989)	Missouri residents			% lymphocytes			
	< 20 ng/kg[g]	16	2200	830 / 32	–	–	
	20–60 ng/kg[g]	12	2300	600 / 32			
	> 60 ng/kg[g]	12	2200	720 / 28			
Jennings *et al.* (1988)	2,4,5-T production workers exposed 17 years earlier	18	1980	840	15	2020	470

Table 51 (contd)

Reference	Population	Exposed				Unexposed			
		No.	Mean level[a]	SD		No.	Mean level[a]	SD	
Ott et al. (1994)	BASF accident cohort	133	1978	805	% lymphocytes 33.4 (± 9.4)	42	2268	838	% lymphocytes 36 (± 12.4)

[a] Units, lymphocyte per mm^3
[b] Serum 2,3,7,8-TCDD level in ng/kg of lipid
[c] Comparison: current dioxin ≤ 10 ng/kg of lipid; background: current dioxin > 10 ng/kg; low: current dioxin > 10 ng/kg, 10 ng/kg < initial dioxin ≤ 143 ng/kg; high: current dioxin > 10 ng/kg, 10 ng/kg < initial dioxin > 143 ng/kg
[d] Adjusted mean
[e] Odds ratio < reference range
[f] Odds ratio > reference range
[g] Adipose tissue 2,3,7,8-TCDD level in ng/kg of lipid

Table 52. B1 Lymphocytes in 2,4,5-T production workers, Missouri residents, Viet Nam veterans, BASF accident cohort and extruder personnel

Reference	Population	Exposed				Unexposed		
		No.	Mean level[a]	SD		No.	Mean level[a]	SD
Roegner et al. (1991)	Ranch Hand personnel							
	Unknown: ≤ 10[b]	127	176	—		301	172	—
	Low: 1.5 ≤ 33.3[b]	71	183	—				
	High: > 33.3[b]	73	191	—				
Grubbs et al. (1995)	Ranch Hand personnel							
	Background[c]	140	245[d]	—		400	214	—
	Low[c]	95	224	—				
	High[c]	106	220	—				
CDC Vietnam Experience Study (1988a)	United States Army Viet Nam veterans	2490	240[e]	—	1.1[f] 1.2[g]	1972	230[e]	—
Webb et al. (1989)	Missouri residents				% B1 cells			
	< 20 ng/kg[h]	16	190	865	9.1	—	—	—
	20–60 ng/kg[h]	12	189	983	8.3			
	> 60 ng/kg[h]	12	171	573	7.8			
Jennings et al. (1988)	2,4,5-T production workers exposed 17 years earlier	18	210	110		15	160	80

Table 52 (contd)

Reference	Population	Exposed			Unexposed		
		No.	Mean level[a]	SD	No.	Mean level[a]	SD
Ott et al. (1994)	BASF accident cohort	133	10.4[i]	6.0	42	12.3[i,j]	5.1

[a] Units, cell/mm^3
[b] Serum 2,3,7,8-TCDD level in ng/kg of lipid
[c] Comparison: current dioxin > 10 ng/kg; low: current dioxin > 10 ng/kg, background: current dioxin ≤ 10 ng/kg of lipid; 10 ng/kg < initial dioxin ≤ 143 ng/kg; high: current dioxin > 10 ng/kg, 10 ng/kg < initial dioxin > 143 ng/kg
[d] Adjusted mean
[e] Geometric mean
[f] Odds ratio < reference range
[g] Odds ratio > reference range
[h] Adipose tissue 2,3,7,8-TCDD level in ng/kg of lipid
[i] % B1 cells
[j] From Zober et al. (1992)

Table 53. CD4 Lymphocytes in production workers, Missouri residents, Viet Nam veterans and BASF accident cohort

Reference	Population	Exposed				Unexposed			
		No.	Mean level[a]	SD		No.	Mean level[a]	SD	
Roegner *et al.* (1991)	Ranch Hand personnel								
	Unknown: ≤ 10 ng/kg[b]	127	867	—		301	907	—	
	Low: 1.5 ≤ 33.3 ng/kg[b]	72	945	—					
	High: > 33.3 ng/kg[b]	72	929	—					
Grubbs *et al.* (1995)	Ranch Hand personnel								
	Background[c]	141	961[d]	—		403	923	—	
	Low[c]	95	917	—					
	High[c]	108	962	—					
CDC Vietnam Experience Study (1988a)	United States Army Viet Nam veterans	2490	1020[e]	—	1.0[f] 1.4[g]	1972	990[e]	—	
Hoffman *et al.* (1986)	Missouri residents in mobile home park	135	1021	353	% abnormal, 0.7	142	1033	346	% abnormal, 0.0
Webb *et al.* (1989)	Missouri residents				% CD4 cells				
	< 20 ng/kg[h]	16	1084	485	48	—	—		
	20–60 ng/kg[h]	12	1198	391	51				
	> 60 ng/kg[h]	12	963	403	42				
Jennings *et al.* (1988)	2,4,5-T production workers exposed 17 years earlier	18	950	340		15	1040	290	
Tonn *et al.* (1996)	2,4,5-TCP production and maintenance workers	11	—		% CD4 cells, 47.6 (± 8.1)	10	—		% CD4 cells, 48.5 (± 10.6)

Table 53 (contd)

Reference	Population	Exposed			Unexposed		
		No.	Mean level[a]	SD	No.	Mean level[a]	SD
Ott et al. (1994)	BASF accident cohort	133	–	% CD4 cells, 42.5 (± 10.4)	42[i]	–	% CD4 cells, 45.1 (± 8.9)

[a] Units, cells/mm³
[b] Serum 2,3,7,8-TCDD in ng/kg of lipid
[c] Comparison: current dioxin ≤ 10 ng/kg of lipid; background: current dioxin > 10 ng/kg; low: current dioxin > 10 ng/kg, 10 ng/kg < initial dioxin ≤ 143 ng/kg; high: current dioxin > 10 ng/kg, 10 ng/kg < initial dioxin > 143 ng/kg
[d] Adjusted mean
[e] Geometric mean
[f] Odds ratio < reference range
[g] Odds ratio > reference range
[h] Adipose tissue 2,3,7,8-TCDD level in ng/kg of lipid
[i] From Zober et al. (1992)

Table 54. CD8 Lymphocytes in production workers, Missouri residents, Viet Nam veterans and BASF accident cohort

Reference	Population	Exposed				Unexposed			
		No.	Mean level[a]	SD		No.	Mean level[a]	SD	
Roegner et al. (1991)	Ranch Hand personnel								
	Unknown: ≤ 10 ng/kg[b]	126	485	–		301	473	–	
	Low: 1.5 ≤ 33.3 ng/kg[b]	71	465	–					
	High: > 33.3 ng/kg[b]	73	475	–					
Grubbs et al. (1995)	Ranch Hand personnel								
	Background[c]	140	645[d]	–		400	634	–	
	Low[c]	95	606	–					
	High[c]	106	618	–					
CDC Vietnam Experience Study (1988a)	United States Army Viet Nam veterans	2490	560[e]	1.0[f] / 0.9[g]		1972	550	–	
Hoffman et al. (1986)	Missouri residents in mobile home park	135	592	223	% abnormal, 1.5	142	578	198	% abnormal, 0.0
Webb et al. (1989)	Missouri residents				% CD8 cells				
	< 20 ng/kg[h]	16	562	215	26	–	–		
	20–60 ng/kg[h]	12	645	225	28				
	> 60 ng/kg[h]	12	807	381	35				
Jennings et al. (1988)	2,4,5-T production workers exposed 17 years earlier	18	630	280	–	15	590	230	

Table 54 (contd)

Reference	Population	Exposed			Unexposed		
		No.	Mean level[a]	SD	No.	Mean level[a]	SD
Ott et al. (1994)	BASF accident cohort	132	–	% CD8 cells, 31.9 (± 10.4)	42[i]	–	% CD8 cells, 32.0 (± 7.1)

[a] Units, cells/mm^3
[b] Serum 2,3,7,8-TCDD level in ng/kg of lipid
[c] Comparison: current dioxin ≤ 10 ng/kg of lipid; background: current dioxin > 10 ng/kg; low: current dioxin > 10 ng/kg, 10 ng/kg < initial dioxin ≤ 143 ng/kg; high: current dioxin > 10 ng/kg, 10 ng/kg < initial dioxin > 143 ng/kg
[d] Adjusted mean
[e] Geometric mean
[f] Odds ratio < reference range
[g] Odds ratio > reference range
[h] Adipose tissue 2,3,7,8-TCDD level in ng/kg of lipid
[i] From Zober et al. (1992)

Table 55. IgG levels in Missouri residents, Viet Nam veterans and BASF accident cohort

Reference	Population	Exposed			Unexposed		
		No.	Mean level[a]	SD	No.	Mean level[a]	SD
Roegner *et al.* (1991)	Ranch Hand personnel						
	Unknown: ≤ 10[b]	335	1087	–	757	1120	–
	Low: 1.5 ≤ 33.3[b]	190	1122	–			
	High: > 33.3[b]	175	1122	–			
Grubbs *et al.* (1995)	Ranch Hand personnel						
	Background[c]	364	1126[d]	–	1035	1113.9	–
	Low[c]	243	1111	–			
	High[c]	251	1115	–			
CDC Vietnam Experience Study (1988a)	United States Army Viet Nam veterans	2490	1078[e]	–	1.0[f] 1972	1077[e]	–
					1.0[g]		
Webb *et al.* (1989)	Missouri residents						
	< 20 ng/kg[h]	16	1064[i]	273	–	–	
	20–60 ng/kg[h]	12	1146	193			
	> 60 ng/kg[h]	12	1151	223			
Ott *et al.* (1994)	BASF accident cohort	132	1200[d]	262	194	1183	310

[a] Units, mg/dL

[b] Serum 2,3,7,8-TCDD in ng/kg of lipid

[c] Comparison: current dioxin ≤ 10 ng/kg of lipid; background: current dioxin > 10 ng/kg, 10 ng/kg < initial dioxin ≤ 143 ng/kg; high: current dioxin > 10 ng/kg, 10 ng/kg < initial dioxin > 143 ng/kg

[d] Significant positive relationship between IgG and current 2,3,7,8-TCDD level and back-extrapolated 2,3,7,8-TCDD ($p < 0.01$)

[e] Geometric mean

[f] Odds ratio < reference range

[g] Odds ratio > reference range

[h] Adipose tissue 2,3,7,8-TCDD in ng/kg of lipid

[i] $p < 0.05$ trend

Table 56. IgM levels in Missouri residents, Viet Nam veterans and BASF accident cohort

Reference	Population	Exposed				Unexposed			
		No.	Mean level[a]	SD	Ratio	No.	Mean level[a]	SD	Ratio
Roegner et al. (1991)	Ranch Hand personnel								
	Unknown: ≤ 10 ng/kg[b]	335	107	–	–	757	103	–	–
	Low: 1.5 ≤ 33.3 ng/kg[b]	190	96	–					
	High: > 33.3 ng/kg[b]	175	106	–					
CDC Vietnam Experience Study (1988a)	United States Army Viet Nam veterans	2490	121[c]	–	1.0[d] 1.0[e]	1972	121[c]	–	–
Webb et al. (1989)	Missouri residents								
	< 20 ng/kg[f]	16	128	90	–	–	–		
	20–60 ng/kg[f]	12	157	57					
	> 60 ng/kg[f]	12	114	44					
Ott et al. (1994)	BASF accident cohort	132	140	65	–	192	135	70	–

[a] Units, mg/dL
[b] Serum 2,3,7,8-TCDD in ng/kg of lipid
[c] Geometric mean
[d] Odds ratio < reference range
[e] Odds ratio > reference range
[f] Adipose tissue 2,3,7,8-TCDD in ng/kg of lipid

Table 57. Levels of natural killer cells in Missouri residents, Viet Nam veterans and extruder personnel

Reference	Population	Exposed			Unexposed		
		No.	Mean level	SD	No.	Mean level	SD
Roegner et al. (1991)	Ranch Hand personnel						
	Unknown ≤ 10 ng/kg[a]	126	455[b,c]		291	414[b]	
	Low 15–≤ 33.3 ng/kg[a]	70	378				
	High > 33.3 ng/kg[a]	72	386				
Grubbs et al. (1995)	Ranch Hand personnel		CD16+CD56				
	Background[d]	139	242[b,e]	–	399	248[b,e]	
	Low[d]	94	219	–			
	High[d]	106	237	–			
Tonn et al. (1996)	2,4,5-TCP production and maintenance workers	11	% CD56 5.4	1.9	10	% CD56 5.5	1.6
Jennings et al. (1988)	2,4,5-T production workers exposed 17 years earlier	18	400[b]	210[f]	15	190[b]	150

[a] Serum 2,3,7,8-TCDD in ng/kg of lipid
[b] Units, cells/mm^3
[c] Net response
[d] Comparison: current dioxin ≤ 10 ng/kg of lipid.; background: current dioxin > 10 ng/kg; low: current dioxin > 10 ng/kg, 10 ng/kg < initial dioxin ≤ 143 ng/kg; high: current dioxin > 10 ng/kg, 10 ng/kg < initial dioxin > 143 ng/kg
[e] Adjusted mean
[f] $p < 0.05$

Levels of IgA, IgG, IgM and complement C4 and C3 were higher in exposed workers than in the unexposed control population in the BASF accident study (Ott et al., 1994).

Flow cytometric analysis of lymphocytes from workers with moderately increased serum 2,3,7,8-TCDD (25–140 ng/kg fat) and other PCDDs/PCDFs (maximum, 522 ng I-TEQ/kg fat) did not indicate any decrease of specific cellular components of the immune system (Neubert et al., 1993a, 1995). Moderate increases in the 2,3,7,8-TCDD body burden did not induce any medically significant change in the capacity for proliferation of lymphocytes, measured as [^{3}H]thymidine incorporation (Neubert et al., 1995).

Tonn et al. (1996) examined lymphocyte function among 11 workers employed between 1966 and 1976 in TCP production. Lipid-adjusted serum 2,3,7,8-TCDD levels, measured in 1989–92, ranged from 43 to 874 ng/kg. Although the numbers of lymphocyte subsets were normal, there was a small but significant difference in the response to alloantigen challenge of T-cells and their proliferative response to interleukin (IL)-2. In addition, compared with unexposed controls, the lymphocytes of the exposed workers displayed a suppressive activity that inhibited an on-going allo-response of HLA-unrelated lymphocytes.

Two studies extensively evaluated parameters of the immune system in Viet Nam veterans. No significant differences were detected between United States Army ground troops and the comparison population in lymphocyte subset populations, T-cell populations or serum immunoglobulins (**Tables 50–57**) (Centers for Disease Control Vietnam Experience Study, 1988a). In the United States Air Force Ranch Hand Study (Roegner et al., 1991), significant positive associations were found between IgA and serum 2,3,7,8-TCDD levels. The authors suggest that the rise in IgA is consistent with a subclinical inflammatory response of unspecified origin.

One report (Weisglas-Kuperus et al., 1995) examined direct and surrogate measures of immune status in 207 babies in Rotterdam. The surrogate measures were derived from questionnaires given to the mothers, that covered incidence of rhinitis, bronchitis, tonsillitis and otitis in children up to 18 months of age. Almost all of the children (205) were vaccinated against measles, rubella and mumps; the children's antibody levels were subsequently measured to assess humoral immunity. No relationship was found between pre- and postnatal PCB/PCDD exposure and respiratory tract symptoms (i.e., number of periods with rhinitis, bronchitis, tonsillitis and otitis) or humoral antibody production. However, high prenatal exposure, estimated by cord blood levels, was associated with alterations in T-cell subsets. All values were within clinically normal ranges, and the small changes observed do not necessarily mirror alterations in the cell composition of lymphoid and non-lymphoid organs, nor do they necessarily reflect functional defects. The long-term effects of such subtle shifts in the distribution of outcome measures remain unknown.

(g) Neurological effects

Adults: Several studies have evaluated the relationship between neurobehavioural and neurological function among chemical production workers and community residents exposed to 2,3,7,8-TCDD (Sweeney et al., 1989). Two studies have reported significant neuropathy in Seveso residents (Filippini et al., 1981) and in TCP production workers

(Moses *et al.*, 1984), but these findings have not been reproduced in subsequent studies of the same populations. Studies of TCP production workers and Viet Nam veterans have found no neurological disorder associated with PCDD exposure (Suskind & Hertzberg, 1984; Assennato *et al.*, 1989; Hoffman *et al.*, 1986; Centers for Disease Control Vietnam Experience Study, 1988a,b; Assennato *et al.*, 1989; Webb *et al.*, 1989; Sweeney *et al.*, 1993).

Infants: A series of studies of infants born in either Rotterdam or Groningen in the Netherlands evaluated their neurological and behavioural development in a series of tests conducted at two weeks and three, seven and 18 months, in relation to breast milk levels of PCBs, PCDDs and PCDFs (see **Table 31**). Exposed infants were breast-fed; the controls were formula-fed. Neurological status of 418 neonates (10–21 days) measured using the Prechtl neonatal neurological examination (Huisman *et al.*, 1995a) was related to total I-TEQ (odds ratio, 3.2; 95% CI, 1.4–7.5) and specifically to higher chlorinated PCDDs, 2,3,7,8-TCDF and 2,3,4,7,8-PeCDF. Multiple tests were conducted in the 207 Groningen children at three, seven and 18 months to evaluate psychomotor development (Bayley Scales of Infant Development) (Koopman-Esseboom *et al.*, 1996) and visual recognition memory (Fagan Test of Infant Intelligence) at three and seven months (Koopman-Esseboom *et al.*, 1995a,b). Results of the Fagan Tests and the psychomotor and mental developmental indices were no different in breast-fed or formula-fed infants. Similarly, the neurological status of children at 18 months was not significantly affected by PCB/PCDD exposure through breast milk (Huisman *et al.*, 1995b).

(*h*) Circulatory system

Several studies have described mortality from diseases affecting the circulatory system among populations exposed to 2,3,7,8-TCDD (Bond *et al.*, 1987; Bertazzi *et al.*, 1989; Zober *et al.*, 1990; Coggon *et al.*, 1991; Fingerhut *et al.*, 1991b; Bertazzi *et al.*, 1992; Bueno de Mesquita *et al.*, 1993; Collins *et al.*, 1993; Flesch-Janys *et al.*, 1995) (**Table 58**).

Mortality from all diseases of the circulatory system was similar to that of general populations in studies of workers from the Netherlands (Plant A) (Bueno de Mesquita *et al.*, 1993), the United States (Nitro, West Virginia) (Collins *et al.*, 1993) and the United Kingdom (Coggon *et al.*, 1991). In two studies of workers with chloracne, mortality was not significantly different from that of the national comparison groups (Bond *et al.*, 1987; Zober *et al.*, 1990). However, in a study of German chemical workers who manufactured TCP and 2,4,5-T in addition to chemicals contaminated with higher chlorinated PCDDs and PCDFs (Flesch-Janys *et al.*, 1995), mortality from all circulatory diseases was positively related to estimated 2,3,7,8-TCDD levels and significantly related to estimated total I-TEQ concentrations above 39 ng/kg (lipid-adjusted).

Mortality from more specific endpoints, including ischaemic heart disease and cerebrovascular disease, has been reported in some studies of TCP production workers (Bond *et al.*, 1987; Bueno de Mesquita *et al.*, 1993; Fingerhut *et al.*, 1991b; Flesch-Janys *et al.*, 1995). With the exception of an increase in risk for ischaemic heart disease with

Table 58. Mortality from diseases of the circulatory system in populations exposed to 2,3,7,8-TCDD

Reference	Population	Outcome	No. of deaths	SMR[a]	95% CI	Cohort size	Years of follow-up
Fingerhut et al. (1991b)	TCP and 2,4,5-T production workers, United States	Diseases of the heart (ICD 390–398, 402–404, 410–414, 420–429)	393	1.0	0.9–1.1	5172	1942–87
		Diseases of the circulatory system (ICD 401, 403, 405, 415–417, 430–438, 440–459)	67	0.8	0.6–1.0		
Zober et al. (1990)	2,4,5-T production workers with chloracne, Germany	Diseases of the circulatory system (ICD 390–458)		1.2	0.8–1.7[b]	127	1953–87
Coggon et al. (1991)	2,4,5-T synthesis or formulation, United Kingdom	Diseases of the circulatory system	74	1.2	0.9–1.5	2239	1975–87
Bond et al. (1987)	United States chemical production workers with chloracne (TCP + 2,4,5-T) (Michigan)	Diseases of the circulatory system	19	1.0	0.6–1.6	322	1940–82
		Atherosclerotic heart disease	13	1.0	0.5–1.6		
		Vascular lesions of CNS	4	2.1	0.6–5.4		
	United States chemical production: workers without chloracne (TCP + 2,4,5-T) (Michigan)	Diseases of the circulatory system	130	1.0	0.8–1.1	2026	1940–82
		Atherosclerotic heart disease	106	1.1	0.9–1.3		
		Vascular lesions of CNS	10	0.6	0.3–1.2		
Bueno de Mesquita et al. (1993)	TCP and 2,4,5-T production workers, The Netherlands	Diseases of the circulatory system (ICD 390–458)	28	1.0	0.7–1.4	549	1955–85
		Ischaemic heart disease (ICD 410–414)	20	1.0	0.6–1.6		
		Cerebrovascular disease (ICD 430–438)	5	1.2	0.4–2.7		

Table 58 (contd)

Reference	Population	Outcome	No. of deaths	SMR[a]	95% CI	Cohort size	Years of follow-up
Asp et al. (1994)	Herbicide sprayers, 2,4,5-T and 2,4-D, Finland	Ischaemic heart disease Other heart disease Cerebrovascular disease Other vascular disease	148 20 26 9	0.9 1.0 0.7 0.7	0.8–1.1 0.6–1.6 0.5–1.0 0.3–1.4	1909	1972–89
Michalek et al. (1990)	United States Air Force Ranch Hand personnel	Diseases of the circulatory system	25	1.0	0.8–1.7	1261	1961–87
CDC Vietnam Experience Study (1988c)	United States Army Viet Nam veterans	Diseases of the circulatory system (ICD 390–459)	12	0.5[c]	0.3–1.0	9324	1965–83
Fett et al. (1987b)	Australian Viet Nam veterans; served > 12 months	Diseases of the circulatory system	20[c]	1.7	0.9–3.0	19 205 Viet Nam veterans 25 677 Non-Viet Nam veterans	1966–85
Bertazzi et al. (1989)	Residents of Seveso, Italy, aged 20–74, Zone A (high TCDD region)	Diseases of the circulatory system (ICD 390–459) Ischaemic heart disease Cerebrovascular disease	11 6 2 5	M: 1.8[c] F: 1.9[c] M: 1.3[c] M: 3.3[c]	1.0–3.2 0.8–4.2 0.5–3.3 1.4–8.0	556[d]	1976–86
Bertazzi et al. (1992)	Residents of Seveso, Italy, aged 1–19 years, Zone A (high TCDD region)	Diseases of the circulatory system (ICD 390–459)	0 2	M: NR F: 1.6[d]	– 0.3–8.1	306[d]	1976–86

Table 58 (contd)

Reference	Population	Outcome	No. of deaths	SMR[a]	95% CI	Cohort size	Years of follow-up
Flesch-Janys et al. (1995)	2,4,5-T, TCP, Bromophos and lindane production workers, Hamburg, Germany	**Cardiovascular disease** (ICD 390–459) Estimated 2,3,7,8-TCDD (ng/kg of blood fat)	414			1189	1952–92
		0–2.8		1.2[c]	0.8–1.8		
		2.81–14.4		0.9	0.5–1.4		
		14.5–49.2		1.4	0.9–2.0		
		49.3–156.7		1.6	1.1–2.4		
		156.8–344.6		1.5	1.0–2.4		
		344.7–3890.2		2.0	1.2–3.3		
		Ischaemic heart disease Estimated 2,3,7,8-TCDD (ng/kg of blood fat)					
		0–2.8		1.4	0.8–2.4		
		2.81–14.4		0.8	0.4–1.6		
		14.5–49.2		1.2	0.7–2.2		
		49.3–156.7		0.9	0.5–1.8		
		156.8–344.6		1.6	0.9–3.0		
		344.7–3890.2		2.5	1.3–4.7		

Table 58 (contd)

Reference	Population	Outcome	No. of deaths	SMR[a]	95% CI	Cohort size	Years of follow-up
		Cardiovascular disease (ICD 390–459) Estimated total TEQ levels (ng/kg of blood fat)	414				
		1.0–12.2		0.9	0.6–1.5		
		12.3–39.5		0.9	0.6–1.5		
		39.6–98.9		1.5	1.0–2.2		
		99.0–278.5		1.6	1.1–2.2		
		278.6–545.0		1.6	1.0–2.6		
		545.1–4361.9		2.1	1.2–3.5		
		Ischaemic heart disease Estimated total TEQ levels (ng/kg of blood fat)					
		1.0–12.2		1.0	0.5–2.0		
		12.3–39.5		1.0	0.5–1.8		
		39.6–98.9		1.0	0.5–1.8		
		99.0–278.5		1.1	0.6–2.0		
		278.6–545.0		1.7	0.9–3.3		
		545.1–4361.9		2.7	1.5–5.0		
Collins *et al.* (1993)	TCP and 2,4,5-T production workers, USA	Diseases of the circulatory system (ICD 390–458)	188	0.9	0.8–1.0	754	1949–87

[a] SMR, Standardized mortality ratio
[b] 90% confidence interval
[c] Relative risk
[d] Zone A males and females combined

levels of 2,3,7,8-TCDD exposure in one study (Flesch-Janys *et al.*, 1995), ischaemic heart disease mortality was consistent with background population rates.

The SMRs for circulatory system diseases reported in the various mortality studies are close to 1.00, suggesting that the 'healthy worker effect' is not seen in these studies. Because employed workers are usually healthier than the general population, the SMR for cardiovascular disease in employed populations tends to be lower than 1.00 (Fox & Collier, 1976; McMichael, 1976). The absence of a healthy worker effect, in the light of the positive results of experiments with animals, suggests that more detailed analyses should be conducted for cardiovascular outcomes in the exposed populations.

Studies of Viet Nam veterans have reported nonsignificant increases in the relative mortality ratio for circulatory diseases (Fett *et al.*, 1987b; Michalek *et al.*, 1990; Wolfe *et al.*, 1994).

Bertazzi *et al.* (1989, 1992) reported increased circulatory disease mortality among residents of Seveso Zone A (the most highly contaminated region) in both men (RR, 1.8; 95% CI, 1.0–3.2) and women (RR, 1.9; 95% CI, 0.8–4.2). The study was limited by the small number of subjects and the crude measure of 2,3,7,8-TCDD exposure.

Several other effects of 2,3,7,8-TCDD on the cardiovascular system have been reported (Bond *et al.*, 1983; Moses *et al.*, 1984; Suskind & Hertzberg, 1984; Centers for Disease Control Vietnam Experience Study, 1988a; Roegner *et al.*, 1991; Grubbs *et al.*, 1995). Statistically significant associations with 2,3,7,8-TCDD exposure were found only in the Ranch Hand study for diastolic blood pressure, arrhythmias detected on the electrocardiogram and peripheral pulse abnormalities (Roegner *et al.*, 1991). Significant increases in blood pressure were found in subjects with serum 2,3,7,8-TCDD levels from 15 to 33.3 ng/kg, but not in those with higher levels.

(i)   *Pulmonary effects*

There is conflicting evidence from controlled epidemiological studies regarding an association between chronic respiratory system effects and human exposure to substances contaminated with 2,3,7,8-TCDD. One study of workers involved in production of TCP and 2,4,5-T suggested that 2,3,7,8-TCDD exposure increases the risk for abnormal ventilatory function (Suskind & Hertzberg, 1984). This study found statistically significant decreases in pulmonary function as measured by spirometric evaluation. However, the exposed workers were, on average, 10 years older than controls and therefore had greater potential exposure to 2,4,5-T formulated in powder form, as used in earlier periods of production, which may have presented a greater risk of impaired lung function than the liquid form used later.

No association between ventilatory function and serum 2,3,7,8-TCDD was found in the NIOSH study (Calvert *et al.*, 1991). The Ranch Hand study found significant declines in the mean FEV_1 and the mean FVC for subjects with serum 2,3,7,8-TCDD levels above 33.3 ng/kg (adjusted mean FEV_1, 91.3%; mean FVC, 87.4%) compared with an unexposed comparison group (adjusted mean FEV_1, 93.5%; mean FVC, 91.7%) (Roegner *et al.*, 1991). Smoking appeared to have a greater influence on lung function than 2,3,7,8-TCDD exposure. In a follow-up examination conducted in 1992, no consistent relationship was found between serum 2,3,7,8-TCDD concentration and respiratory parameters (Grubbs *et al.*, 1995).

(j)   Renal effects

There is little evidence in the human data to suggest that exposure to 2,3,7,8-TCDD is related to renal or bladder dysfunction. No major renal or bladder dysfunction was noted among Ranch Hand veterans (Roegner *et al.*, 1991) or among TCP production workers from West Virginia (Suskind & Hertzberg, 1984) or New Jersey (Poland *et al.*, 1971).

4.2.2   Experimental systems

(a)   Species comparisons of toxic effects

(i)   Lethality and other major effects

2,3,7,8-TCDD-induced mortality does not occur immediately after exposure, but only after several days or several weeks, and it is therefore not reasonable to perform animal experiments studying specific organ functions during the lag phase between exposure to potentially lethal doses and death.

A very large number of studies on the acute, subchronic and chronic toxicity of PCDDs and PCDFs has revealed that the toxic outcome of treatment with a certain congener or with a mixture of congeners strongly depends on the species, strain and toxicological endpoint investigated. Furthermore, there are remarkable differences in the potency of individual PCDD or PCDF congeners. The situation is further complicated by the fact that the relative potency, and probably the dose–response relationship, of a given congener varies with the experimental system and the parameters of toxicity measured. Finally, the large differences in doses or dose ranges used contribute to the sometimes considerable uncertainty when an 'effect' of PCDDs/PCDFs on a certain biological parameter is discussed.

However, there is no doubt that potent PCDDs/PCDFs have a number of characteristic toxic effects in common, which make them an almost unique example for a distinct class of toxic substances. Among the toxic responses consistently observed in all mammalian species tested so far are a progressive loss of body weight, a reduced intake of food, atrophy of the thymus, gastrointestinal haemorrhage and delayed lethality (Safe, 1986; Vanden Heuvel & Lucier, 1993). Other characteristic signs of toxicity are frequently found in the liver, skin and organs of the endocrine system (see **Tables 59** and **60** for 2,3,7,8-TCDD data). The most sensitive endpoints for 2,3,7,8-TCDD effects are listed in **Table 61**.

An early report on the acute toxicity of 2,3,7,8-TCDD, 2,7-DCDD, an unspecified HxCDD and OCDD in animals was published by Schwetz *et al.* (1973). The authors reported the much higher acute toxicity of 2,3,7,8-TCDD compared with HxCDD or OCDD in guinea-pigs and rabbits. Furthermore, the acnegenic, teratogenic and hepatotoxic properties of 2,3,7,8-TCDD and HxCDD were described.

Table 59. Acute lethality of 2,3,7,8-TCDD in various animal species and strains

Species/strain (sex)	Administration	LD_{50} (μg/kg)	Time of death (days after exposure)	Follow-up (days)	Body weight loss[a] (%)	References
Guinea-pig/Hartley (male)	Oral	0.6–2.0	5–34	NR	50	Schwetz et al. (1973); McConnell et al. (1978a); DeCaprio et al. (1986)
Mink/NR (male)	Oral	4.2	7–17	28	31	Hochstein et al. (1988)
Chicken/NR	Oral	< 25	12–21	NR	NR	Greig et al. (1973)
Rhesus monkey (female)	Oral	c. 70	14–34	42–47	13–38	McConnell et al. (1978b)
Rat/Long-Evans (male)	Intraperitoneal	c. 10	15–23	48–49	39	Tuomisto & Pohjanvirta (1987)
Rat/Sherman, Spartan (male) (female)	Oral	22 13–43	9–27	NR	NR	Schwetz et al. (1973)
Rat/Sprague-Dawley (male)	Oral	43	28–34	30 or until death	NR	Stahl et al. (1992a)
Rat/Sprague-Dawley (male) (female) (weanling male)	Intraperitoneal	60 25 25	NR	20	NR	Beatty et al. (1978)
Rat/Fischer Harlan (male)	Oral	340	28[b]	30	43	Walden & Schiller (1985)
Rat/Han-Wistar (male)	Intraperitoneal	> 3000	23–34	39–48	40–53	Pohjanvirta & Tuomisto (1987); Pohjanvirta et al. (1987)

Table 59 (contd)

Species/strain/sex	Administration	LD$_{50}$ (µg/kg)	Time of death (days post-exposure)	Follow-up (days)	Body weight loss[a] (%)	References
Mouse C57BL/6 (male) DBA2/2J (male) B6D2F1 (male)	Oral	181 2570 296	24[b] 21[b] 25[b]	30	25 33 34	Chapman & Schiller (1985)
Mouse C57BL/6 DBA2 B6D2F1	Intraperitoneal	132 620 300	NR	NR	NR	Neal et al. (1982)
Rabbit/New Zealand White (male and female)	Oral Dermal	115 275	6–39 12–22	NR 22	NR NR	Schwetz et al. (1973)
Rabbit/New Zealand White (male and female)	Intraperitoneal	ca. 50	7–10	10–20	14.5	Brewster et al. (1988)
Syrian hamster (male and female)	Oral	1157–5051	2–43	50	NR	Henck et al. (1981)
Syrian hamster (male and female)	Intraperitoneal	> 3000	14–32	50	1[c]	Olson et al. (1980)

[a] Of dead animals
[b] Mean time to death
[c] Data from five animals
NR, not reported

Table 60. Acute toxic responses following exposure to 2,3,7,8-TCDD: species differences[a]

Response	Rhesus monkey	Guinea-pig	Mink	Rat	Mouse	Rabbit[b]	Chicken[b]	Syrian hamster
Hyperplasia or metaplasia								
Gastric mucosa	++	0	+	0	0			0
Intestinal mucosa	+		±					++
Urinary tract	++	++		0	0			
Bile duct and/or gall-bladder	++	0			++			0
Lung: focal alveolar				++				
Skin	++	0		0	0	++		0
Hypoplasia, atrophy, or necrosis								
Thymus	+	+		+	+		+	+
Bone marrow	+	+			±		+	
Testicle	+	+		+	+		+	+
Other lesions								
Liver lesions	+	±		+	++	+	+	±
Porphyria	0	0		+	++		+	0
Oedema	+	0		0	+		++	+
Haemorrhage	+	+	+	+	+		+	+

0, lesion not observed; +, lesion observed; ++, severe lesion observed; ±, lesion observed to a very limited extent; blank, no evidence reported in the literature.

[a] References: Kimmig & Schulz (1957a); Allen & Lalich (1962); Vos & Koeman (1970); Vos & Beems (1971); Greig et al. (1973); Gupta et al. (1973); Norback & Allen (1973); Schwetz et al. (1973); Vos et al. (1974); Allen et al. (1977); Kociba et al. (1976, 1978); McConnell et al. (1978a,b); Kociba et al. (1979); Moore et al. (1979); McConnell (1980); Olson et al. (1980); Henck et al. (1981); Turner & Collins (1983); Hochstein et al. (1988)

[b] Responses followed exposure to 2,3,7,8-TCDD or structurally related chlorinated hydrocarbons.

Table 61. No observed-effect and lowest-observed-effect levels (NOEL and LOEL) of 2,3,7,8-TCDD for mammalian species

Species	Experimental design	NOEL	LOEL	Effect	Reference
Rhesus monkey	0.5 µg/kg in food, 9 months		12 ng/kg/d	Death	Allen et al. (1977)
	2 µg/kg in food, 61 days		50 ng/kg/d	Death	McNulty (1977)
	0.05 µg/kg in food, 20 months		1.5 ng/kg/d	Hair loss	Schantz et al. (1979)
	5 and 25 ng/kg in food to mother, 4 years		0.126 ng/kg/d	Object recognition, juvenile	Bowman et al. (1989b)
	5 and 25 ng/kg in food to mother, 4 years		0.642 ng/kg/d	Prenatal death	Bowman et al. (1989a); Hong et al. (1989)
	9 × 22–111 ng/kg to mother, days 20–40 of pregnancy		9 ×111 ng/kg	Prenatal death	McNulty (1984)
	25 ng/kg in food to mother, 4 years		0.642 ng/kg/d	Change in lymphocytes	Hong et al. (1989)
	5 and 25 ng/kg in food to mother, 4 years		0.126 ng/kg/d	Endometriosis	Rier et al. (1993)
Marmoset	3 ng/kg, 1 × orally		3 ng/kg	Induction of CYP1A2	Krueger et al. (1990)
	0.3 ng/kg/wk × 24 wk		0.135 ng/kg/d chronic.[a]	Change in lymphocytes	Neubert et al. (1992)
	1.5 ng/kg/wk × 6 wk + 0 × 12 wk				
Sprague-Dawley rat	2 ng/kg, 1 × orally	0.6 ng/kg	2 ng/kg	Induction of CYP1A1	Kitchin & Woods (1979)
	1–100 ng/kg/d, orally, 2 years	1 ng/kg/d	10 ng/kg/d	Porphyria	Kociba et al. (1978)
	14–1024 ng/kg/d, orally, 3 months	<14 ng/kg/d	14 ng/kg/d	Less vitamin A	van Birgelen et al. (1995a)
	14–1024 ng/kg/d, orally, 3 months	0.3 ng/kg/d[a]	14 ng/kg/d	Induction of CYP1A1	van Birgelen et al. (1995a)
	14–1024 ng/kg/d, orally, 3 months	0.5 ng/kg/d[a]	14 ng/kg/d	Induction of CYP1A2	van Birgelen et al. (1995a)
	1–100 ng/kg to mother, chronic	1 ng/kg/d mth	10 ng/kg/d	Prenatal death	Murray et al. (1979)
	30 ng/kg/d to mother, days 6–15 of pregnancy	30 ng/kg/d mth		Prenatal death	Sparchu et al. (1971)

Table 61 (contd)

Species	Experimental design	NOEL	LOEL	Effect	Reference
Sprague-Dawley rat	100–10 000 ng/kg/d, 30 d		100 ng/kg/d	Lower serum glucose	Zinkl et al. (1973)
	Calculated with data from Tritscher et al. (1992) and Sewall et al. (1993); 3.5-10, 7–35, 7–125 ng/kg/d, 30 wk	0.01 ng/kg/d 0.1 ng/kg/d 0.1 ng/kg/d 0.1 ng/kg/d 0.1 ng/kg/d	0.1 ng/kg/d 1 ng/kg/d 1 ng/kg/d 1 ng/kg/d 1 ng/kg/d	CYP1A induction CYP1A2 induction Ah receptor induction EGF receptor induction Oestrogen receptor induction	Kohn et al. (1993)
Holtzmann rat	64 ng/kg/d to mother, day 15 of pregnancy		64 ng/kg/d	Decrease in male reproductive capacity	Mably et al. (1992a,b)
C57BL/6 mouse	1 ng/kg/wk, 4 wk intraperitoneally		1 ng/kg/wk	Immunosuppression, low CTL generation	Clark et al. (1983)
B6C3F1 mouse	10 ng/kg, 7 days after fertilization		10 ng/kg, d 7	Increase in viral infection	Lebrec & Burleson (1994)
Guinea-pig	8–200 ng/kg/wk, 8 wk		8 ng/kg/wk 200 ng/kg/wk	Immunosuppression Lower response to tetanus toxin	Vos et al. (1973)

wk, week(s); d, day(s); EGF, epidermal growth factor; CTL, cytotoxic T-lymphocyte

[a]Calculated

Guinea-pig

Guinea-pigs are among the most sensitive species towards 2,3,7,8-TCDD and other PCDDs and PCDFs, with regard to lethality (Plüss *et al.*, 1988a), with 90% dying from a single 3 µg/kg dose (Harris *et al.*, 1973). The mean time interval until death was 18 days, and a large weight loss over a period of days preceded death. Thymic atrophy was observed after treatment with weekly doses of 0.008 µg/kg 2,3,7,8-TCDD over four to five weeks (Gupta *et al.*, 1973). Other lesions were haemorrhages, hyperplasia of the urinary bladder mucosa and atrophy of the adrenal zona glomerulosa. In a subchronic study, DeCaprio *et al.* (1986) treated guinea-pigs with various doses of 2,3,7,8-TCDD in the diet for up to 90 days. At a total dose of 0.44 µg/kg, animals exhibited a decreased rate of body weight gain and increased relative liver weights. Male animals also displayed a reduction in relative thymus weights and elevated serum levels of triglycerides, while females showed hepatocellular cytoplasmic inclusion bodies and lowered serum ALT activities. A no-observed-effect level of approximately 0.65 ng/kg per day for prolonged exposure was calculated for these lesions.

After a single lethal dose of ≥ 10 µg/kg 2,3,7,8-TCDD, there was a marked reduction in the size of the thymus, loss of body fat and reduction of muscle mass in guinea-pigs. Histopathological examination revealed epithelial hyperplasia in the renal pelvis, ureter and urinary bladder, hypocellularity of the bone marrow and seminiferous tubules and loss of lymphocytes in thymic cortex, spleen and Peyer's patches, whereas no marked pathological alterations of the liver were evident (Moore *et al.*, 1979). After treatment of guinea-pigs with 20 µg/kg 2,3,7,8-TCDD, hepatocellular hypertrophy, steatosis, focal necrosis and hyalin-like cytoplasmic bodies as well as hepatic focal necrosis were observed in a study by Turner and Collins (1983).

Rat

The single oral LD_{50} value of four PCDDs in male Sprague-Dawley rats was determined to be 43 µg/kg for 2,3,7,8-TCDD, 206 µg/kg for 1,2,3,7,8-PeCDD, 887 µg/kg for 1,2,3,4,7,8-HxCDD and 6325 µg/kg for 1,2,3,4,6,7,8-HpCDD (Stahl *et al.*, 1992a). A mixture containing all four congeners in a predicted equitoxic amount showed strictly additive toxic effects.

The discovery of a more than 300-fold difference in acute LD_{50} values for 2,3,7,8-TCDD between the Long-Evans and Han/Wistar rat strains led to a number of studies aimed at elucidating the biochemical basis of this difference. Han/Wistar rats are extraordinarily resistant towards 2,3,7,8-TCDD (Pohjanvirta & Tuomisto, 1987). Doses of 125–1400 µg/kg resulted in marked decreases in food consumption, and in a decrease of 20–25% in body weight. However, the lethality to the animals was low (two of 40 died). A similar strain difference exists for 1,2,3,7,8-PeCDD, whereas it was much less pronounced for 1,2,3,4,7,8-HxCDD (Pohjanvirta *et al.*, 1993). Genetic crossings between Long-Evans and Han/Wistar rats suggest that 2,3,7,8-TCDD resistance is the dominant trait in the rat. Two (or possibly three) genes seem to regulate resistance (Pohjanvirta, 1990). However, even within a given rat strain, such as Long-Evans or Han/Wistar, substrains with markedly differing sensitivity towards 2,3,7,8-TCDD may exist.

Therefore, a critical analysis of 2,3,7,8-TCDD sensitivity in the used animals is required (Pohjanvirta & Tuomisto, 1990a). Most toxic effects are similar in both strains, the Long-Evans strain, however, being more sensitive. In the livers of Long-Evans rats, a (lethal) dose of 50 μg/kg bw 2,3,7,8-TCDD caused marked hepatocyte swelling, vacuoles probably containing fat in the cytoplasm, multinuclear cells (up to eight nuclei) and accumulation of inflammatory cells in hepatic sinusoids (Pohjanvirta et al., 1989a). At the same dose, Han/Wistar rats showed slight cytoplasmic swelling and irregular haema-toxylin–eosin staining. Thymic atrophy was seen in both strains, the Long-Evans strain being about 10-fold more sensitive than the Han/Wistar strain. Furthermore, pronounced reduction in serum T4 and increases in TSH, corticosterone and free fatty acids were observed in Long-Evans rats.

In CD rats, moderate thymic atrophy was observed after treatment with 1 μg/kg per day over four to five weeks (Gupta et al., 1973). Other effects were haemorrhages, degenerative changes in kidney and thyroid, increase in megakaryocytes in spleen, lymphoid depletion of the spleen and lymph nodes and severe liver lesions. Female CD rats were slightly more sensitive than males (Harris et al., 1973). A more sensitive indicator of 2,3,7,8-TCDD exposure than body weight reduction was a decrease in thymus weight. Blood coagulation was not significantly affected in five-week-old rats that had received 1 μg/kg 2,3,7,8-TCDD (Bouwman et al., 1992).

In a 13-week oral toxicity study in adult Sprague-Dawley rats (Kociba et al., 1976; Goodman & Sauer, 1992), 1 μg/kg 2,3,7,8-TCDD per day caused some mortality, inactivity, decreased body weights and food consumption, icterus, pathomorphological changes in the liver, lymphoid depletion of the thymus and other lymphoid organs and minimal alterations of some haematopoietic components. Doses of 0.1 μg/kg 2,3,7,8-TCDD per day also caused decreased body weights and food consumption and lymphoid depletion. Effects seen only in males given this dose level included a depression in packed blood cell volume, red blood cells and haemoglobin. Lower doses (0.01 or 0.001 μg/kg 2,3,7,8-TCDD per day) did not affect any of the measured parameters, except for a slight increase in the mean liver-to-body weight ratio in rats given 0.01 μg/kg 2,3,7,8-TCDD per day. A single dose of 1 or 10 μg/kg 2,3,7,8-TCDD led to a pronounced reduction in blood glucose. In female Sprague-Dawley rats, chronic daily intake of 47 ng/kg 2,3,7,8-TCDD resulted in a decrease in plasma concentration of thyroid hormone (total T4) and body weight. More sensitive parameters influenced at 14 ng/kg per day were a decrease in relative thymus weight, loss of hepatic retinoids and induction of CYP1A1 and CYP1A2 activities in the liver (van Birgelen et al., 1995a). Hepatic CYP1A1 and CYP1A2 were induced at comparable doses of 2,3,7,8-TCDD in both mice and rats (Smialowicz et al., 1994).

Hamster

In the Syrian hamster, 2,3,7,8-TCDD treatment led to loss of body weight and thymic atrophy, while no histopathological changes were seen in the liver, spleen, kidney adrenals or heart (Olson et al., 1980). Oral treatment resulted in moderate to severe ileitis and peritonitis in many animals, associated with marked hyperplasia with mild to severe haemorrhage and necrosis of the mucosal epithelium.

Inter-species rodent comparisons

In a comparative study in rats, mice and guinea-pigs (Zinkl *et al.*, 1973), 2,3,7,8-TCDD was found to cause acute/subacute increases in serum levels of alanine amino-transferase (ALT, previously SGPT) and aspartate aminotransferase (AST, previously SGOT), cholesterol and bilirubin in rats after a single dose of 1 or 10 μg/kg bw. Histo-pathological examination also suggested that the liver is highly sensitive to 2,3,7,8-TCDD in rats but not in guinea-pigs and mice. Furthermore, significant reductions in numbers of platelets in the peripheral blood of rats and guinea-pigs, and lymphopenia in mice and guinea-pigs were evident.

In male C57BL/6 mice (Gasiewicz *et al.*, 1980) and guinea-pigs, various PCDD congeners were administered as a single oral dose (McConnell *et al.*, 1978a). LD_{50}s of 2 μg/kg in guinea-pigs and 283.7 μg/kg in mice were determined for 2,3,7,8-TCDD. The acute toxicity of 2,3,7,8-substituted PCDD was in the following rank order: 1,2,3,4,6,7,8 < 1,2,3,7,8,9 = 1,2,3,6,7,8 = 1,2,3,4,7,8 < 1,2,3,7,8 < 2,3,7,8. In both species, 2,3,7,8-TCDD strongly reduced the thymus weight due to a reduction in cortical lymphocytes. Significant macroscopic or histopathological hepatic effects including porphyria were observed only in the mouse. Hyperplasia of the transitional epithelium in the urinary tract was found in guinea-pigs.

The relative toxicity of four different congeners was found by Rozman *et al.* (1993) to be similar in guinea-pigs and Sprague-Dawley rats following acute, subchronic or chronic dosing. Furthermore, the dose–response relationships for 2,3,7,8-TCDD concerning the endpoints mortality, porphyria and carcinogenicity were very similar. Therefore, the authors suggested that the product of average tissue concentration and time can describe the toxicity for a given congener.

Rhesus monkey

In rhesus monkeys (*Macaca mulatta*) fed toxic fat containing 2,3,7,8-TCDD, gastric hyperplasia and ulceration, hydropericardium, ascites, reduced spermatogenesis, focal liver necrosis, decreased haematopoiesis, skin lesions and eventual mortality were observed (Allen *et al.*, 1977). In an earlier study (Norback & Allen, 1973), atrophy of the lymph tissue, liver enlargement and a reduction in the number of spermatocytes in the testes were also reported.

Following administration of a single dose of 70 μg/kg 2,3,7,8-TCDD by gastric instil-lation to rhesus monkeys, McConnell *et al.* (1978b) observed weight loss, blepharitis, loss of fingernails and eyelashes, facial alopecia with acneform eruptions, mild anaemia, neutrophilia, lymphopenia and a decrease in serum cholesterol with an increase in serum triglyceride concentrations. The liver, adrenal gland and kidney showed increased relative organ weight, whereas the thymus was dramatically reduced in size due to a loss of cortical lymphocytes. Histopathological examination revealed hyperplastic and meta-plastic changes in sebaceous glands, especially in the eyelid (meibomian glands) and ear canal, together with epithelial hyperplasia in the renal pelvis, stomach, gall-bladder and bile duct, whereas the histology of the liver parenchyme was relatively normal.

Cachexia

One of the most striking effects of 2,3,7,8-TCDD in all mammalian species tested so far is body weight loss combined with a reduced intake of food. From a pair-feeding experiment, hypophagia was suggested to be the major factor leading to wasting in guinea-pigs, Fischer 344 rats and C57BL/6 mice (Kelling *et al.*, 1985). However, lethality was only partially due to body weight loss, since the lethality, in particular in rats and mice, was significantly lower among pair-fed controls than among 2,3,7,8-TCDD-treated animals. Similarly, total parenteral nutrition, preventing the body weight loss associated with 2,3,7,8-TCDD toxicity in rats after a single dose of 100 µg/kg bw, did not prevent death (Gasiewicz *et al.*, 1980).

Seefeld *et al.* (1984a) reported that 2,3,7,8-TCDD-treated rats maintained their body weight at a lower, nearly constant percentage of that of control rats fed *ad libitum*. The authors concluded from this and a number of additional experiments that the target level for body weight is reduced under the influence of 2,3,7,8-TCDD. Hypophagia relative to untreated animals was suggested to be the key symptom of this down-regulation of body weight, whereas malabsorption or less efficient feed utilization did not play a decisive role (Seefeld *et al.*, 1984b). The role of hypophagia in weight loss, and the changes in carbohydrate and lipid metabolism observed after 2,3,7,8-TCDD treatment, were questioned by Chapman and Schiller (1985), who found no influence of 2,3,7,8-TCDD on the cumulative amount of feed consumption by C57BL/6 mice until the animals became moribund. In addition, the alterations in serum glucose and lipid concentrations in fasted mice were very different from those induced by 2,3,7,8-TCDD exposure. In DBA/2J mice bearing a low-affinity Ah receptor, dose–response experiments showed comparable changes in glucose and lipid parameters when the animals were exposed to 10-fold higher doses of 2,3,7,8-TCDD than C57BL/6 mice.

In a series of experiments, Pohjanvirta and Tuomisto (1990b) administered sodium chloride, 2-deoxy-D-glucose, sodium mercaptoacetate, insulin, naloxone, glucose or fructose to 2,3,7,8-TCDD-treated or control rats. 2,3,7,8-TCDD caused an attenuation of feeding responses to metabolic deficits, resulting, for example, in severe hypoglycaemia (Pohjanvirta *et al.*, 1991a), but induced hypersensitivity to peripheral satiety signals. The central nervous system was suggested to play a crucial role in these effects. Transfusion of blood from rats with 2,3,7,8-TCDD-induced appetite suppression into untreated rats did not affect their feed intake, whereas transfusion of blood from normally sated rats did (Rozman *et al.*, 1991). This indicated that 2,3,7,8-TCDD treatment does not increase a satiety-signalling factor in blood but may rather suppress the formation of hunger-related signals. Evidence for the involvement of a serotonergic mechanism was derived from the finding that 2,3,7,8-TCDD increased the levels of tryptophan and its metabolites serotonin and 5-hydroxyindoleacetic acid in blood and brain.

2,3,7,8-TCDD treatment also produced a longer-lasting suppression of feed intake after oral treatment with glucose than in untreated rats (Pohjanvirta *et al.*, 1991b) and induced aversion to eating energy-providing food, irrespective of its type (Pohjanvirta & Tuomisto, 1990c). From another series of experiments in rats, including behavioural, biochemical and antiemetic approaches, it was concluded that nausea cannot explain the lethal wasting syndrome (Pohjanvirta *et al.*, 1994a). Food intake and body weight loss after 2,3,7,8-TCDD treatment of Long-Evans rats did not change after either vagotomy or portocaval anastomosis resulting in a circumvention of the liver and a direct blood flow from the intestine to extrahepatic organs (Tuomisto *et al.*, 1995).

Cachexia observed after 2,3,7,8-TCDD treatment can also be induced with certain cytokines such as the endotoxin-responsive tumour necrosis factor α (TNFα) (Döhr *et al.*, 1994), which led to the suggestion that TNFα might mediate the acute toxicity of 2,3,7,8-TCDD. In fact, mortality following a single 2,3,7,8-TCDD dose of 300 µg/kg in male C57BL/6J mice was significantly reduced by treatment with the anti-inflammatory corticoid dexamethasone or with anti-TNFα antibodies (Taylor *et al.*, 1992). In endo-toxin-non-responsive C3H/HeJ mice, Clark and Taylor (1994) found no trend in body weight loss after a single 2,3,7,8-TCDD dose of 350 µg/kg, while endotoxin-responsive C57BL/6 mice demonstrated a statistically significant decline in body weight. However, pathological effects, such as peritoneal infiltration and hepatotoxicity, were also observable in C3H/HeJ mice.

Mechanistic studies of toxicity

Early attempts to investigate the mechanism of action of 2,3,7,8-TCDD in cell culture were made by Knutson and Poland (1980). In 23 cultured cell types including rat hepatoma cells and primary hepatocytes, mouse fibroblasts and human epithelial cell lines, no morphological abnormalities were observed with 10^{-7}–10^{-11} M 2,3,7,8-TCDD. Analysis of trypan blue exclusion or cell proliferation in a number of cell types also failed to show any toxicity. Also, aryl hydrocarbon hydroxylase activity was inducible only in a subgroup of cell types including most hepatoma cell lines, some mouse embryo cell lines and primary rat and chicken hepatocytes.

The fundamental role of the Ah receptor for the toxicity of 2,3,7,8-TCDD (see Section 4.3) was demonstrated by Poland and Glover (1979). DBA/2J mice, which have a low-affinity receptor, were approximately 10-fold less sensitive to thymic involution after 2,3,7,8-TCDD treatment than C57BL/6J mice, a result that precisely matches the 10-fold difference in affinity of 2,3,7,8-TCDD for the Ah receptor (Ema *et al.*, 1994). Furthermore, the capacity of other halogenated aromatic hydrocarbons to produce thymic atrophy corresponded to their capacity to bind to the receptor. The same dependence on receptor affinity applied to the production of cleft palate and to the reduction of the adipose-type (type 4) glucose transporter (GLUT) in adipose tissue and of the brain-type transporter GLUT1 in brain (Liu & Matsumura, 1995).

Comparison of low-affinity Ah receptor (Ah^d/Ah^d) with congenic wild-type high-affinity (Ah^b/Ah^b) Ah receptor mice revealed LD$_{50}$ values for 2,3,7,8-TCDD of 3351 and 159 µg/kg, respectively. A similar difference in dose–response was found for the decrease in body weight, increase in liver weight and decreases in the weight of thymus, spleen, testes and epididymal fat pad (Birnbaum *et al.*, 1990). Okey *et al.* (1995) pointed out the strong genetic link between the Ah receptor and the sensitivity of different mouse strains towards a wide variety of toxic outcomes *in vivo* such as thymic atrophy, induction of cleft palate and porphyria (Jones & Sweeney, 1980; Poland & Knudson, 1982).

It has been claimed, however, that the discrepancy between the Han/Wistar and Long-Evans rats cannot be explained on the basis of Ah receptor concentration, and that differences in the acute toxicity of 2,3,7,8-TCDD between Long-Evans and Sprague-Dawley rats are not related to Ah receptor-mediated induction of ethoxyrufin-O-deethylase activity (Fan & Rozman, 1994). In a reply, Okey *et al.* (1995) pointed out that the very diversity of tissue-selective and species-selective responses elicited by 2,3,7,8-TCDD almost requires that the receptor is part of a multicomponent system. Therefore, it is unlikely that the differences in dose–response are related solely to differences in Ah receptor concentrations or affinities in various species or tissues. In particular, conclusions on the relative susceptibility of different species cannot be drawn on the basis of receptor data only.

Fernandez-Salguero *et al.* (1995) demonstrated that Ah receptor-deficient mice are relatively unaffected by doses of 2,3,7,8-TCDD (2000 µg/kg) 10-fold higher than those found to induce severe toxic and pathological effects in litter mates expressing a functional Ah receptor.

(ii)   *Skin*

The occurrence of cutaneous lesions after treatment with 2,3,7,8-TCDD and related compounds has been described primarily in humans and non-human primates; most rodent species do not represent suitable experimental models for the study of such lesions. The development of a strain of hairless mice susceptible to the skin toxicity of 2,3,7,8-TCDD was an important first step to provide such a model.

In haired and hairless newborn and adult mice, skin application of 2,3,7,8-TCDD caused an involution of sebaceous glands (Puhvel & Sakamoto, 1988). Epidermal hyperplasia and hyperkeratinization, however, were induced in the hairless mice only. The density of inflammatory cell infiltrates in the skin was not reduced by topical treatment with anti-inflammatory agents. The distinct pattern of chloracne observable in hairless mice (Puhvel *et al.*, 1982) did not include the hyperkeratinization of the sebaceous follicles that is typical of human chloracne. Histopathological changes observed with all acnegenic compounds were epidermal hyperkeratosis and hyperplasia, loss of sebaceous glands, keratinization of intradermal pilar cysts and diffuse lymphohistiocytic infiltration of the dermis. Atrophy or complete absence of the hair follicles was evident in severe lesions (Hébert *et al.*, 1990b). In these cases, the epidermis was atrophic with keratinization.

Skin application of 2,3,7,8-TCDD to hairless mice produced an increase in relative liver weight after treatment with 5 ng per week, and a decrease in relative thymus weight after treatment with 20 ng per week over 20 weeks (Hébert *et al.*, 1990a).

Connor *et al.* (1994) showed that the acute systemic toxicity of 2,3,7,8-TCDD is even higher in mice bearing the recessive mutation hairless (hr). Vitamin A deficiency enhanced the dermal but not the systemic toxicity of 2,3,7,8-TCDD after dermal application to hairless mice (Puhvel *et al.*, 1991). 2,3,7,8-TCDD treatment did not affect cutaneous vitamin A levels. Using an ear bioassay for acnegenic activity, Schwetz *et al.* (1973) showed that the rabbit is highly sensitive to the acnegenic effect of 2,3,7,8-TCDD; a single treatment with a solution containing 4 ng/mL 2,3,7,8-TCDD led to a positive result. In rhesus monkeys, a single dose of 1000 ng/kg bw 2,3,7,8-TCDD induced chloracne (McNulty, 1975).

The ability of 2,3,7,8-TCDD and 1,2,4,7,8-PeCDD to induce a flat, cobblestone-like morphology was studied in a non-keratinizing derivative (XBF) of the keratinizing XB mouse epithelial cell line cocultured with irradiated 3T3 feeder cells. The minimal concentrations required to produce these changes from the normal spindle-shape cells, over a 14-day exposure period, were 0.0032 μg/L (ppb) for 2,3,7,8-TCDD and 0.359 μg/L for 1,2,4,7,8-PeCDD (Gierthy & Crane, 1985).

The growth inhibitory effect of transforming growth factor (TGF) β1 in the human squamous carcinoma cell lines, SCC-15G and SCC-25, was not affected by 10^{-8} M 2,3,7,8-TCDD (Hébert *et al.*, 1990b). Furthermore, 2,3,7,8-TCDD had no effect on binding of ^{125}I-labelled TGFβ1 to SCC-15G cells or secretion of TGFβ1 by them, while TGFβ1 suppressed the induction of 7-ethoxyresorufin *O*-deethylase (EROD) activity. The authors concluded that 2,3,7,8-TCDD and TGFβ1 exert their opposite effects on proliferation of the SCC lines by independent mechanisms.

In two human squamous carcinoma cell lines, 0.1 or 1 nM 2,3,7,8-TCDD induced proliferation (Hébert *et al.*, 1990c). This effect was detectable only in cells exposed at subconfluent density, indicating that 2,3,7,8-TCDD prevented normal density-dependent growth arrest. In addition, 2,3,7,8-TCDD inhibited differentiation, measured as keratin staining, and envelope formation in the presence of calcium ionophore. When XB cells derived from a mouse teratoma were cultured at high density, cocultured with irradiated 3T3 feeder-cells, 5×10^{-11} M 2,3,7,8-TCDD produced maximal keratinization (Knutson & Poland, 1980). The potency of other Ah receptor agonists to induce keratinization correlated with their binding affinities to the receptor.

In human cultured epidermal cells, 2,3,7,8-TCDD decreased the number of small (basal) cells and DNA synthesis, while increasing the number of cells containing spontaneous envelopes (which consist of insoluble cross-linked proteins beneath the plasma membrane; an indicator of terminal differentiation of epidermal keratinocytes), as well as the number of envelope-competent cells (Osborne & Greenlee, 1985). On the basis of these findings, it was proposed that 2,3,7,8-TCDD enhances terminal differentiation in epidermal basal cells (Hudson *et al.*, 1986), leading, for example, to hyperkeratinization. T3 and T4 did not produce hyperkeratinization in human epidermal cells or in the SCC-12F human keratinocyte cell line, indicating that 2,3,7,8-TCDD and thyroid hormone effects on the skin are mediated by different mechanisms (Osborne *et al.*, 1987).

In non-transformed human keratinocytes, 2,3,7,8-TCDD treatment caused an increase in the state of differentiation, as judged by an increase in cross-linked envelope formation, and an increase in stratification and keratin staining (Gaido & Maness, 1994).

(iii) *Nervous system*

The possible links between the anorexigenic potency of 2,3,7,8-TCDD and biogenic amines at central nervous sites controlling body weight and food intake were investigated in a number of reports. After measuring noradrenaline, dopamine, dihydroxyphenylacetic acid, homovanillic acid, 5-hydroxytryptamine, 5-hydroxyindoleacetic acid, tryptophan and histamine in the brain and pituitary gland of 2,3,7,8-TCDD-treated male Long-Evans rats, Tuomisto *et al.* (1990) concluded that 2,3,7,8-TCDD caused minor changes in brain neurotransmitter systems, which were not likely to cause 2,3,7,8-TCDD-induced hypophagia. Eight days after intraperitoneal injection with 1000 µg/kg 2,3,7,8-TCDD, a significant increase in tryptophan concentration of about 20% was found in the lateral hypothalamic area and in lateral and medial accumbens nuclei (Unkila *et al.*, 1993a). Furthermore, a slight tendency to diminished dopamine, serotonin and/or 5-hydroxy-indoleacetic acid levels in various brain sites was found during the first day after exposure. Histamine concentrations were not changed in a number of discrete brain nuclei but in the median eminence, 25 h after a single intraperitoneal dose of 1000 µg/kg 2,3,7,8-TCDD (Tuomisto *et al.*, 1991). Unkila *et al.* (1994a) found a selective increase in brain serotonin turnover in 2,3,7,8-TCDD-susceptible Long-Evans but not in 2,3,7,8-TCDD-resistant Han/Wistar rats. The authors related this to increased plasma levels of tryptophan, possibly resulting from inhibited tryptophan catabolism in the liver. Direct application of 2,3,7,8-TCDD into the lateral cerebral ventricle of rats, leading to much higher brain concentrations than intravenous administration of the same dose, did not cause appetite suppression or loss of body weight, whereas animals treated intravenously displayed the cachectic syndrome (Stahl & Rozman, 1990). In contrast, Pohjanvirta *et al.* (1989b) reported that intracerebroventricular injection of 2,3,7,8-TCDD into male Han/Wistar or Long-Evans rats depressed food intake more severely than subcutaneous administration.

Hanneman *et al.* (1996) recently reported that 2,3,7,8-TCDD induces rapid calcium uptake in rat hippocampal neuronal cells, accompanied by decreased mitochondrial membrane potential and increased neuronal membrane protein kinase C activity.

In young male Han/Wistar rats, a single intraperitoneal dose of 1000 µg/kg 2,3,7,8-TCDD did not lead to changes in behaviour or motility (Sirkka *et al.*, 1992). In particular, spontaneous motor activity, anxiety scores, passive avoidance learning, motor coordination and nociception were not altered markedly. A slowing of sensory and motor conduction velocities was observed in male Wistar rats 10 months after a single intra-venous injection of 2.2 µg/kg 2,3,7,8-TCDD. Histopathological examination of peripheral nerves revealed a progressive, and proximally accentuated neuropathy (Grehl *et al.*, 1993).

(iv) *Liver*

In male rhesus monkeys, an oral dose of 5 µg/kg bw 2,3,7,8-TCDD caused an initial mild increase in indocyanine green blood clearance followed by a slight decrease (Seefeld *et al.*, 1979). Serum glutamic pyruvate transaminase and sorbitol dehydrogenase levels were increased. Light microscopy of the livers revealed fatty infiltration with minimal hepatocellular necrosis. In rats, hepatotoxic reactions were characterized by swelling of hepatocytes, fatty metamorphosis and ultimately necrosis after treatment with 10 µg/kg 2,3,7,8-TCDD per day over 10–13 days (Gupta *et al.*, 1973). At this time, there was also an increase in serum transaminase activities. Thereafter, the hepatic lesions progressed and more parenchymal tissue was destroyed. Besides these degenerative lesions, large multinucleated giant hepatocytes were also seen.

A high dose of 2,3,7,8-TCDD (25 µg/kg bw) led to impairment of the clearance and biliary excretion of phenol-3,6-dibromophthalein and sulfobromophthalein, reduced bile flow, swelling and occasional necrosis of hepatocytes and infiltration of mononuclear inflammatory cells in the liver of male Holtzman rats (Yang *et al.*, 1977). Twenty-five days after treatment with 10 µg/kg bw, however, an enhancement of biliary excretion of the bromophthaleins was observed.

In 2,3,7,8-TCDD-sensitive C57BL/6J mice, 3 µg/kg bw 2,3,7,8-TCDD caused mild to moderate hepatic lipid accumulation in the absence of both inflammation and necrosis (Shen *et al.*, 1991), while severe fatty change and mild inflammation and necrosis occurred after treatment with 150 µg/kg. In contrast, DBA mice exposed to 30 µg/kg 2,3,7,8-TCDD developed hepatocellular necrosis and inflammation without any fatty change. The authors concluded that the Ah locus plays a role in determining the sensitivity of mice to the steatotic effects of 2,3,7,8-TCDD in the liver. In female CD1 mice, 2,3,7,8-TCDD produced a centrilobular pattern of hepatocellular degeneration and necrosis with perivascular infiltration of inflammatory cells (MacKenzie *et al.*, 1992). This effect was potentiated by tamoxifen, which is possibly associated with decreased hepatic excretion of 2,3,7,8-TCDD.

A single low-lethality oral dose of 75 µg/kg 2,3,7,8-TCDD induced hepatic porphyria in both male and female C57BL/10 mice (Smith *et al.*, 1981), which was associated with decreased activity of hepatic uroporphyrinogen decarboxylase. DBA/2 mice, bearing a low-affinity Ah receptor, were much less sensitive to these effects of 2,3,7,8-TCDD. In male C57BL/6 mice, chronic administration of 25 µg/kg 2,3,7,8-TCDD per week resulted in hepatic porphyrin accumulation and inhibition of porphyrinogen decarboxylase activity (Cantoni *et al.*, 1984). Partial antagonism of 2,3,7,8-TCDD-induced hepatic porphyrin accumulation in male C57BL/6 mice with 6-methyl-1,3,8-trichlorodibenzofuran was not related to suppression of induction of CYP1A activities or to a less pronounced suppression of uroporphyrinogen decarboxylase (Yao & Safe, 1989). In female Sprague-Dawley rats, administration of 1 µg/kg 2,3,7,8-TCDD per week over 16 weeks also resulted in hepatic porphyria (Goldstein *et al.*, 1982). After the administration period, recovery from the porphyrogenic effects of 2,3,7,8-TCDD was very slow and did not correlate with the biological half-life of 2,3,7,8-TCDD. In female Sprague-Dawley rats treated with 2,3,7,8-TCDD and various PCBs, a significant correlation was observed between CYP1A2 activities and hepatic porphyrin levels. In addition, the non-dioxin-like 2,2',4,4',5,5'-hexachlorobiphenyl caused a strong synergistic effect on 2,3,7,8-TCDD-induced hepatic porphyric (800 times) (van Birgelen *et al.*, 1996a,b). An interaction between 2,3,7,8-TCDD and iron was noted by Jones *et al.* (1981). In iron-deficient mice, the liver toxicity of 2,3,7,8-TCDD (25 µg/kg per week over 12 weeks) was much less pronounced than in iron-supplemented animals, while extrahepatic effects of 2,3,7,8-TCDD were not affected.

A somewhat controversial issue is the effect of 2,3,7,8-TCDD on the proliferation of hepatocytes *in vivo* and *in vitro*. In male and female Harlan-Sprague-Dawley rats, Dickins *et al.* (1981) observed a significantly higher increase in liver DNA synthesis after a one-third hepatectomy when the animals were treated with 2,3,7,8-TCDD

(5 μg/kg bw) five days before surgery. Interestingly, the effect was also observable after laparotomy only (Christian & Peterson, 1983). In female CD (Sprague-Dawley) rats and in male B6C3F1 mice, 2,3,7,8-TCDD caused an acute 1.5–1.7-fold increase in liver DNA synthesis (Büsser & Lutz, 1987), while no increase in total hepatic BrdU labelling index was observed in male or female Sprague-Dawley rats one and two weeks after 2,3,7,8-TCDD treatment designed to achieve quasi-steady-state liver concentrations of 0.03, 30 or 150 ng/g liver (Fox et al., 1993). However, a slight increase was seen in the periportal hepatocyte proliferation pattern. Inhibition of hepatocellular proliferation, stimulated by a two-thirds hepatectomy, was also observed in female Sprague-Dawley rats after 14 days of a dosing regimen designed to achieve and maintain a steady-state concentration of 30 ng 2,3,7,8-TCDD/g liver (Bauman et al., 1995). Furthermore, 2,3,7,8-TCDD induced a periportal pattern of cell proliferation as compared to the pan-lobular pattern in the control partial hepatectomy group.

In female Sprague-Dawley rats either ovariectomized or sham-operated, and then treated first with N-nitrosodiethylamine (NDEA) and, from one week later, with 100 ng/kg 2,3,7,8-TCDD per day (for details, see Section 3.6.3(b)), 2,3,7,8-TCDD-induced cell proliferation was observed in the intact rats (Lucier et al., 1991). The average BrdU labelling index values were 6.0 and 7.3 in intact rats treated with 2,3,7,8-TCDD alone and with NDEA followed by 2,3,7,8-TCDD. Control values were 0.32 in intact rats and 1.09 in ovariectomized rats. The average BrdU labelling index values were 0.97 in rats treated with 2,3,7,8-TCDD alone and 1.15 in rats treated with NDEA followed by 2,3,7,8-TCDD. Intact rats treated with NDEA alone had a slightly higher labelling index (0.8) than untreated controls. Large interindividual variations were observed in the effects of 2,3,7,8-TCDD on cell proliferation. Similarly, large interindividual variations were seen for the development of GGT- and GSTP-positive foci. Livers from animals undergoing more rapid cell proliferation had the greatest number of GSTP-positive foci. The correlation coefficient for the two parameters was 0.85 ($p = 0.007$). A similar positive correlation was seen for GGT-positive foci and cell proliferation ($r = 0.67$; $p = 0.05$). The volume percentage of PGST-positive foci of the livers having the four highest proliferation rates was 1.9, whereas the corresponding value for the four lowest was 0.7.

A further series of female Sprague-Dawley rats were given similar treatment using a range of 2,3,7,8-TCDD doses (for details, see Section 3.6.3(b)). For all rats treated only with NDEA, BrdU[+] S-phase nuclei were randomly distributed throughout the hepatic lobules. In contrast, there was a periportal distribution of BrdU[+] S-phase nuclei in several non-NDEA-treated, 2,3,7,8-TCDD-treated rats. Overall, there was a statistically significant increasing trend in labelling index as a function of dose of 2,3,7,8-TCDD, with an interaction between 2,3,7,8-TCDD and NDEA. This trend suggests dose-dependence, but the results in comparison to the controls were not statistically significant. The trend in increasing labelling index was stronger in initiated rats than in non-initiated rats. There was a significant decrease in labelling index in the low-dose group of initiated rats (Maronpot et al., 1993).

Groups of female Wistar rats were pretreated with NDEA, then given either a single ('acute') or repeated ('chronic') treatment with 2,3,7,8-TCDD (for details, see Section 3.6.3(*b*)). Proliferation as measured by BrdU labelling index was not significantly increased (NDEA, 6.7%; NDEA + 'acute' 2,3,7,8-TCDD, 8.8%; NDEA + 'chronic' 2,3,7,8-TCDD, 9.5%). However, apoptosis was markedly decreased (NDEA, 6.2%; NDEA + 'acute' 2,3,7,8-TCDD, 3.7%; NDEA + 'chronic' 2,3,7,8-TCDD, 0.8%) (Stinchcombe *et al.*, 1995). [The Working Group noted that measurement of apoptosis by the fluorescent method used in this study has not been validated.]

In rodent hepatocytes in primary culture, Schrenk *et al.* (1992, 1994b) found that 2,3,7,8-TCDD concentrations between 10^{-12} M and 10^{-9} M did not affect DNA synthesis. However, the response of DNA synthesis to the epidermal growth factor (EGF) was enhanced at low and attenuated at high 2,3,7,8-TCDD concentrations, also depending on cell density. Hepatocytes from Ah^d/Ah^d (low-affinity receptor) C57BL/6J mice were about 10-fold less sensitive than those from Ah^b/Ah^b (high-affinity receptor) mice, consistent with the involvement of the Ah receptor in these effects. In rat hepatocytes, the enhancement of the EGF response by 2,3,7,8-TCDD was further increased when ethinyloestradiol was added to the cultures. A synergistic effect of 2,3,7,8-TCDD on DNA synthesis in cultured rat hepatocytes stimulated with EGF or insulin was also reported by Wölfle *et al.* (1993). In contrast, Hushka and Greenlee (1995) did not detect a 2,3,7,8-TCDD-mediated increase in proliferation of either untreated or EGF-treated cultured hepatocytes from male or female Sprague-Dawley rats. 2,3,7,8-TCDD rather caused an inhibition of DNA synthesis, with an EC_{50} of 10^{-11} M.

In 5L cells derived from the rat hepatoma cell line H4IIEC3, 2,3,7,8-TCDD reduced proliferation by about 50%, with half-maximal inhibition at $1-3 \times 10^{-10}$ M (Göttlicher & Wiebel, 1991; Wiebel *et al.*, 1991), while the parental line was insensitive to the growth-inhibitory effect of 2,3,7,8-TCDD. Flow cytometric analysis revealed that 2,3,7,8-TCDD blocked the entry of 5L cells into S-phase, without affecting their progression through S and G_2/M to the G_1 phase. This effect is associated with the presence of the Ah receptor (Göttlicher *et al.*, 1990). In WB-F344 rat liver epithelial cells, however, 10^{-9} M 2,3,7,8-TCDD increased DNA synthesis two- to three-fold (Münzel *et al.*, 1996).

(v) *Endocrine system*

Studies on the interactions of 2,3,7,8-TCDD with a variety of hormone systems have demonstrated that a number of links exist, in particular to the sex steroids, corticosteroids and thyroid hormones.

The effects on gonads and on levels and function of gonadal steroids are described in Section 4.4.

A target organ for 2,3,7,8-TCDD is the pituitary, where it disrupted the normal feedback mechanisms between plasma testosterone, 5α-dihydrotestosterone or 17β-oestradiol and luteinizing hormone (LH) secretion (Bookstaff *et al.*, 1990a). In male Sprague-Dawley rats, an oral dose of 20 μg/kg 2,3,7,8-TCDD (ED_{50}) inhibited the compensatory increases in pituitary gonadotropin-releasing hormone (GnRH) receptor number, and the LH secretory responsiveness of the pituitary to GnRH and plasma LH concentrations which should have occurred in response to 2,3,7,8-TCDD-induced decreases in plasma testosterone concentration (Bookstaff *et al.*, 1990b).

A single oral dose of 2,3,7,8-TCDD (50 µg/kg) resulted in a significant and sustained increase in plasma adrenocorticotropin in male Sprague-Dawley rats (Bestervelt *et al.*, 1993a). Plasma corticosterone levels were slightly but significantly increased at days 1–5, but were below those of untreated controls at days 10 and 14, indicating that the pituitary–adrenal axis was disturbed at these later time points. This conclusion was supported by in-vitro findings using primary cultures of rat anterior pituitary cells and adrenal cells (Bestervelt *et al.*, 1993b).

Neal *et al.* (1979) concluded from determinations of the corticosteroid-inducible tyrosine aminotransferase that 2,3,7,8-TCDD (200 µg/kg bw) does not mimic gluco-corticoid activity. No direct interference with T3 was found, although application of T3 caused a delay of up to 50% in 2,3,7,8-TCDD mortality. In a receptor-binding experiment using rat liver cytosol, 2,3,7,8-TCDD did not displace dexamethasone from the glucocorticoid receptor.

The hypothalamic/endorphin concentration initially increased after 2,3,7,8-TCDD treatment (50 µg/kg) of male Sprague-Dawley rats and then was depressed (Bestervelt *et al.*, 1991), while brain mu opioid receptor number was increased by 60%.

2,3,7,8-TCDD also affects serum melatonin levels in rats, changing the concentration of this hormone in the pineal gland (Pohjanvirta *et al.*, 1989c; Linden *et al.*, 1991; Pohjanvirta *et al.*, 1996). This response appears to be related to increased extrahepatic metabolism of melatonin (Pohjanvirta *et al.*, 1996).

Total T4, T3, TSH serum levels and uridine diphosphate-glucuronosyl transferase (UDP-GT) activity were measured in 21-day-old Sprague-Dawley rats whose mothers had been treated with 2,3,7,8-TCDD doses of 0.025 or 0.10 µg/kg bw per day on days 10–16 of gestation (Seo *et al.*. 1995). With regard to total T4, no difference between the undivided groups was observed; however, a small (20.4%), but significant reduction in total T4 was found in female but not male rats derived from the high-dose group. Neither total T3 nor TSH was affected by treatment. Significant increases were observed in both low- and high-dose-derived weanling rats, with regard to hepatic UDP-GT activity (310% in the high-dose group); there was no evidence of a sex difference.

Administration of 2,3,7,8-TCDD by gastric instillation to 12-week-old female Sprague-Dawley rats once every two weeks for 30 weeks induced a dose-dependent decrease in serum T4 level that was significant at daily dose equivalents of 0.035 µg/kg bw or more. Total T3 levels were not significantly affected, but TSH was increased 2–3-fold at a daily dose equivalent of 0.125 µg/kg bw. In this same dose group, the hepatic mRNA levels for a UDP-GT (UGT1A1) and a cytochrome P450 (CYP1A1) were increased about 2.5- and 250-fold respectively (Sewall *et al.*, 1995). Decreases in total T4 plasma level following treatment of rats with 2,3,7,8-TCDD were related to the induction of UGT1A1, which catalyses the conjugation of T4 and thereby facilitates its excretion (van Birgelen *et al.*, 1995b). The resulting elevation of TSH level has been suggested to lead to the follicular cell hyperplasia and hypertrophy observed in 2,3,7,8-TCDD-treated rats (Sewall *et al.*, 1995).

A pronounced reduction in serum T4 level was observed (Potter *et al.*, 1983) along with decreases in blood levels of insulin and glucose in male Sprague-Dawley rats treated with 45 μg/kg 2,3,7,8-TCDD. Furthermore, the body temperature of the animals dropped to 34.5 °C. In pair-fed controls, no hypothyroxinaemia, hypothermia or hypoglycaemia was observed. 2,3,7,8-TCDD did not cause significant alterations in serum glucagon or somatostatin levels. A dose-dependent decrease in serum T4 (free and total), but not in TSH or T3, was also observed by Górski and Rozman (1987); T4 levels returned to normal 32 days after 2,3,7,8-TCDD dosage. Other effects of 2,3,7,8-TCDD were a decrease in serum levels of insulin and glucose after high dosage. The hypoinsulinaemic rats were hypersensitive towards insulin, so that otherwise non-toxic insulin doses were lethal. The authors concluded that hypoinsulinaemia is part of an adaptive response of the organism to reduce toxicity after 2,3,7,8-TCDD exposure.

Thyroidectomy with ^{131}I has been shown to protect male Sprague-Dawley rats (10 per group) from the acute toxicity of 2,3,7,8-TCDD at a dose of 100 μg/kg bw, whereas substitution of T4 re-established sensitivity towards 2,3,7,8-TCDD. Percentage mortality figures after 45 days in non-thyroidectomized rats, thyroidectomized + T4 rats and thyroidectomized rats were 78%, 70% and 0%, respectively (Rozman *et al.*, 1984). The authors concluded that thyroid hormone(s) play(s) an important role in mediating the toxicity of 2,3,7,8-TCDD. Radiothyroidectomy protected rats against the 2,3,7,8-TCDD-induced immunotoxicity, as assessed by the spleen anti-sheep red blood cell (SRBC) plaque-forming assay (Pazdernik & Rozman, 1985). The authors suggested that the T4 decrease induced by 2,3,7,8-TCDD may also represent a protective response of the organism to reduce 2,3,7,8-TCDD toxicity including immunotoxicity.

(vi) *Other systems*

Treatment of rats with 2,3,7,8-TCDD (50–100 μg/kg bw) led to a significant increase in serum levels of gastrin (Mably *et al.*, 1990; Theobald *et al.*, 1991).

High, generally toxic doses of 2,3,7,8-TCDD alter cardiac function and morphology, as shown in several animal species (Buu-Hoï *et al.*, 1972; Gupta *et al.*, 1973; Allen *et al.*, 1977; Kociba *et al.*, 1979; Poland & Knutson, 1982; Rifkind *et al.*, 1984; Kelling *et al.*, 1987).

Rozman (1984) suggested that the brown adipose tissue was a target for 2,3,7,8-TCDD toxicity. In fact, 2,3,7,8-TCDD induced a progressive lipid depletion in the brown adipose tissue followed by alterations in glycogen, widening of intercellular spaces, mitochondrial swelling and enhanced lysosomal activity (Rozman *et al.*, 1986). In 3T3-L1 cells, 10 nM 2,3,7,8-TCDD suppressed differentiation into fat cell colonies induced by dexamethasone and isobutylmethylxanthine (Phillips *et al.*, 1995). In contrast, 2,3,7,8-TCDD had no effect on the maintenance of the adipose phenotype in differentiated cells.

(b) *Immunological responses*

Immunological responses induced by PCDDs and PCDFs in mammals have been observed for the last 25 years with doses varying over many orders of magnitude. Initial studies were performed with doses in the mg/kg and μg/kg range in mice and rats, but it is now known that alterations of some immune responses can be observed after exposure to ng/kg doses of 2,3,7,8-TCDD in mice and non-human primates.

Immunological responses observed after treatment with doses which cause overt toxicity or even mortality are without relevance to the human situation in relation to environmental or occupational exposures.

Studies in mice and rats performed at doses which induce thymic atrophy should be interpreted with great caution.

(i)   Effects of 2,3,7,8-TCDD

The effects of 2,3,7,8-TCDD and other polyhalogenated dibenzo-*para*-dioxins and polyhalogenated dibenzofurans on the mammalian immune system have been reviewed several times. 2,3,7,8-TCDD causes suppression of both cell-mediated and humoral immunity, but little is known about the underlying mechanisms (Vos & Luster, 1989; Holsapple *et al.*, 1991a,b; Vos *et al.*, 1991; Kerkvliet, 1994; Kerkvliet & Burleson, 1994; Holsapple, 1995).

Effects on thymus and role of Ah receptor

Poland and Glover (1979) studied the dose–response relationship for thymic atrophy produced by 2,3,7,8-TCDD in two strains of mice. C57BL/6 mice, which have a high-affinity Ah receptor, were approximately 10-fold more sensitive to thymic involution than DBA/2 mice, which have a lower-affinity receptor.

Germolec *et al.* (1996) have described CYP1A1 induction in lymphoid tissues from Fischer 344 rats exposed to a single oral dose of 100 µg/kg bw 2,3,7,8-TCDD. Immuno-histochemical localization of CYP1A1 in immune tissues indicated that cells other than the lymphoid populations are responsible for the increased CYP1A1 expression.

The presence of the Ah receptor and the protein Arnt was demonstrated in T cells, and a combined exposure to 2,3,7,8-TCDD and the T-cell activator anti-CD3 caused the Ah receptor to translocate to the nucleus, but DNA binding activity of the murine T-cell Ah receptor was not detected (Lawrence *et al.*, 1996).

Ah receptor-deficient mice showed decreased accumulation of lymphocytes in the spleen and lymph nodes, but not in the thymus (Fernandez-Salguero *et al.*, 1995). However, corresponding results were not observed in Ahr⁻/Ahr⁻ mice generated by another group (Schmidt *et al.*, 1996).

Kerkvliet and Brauner (1990) showed that, in C57BL/6 mice treated with 2 µg/kg bw 2,3,7,8-TCDD, the percentage of double positive CD4$^+$CD8$^+$ (DP) thymocytes was decreased, whereas the percentage of double negative CD4$^-$ CD8$^-$ (DN) thymocytes was increased.

In C57BL/6 mice treated with a single intraperitoneal injection of 50 µg/kg bw 2,3,7,8-TCDD, a decrease was seen in cell number in the thymus mainly of the DP and DN populations (Lundberg *et al.*, 1990a; Lundberg, 1991).

Silverstone *et al.* (1994a) showed that thymic atrophy after a single intraperitoneal dose of 30 µg/kg bw 2,3,7,8-TCDD in BALB/c mice resulted from a proportional loss of all classes of thymocytes. There was no significant relative reduction in terminal deoxynucleotidyl transferase (TdT)[+] recombinase activating gene (RAG-1)[+] cells in the thymus, but a slow and persistent reduction of TdT and RAG-1 in bone marrow [TdT and RAG-1 are markers for lymphocyte stem cells].

A single intraperitoneal 2,3,7,8-TCDD dose of 30 μg/kg bw to sham-operated or neonatally thymectomized BALB/c mice reduced the bone marrow levels of mRNA for TdT and RAG-1. Thus, neonatal thymectomy had no effect on the 2,3,7,8-TCDD-elicited reduction of TdT or RAG-1 mRNAs. Corresponding effects of 2,3,7,8-TCDD were also observed in athymic nu/nu mice (Frazier *et al.*, 1994a).

Severe combined immunodeficient C.B-17 *scid/scid* (SCID) mice engrafted with human fetal thymus and liver tissue fragments (SCID-hu mice) were used to assess the sensitivity of the human thymus to 2,3,7,8-TCDD. The relative size of the cortex showed a dose-dependent decrease in grafted human thymus as well as in rat thymus, which was significant after exposure to 25 μg/kg 2,3,7,8-TCDD. A dose-dependent increase in keratinization of Hassal's corpuscles in the medullary areas of the thymus grafts was observed (de Heer *et al.*, 1995)

Muralidhara *et al.* (1994) observed decreased activity of the enzyme adenosine deaminase in thymic tissue of BALB/c mice (but not in DBA/2 mice) after treatment with a single intraperitoneal injection of 28.8, 57.5 or 115 μg/ kg bw 2,3,7,8-TCDD or more. The lowest dose tested (11.5 μg/kg) did not cause a significant reduction in the enzyme activity.

Thymocytes from 15-day-old C57BL/6 mice, treated with 50 μg/kg bw 2,3,7,8-TCDD four days before sacrifice, showed an earlier response and a higher maximal cell proliferation than thymocytes from control mice upon stimulation with concanavalin A *in vitro* (Lundberg *et al.*, 1990b).

The effects of 2,3,7,8-TCDD on the murine fetal thymus were studied in an organ culture system. A concentration of 5×10^{-10} M caused a 50% inhibition of lymphoid development. At 10^{-9} M, reduction of DP cells was most pronounced (Dencker *et al.*, 1985; d'Argy *et al.*, 1989; Lundberg *et al.*, 1990a).

Greenlee *et al.* (1985) studied the effects of 2,3,7,8-TCDD on primary cultures of thymic epithelial cells from C57BL/6 mice. Treatment of the cultures with 10 nM 2,3,7,8-TCDD resulted in altered maturation of cocultured thymocytes as judged by the suppression (40% of control) of thymic epithelium-dependent responsiveness of thymocytes to the mitogens concanavalin A and phytohaemagglutinin.

With human thymic epithelial cells, marked differences were seen in the sensitivity of the cells from different donors to 2,3,7,8-TCDD. Cytochrome P450 activities were inducible in these cells *in vitro* (EC_{50} value, approximately 1 nM), with maximal increases in 7-ethoxycoumarin-*O*-deethylase (ECOD) and EROD activities of 3–400-fold and 1–21-fold, respectively (Cook *et al.*, 1987).

Thymic atrophy in rats following exposure to 2,3,7,8-TCDD (at doses of 1 and 10 mg/kg bw) was first described in the Wistar strain by Buu-Hoï *et al.* (1972).

In Fischer 344 rats, Rice *et al.* (1995) observed a significant reduction in the relative thymus weight (thymus weight/body weight) after a single intraperitoneal injection of 0.3 μg/kg bw 2,3,7,8-TCDD.

de Heer *et al.* (1994a,b) reported a significant reduction in the number of immature CD4⁺CD8⁺ thymocytes after single oral doses of 1 µg/kg bw 2,3,7,8-TCDD or more in Wistar rats. Numbers of mature CD3 medullary thymocytes were not affected at doses of up to 25 µg/kg bw 2,3,7,8-TCDD. A detailed study of the time course of the effect after treatment with 25 µg/kg 2,3,7,8-TCDD revealed a recovery in proliferative activity in the thymic cortex (after six days) and an increase in cellularity after day 13.

Kurl *et al.* (1993) studied the time course of events which precede 2,3,7,8-TCDD-induced thymic apoptosis. They showed that, in thymocytes from immature rats incubated *in vitro*, nuclear accumulation of 2,3,7,8-TCDD reaches maximal levels within 60 min, paralleling 2,3,7,8-TCDD-induced increases in RNA synthesis and poly(A)polymerase activity.

Pronounced thymic atrophy was induced in PVG rats by treatment with a single dose of 50 µg/kg bw 2,3,7,8-TCDD. Thymus lobes were transplanted into control rats and evaluated 20 days later, when they did not differ from controls, indicating that the 2,3,7,8-TCDD-induced damage in rat thymus is rapidly reversible (van Loveren *et al.*, 1991).

de Waal *et al.* (1992, 1993) investigated rat thymus by immunohistochemistry and electron microscopy after treatment with single doses of 50 and 150 µg/kg bw 2,3,7,8-TCDD. They observed changes which mainly affected the cortical epithelial cells, but, because both dose levels used in this study were lethal to the animals, the relevance of the results is doubtful.

Cytotoxic T-cells

Doses of 4 ng/kg bw 2,3,7,8-TCDD altered the ability of adult male C57BL/6 mice to generate cytotoxic T-lymphocytes (CTL) in response to alloantigen challenge. The cellular basis of the 2,3,7,8-TCDD-induced suppression was shown to be an enhanced suppressor T-cell activity of CTL responses, whereas CTL precursers and IL-2 production appeared to be intact in 2,3,7,8-TCDD-exposed mice. CTL activity generated *in vitro* following allogenic stimulation was not impaired when spleen cells from 2,3,7,8-TCDD-treated DBA/2 mice were used (Clark *et al.*, 1981, 1983; Nagarkatti *et al.*, 1984). However, these results at very low dose levels could not be corroborated by other investigators.

Hanson and Smialowicz (1994) specifically designed a study to re-evaluate the effect of 2,3,7,8-TCDD on CTL response as described by Clark *et al.* (1981). Neither the in-vivo- nor the in-vitro-generated CTL response was altered following a single intraperitoneal injection of 2,3,7,8-TCDD at doses ranging from 0.24 to 7.2 µg/kg bw. Also, no effect was observed on the in-vivo-generated CTL response following four weekly exposures to 2,3,7,8-TCDD at doses of 0.01 to 3.0 µg/kg bw. Similarly, 2,3,7,8-TCDD did not alter the in-vitro-generated CTL response at these dose levels. [The Working Group noted that the sex of the C57BL/6 mice was different (female instead of male), but it is unlikely that this accounts for the discrepancy in the results.]

Kerkvliet *et al.* (1990a) observed a significant suppression of CTL response in C57BL/6 mice (Ah^b/Ah^b) at doses of 5–20 µg/kg bw 2,3,7,8-TCDD. Ah^d/Ah^d mice were less susceptible.

Single oral doses of 2.5–40 µg/kg 2,3,7,8-TCDD suppressed the activity of CTL in C57BL/6 mice with a calculated ID$_{50}$ (50% immunosuppressive dose) of 7.2 µg/kg. Glucocorticoid levels (corticosterone) were not altered at doses below 40 µg/kg, indicating that 2,3,7,8-TCDD-induced CTL suppression is not dependent on elevated glucocorticoid levels (de Krey & Kerkvliet, 1995).

Rice *et al.* (1995) treated Fischer 344 rats with single oral doses of 2,3,7,8-TCDD up to 30 µg/kg bw and examined CTL activities 24 days following treatment. Syngenic invivo tumour-specific CTL were generated that model cell-mediated immune reactions against neoplastically transformed self antigens. Under these conditions, CTL activity showed no significant dose-dependent alteration due to 2,3,7,8-TCDD exposure, but relative thymus weight was significantly decreased at the lowest dose studied (0.3 µg/kg bw).

Effects on lymphocytes in vivo

Oughton *et al.* (1995) studied the effects of 2,3,7,8-TCDD on lymphocytes by flow cytometry. Female C57BL/6 mice were treated weekly with 200 ng/kg bw 2,3,7,8-TCDD for 14–15 months. Besides an age-matched vehicle control, a group of four-month-old mice was evaluated to assess alterations associated with ageing. In the thymus of the 2,3,7,8-TCDD-treated mice, the proportion of CD4$^-$CD8$^-$ cells was increased, as was the proportion of *gamma-delta*$^+$ thymocytes. The most definite change in 2,3,7,8-TCDD-treated mice was a decrease in the frequency of memory T helper cells, defined as CD4$^+$Pgp-1^{hi}CD45RB^{lo}, with a concomitant increase in the proportion of naive T helper cells identified as CD4$^+$Pgp-1^{lo}CD45RB^{hi}. [Pgp-1 and CD45RB are the murine analogues to the human markers CD29 and CD45RA. The results of this paper are consistent with the findings in marmosets described below.]

Following a single subcutaneous injection of 10 ng/kg bw 2,3,7,8-TCDD into four mature female marmosets, a pronounced decrease was observed in the number of cells from a defined lymphocyte subpopulation carrying both the CD4 and the CD29 epitopes ('helper-inducer' or memory cells). Also, the percentage of pan-B cells (B1, CD20$^+$) was clearly lower than that in the controls (Neubert *et al.*, 1990b).

In a 42-week study with lower doses, an opposite effect was initially observed, whereas the results of the first study were confirmed after an increase of the weekly dose. The study consisted of three parts: (*a*) weekly subcutaneous doses of 0.3 ng/kg bw 2,3,7,8-TCDD were given to seven marmosets for 24 weeks; (*b*) the weekly dose was then raised to 1.5 ng/kg bw 2,3,7,8-TCDD for another six weeks; (*c*) finally, this was followed by a dose-free period of 12 weeks. An increase in the percentage as well as the absolute number of CD4$^+$CD29$^+$ cells was observed after the 24-week treatment period with weekly injections of 0.3 ng/kg bw 2,3,7,8-TCDD. In the second part of the study, this lymphocyte subpopulation decreased after weekly injections of 1.5 ng/kg bw 2,3,7,8-TCDD. The effect was completely reversed during the 12-week recovery period. In addition, several changes were observed in other lymphocyte subpopulations: there was a change in CD4$^+$CD45R$^+$ cells contrary to that of the helper-inducer cells. Furthermore, a transient increase in CD8$^+$CD56$^+$ cells ('cytotoxic T-cells') was found, and a decrease in pan-B cells (CD20$^+$), which were again reversible after discontinuation of the dosing (Neubert et al., 1992a,b).

After subcutaneous injection of a single dose of 300 ng/kg bw 2,3,7,8-TCDD into three marmosets, the number of total lymphocytes decreased and at doses of 1 µg/kg or more the number of total leukocytes in peripheral blood of two marmosets was significantly reduced (Neubert et al., 1993b).

Effects on lymphocytes in vitro

Neubert et al. (1991) studied the effects of 2,3,7,8-TCDD on pokeweed mitogen-stimulated proliferation and differentiation of peripheral lymphocytes in vitro with cells from a marmoset and from two healthy human donors. They observed a pronounced decrease in the percentage of B-cells (CD20$^+$) and CD4$^+$ cells and a concomitant increase in the percentage of CD8$^+$ cells at dose levels as low as 10^{-12}–10^{-14} M 2,3,7,8-TCDD.

Using a similar experimental approach, Lang et al. (1994) exposed human lymphocytes from peripheral blood in vitro to concentrations of 10^{-7}–10^{-14} M 2,3,7,8-TCDD. Cells were stimulated by pokeweed mitogen or anti-CD3 monoclonal antibody. Analysis of surface markers (e.g., CD4$^+$, CD29$^+$, CD19$^+$) by flow cytometry showed no significant alterations under the given conditions.

Effects on antibody-producing cells in vivo

Intraperitoneal injections of single 2,3,7,8-TCDD doses ranging from 1.2 to 30 µg/kg bw suppressed primary antibody production to SRBC plaque-forming cell (PFC) response in C57BL/6J and in less sensitive DBA/2 mice (Vecchi et al., 1980, 1983).

A single oral 2,3,7,8-TCDD dose ranging from 0.2 to 5 µg/kg bw given two days before SRBC sensitization produced a suppression of anti-SRBC PFC response on day 5 in C57BL/6 mice; the ID$_{50}$ was 0.74 µg/kg (Kerkvliet & Brauner, 1990).

Narasimhan et al. (1994) determined the splenic antibody PFC response to SRBC nine days after administration of 2,3,7,8-TCDD to B6C3F1 mice. Suppression of PFC response expressed per spleen or per 10^6 cells was observed at 100 ng/kg bw 2,3,7,8-TCDD and higher doses (results with 50 ng/kg bw 2,3,7,8-TCDD were not significantly different from controls).

Kerkvliet et al. (1990b) compared the effects of 2,3,7,8-TCDD in two congenic strains of C57BL/6 mice that differed at the Ah locus. Using the haemolytic antibody isotope release assay, both Ah^b/Ah^b and Ah^d/Ah^d mice exhibited dose-dependent suppression of the anti-trinitrophenyl (TNP) response following 2,3,7,8-TCDD exposure (T-cell-independent). The ID$_{50}$ values were 7.0 µg/kg (Ah^b/Ah^b mice) and 30.8 µg/kg (Ah^d/Ah^d mice). Suppression of the antibody response to the T-cell-dependent antigen SRBC occurred at lower doses (0.6 µg/kg bw 2,3,7,8-TCDD in Ah^b/Ah^b mice) and the reaction in Ah^d/Ah^d mice showed an apparent biphasic dose–response relationship.

When spleen cells from mice treated two days previously with 5 µg/kg bw 2,3,7,8-TCDD were transferred to an irradiated host, no suppression of the PFC response to SRBC was observed, while a similar dose in a non-irradiated animal produced profound suppression of the PFC response. Cultures of spleen cells from SRBC-primed 2,3,7,8-TCDD-treated (5 µg/kg) C57BL/6 mice produced fewer anti-TNP PFC when immunized with TNP-SRBC, as compared to cells from primed vehicle-treated controls (Tomar & Kerkvliet, 1991).

Dooley and Holsapple (1988) showed that the B lymphocyte is the primary target for suppression of the T-dependent antibody response in B6C3F1 mice by demonstrating that the suppression of several humoral responses (the polyclonal response to lipopolysaccharide (LPS), the T-cell-independent response to dinitrophenyl (DNP)–Ficoll and the T-cell-dependent response to SRBC) was characterized by dose–response–effect curves that were approximately parallel. They used separation/reconstitution assay techniques to show that the suppression of antibody responses to 2,3,7,8-TCDD is the predominant result of a specific effect on the functional capacities of the B-cell.

Dooley *et al.* (1990) treated B6C3F1 mice orally on five consecutive days with daily doses of 1 µg/kg bw 2,3,7,8-TCDD. They observed no effect of 2,3,7,8-TCDD exposure on [³H]thymidine uptake in splenocytes of these mice 24 h after in-vitro stimulation with the T-cell mitogen concanavalin A. Titration of T-cells from 2,3,7,8-TCDD-treated mice into naïve splenocyte cultures did not suppress the humoral response to either a T-cell-dependent (SRBC) or -independent (DNP–Ficoll) antigen. Data suggest that an alteration of T-cell function following 2,3,7,8-TCDD exposure does not play a role in the suppression of the antibody response elicited by antigen stimulation of splenocytes from B6C3F1 mice.

Morris *et al.* (1992) showed that the sensitivity of DBA/2 mice to suppression of the antibody response increased significantly when 2,3,7,8-TCDD was administered daily over two weeks rather than as an acute exposure. This change in sensitivity was not paralleled by a shift in the sensitivity to other effects of 2,3,7,8-TCDD, including thymic atrophy and liver enzyme induction.

Smialowicz *et al.* (1994) studied the effects of 2,3,7,8-TCDD on the antibody PFC response to SRBC comparatively in B6C3F1 mice and in Fischer 344 rats. Their data for mice were in agreement with the results from other laboratories (ED$_{50}$, 0.7 µg/kg bw 2,3,7,8-TCDD). In contrast, 2,3,7,8-TCDD failed to suppress, and in fact enhanced, the PFC response to SRBC in rats at doses of 3 and 30 µg/kg bw. Flow cytometric analysis of thymocytes and splenic lymphocytes from 2,3,7,8-TCDD-dosed (3, 10 and 30 µg/kg bw) and SRBC-immunized mice and rats revealed that CD4⁻CD8⁺ splenocytes were reduced and IgM⁺ splenocytes were increased in a dose-related manner in rats only.

Corresponding experiments were performed with a T-cell-independent antigen TNP-LPS in B6C3F1 mice and in Fischer 344 rats. The dose of 2,3,7,8-TCDD required to suppress the immune response in rats was higher (30 µg/kg) than in mice (10 and 30 µg/kg). Thus, species differences were demonstrable also under these conditions; however, they were not as pronounced as with the T-cell-dependent antigen SRBC (Smialowicz *et al.*, 1996).

Harper *et al.* (1993) studied the effects of a single intraperitoneal injection of 2,3,7,8-TCDD on the suppression of the splenic PFC response to the T-cell-independent antigen

TNP-LPS in C57BL/6 and DBA/2 mice. The ED_{50} values (PFC/10^6 viable cells) were 1.5 μg/kg bw (C57BL/6 mice) and 9.7 μg/kg bw (DBA/2 mice).

Effects on antibody-producing cells in vitro

Tucker *et al.* (1986) observed a direct effect of 2,3,7,8-TCDD on cultured lymphcytes resulting in a selective inhibition of the differentiation of B-cells into antibody-secreting cells. Using lymphocytes from congenic mice differing only at the Ah locus, it was determined that the Ah^b/Ah^b-derived cells were inhibited by 2,3,7,8-TCDD *in vitro*, whereas the Ah^d/Ah^d-derived cells were not.

Holsapple *et al.* (1986a) reported a reduction in the number of antibody-producing murine spleen cells which developed in response to LPS, DNP–Ficoll and SRBC with 2,3,7,8-TCCD at concentrations ranging from 5 to 20 nM. Direct addition of 2,3,7,8-TCDD had no effect on mitogen-induced proliferation. There was no suppression when 2,3,7,8-TCDD was added to the medium 3 h after LPS (200 μg/mL). 2,3,7,8-TCDD suppressed the antibody response of cells from DBA/2 mice at concentrations similar to those required to suppress the cells from B6C3F1 mice, suggesting that the observed effect is independent of the Ah locus.

In agreement with these results, Davis and Safe (1991) reported that 2,3,7,8-TCDD and other congeners produced a similar concentration-dependent suppression of the in-vitro anti-SRBC response using cells from either C57BL/6 mice or DBA/2 mice.

Morris *et al.* (1991) showed that, with spleen cells from B6C3F1 mice, the suppression of the in-vitro T-cell-dependent humoral immune response by 2,3,7,8-TCDD is dependent on the lot of serum used. Only three of 23 commercial lots supported a full dose-responsive suppression.

Morris *et al.* (1994) compared the influence of calf serum and mouse serum on the results of in-vitro splenocyte antibody response experiments with cells derived from B6C3F1 or DBA/2 mice. With calf serum, a similar degree of suppression of antibody responses by 2,3,7,8-TCDD in splenocytes from both strains was found. In contrast, responses in the presence of mouse serum showed an Ah receptor-dependence that was characterized by a dose-related suppression of antibody responses by B6C3F1 splenocytes only.

Morris and Holsapple (1991) observed an increase in proliferation of dense resting B-cells in the presence of 30 and 60 nM 2,3,7,8-TCDD in the medium.

When 2,3,7,8-TCDD was added at concentrations between 0.3 and 30 nM to activated low-density B-cells isolated from whole spleen cell suspensions from B6C3F1 mice, suppression of cell proliferation and antibody response was observed. In contrast, neither the proliferation nor the antibody response of high-density B-cells (small resting cells) stimulated with LPS was affected by 2,3,7,8-TCDD (Morris *et al.*, 1993).

Wood *et al.* (1992) studied the effects of 2,3,7,8-TCDD on cultured murine splenocytes ((C57BL/6 × C3H)F1 mice) and compared the effects with those seen with human tonsillar lymphocytes. 2,3,7,8-TCDD at concentrations between 0.3 and 30 nM caused a significant reduction in the proliferation of both human and murine cells;

however, the substance had no effect on pokeweed mitogen-induced proliferation or antibody production.

In low-density human B-cells (isolated from human tonsils), 2,3,7,8-TCDD suppressed background proliferation and IgM secretion at concentrations between 0.3 and 30 nM. 2,3,7,8-TCDD-induced suppression was less pronounced when cells were stimulated with LPS or T-cell replacing factor. 2,3,7,8-TCDD did not alter background or stimulated proliferation of high-density human B-cells (Wood *et al.*, 1993).

Wood and Holsapple (1993) examined the effects of 2,3,7,8-TCDD upon human tonsillar lymphocytes stimulated with toxic shock syndrome toxin-1. 2,3,7,8-TCDD at concentrations < 30 nM had no effect upon T-cell or B-cell proliferation, but B-cell differentiation, as manifested by IgM secretion, was significantly suppressed at all concentrations tested (0.3–30 nM). The sensitivity to 2,3,7,8-TCDD varied considerably, with IC_{50} values ranging from < 0.3 nM to 25 nM with cells from four different donors.

Karras and Holsapple (1994a,b) observed inhibitory effects of 2,3,7,8-TCDD on proliferative responses of murine low-density B-cells to activation by anti-IgM.

In another study, Karras *et al.* (1996) reported that 2,3,7,8-TCDD suppressed murine B-cell IgM secretion induced by either soluble or insolubilized anti-IgM plus lymphokines, but did not affect IgM secretion stimulated by activated T_H-cells and lymphokines. Their data indicate that 2,3,7,8-TCDD elevates resting intracellular calcium levels in murine B-cells and may selectively inhibit calcium-dependent signalling pathways linked to surface immunoglobulin.

Karras *et al.* (1995) investigated whether the immunosuppression mediated by direct exposure of murine B-cells to 2,3,7,8-TCDD *in vitro* is due to an IL-4-like biological activity. However, 2,3,7,8-TCDD failed to demonstrate any of the activities of IL-4 observed in parallel cultures.

Masten and Shiverick (1995) found that 25 nM 2,3,7,8-TCDD decreased steady-state levels of CD19 mRNA by 67% in a human B-lymphocyte cell line (IM-9). They identified a DNA-binding complex in nuclear extracts that appeared to be the Ah receptor. The Ah receptor complex recognized a DNA-binding site for B-cell lineage-specific activator protein in the promoter region of the human CD19 gene that was similar to the Ah receptor DNA-binding site.

Effects on macrophages, neutrophils and natural killer (NK) cells

Mantovani *et al.* (1980) found no alteration in macrophage-mediated or NK cell-mediated cytotoxicity in C57BL/6J mice after treatment with single doses of up to 30 µg/kg bw 2,3,7,8-TCDD.

Kerkvliet and Oughton (1993) showed that, in C57BL/6 mice, the inflammatory response following intraperitoneal injection of SRBC was aggravated when mice were treated with 5 µg/kg bw 2,3,7,8-TCDD compared with vehicle-treated controls. The increased number of peritoneal cells reflected significant increases in both neutrophils and macrophages. 2,3,7,8-TCDD treatment did not significantly alter expression of the macrophage activation markers F4/80 or I-A on Mac-1[+] cells. The antigen-presenting function of the peritoneal exudate cells was unaltered by 2,3,7,8-TCDD.

Ackermann *et al.* (1989) observed a reduced cytolytic and cytostatic activity of polymorphonuclear neutrophils (PMN) from B6C3F1 mice (but not those from DBA/2 mice) after a single oral exposure to 5 or 10 μg/kg bw 2,3,7,8-TCDD. Supernatants recovered from PMN cell cultures of B6C3F1 mice (but not those of DBA/2 mice) showed reduced killing capacity for actinomycin D-treated L929 tumour cells.

Funseth and Ilbäck (1992) treated male A/J mice with a loading dose of 5 μg/kg bw 2,3,7,8-TCDD and three weekly maintenance doses of 1.42 μg/kg, given intraperitoneally. NK cell activity increased significantly in blood and spleen (3.4-fold and 2.2-fold, respectively). The effects were still present on day 120 after the treatment.

Effects on popliteal lymph nodes after local stimulation

In C57BL/6 mice, a single intraperitoneal injection of 50 μg/kg bw 2,3,7,8-TCDD suppressed the normal immune response in popliteal and inguinal lymph nodes to ovalbumin injected into the hind foot pads four days after 2,3,7,8-TCDD treatment. Increase of the lymph node cell number was inhibited and a reduced frequency of antigen-specific B-cells was observed. The antigen-specific T-cell proliferation and IL-2 production in response to ovalbumin were significantly suppressed by 2,3,7,8-TCDD (Lundberg *et al.*, 1991, 1992).

An anti-CD3 monoclonal antibody was injected into both rear footpads of female C57BL/6 mice and the draining popliteal and inguinal lymph nodes were removed 24 h later. 2,3,7,8-TCDD enhanced anti-CD3-induced [^{3}H]thymidine incorporation and increased the percentage of both CD4$^+$ and CD8$^+$ cells cycling in S and G$_2$M phases. The authors concluded that 2,3,7,8-TCDD appeared to be targeting T-cells undergoing activation rather than resting cells (Neumann *et al.*, 1993).

Schmidt *et al.* (1992) treated NMRI mice with single subcutaneous injections of up to 3 μg/kg bw 2,3,7,8-TCDD. One week later they injected streptozotocin or other stimulants into one hind foot pad of the animals. Lymph node enlargement (weight or cell number) in 2,3,7,8-TCDD-treated mice was not significantly different from that of controls.

Korte *et al.* (1991a) and Stroh *et al.* (1992) used the popliteal lymph node assay to investigate effects of 2,3,7,8-TCDD on immune reactions in Wistar rats. Animals were treated with single subcutaneous injections of 2,3,7,8-TCDD at doses of up to 600 ng/kg or 3 μg/kg bw, respectively. Seven days later, either erythrocytes or streptozotocin were injected into one hind foot pad and the weight and cell number of the lymph node were determined after a further seven days. 2,3,7,8-TCDD had no significant effect on the results of this test under the given conditions.

Fan *et al.* (1995) injected 2,3,7,8-TCDD directly into one foot pad of Sprague-Dawley rats (approximately 10 μg/kg bw) and observed a slightly increased weight index (1.59 ± 0.2 versus 1.07 ± 0.2 in controls; mean ± SEM; $n = 4$ and 6).

Theobald *et al.* (1983) first reported that the paw oedema formation after subplantar injection of carrageenan was enhanced in Sprague-Dawley rats treated with 2,3,7,8-TCDD. The ED$_{50}$ of 2,3,7,8-TCDD for this effect was 6 μg/kg bw.

Katz *et al.* (1984) injected various irritants into the subplantar surface of one hind paw of Sprague-Dawley rats or C57BL/6 mice pretreated with 10 µg/kg bw 2,3,7,8-TCDD. 2,3,7,8-TCDD increased the oedemagenic potency of carrageenan, dextran, bradykinin and histamine, but not that of prostaglandin E2 or serotonin.

Effects on complement

Treatment of B6C3F1 mice with daily doses of 0.01–2.0 µg/kg bw 2,3,7,8-TCDD for two weeks suppressed serum total haemolytic complement activity (CH50). Serum levels of complement component C3 were decreased at daily doses of 0.5 µg/kg or more. Immediately after treatment with single doses of 10–40 µg/kg bw 2,3,7,8-TCDD, a rapid, but transient, dose-dependent increase in liver intracellular C3 levels was observed. No inhibitory effect of 2,3,7,8-TCDD on C3 production was detected when cells of a hepatoma cell line (Hepa 1c1c7) were exposed to 2,3,7,8-TCDD (White *et al.*, 1986; Lin & White, 1993a,b,c).

Host resistance assays

Host resistance assays are often used for assessing effects of xenobiotics on the mammalian immune system, because more than one aspect of the specific and non-specific defence mechanisms are included. Several authors have described the potential of PCDDs to suppress resistance to bacterial, viral, parasitic and neoplastic challenges in mice.

Acute exposure of adult mice to 2,3,7,8-TCDD results in hypersensitivity to endo-toxin (Vos *et al.*, 1978; Rosenthal *et al.*, 1989). Clark *et al.* (1991b) investigated the effects of 2,3,7,8-TCDD on the endotoxin-induced release of TNFα. They observed a significant increase in TNFα in the serum of endotoxin-exposed mice (Ah^b/Ah^b) after exposure to a single oral dose of 10 µg/kg bw 2,3,7,8-TCDD.

Studies of effects of 2,3,7,8-TCDD on host resistance in mice are summarized in **Table 62**. To date, the finding of Burleson *et al.* (1996), that a single dose of 2,3,7,8-TCDD at 0.1, 0.05 or 0.01 µg/kg bw resulted in an increase in mortality from Hong Kong influenza virus when B6C3F1 mice were challenged seven days after 2,3,7,8-TCDD administration, represents the most sensitive adverse effect yet reported for 2,3,7,8-TCDD.

Only a few host resistance studies have been performed with PCDDs in rats.

Virus-augmented NK activity assessed 48 h after infection in the lung was signi-ficantly suppressed in Fischer 344 rats treated with 3, 10 or 30 µg/kg bw 2,3,7,8-TCDD. Significantly higher virus titres were observed on days 2, 3 and 4 after infection in the lungs of rats treated with 10 µg/kg bw (Yang *et al.*, 1994).

Using the parasite *Trichinella spiralis* in five-week-old Wistar rats that were exposed perinatally to 2,3,7,8-TCDD (one subcutaneous injection of 0.3 or 3 µg/kg bw on day 19 of gestation), no differences were found in the antibody titres or the number of *T. spiralis* larvae in muscle (Korte *et al.*, 1991b).

In Fischer 344 rats treated with single doses of 30 µg/kg bw 2,3,7,8-TCDD, no evidence for an immunosuppressive effect was seen in the *T. spiralis* host resistance assay, but proliferative responses of lymphocytes cultured with parasite antigen were

Table 62. Effects of 2,3,7,8-TCDD on host resistance in mice

Strain	Effect	Dose	No./time of exposures	Reference
C57BL/6	No effect on resistance to *Herpes suis*	20 µg/kg p.o.	once a week/4 weeks	Thigpen *et al.* (1975)
C57BL/6	Reduced resistance to *Salmonella bern*	1 µg/kg p.o.	once a week/4 weeks	Thigpen *et al.* (1975)
C57BL/6	Reduced resistance to Herpes simplex type II	0.04 µg/kg i.p.	once a week/4 weeks	Clark *et al.* (1983)
Swiss	Reduced resistance to endotoxin	1.5 µg/kg p.o.	once a week/4 weeks	Vos *et al.* (1978)
Swiss	Reduced resistance to endotoxin	1 µg/kg diet	pre/postnatal	Thomas & Hinsdill (1979)
Swiss	No effect on resistance to *Listeria monocytogenes*	10 µg/kg diet	pre/postnatal	Thomas & Hinsdill (1979)
Swiss	Reduced resistance to *Salmonella* and *Listeria*	50 µg/kg diet	5 weeks	Hinsdill *et al.* (1980)
B6C3F1	Reduced resistance to *Listeria monocytogenes*	5 µg/kg p.o.	4 times (pre/postnatal)[a]	Luster *et al.* (1980)
B6C3F1	Reduced resistance to *Plasmodium yoelli*	5 µg/kg p.o.	once	Tucker *et al.* (1986)
B6C3F1	Reduced resistance to *Streptococcus pneumoniae*	1 µg/kg p.o.	once a day/2 weeks	White *et al.* (1986)
B6C3F1	No effect on resistance to *Listeria monocytogenes*	10 µg/kg i.p.	once	House *et al.* (1990)
B6C3F1	Reduced resistance to influenza virus	0.1 µg/kg i.p.	once	House *et al.* (1990)
B6C3F1	Reduced resistance to *Trichinella spiralis*	10 µg/kg i.p.	once	Luebke *et al.* (1994)
B6C3F1	Reduced resistance to influenza virus	0.01 µg/kg p.o.	once	Burleson *et al.* (1996)

p.o., oral; i.p., intraperitoneal

[a] Day 14 of gestation and days 1, 7 and 14 after birth

enhanced (Luebke *et al.*, 1995). This is in contrast to results obtained with the *T. spiralis* test in mice from the same laboratory (**Table 62**). It was shown in this study that infection delayed elimination from the host: infected mice had higher 2,3,7,8-TCDD levels than non-infected mice (Luebke *et al.*, 1994).

A/J mice infected with Coxsackievirus B3 (CB3) had increased tissue concentrations of 2,3,7,8-TCDD in the brain, pancreas, heart, spleen and liver compared with uninfected controls (Funseth & Ilbäck, 1994).

Direct exposure of isolated human erythrocytes to 10 nM 2,3,7,8-TCDD caused a two-fold increase in the infectivity of *Plasmodium falciparum* after 48 h, when the parasites were in a synchronized state of growth. Additional treatment with sodium orthovanadate, an inhibitor of plasma membrane Ca-ATPase and phosphotyrosine phosphatase, completely blocked the 2,3,7,8-TCDD-induced increase in parasitaemia (Kim *et al.*, 1994).

Pre- and perinatal exposure

Vos and Moore (1974) treated female Fischer 344 rats and C57BL/6 mice with doses of up to 5 µg/kg bw 2,3,7,8-TCDD pre- and postnatally (rats: gestation days 11 and 18, postnatally on days 4, 11 and 18; mice: gestation days 14 and 17, postnatally on days 1, 8 and 15). The high-dose regimen was lethal to 31/34 rat offspring. The authors observed a depletion of lymphocytes in the thymic cortex of the offspring which, histologically evaluated, was not due to lymphocyte destruction. Cellular immunity was impaired. Allograft rejection times were prolonged in rats and mice. Graft-versus-host activity of spleen cells was reduced, as well as the response of rat thymus and spleen cells to phytohaemagglutinin. In four-month-old mice treated with six weekly doses of 25 µg/kg bw 2,3,7,8-TCDD, these effects were not observed.

Fine *et al.* (1988, 1990a,b) studied the effects of 2,3,7,8-TCDD on lymphocyte stem cell function in BALB/c mice following direct or perinatal exposure (maternal treatment with 10 or 15 µg/kg bw 2,3,7,8-TCDD on day 14 of gestation). In the fetus and the neonate, significant reductions were found in both the biosynthesis and mRNA levels of the lymphocyte stem cell-specific DNA polymerase TdT. Thymic biosynthesis was relatively unaffected, suggesting that alterations of early events of T-cell lymphopoiesis (prothymocytes) can contribute to 2,3,7,8-TCDD-induced thymic atrophy. A slight reduction in the expression of the thymocyte surface marker Lyt-2$^+$L3T4$^+$ was demonstrated by flow cytometry.

Holladay *et al.* (1991) and Blaylock *et al.* (1992) treated pregnant C57BL/6 mice on nine consecutive days (gestation days 6–14) with daily doses of 1.5 or 3.0 µg/kg bw 2,3,7,8-TCDD by gastric instillation (total doses of 13.5 and 27 µg/kg bw 2,3,7,8-TCDD). 2,3,7,8-TCDD treatment (both groups) resulted in significant decreases in fetal thymic weight and the percentage of CD4$^+$CD8$^+$ fetal thymocytes (DP), as well as significantly increased CD4$^-$CD8$^-$ (DN) and CD4$^-$CD8$^+$ thymocytes on gestation day 18 as analysed by flow cytometry. 2,3,7,8-TCDD induced a significant shift in T-cell receptor (TCR) expression of thymocytes with a decrease in alpha-beta-TCR and a concomitant increase in gamma-delta-TCR expression. On postnatal day 6, no significant differences were detectable by flow cytometry; however, a significantly depressed CTL activity was demonstrable until eight weeks postnatally (offspring had been cross-fostered to avoid exposure via milk). There were no significant differences at postnatal weeks 7–8 between controls and 2,3,7,8-TCDD-exposed mice in lymphocyte proliferation to mitogens or antibody PFC response.

Faith and Moore (1977) showed that when Fischer 344 rats were exposed to 2,3,7,8-TCDD prenatally (day 18 of gestation) and postnatally (days 0, 7, 14 of lactation), body weight and thymus/body weight ratios were suppressed up to 145 days. The effects were less pronounced when the rats were exposed only postnatally (days 0, 7, 14 of lactation).

Badesha *et al.* (1995) fed a 2,3,7,8-TCDD-containing diet to lactating Leeds rats starting on postnatal day 1. Total doses of 0.2, 1.0 or 5.0 µg/kg were administered over a period of 18 days. At the age of 130 days, body weights remained significantly reduced in all three groups of female offspring and the two highest-dose groups of males. Immunocompetence of the offspring was affected: in-vitro T-cell-dependent and T-cell-independent responses and mitogen-induced in-vitro production of IL-1 and IL-2 were suppressed at postnatal day 130.

(ii)   *Effects of other PCDDs*

Only seven of 75 possible PCDD congeners and five out of 135 PCDF congeners have been studied for their effects on the mammalian immune system (Holsapple, 1995).

Mason *et al.* (1986) demonstrated that in immature male Wistar rats 2,3,7,8-TCDD was the most active congener out of a series of six compounds with respect to their potency to induce thymic atrophy after intraperitoneal injection. The ED_{50} values (dose that caused a 50% decrease in thymus/body weight ratio compared with control rats) were: 0.09 µmol/kg for 2,3,7,8-TCDD, 0.17 µmol/kg for 1,2,3,7,8-PeCDD, 1.07 µmol/kg for 1,2,3,4,7,8-HxCDD, 11.2 µmol/kg for 1,2,4,7,8-PeCDD, 98.1 µmol/kg for 2,3,7-triCDD and 100 µmol/kg for 1,3,7,8-TCDD.

The effects of 1,2,3,4,6,7,8-HpCDD on antibody responses to T-helper cell-dependent (SRBC) and T-helper cell-independent antigens (TNP-LPS and DNP-Ficoll) were studied in C57BL/6 mice. The results indicated that sensitivity to HpCDD-induced suppression directly correlated with the sensitivity of the response to T-cell regulation. T-cell deficient nu/nu mice were significantly more resistant to the immunosuppressive effects of 1,2,3,4,6,7,8-HpCDD as compared with their nu/+ littermates. Following treatment with 100 µg/kg bw 1,2,3,4,6,7,8-HpCDD, the response of nu/nu mice was unaffected, whereas the response of nu/+ mice was significantly suppressed, indicating that the primary immunological defect induced by the substance is at the level of regulatory T-cells. However, after treatment with a dose of 500 µg/kg bw 1,2,3,4,6,7,8-HpCDD, the response of nu/nu mice was also suppressed (Kerkvliet & Brauner, 1987).

Holsapple *et al.* (1986b) compared the effects of 2,3,7,8-TCCD, 2,7-DCDD and OCDD on the antibody response to SRBC and to DNP-Ficoll in B6C3F1 mice. 2,3,7,8-TCDD and 2,7-DCDD suppressed antibody responses to both antigens (compared with 2,3,7,8-TCDD, 10-fold higher doses of 2,7-DCDD induced less pronounced effects). OCDD was without effect.

Treatment of B6C3F1 mice with daily doses of 0.01 µg/kg bw 2,3,7,8-TCDD for two weeks or more suppressed serum total haemolytic complement activity (CH50). 1,2,3,6,7,8-HxCDD was less active than 2,3,7,8-TCDD. Suppression of complement activity was seen after multiple doses of 0.1 to 10 µg/kg bw with decreased C3 levels at 10 µg/kg. Recovery studies showed that complement activity in animals treated with 2,3,7,8-TCDD (1 µg/kg) or 1,2,3,6,7,8-HxCDD (10 µg/kg) was suppressed until 50 days after treatment. Interestingly, CH50 levels were elevated after low doses (0.1 and 1.0 µg/kg) of 1,2,3,6,7,8-HxCDD (White *et al.*, 1986).

4.3 Interactions with Ah receptors and their early molecular consequences and other biochemical responses

The toxic effects elicited by 2,3,7,8-TCDD and other PCDDs are accompanied by modulation of numerous biochemical responses in target tissues and organs. Although there is extensive support for the role of the intracellular dioxin or aryl hydrocarbon (Ah) receptor in mediating PCDD-induced biochemical and toxic effects, the direct link between a series of biochemical alterations and any specific toxicity is unclear. This section highlights the effects of 2,3,7,8-TCDD and other PCDDs on various biochemical parameters, interactions of these compounds with the Ah receptor and the molecular consequences of these reactions.

As outlined below, intracellular signal transduction by PCDDs and PCDFs, most notably 2,3,7,8-TCDD and 2,3,7,8-TCDF, is mediated by the Ah receptor. This protein is a ubiquitous regulatory factor that binds 2,3,7,8-TCDD and its planar aromatic congeners in a saturable manner and with high affinity (in the case of 2,3,7,8-TCDD and 2,3,7,8-TCDF with dissociation constants (K_d, a measure of binding affinity) in the subnanomolar range; reviewed by Poland & Knutson, 1982; Safe, 1986; Bradfield *et al.*, 1988; Gillner *et al.*, 1993). At the molecular level, high-affinity Ah receptor ligands such as 2,3,7,8-TCDD and 2,3,7,8-TCDF are very potent inducers of transcription of a distinct network of target genes encoding xenobiotic-metabolizing enzymes such as cytochrome P4501A1 (CYP1A1), P4501A2 (CYP1A2) and glutathione *S*-transferase Ya (for recent reviews, see Fujii-Kuriyama *et al.*, 1992; Swanson & Bradfield, 1993; Whitlock, 1994; Hankinson, 1994; Poellinger, 1995). Although there is a paucity of data regarding primary Ah receptor target genes that do not encode drug-metabolizing enzymes, 2,3,7,8-TCDD has been reported to modulate expression of the growth modulatory genes for IL-1β and plasminogen activator inhibitor-2 (PAI-2) (Sutter *et al.*, 1991). (See the section below on modulation of growth factors, growth factor receptors, lymphokines and related factors.)

Binding affinities of individual PCDDs to the Ah receptor are strongest for those congeners having a 2,3,7,8-chlorine substitution pattern, with 2,3,7,8-TCDD being the most potent. Within this group of congeners, increasing chlorination on the 1, 4, 6 and 9 positions leads to a significant decrease in the binding affinity of up to several orders of magnitude (Poland & Knutson, 1982; Safe, 1990).

The binding affinity (K_d) of PCDDs for the rat hepatic Ah receptor ranges between 10^{-10} and 10^{-5} M or higher. Across and within species, the Ah-receptor binding affinities for, e.g., 2,3,7,8-TCDD can vary by one or two orders of magnitude. For example, in both man and mouse, two forms of Ah receptor have been identified which show a 5–10-fold difference in binding affinity for 2,3,7,8-TCDD. In the human forms, one has a K_d for 2,3,7,8-TCDD of 0.4 nM, while the other form has a K_d of about 2 nM. In addition, variability in Ah-receptor binding is influenced by the cell type, tissue, sex, age, experimental conditions and assay used (Okey *et al.*, 1989; Bradfield *et al.*, 1988; Safe, 1990; Poland & Knutson, 1982).

4.3.1   *The Ah receptor*

The Ah receptor is a member of the basic helix–loop–helix (bHLH) family of gene regulatory proteins (Burbach *et al.*, 1992; Ema *et al.*, 1992). The bHLH motif represents a well studied dimerization and DNA-binding domain common to a large group of regulatory factors that are generally involved in cell growth and differentiation and include the proto-oncogene c-*myc* and the muscle developmental factor MyoD (reviewed by Jan & Jan, 1993; Weintraub, 1993; Dorschkind, 1994). Thus, the Ah receptor is distinct from the superfamily of ligand-activated nuclear receptors that encompasses steroid hormone, thyroid hormone, vitamin D and retinoic acid receptors and contains the structurally well characterized 'zinc finger' DNA binding motif (see Gronemeyer & Laudet, 1995, for a comprehensive review).

The receptor functions as a ligand-dependent transcription factor that, upon exposure to ligand, recognizes DNA of target genes as a heterodimeric complex with the structurally related factor Arnt (Reyes *et al.*, 1992; Dolwick *et al.*, 1993; Matsushita *et al.*, 1993; Whitelaw *et al.*, 1993a). Both the Ah receptor and Arnt (Hoffman *et al.*, 1991) belong to a distinct subgroup, bHLH/PAS (Per–Arnt–Sim homology region) (Littlewood & Evan, 1995), of the bHLH family transcription factors, and are characterized by an N-terminal arrangement of the bHLH DNA-binding motif contiguous with a second structural motif, PAS. The PAS domain of about 250 amino acids contains two imperfect repeats and is also conserved in the product of the *Drosophila* gene *period* (Per) (Takahashi, 1992 and references therein), that is involved in circadian rhythm regulation, the *Drosophila* neurodevelopmental factor *single-minded* (Sim) (Nambu *et al.*, 1991), the *Drosophila* factor *trachealess*, important for insect tubulogenesis (Isaac & Andrew, 1996; Wilk *et al.*, 1996), as well as the hypoxia-inducible factor (HIF-1α) and E-PAS of mammals (Wang *et al.*, 1995; Gradin *et al.*, 1996; Tian *et al.*, 1997) and a human *single-minded* homologue identified as a putative Down syndrome-critical factor (Dahmane *et al.*, 1995). In addition, a mammalian factor, Arnt 2, closely related to Arnt (Drutel *et al.*, 1996; Hirose *et al.*, 1996) has recently been cloned. This factor supports Ah receptor functions in hepatoma cells deficient in Arnt (Hirose *et al.*, 1996).

Ligand-dependent activation of Ah receptor function is a multi-step process. In the absence of ligand, the latent, non-DNA-binding form of the receptor is recovered in cytosolic cellular extracts as a ~300 kDa heteromeric complex associated with the molecular chaperone hsp90 (heat shock protein 90) (Denis *et al.*, 1988; Perdew, 1988; Wilhelmsson *et al.*, 1990; Chen & Perdew, 1994). 2,3,7,8-TCDD and other known receptor ligands induce nuclear import of the Ah receptor (Jain *et al.*, 1994; Pollenz *et al.*, 1994, and references therein) and release of the hsp90 chaperone (Wilhelmsson *et al.*, 1990) and regulate dimerization with Arnt (Whitelaw *et al.*, 1993a), enabling both proteins to bind to DNA (Reyes *et al.*, 1992; Dolwick *et al.*, 1993; Matsushita *et al.*, 1993; Whitelaw *et al.*, 1993a). The ligand-activated Ah receptor–Arnt complex induces transcription of target promoters via potent transactivation domains that are contained within the C-terminus of both the Ah receptor and Arnt (Jain *et al.*, 1994; Li *et al.*, 1994; Whitelaw *et al.*, 1994). The Ah receptor may also modulate biochemical and cellular responses via non-DNA dependent mechanisms (Matsumura, 1994; Birnbaum, 1995a; Weiss *et al.*, 1996).

In the absence of ligand, it appears that hsp90 blocks receptor–Arnt dimerization (Whitelaw *et al.*, 1993a), resulting in repression of receptor function. Ligand-induced release of hsp90 is facilitated *in vitro* by concomitant dimerization of the receptor with Arnt (McGuire *et al.*, 1994), indicating that these two processes are functionally inter-digitated. Ligand (Dolwick *et al.*, 1993; Whitelaw *et al.*, 1993b) and hsp90 (Whitelaw *et al.*, 1993b) binding activities of the receptor are co-localized within the PAS domain. In contrast, the PAS domain of Arnt does not mediate association with hsp90 (Probst *et al.*, 1993; McGuire *et al.*, 1994). In-vitro ligand-binding experiments indicate that hsp90 chaperones a high-affinity ligand-binding conformation of the receptor (Pongratz *et al.*, 1992). Consistent with this model, ligand responsiveness of the Ah receptor is severely impaired upon expression in a yeast strain in which hsp90 expression levels are down-regulated to about 5% of wild-type levels (Carver *et al.*, 1994; Whitelaw *et al.*, 1995). Taken together, these data indicate that hsp90 may be critical for folding of a functional, ligand-responsive form of the Ah receptor.

All known ligands of the Ah receptor are of xenobiotic origin, and a physiological receptor ligand has not yet been identified (reviewed by Poland & Knutson, 1982; Poellinger *et al.*, 1992). Given the critical roles of the majority of bHLH factors in general (Jan & Jan, 1993; Weintraub, 1993; Dorschkind, 1994), and bHLH-PAS factors in particular (Nambu *et al.*, 1991; Isaac & Andrew, 1996; Wilk *et al.*, 1996; Tian *et al.*, 1997) for embryonic development, it is plausible that a physiological function (and possibly a ligand-dependent regulatory strategy) of the Ah receptor is to be found in developmental processes. Ah⁻/Ah⁻ mice were found to be viable and fertile, but showed hepatic defects that indicate a role for the Ah receptor in normal liver growth (Fernandez-Salguero *et al.*, 1995; Schmidt *et al.*, 1996). Thus, the exact role of the Ah receptor in mammalian development remains unclear.

4.3.2   *Induction of drug-metabolizing enzymes*

CYP1A1. The induction of *CYP1A1* gene expression and associated enzyme activities by 2,3,7,8-TCDD and other PCDDs is a common result of exposure to these chemicals and is readily demonstrated in laboratory animals and cells in culture. There is relatively low constitutive expression of CYP1A1 in most tissues and cells; however, after treatment with 2,3,7,8-TCDD, the Ah receptor complex rapidly accumulates in the nucleus, and this is accompanied by the sequential induction of CYP1A1 mRNA levels followed by induction of CYP1A1-dependent enzyme activity and immunoreactive protein (Tukey *et al.*, 1982; Zacharewski *et al.*, 1989; Harris *et al.*, 1990; Pendurthi *et al.*, 1993). The mechanism of this response has been extensively investigated (González & Nebert, 1985; Jones *et al.*, 1985, 1986a,b; Sogawa *et al.*, 1986; Fujisawa-Sehara *et al.*, 1986, 1988; Neuhold *et al.*, 1989) and involves interaction of the Ah receptor complex with functional xenobiotic-responsive enhancers (XREs; also referred to as dioxin-responsive enhancers (DREs)) in the 5′-promoter region of *CYP1A1* genes (Denison *et al.*, 1988; Fujisawa-Sehara *et al.*, 1988; Hapgood *et al.*, 1991). Thus, the Ah receptor functions as a ligand-activated DNA-binding protein directly communicating with its target genes.

Species-, age-, sex- and organ-dependent differences in induction of *CYP1A1* gene expression and dependent enzyme activities have been reported in laboratory animals, mammalian cells in culture, and in humans, and these data have been extensively reviewed (Poland & Knutson, 1982; Whitlock, 1986, 1987; Okey, 1990; Safe, 1990; Whitlock, 1990; Kohn *et al.*, 1993; Whitlock, 1993; Okey *et al.*, 1994; Denison & Whitlock, 1995; Safe, 1995).

The induction of *CYP1A1* gene expression is also influenced by a number of other factors. For example, in wild-type and mutant Hepa-1 cells, treatment with 2,3,7,8-TCDD results in binding of the nuclear Ah receptor complex to enhancer sequences and binding of other proteins to promoter DNA (Watson & Hankinson, 1992; Wu & Whitlock, 1993). The enhancer/promoter sequence in uninduced cells forms a nucleo-somal structure; after addition of 2,3,7,8-TCDD, alterations of chromatin structure and nucleosome disruption are observed (Durrin & Whitlock, 1987; Morgan & Whitlock, 1992; Wu & Whitlock, 1992). Induction of *CYP1A1* gene expression and formation of the nuclear Ah receptor complex have also been observed in human keratinocytes and mouse Hepa 1c1c7 cells suspended in solid medium containing methyl cellulose or Percoll solution (Sadek & Allen-Hoffmann, 1994a,b).

Protein kinase C-dependent phosphorylation is important for 2,3,7,8-TCDD activation of the Ah receptor and Arnt proteins (Carrier *et al.*, 1992; Reiners *et al.*, 1992, 1993; Berghard *et al.*, 1993). In human keratinocytes and mouse Hepa-1 cells, phorbol esters and protein kinase C inhibitors blocked 2,3,7,8-TCDD-dependent formation of the transformed Ah receptor complex (Berghard *et al.*, 1993), and similar results were observed in C57BL/6 mice co-treated with 2,3,7,8-TCDD plus phorbol esters (Okino *et al.*, 1992). In contrast, in-vitro transformation of the Ah receptor of guinea-pig, mouse and rat hepatic cytosol is not affected by inhibitors of protein kinase C (Schaefer *et al.*, 1993) and staurosporine, a protein kinase C inhibitor, did not affect nuclear translocation of the Ah receptor in mouse Hepa-1 cells in culture (Singh & Perdew, 1993). Moreover, in MCF-7 human breast cancer cells in which protein kinase C activity was depleted as a result of prolonged treatment with phorbol esters, 2,3,7,8-TCDD caused superinducibility of *CYP1A1* gene expression, and this was accompanied by a two- to three-fold increase in levels of the nuclear Ah receptor complex (Moore *et al.*, 1993). These observations indicate that the role of protein phosphorylation of the Ah receptor complex may vary among different cell lines or target tissues.

Several other factors which inhibit the 2,3,7,8-TCDD-dependent induction of *CYP1A1* and *CYP1A2* gene expression include IL-1β, insulin, EGF, rat hepatocytes (Barker *et al.*, 1992) and TGFβ in squamous carcinoma cells (Hébert *et al.*, 1990b) and human A549 lung cancer cells (Vogel *et al.*, 1994).

CYP1A2. Expression of the *CYP1A2* gene and related enzyme activities is also induced by 2,3,7,8-TCDD and related Ah receptor agonists (Koga *et al.*, 1990; DeVito *et al.*, 1994; Narasimhan *et al.*, 1994; Paroli *et al.*, 1994; De Jongh *et al.*, 1995; Diliberto *et al.*, 1995). In laboratory animals and humans, *CYP1A2* is expressed primarily in liver and is inducible, together with *CYP1A1*, by 2,3,7,8-TCDD in primary cultures of human hepatocytes (Schrenk *et al.*, 1995), whereas in most cell lines, the gene is not expressed (Fagan *et al.*, 1986; Kimura *et al.*, 1986; Silver & Krauter, 1988; Ikeya *et al.*, 1989). CYP1A2 catalyses oxidation of aromatic amines and 17β-oestradiol and may also be important in 4-hydroxylation of tamoxifen (Kupfer *et al.*, 1994). The hydroxylation of 17β-oestradiol by CYP1A2 to catechols has been suggested to play a role in 2,3,7,8-TCDD-induced carcinogenesis (Liehr, 1990; Liehr & Roy, 1990; Lucier *et al.*, 1991; Yager & Liehr, 1996). In addition, PCDDs can bind strongly to this isoenzyme and also function as competitive binding inhibitors (Voornan & Aust, 1987; Poland *et al.*, 1989). Deletion analyses of the CYP1A2 promoter from the human *CYP1A2* gene have revealed XRE core sequences at -2259 to -1970 and -2888 to -2903 (Quattrochi & Tukey, 1989; Quattrochi *et al.*, 1994). Transfected cells with deletion plasmids containing the core (-2888 to -2903) XRE sequence were Ah-receptor responsive in human Hep G2 but not MCF-7 cells, suggesting that *CYP1A2* gene expression is regulated by multiple factors in addition to the Ah receptor complex (Quattrochi *et al.*, 1994).

CYP1B1. 2,3,7,8-TCDD also induces another cytochrome P450, CYP1B1, that occurs in humans and rodents (Sutter *et al.*, 1991; Savas *et al.*, 1994; Shen *et al.*, 1994a,b; Sutter *et al.*, 1994; Bhattacharyya *et al.*, 1995; Walker *et al.*, 1995). CYP1B1 is expressed in a variety of human tissues (Sutter *et al.*, 1994; Hayes *et al.*, 1996) and inducible by 2,3,7,8-TCDD in numerous human cell types (Sutter *et al.*, 1991; Spink *et al.*, 1994; Sutter *et al.*, 1994) and rodent tissues including liver, lung and kidney (Walker *et al.*, 1995). CYP1B1 is active in the metabolism of numerous polycyclic aromatic hydrocarbons and aryl-amines (Pottenger & Jefcoate, 1990; Pottenger *et al.*, 1991; Otto *et al.*, 1992; Shimada *et al.*, 1996) and can catalyse the 4-hydroxylation of 17β-oestradiol in humans cells (Hayes *et al.*, 1996). Further studies are needed to elucidate the role of CYP1B1 in 2,3,7,8-TCDD-induced toxicity and the mechanisms associated with this induced response.

Aldehyde-3-dehydrogenase. 2,3,7,8-TCDD induces aldehyde-3-dehydrogenase activity (Takimoto *et al.*, 1992; Unkila *et al.*, 1993b; Germolec *et al.*, 1996), and analysis of the promoter region has identified XRE sequences (Hempel *et al.*, 1989; Takimoto *et al.*, 1991; Asman *et al.*, 1993). Deletion analysis of the 5'-flanking region revealed DNA sequences which both enhance and decrease activity of chimeric genes, and an XRE core binding sequence (GCGTG) was also identified (Takimoto *et al.*, 1994).

Glutathione S-transferase Ya. 2,3,7,8-TCDD and related compounds induce GST activities and gene expression in laboratory animals and mammalian cells (Paulson *et al.*,

1990; Rushmore et al., 1990; Aoki et al., 1992; Pimental et al., 1993; Rushmore & Pickett, 1993). Analysis of the 5'-promoter region of the rat GST Ya gene has revealed several genomic regulatory sequences including an XRE sequence containing the core 5'-GCGTG-3' sequence which binds the Ah receptor complex. Deletion and mutational analysis studies showed the requirement of XRE for Ah-responsiveness. Pimental et al. (1993) have also demonstrated binding of the constitutive protein, C/EBPα, to the XRE and shown that Ah receptor-mediated induction of constructs containing the XRE may involve cooperative protein–protein interactions between C/EBPα and the Ah receptor complex. GSTP-1 is also induced by PCDDs (Aoki et al., 1992, 1993), and this response can be inhibited by glucocorticoids and protein kinase C inhibitors.

Glucuronosyl transferase. UDP-GT activity is also induced by 2,3,7,8-TCDD and other Ah receptor agonists (Owens, 1977), and recent studies with the rat *UGT1A1* gene have identified a functional XRE sequence (-134 to -139) in the 5'-promoter region of this gene (Emi et al., 1995, 1996). 2,3,7,8-TCDD also induced UGT1A1 levels in a human cell line (Abid et al., 1995), although induction in humans *in vivo* has not been proven.

NAD(P)H:quinone oxidoreductase. NAD(P)H:quinone oxidoreductase (or DT dia-phorase) activity is also induced by Ah receptor agonists, and the human gene structure, activity and tissue-specific expression have been reported (Shaw et al., 1991; Jaiswal, 1994). The sequence of the 5'-flanking region contains binding sites for several nuclear proteins, and these include an XRE 5'-GCGTG-3' sequence between -708 and -704; plasmids containing the XRE sequences are inducible by 2,3,7,8-TCDD and β-naphtho-flavone in transient assays. The gene is widely expressed in human tissues, but the role of 2,3,7,8-TCDD-induced expression of NAD(P)H:quinone oxidoreductase in the toxic responses elicited by this compound is unknown.

Prostaglandin endoperoxide H synthase-2 (PGHS-2). The *PGHS-2* gene was recently identified as a 2,3,7,8-TCDD-regulated gene in a canine kidney cell line (Kraemer et al., 1996). Its induction by 2,3,7,8-TCDD in human cells has not been investigated.

4.3.3 Modulation of growth factors, growth factor receptors, transcription factors, lymphokines and related factors

2,3,7,8-TCDD and related compounds decrease epidermal growth factor (EGF) receptor binding and/or autophosphorylation in several cells or organs, including human keratinocytes in culture (Hudson et al., 1985), mouse hepatoma cells (Kärenlampi et al., 1983), mouse, rat and guinea-pig liver (Madhukar et al., 1984, 1988; Ryan et al., 1989b; Lin et al., 1991a; Sewall et al., 1993), fish liver (Newsted & Giesy, 1993) and rat uterus (Astroff et al., 1990). In contrast, EGF receptor binding was increased in palatal medial epithelial cells from mouse embryo (Abbott et al., 1989). Support for the role of the Ah receptor in mediating down-regulation of the EGF receptor has been supported by structure–activity studies in mice (Ryan et al., 1989b) and the differential responsiveness of congenic mice differing only in the structure of the Ah receptor gene (Lin et al., 1991b). It has been suggested that decreased EGF receptor binding may play a role in the development of hepatocellular carcinomas in female rats treated with 2,3,7,8-TCDD

(Sewall *et al.*, 1993), since development of preneoplastic hepatic lesions and decreased hepatic EGF receptor binding was observed only in unovariectomized 2,3,7,8-TCDD treated animals. 2,3,7,8-TCDD also induces TGFα, IL-1β and TGFβ mRNA levels in some cells (Abbott & Birnbaum, 1990a; Choi *et al.*, 1991; Sutter *et al.*, 1991; Gaido *et al.*, 1992; Döhr *et al.*, 1994; Lee *et al.*, 1996). Expression of PAI-2 is induced in the human keratinocyte cell line SCC-12F (Sutter *et al.*, 1991) and in human hepatocytes in primary culture (Gohl *et al.*, 1996). 2,3,7,8-TCDD has been shown to alter transcription factors involved in growth and differentiation. Both *in vivo* and *in vitro*, 2,3,7,8-TCDD causes a rise in the expression of *ras* and *erbA*, both proto-oncogenes (Matsumura, 1994). In-vitro studies have shown an increase in the expression of c-*fos* and c-*jun*, as well as an increase in AP1 (Puga *et al.*, 1992).

4.3.4 *Modulation of thyroid hormones, vitamin A and retinoids*

Interactions between 2,3,7,8-TCDD and thyroid hormones (T4 and T3) and the effects of altered thyroid hormone levels on the toxicity of 2,3,7,8-TCDD have been extensively studied (see also Section 4.2.1(*d*)). Daily injections of T3 increased survival times of animals treated with 2,3,7,8-TCDD (Neal *et al.*, 1979) and thyroidectomy offered some protection from 2,3,7,8-TCDD-induced mortality and immunotoxicity in rats (Pazdernik & Rozman, 1985; Rozman *et al.*, 1985a, 1987). In mice treated with 2,3,7,8-TCDD plus T3 or T4, there was an increased incidence of cleft palate (Lamb *et al.*, 1986). Decreased serum T4 levels have been observed in some laboratory animals after treatment with 2,3,7,8-TCDD (Bastomsky, 1977; McKinney *et al.*, 1985; Pazdernik & Rozman, 1985; Rozman *et al.*, 1985b; Henry & Gasiewicz, 1987; Jones *et al.*, 1987; Sewall *et al.*, 1995) and this may be related to increased rates of thyroxine glucuronidation. However, in other studies, thyroid hormone levels were unchanged or increased after treatment with 2,3,7,8-TCDD (Potter *et al.*, 1983; McKinney *et al.*, 1985; Potter *et al.*, 1986; Henry & Gasiewicz, 1987). The decrease in serum T4 levels in rats treated with 2,3,7,8-TCDD was preceded by an initial decrease in serum prolactin levels (within 4 h) which were then significantly increased seven days after the initial exposure (Jones *et al.*, 1987). Hydroxylated PCDDs have been found to bind to the thyroid hormone-binding proteins in in-vitro experiments using human TBG (Lans *et al.*, 1993, 1994). For PCDDs, it has not been shown that the observed decreased T 4 levels in in-vivo experiments were caused by these hydroxylated metabolites. In view of the extremely low biotransformation rate of most 2,3,7,8-PCDDs, other mechanisms might be involved (Van den Berg *et al.*, 1994; van Birgelen *et al.*, 1995b).

The similarities between some 2,3,7,8-TCDD-induced toxic responses and hypovitaminosis A, and the synergistic interactions between 2,3,7,8-TCDD- and retinoic acid-induced cleft palate (Abbott & Birnbaum, 1989a,b; Birnbaum *et al.*, 1989) have stimulated several studies on the biochemical responses associated with these interactions. Several studies have reported that 2,3,7,8-TCDD markedly decreases hepatic retinol levels in various laboratory animal species, the guinea-pig being the most sensitive. Modulation of serum retinol levels and of concentrations in other organs was species-dependent (Thunberg *et al.*, 1980; Thunberg & Håkansson, 1983; Rozman *et al.*, 1987;

Brouwer *et al.*, 1989; Håkansson & Hanberg, 1989; Jurek *et al.*, 1990; Pohjanvirta *et al.*, 1990; Håkansson *et al.*, 1991a,b; Hanberg *et al.*, 1996). In 2,3,7,8-TCDD-exposed rats, a pronounced, rapid and long-lasting increase in renal vitamin A was observed. Feeding vitamin A-supplemented diet to male Sprague-Dawley rats did not result in a consistent reduction in 2,3,7,8-TCDD toxicity (Håkansson *et al.*, 1990). Hepatic stellate cells are a major storage site for vitamin A (retinyl ester form) and treatment with 2,3,7,8-TCDD markedly reduces retinol and retinyl palmitate levels in these cells; however, this is not accompanied by decreased cell number or transformation (Hanberg *et al.*, 1996). 2,3,7,8-TCDD also affects retinoic acid metabolism and tissue-specific accumulation of various metabolites (Fiorella *et al.*, 1995), and it has been suggested that 2,3,7,8-TCDD-induced toxicity may be related to altered metabolism of retinoic acid. 2,3,7,8-TCDD also decreases retinoic acid-induced gene expression in mouse embryonic cells (Weston *et al.*, 1995), and both retinoic acid and retinol inhibit 2,3,7,8-TCDD-induced terminal differentiation in human keratinocytes (Berkers *et al.*, 1995). The significance of vitamin A depletion for the chronic toxicity of 2,3,7,8-TCDD is unclear.

4.3.5   *Modulation of protein phosphorylation*

Kinase-dependent protein phosphorylation plays a central role in cell signalling, and 2,3,7,8-TCDD alters both protein phosphorylation patterns and kinase activities. For example, treatment with 2,3,7,8-TCDD stimulates protein kinase C activity in rat splenocytes, hepatocytes, thymocytes, hippocampal cells and rat and guinea-pig hepatic plasma membranes (Bombick *et al.*, 1985; DePetrillo & Kurl, 1993; Wölfle *et al.*, 1993; Zorn *et al.*, 1995; Hanneman *et al.*, 1996). 2,3,7,8-TCDD also induces tyrosine phosphorylation in many of these same cell types (Kramer *et al.*, 1987; Clark *et al.*, 1991c; Ebner *et al.*, 1993; Ma & Babish, 1993; DeVito *et al.*, 1994; Enan & Matsumura, 1994a,b, 1995a,b). Snyder *et al.* (1993) showed that, in B6C3F1 mice, 2,3,7,8-TCDD-induced phosphorylation of proteins was selective for activated B cells. Purified B cells from both DBA/2 (Ah^d/Ah^d) and C57BL/6 (Ah^b/Ah^b) mice demonstrated equivalent enhancement of phosphorylation in response to 2,3,7,8-TCDD. Administration of human γ-interferon produced a reversal of 2,3,7,8-TCDD-induced suppression of in-vitro antibody responses in splenocytes isolated from B6C3F1 mice. Ma and Babish (1993) demonstrated that 2,3,7,8-TCDD enhances phosphorylation of cyclin-dependent kinases (p34cdc2 and p33cdk2) in mouse liver.

4.3.6   *Modulation of biochemical responses associated with glucose metabolism and transport*

In several rodent species, 2,3,7,8-TCDD decreased phosphoenol pyruvate carboxykinase (PEPCK), glucose-6-phosphatase, GGT and pyruvate carboxylase activities, and the reduced enzyme activities were correlated with decreased gluconeogenesis in the treated animals (Górski *et al.*, 1990; Weber *et al.*, 1991b,c; Stahl *et al.*, 1992b, 1993; Sparrow *et al.*, 1994; Fan & Rozman, 1995; Li & Rozman, 1995; Ryu *et al.*, 1995). 2,3,7,8-TCDD also decreased PEPCK mRNA levels in male Sprague-Dawley rats (Stahl *et al.*, 1993) and the decrease in pyruvate carboxylase activity appears to be Ah receptor-mediated based on studies with congenic Ah-responsive (Ah^b/Ah^b) and less responsive (Ah^d/Ah^d) male C57BL/6 mice (Ryu *et al.*, 1995). A comparison of the effects of 2,3,7,8-TCDD in guinea-pigs (0.3–2.7 µg/kg) and hamsters (900–4600 µg/kg) showed that hepatic PEPCK was decreased in hamsters but not guinea-pigs, suggesting that altered carbohydrate homeostasis does not correlate with species-dependent susceptibility to 2,3,7,8-TCDD-induced lethality (Unkila *et al.*, 1995).

In guinea-pigs, adipose tissue and brain glucose uptake was decreased, whereas in liver, uptake was initially decreased (6–12 h) then increased (24–96 h) (Enan *et al.*, 1992; Enan & Matsumura, 1994a). Decreased glucose transport activity was associated in mice with tissue-specific decreased levels of glucose transporter (Liu & Matsumura, 1995). The relationship between the effects of glucose transport and 2,3,7,8-TCDD-induced toxicity has yet to be determined.

Several studies of rats and rhesus monkeys have shown consistent decreases in serum glucose levels after daily doses of 2,3,7,8-TCDD administered over 30 days (Zinkl *et al.*, 1973) or after a single dose (McConnell *et al.*, 1978b; Gasiewicz *et al.*, 1980; Schiller *et al.*, 1986; Ebner *et al.*, 1988).

4.3.7 *Modulation of oestrogenic responses by PCDDs*

2,3,7,8-TCDD inhibited the following oestrogen-induced responses in the ovariec-tomized or immature female rodent uterus: uterine weight increase, progesterone receptor levels, peroxidase activity, EGF-receptor binding and mRNA levels, and c-*fos* proto-oncogene mRNA levels (Romkes *et al.*, 1987; Astroff & Safe, 1988; Romkes & Safe, 1988; Umbreit *et al.*, 1988, 1989; Astroff & Safe, 1990; Astroff *et al.*, 1990; Astroff & Safe, 1991; Astroff *et al.*, 1991). In 21 day-old weanling rats, inhibition of oestradiol-induced uterine weight increase was not observed in Sprague-Dawley rats (White *et al.*, 1995). In-vitro studies using human breast cancer cell lines have also demonstrated the negative regulation by 2,3,7,8-TCDD of the following oestradiol-induced responses: cell proliferation, [^{3}H]thymidine uptake, postconfluent focus production, secretion of pS2, cathepsin D, procathepsin D and tissue plasminogen activator activity, progesterone receptor binding, and oestrogen receptor, progesterone receptor, pS2, prolactin receptor and cathepsin D gene expression (Gierthy *et al.*, 1987; Gierthy & Lincoln, 1988; Biegel & Safe, 1990; Krishnan *et al.*, 1992; Krishnan & Safe, 1993; Wang *et al.*, 1993; Harper *et al.*, 1994; Moore *et al.*, 1994; Zacharewski *et al.*, 1994; Krishnan *et al.*, 1995; Lu *et al.*, 1996). Moreover, using oestrogen-responsive promoter-reporter constructs derived from the 5′-regions of the pS2 and cathepsin D genes, 2,3,7,8-TCDD also inhibited E2-induced reporter gene activity in transiently transfected MCF-7 cells (Zacharewski *et al.*, 1994; Krishnan *et al.*, 1995). The role of the Ah receptor in mediating the anti-oestro-genic activities of various structural classes of agonists has been confirmed in several studies (Safe, 1995). Structure–activity studies with several Ah receptor agonists indi-cated a role of the Ah receptor in negatively modulatory oestrogenic responses (Krishnan *et al.*, 1994; Zacharewski *et al.*, 1994). In fact, interference between oestrogen- and Ah receptor-dependent signalling pathways has recently been proposed to be mediated by physical interaction between these receptor systems (Kharatt & Saatcioglu, 1996).

Expression of a functional nuclear Ah receptor complex is required for ligand-induced anti-oestrogenicity (Moore *et al.*, 1994). Studies of the cathepsin D gene have shown strategically located Ah receptor-binding sites, which may impair oestrogen-receptor function. A similar mechanism may be operative for inhibition of oestradiol-induced pS2 gene expression (Zacharewski *et al.*, 1994). It should be noted that the above oestrogen receptor modulatory effects of PCDDs are tissue-, age- and species-specific (Safe, 1995).

2,3,7,8-TCDD inhibits aromatase (CYP19) activity in the human choriocarcinoma cell line Jeg-3. The EC_{50} value for inhibition was in the same range as that observed for CYP1A1 induction in this cell type (Drenth *et al.*, 1996). This action could be a cause for the anti-oestrogenic effects of PCDDs; these in-vitro results need to be confirmed in in-vivo experiments.

4.3.8   *Role of oxidative stress in the toxicity of PCDDs*

Exposure of rats to an oral dose of 100 µg/kg bw 2,3,7,8-TCDD (a lethal dose) increased lipid peroxidation in hepatic mitochondria (Stohs *et al.*, 1990). Marked increases in hepatic lipid peroxidation were observed in female Sprague-Dawley rats [males not studied] seven days after treatment with 50 µg/kg 2,3,7,8-TCDD (Wahba *et al.*, 1990). The increase in hepatic lipid peroxidation was suppressed by antioxidants such as butylated hydroxyanisole, vitamin A or *d*-α-tocopherol (Stohs *et al.*, 1984). 2,3,7,8-TCDD also enhanced lipid peroxidation in various other tissues (Bagchi *et al.*, 1993) and altered membrane structure and functions. Enhanced lipid peroxidation after 2,3,7,8-TCDD treatment was suggested to arise as a secondary phenomenon in 2,3,7,8-TCDD toxicity, possibly contributing to lethality (Pohjanvirta *et al.*, 1990c). 2,3,7,8-TCDD depleted glutathione levels, altered calcium homeostasis and increased DNA damage in the form of single strand breaks (Stohs *et al.*, 1990). In addition, 2,3,7,8-TCDD enhances the release of TNFα (Alsharif *et al.*, 1994a) and induces production of stress/heat shock protein 90 (hsp90) (Perdew, 1992; Henry & Gasiewicz, 1993; Abbott *et al.*, 1994a). The use of TNF antibody decreases 2,3,7,8-TCDD-induced DNA damage, lipid peroxidation and macrophage activation.

4.3.9   *Cell cycle regulation and apoptosis*

Exposure to 2,3,7,8-TCDD delays G1-S progression in mouse and rat hepatoma cells in a receptor-dependent manner (Göttlicher & Wiebel, 1991; Ma & Whitlock, 1996; Weiss *et al.*, 1996), whereas 2,3,7,8-TCDD-induced enhancement of cell proliferation has been observed in human squamous carcinoma cell lines in a cell confluence-dependent manner (Hébert *et al.*, 1990b).

Tyrosine phosphorylation and the level of expression of two cyclin-dependent kinases which regulate cell cycle progression have been found to be increased in mouse liver after both acute (Ma & Babish, 1993) and subchronic (DeVito *et al.*, 1994) 2,3,7,8-TCDD dosing. Increased cell proliferation does not necessarily determine that cancer will occur, and hence not all chemicals that cause increased cell proliferation cause cancer (Melnick *et al.*, 1992).

Recent studies have also demonstrated that 2,3,7,8-TCDD modulates programmed cell death (apoptosis) *in vivo* and *in vitro*. In Ah-responsive mice deficient in the apoptosis-inducing ligand Fas, 2,3,7,8-TCDD was less toxic to the thymocytes than in Fas-proficient mice (Rhile *et al.*, 1996). In a study in female BALB/cJ mice treated with a single intraperitoneal dose of 30 µg/kg 2,3,7,8-TCDD, however, no indication of thymocyte apoptosis was obtained (Silverstone *et al.*, 1994b).

Stinchcombe *et al.* (1995) reported suppression of apoptosis in preneoplastic hepatocytes in a two-stage initiation–promotion protocol. Inhibition of apoptosis with 1 nM 2,3,7,8-TCDD was also observed in rat hepatocytes in primary culture pretreated with ultraviolet light or 2-acetylaminofluorene (Wörner & Schrenk, 1996). This effect was linked to negative regulation of expression of the *p53* tumour-suppressor gene.

4.4 Reproductive and developmental effects

4.4.1 *Humans*

Most studies on human reproductive effects of PCDDs concern paternal exposure, usually long after a high exposure occurred. A number of studies evaluated reproductive effects in cohorts with high potential for exposure to 2,3,7,8-TCDD or other PCDDs. These studies include the United States Ranch Hand personnel (Wolfe *et al.*, 1995), the Seveso population (Mastroiacovo *et al.*, 1988), workers who manufactured TCP and 2,4,5-T (Townsend *et al.*, 1982; Suskind & Hertzberg, 1984) and pesticide applicators (Smith *et al.*, 1992b). Only the studies of Ranch Hand personnel and of pesticide applicators measured serum 2,3,7,8-TCDD levels, and the quality of the studies varies. Cohorts of Viet Nam veterans other than Ranch Hand personnel (Stellman *et al.*, 1988; Centers for Disease Control Vietnam Experience Study, 1988b) and of Missouri residents (Stockbauer *et al.*, 1988) have not been proven to have high potential for exposure or the exposure was not well defined.

The study populations mentioned below and their exposures are described more fully in Sections 1.3.1, 1.3.2 and 2.2.

(a) *Endocrine and gonadal effects*

Total serum testosterone, LH and follicle-stimulating hormone (FSH) were measured in 248 TCP production workers and in 231 non-exposed neighbourhood controls matched for age and race (Egeland *et al.*, 1994). In linear regression analyses, current serum levels of 2,3,7,8-TCDD were positively related to LH and FSH and inversely related to total testosterone levels after adjustment for potential confounders (age, body mass index, diabetes mellitus, current alcohol consumption, race and smoking status). Similar results were obtained by multiple logistic regression, showing stronger adverse effects in higher-exposure groups. The presence of both low testosterone and high LH was not observed in the same individuals, therefore, the authors interpreted their findings as being suggestive of more subtle alterations in gonadotropins and testosterone than of primary gonadal failure due to PCDD exposure.

In a random subsample of 571 men, from a total of 4462 who were examined, Viet Nam veterans (n = 324) had significantly lower sperm concentrations than the 247 non-Viet Nam veterans (64.8 million/mL versus 79.8 million/mL) and a lower proportion of 'normal' sperm heads (57.9% versus 60.8%) (Centers for Disease Control Vietnam Experience Study, 1988a). There was also a doubling of the proportion of men with sperm characteristics (concentration, percentage of motile cells, percentage of morphologically 'normal' cells) below the normal range. Ability to father children was not affected. Differences in semen concentration and morphology could not be related to a particular subgroup of veterans or military occupational specialty, to self-reported combat experiences or to herbicide exposure.

In the 1982 examination, 474 Ranch Hand veterans out of 1045 and 532 of the 1224 comparison veterans were included in the analysis of association between serum 2,3,7,8-TCDD and serum testosterone, FSH, LH, testicular abnormality, sperm count, percentage of abnormal sperm and testicular volume. No pattern of consistent or meaningful associations was seen between 2,3,7,8-TCDD body burden and any of the variables studied, when either categorized (% abnormalities) (Henriksen *et al.*, 1996) or analysed as continuous variables (Henriksen & Michalek, 1996). The authors explain that their study and the previous study by Egeland *et al.* (1994) differ in terms of the exposure circumstances and demographics and conclude that 'the Ranch Hand exposure was not sufficient to exhibit the associations similar to those seen in the industrial workers, who have higher dioxin body burdens and were exposed over a longer period of time than the Ranch Hand veterans.'

(b)   *Effects on pregnancy* (**Table 63**)

(i)   *Studies on Viet Nam veterans (United States and Australia)*

Exposure data relating to these groups are described in Section 1.3.1(a)(ii); in general, exposure to PCDDs was low, except in the case of the Ranch Hand Study. In the following studies, exposure to Agent Orange was classified as 'service in Viet Nam'. No direct exposure measurements were made. However, in two studies, exposure indices were based on location of service in Viet Nam. These indices may still misclassify actual exposure to Agent Orange.

Telephone interviews were conducted with 7924 Viet Nam veterans (87% of the eligible) and 7364 non-Viet Nam veterans (84%), randomly selected from the Vietnam-Era United States Army personnel records (Centers for Disease Control Vietnam Experience Study, 1988b). Viet Nam veterans were more likely to report having fathered a pregnancy that ended in a miscarriage than were non-Viet Nam veterans (odds ratio, 1.3; 95% CI, 1.2–1.4). In a birth defects sub-study (1237 Viet Nam veterans and 1045 non-Viet Nam veterans) for which hospital birth records were obtained for all reported births (1791 offspring of Viet Nam veterans and 1575 offspring of non-Viet Nam veterans), no difference in the rates of all birth defects was identified: 72.6 per 1000 births for Viet Nam veterans; 71.1 per 1000 among non-Viet Nam veterans. The rates for major defects were respectively 28.5 per 1000 and 23.5 per 1000. The adjusted odds ratio for total defects among offspring of black veterans was 3.3 (95% CI, 1.5–7.5). The observed

Table 63. Results of studies examining the effect of 2,3,7,8-TCDD on pregnancy outcomes in humans

Reference	Exposed group	Control group	Type of exposure	Data source: exposure/outcome	Outcome	Outcome in exposed (no.)	Outcome in unexposed (no.)	Odds ratio	CI (95% unless indicated)
Studies of cohorts with high potential exposure									
Wolfe et al. (1995)	1006 conceptions among 454 Ranch Hand personnel	1235 conceptions among 570 non-Ranch Hand personnel	Spraying/handling of Agent Orange	Serum 2,3,7,8-TCDD levels/medical records	Spontaneous abortion				
					Comparison		172	1	
					Background exposure	57		1.1	0.8–1.5
					Low exposure	56		1.3	1.0–1.7
					High exposure	44		1.0	0.7–1.3
					Stillbirth				
					Comparison		13	1	
					Background exposure	7		1.8	0.7–4.5
					Low exposure	6		1.8	0.7–4.7
					High exposure	1		0.3	0.0–2.3
					Major birth defects				
					Comparison		56	1	
					Background exposure	17		1.1	0.6–1.8
					Low exposure	23		1.7	1.1–2.7
					High exposure	19		1.2	0.8–2.1
					Developmental delays				
					Comparison		71	1	
					Background exposure	24		1.2	0.8–1.8
					Low exposure	26		1.5	1.0–2.3
					High exposure	21		1.1	0.7–1.7
Mastroiacovo et al. (1988)	2900 births in zones A, B and R, Seveso, Italy, 1977–82	12 391 births in study area outside zones A, B and R	2,3,7,8-TCDD cloud released from chemical plant accident	2,3,7,8-TCDD soil analysis/Seveso Congenital Malformations Registry	Total birth defects	137	605	1.0	0.8–1.1[a]
					Multiple birth defects	10	38	1.1	0.6–2.0[a]
					Syndromes	5	29	0.7	0.3–1.6[a]
					Major birth defects	67	343	0.8	0.7–1.0[a]
					Minor birth defects	70	262	1.1	0.9–1.4[a]

Table 63 (contd)

Reference	Exposed group	Control group	Type of exposure	Data source: exposure/ outcome	Outcome	Outcome in exposed (no.)	Outcome in unexposed (no.)	Odds ratio	CI (95% unless indicated)
Studies of cohorts with high potential exposure (contd)									
Townsend et al. (1982)	Male chemical workers exposed to any PCDDs	Unexposed workers	Chlorophenol and 2,4,5-T production	Company records/ interview	Total conceptuses	737	2031	–[b]	
					All fetal deaths	100	246	1.0	0.8–1.4
					Stillbirth	15	33	1.1	0.5–2.1
					Spontaneous abortions	85	213	1.0	0.8–1.4
					Infant deaths	9	39	0.6	0.3–1.4
					Health defects	52	155	0.9	0.6–1.2
					Congenital malformations	30	87	0.9	0.5–1.4
Suskind & Hertzberg (1984)	189 male chemical workers exposed to 2,4,5-T processes	155 male workers in the same plant not exposed to 2,4,5-T processes	2,4,5-T process	Interview, personal work records/ interview	Pregnancies	655	429		
					Miscarriages	69	51	0.9[c]	NS
					Stillbirths	11	5	1.4[c]	NS
					Dead in 4 weeks	17	6	1.8[c]	NS
					Birth defects	18	11	1.1[c]	NS
Smith et al. (1982b)	548 male pesticide applicators who sprayed 2,4,5-T and other pesticides	441 agricultural contractors	Spraying of 2,4,5-T	Mailed survey/ mailed survey	Total pregnancies	486	401		
					Congenital defect	13	9	1.2	0.6–2.5[a]
					Miscarriage	43	40	0.9	0.6–1.3[a]
					Stillbirth	3	0	–	–
Studies of cohorts with potential for low or undefined exposure									
Stockbauer et al. (1988)	402 births to exposed mothers	804 births to unexposed mothers (matched on maternal age and race, hospital and year of birth, plurality)	Contact with soil sprayed with 2,3,7,8-TCDD for dust control	EPA soil analyses for 2,3,7,8-TCDD/ vital statistics and hospital records	Birth defects - all	17	42	0.8	0.4–1.5
					Major birth defects	15	35	0.8	0.4–1.7
					Multiple birth defects	2	11	0.3	0.0–1.7
					Fetal deaths	4	5	1.6	0.3–7.4
					Infant deaths	5	5	2.0	0.5–8.7
					Perinatal deaths	6	9	1.3	0.4–4.2
					Low birth weight	27	36	1.6	0.9–2.8
					Very low birth weight	1	4	0.5	0.0–5.1

Table 63 (contd)

Reference	Exposed group	Control group	Type of exposure	Data source: exposure/outcome	Outcome	Outcome in exposed (no.)	Outcome in unexposed (no.)	Odds ratio	CI (95% unless indicated)
Studies of cohorts with potential for low or undefined exposure (contd)									
CDC (1988b)	7294 Viet Nam veterans	7364 non-Viet Nam veterans	Viet Nam military service	Military records/self reports	Total birth defects	826	590	1.3	1.2–1.4
					Spontaneous abortion	716	655[a]	1.3	1.2–1.4
					Low birth weight	25	17	1.1	0.8–1.4
					Childhood cancer			1.5	0.8–2.8
CDC (1988b)	1791 offspring of Viet Nam veterans	1575 offspring of non-Viet Nam veterans	Viet Nam military service	Military records/self report and hospital records verification	Total birth defects	130	112	1.0	0.8–1.4
					Major birth defects	51	37	1.1	0.7–1.8
					Minor birth defects	58	54	1.0	0.7–1.5
					Suspected birth defects	21	21	0.9	0.5–1.7
Stellman *et al.* (1988)	2858 Viet Nam veterans	3933 non-Viet Nam veterans	Viet Nam military service	Survey/survey	Difficulty conceiving	349	363	1.3	$p < 0.01$
					Spontaneous abortion	231	195	1.4	$p < 0.01$
Case–control studies									
Erickson *et al.* (1984)	7133 infants from the Metropolitan Atlanta Congenital Defects Program	4246 infants from Georgia Vital Statistics Records	Viet Nam military service	Self-reported and Exposure Opportunity Index/Birth defects registry and vital statistics	Total birth defects (96 subcategories also examined)	428	268	1.0	0.8–1.1
					Spina bifida	NR	NR	1.1	
					Cleft lip without cleft palate	NR	NR	1.1	
Donovan *et al.* (1984)	8517 infants born with congenital anomalies (Australia, 1966–79)	8517 infants without anomalies matched by hospital, period of birth, age of mother, hospital payment category	Past paternal military service in Viet Nam	Military records/hospital records	Congenital anomalies	127	123	1.0	0.8–1.3

Table 63 (contd)

Reference	Exposed group	Control group	Type of exposure	Data source: exposure/outcome	Outcome	Outcome in exposed (no.)	Outcome in unexposed (no.)	Odds ratio	CI (95% unless indicated)
Case–control studies (contd)									
Aschengrau & Monson (1989)	201 spontaneous abortion cases at Boston Hospital for Women	1119 full-term births at Boston Hospital for Women	Viet Nam military service	Military records/ hospital records	Spontaneous abortion	10	60	0.9	0.4–1.9
Aschengrau & Monson (1990)	966 infants with late adverse pregnancy outcomes at Boston Hospital for Women	998 normal term infants at Boston Hospital for Women	Viet Nam military service	Military records/ hospital records	Total birth defects	55	146	1.1	0.7–1.8
					≥ 1 major malformation	18	45	1.7	0.8–3.5
					Minor malformation	11	32	0.9	0.4–2.3
					Stillbirths	5	5	3.2	0.7–14.5
					Neonatal deaths	3	9	1.1	0.2–4.5
Ha et al. (1996)	87 cases of gestational trophoblastic disease at Ho Chi Minh City Gynaecology Hospital	87 surgical controls matched for age and last residence	Cumulative exposure to Agent Orange in the environment	Residence history and US military records/ hospital admissions	Gestational trophoblastic disease (hydatidiform mole or choriocarcinoma)				
					Background exposure	–	–	1.0	
					Highest cumulative exposure	–	–	0.7	0.2–1.8

NS, not stated; NR, not reported
[a] 90% confidence interval
[b] Adjusted for mother's age at time of birth, birth control methods, labour and delivery complications, medical conditions and mediations during pregnancy, smoking and alcohol use during pregnancy, high rob risk and gravidity
[c] Estimated from published results
[d] Referent category: non-Viet Nam veterans

number of cases of central nervous system defects (26) among babies of Viet Nam veterans was within the expected range (18.3–32.4) based on national rates (Birth Defects Monitoring Program) or Metropolitan Atlanta race-specific rates, whereas the observed number (12) among non-Viet Nam veterans was lower than expected (17.0–30.2).

Verified conceptions and births fathered during or after service in south-east Asia in relation to serum 2,3,7,8-TCDD levels were compared in 454 Ranch Hand veterans and 570 air force veterans not involved in Ranch Hand (Wolfe *et al.*, 1995). For the Ranch Hand veterans, three categories of exposure were defined according to the extrapolated initial 2,3,7,8-TCDD level at the time of conception: background, low (≤ 110 ng/kg serum fat) and high (> 110 ng/kg serum fat). There was no significant elevation in risk for spontaneous abortions, stillbirths, major birth defects or delays in development after adjustment for several covariates. [The Working Group noted that, of the studies of pregnancy outcomes, this study presents the best-quality data with biological measurement of exposure and medical reports of reproductive outcomes. However, measurements were made up to 25 years after exposure ended and extrapolation to the initial 2,3,7,8-TCDD level at the time of conception may be imprecise. The power of the study for detecting an increase in the rate of specific birth defects is limited.]

A cross-sectional survey of the health status of Viet Nam veterans was conducted in a random sample of members of the American Legion who served in the United States armed forces during 1961–75 (Stellman *et al.*, 1988). Return rates of the self-administered mail questionnaire ranged from 52.5% to 64.1%. Among the respondents, 42% had served in south-east Asia. Of a total of 3046 live births and miscarriages, 2215 were fathered by veterans who served in south-east Asia; the potential exposure of these veterans to Agent Orange was ranked. The self-reported miscarriage rate among wives of Viet Nam veterans was 7.6% versus 5.8% among wives of non-Viet Nam veterans ($p < 0.01$) and increased with Agent Orange exposure index (7.3% for low exposure, 9.6% for high exposure). In a multivariate model, Agent Orange exposure remained a significant predictor of the rate of miscarriage. [The Working Group noted the low participation rate and low reliability of miscarriage information from male partners. The miscarriage rates reported (5.8% for non-Viet Nam veterans) are in fact very low.]

A case–control study (Erickson *et al.*, 1984) compared the Viet Nam experience of fathers of 7133 babies born with a serious structural congenital malformation with 4246 babies born without defects. Seventy per cent of eligible mothers and 56.3% of eligible fathers completed an interview. An 'exposure opportunity index' (EOI) score was assigned to Viet Nam veterans potentially exposed to Agent Orange. The risk of Viet Nam veterans fathering babies with birth defects was not increased (odds ratio, 1.0; 95% CI, 0.8–1.1); however, there was a slight increase for spina bifida (odds ratio, 1.1; $p > 0.05$), cleft lip with or without cleft palate (odds ratio, 1.1; $p < 0.05$) and congenital neoplasms with the higher EOI scores.

A case–control study was conducted in Australia including 8517 infants born with congenital anomalies between 1966 and 1979 and the same number of matched control children born without an anomaly (Donovan *et al.*, 1984). Viet Nam veterans comprised

127 fathers of cases and 123 fathers of controls, giving an overall odds ratio among veterans for fathering a malformed infant of 1.0 (95% CI, 0.8–1.3). No significant difference was observed for the numbers of discordant pairs for anomalies of the central nervous system, cardiac anomalies and chromosomal anomalies. No other group was more frequent among cases.

A case–control study was conducted in Boston Hospital for Women among 201 women admitted for spontaneous abortion (< 28 weeks of gestation) and 1119 controls (Aschengrau & Monson, 1989). The adjusted odds ratio for spontaneous abortion among Viet Nam veterans' wives was 0.9 (95% CI, 0.4–1.9) and 0.7 (95% CI, 0.5–1.2) for non-Viet Nam veterans' wives, using a group with no known military service as a reference. Odds ratios for early spontaneous abortion (< 13 weeks of gestation) were 1.2 (95% CI, 0.6–2.8) and 0.7 (95% CI, 0.4–1.2) for Viet Nam and non-Viet Nam veterans' wives, respectively.

In a second case–control study conducted at Boston Hospital (Aschengrau & Monson, 1990), 857 cases of congenital anomaly, 61 cases of stillbirth, 48 cases of neonatal death and 998 normal controls were identified. For Viet Nam veterans, the relative risk of fathering an infant with one or more major malformations was slightly elevated when compared with non-Viet Nam veterans (RR, 1.7; 95% CI, 0.8–3.5) and with non-veterans (RR, 2.2; 95% CI, 1.2–4.0). Fathers of babies with major malformations served more often in the Marine Corps and had longer durations of Viet Nam service. No particular type of defect was reported.

(ii) Environmental studies

The Seveso accident has provided a unique opportunity to evaluate the effect of environmental contamination on reproductive outcomes.

The Seveso Congenital Malformations Registry examined all live births and stillbirths that occurred from 1 January 1977 to 31 December 1982 to women who were residents of zones A, B and R and non-ABR (control area) in July 1976 (Mastroiacovo et al., 1988). A total of 15 291 births occurred, out of which 742 malformed were identified (48.5/1000 births). Twenty-six births were recorded in the most highly contaminated area (Zone A); none had any major structural defect and two infants had mild defects. The frequencies of major defects observed in the area of low contamination (Zone B) or very low contamination (Zone R) were 29.9/1000 and 22.1/1000, respectively, compared to 27.7/1000 in the control area. No specific subgroup of malformations was seen in excess in the contaminated areas. The authors did not rule out the possibility that an increase in spontaneous abortions could have obscured an increase in malformations seen at birth. Due to the small number of exposed pregnancies, this study had insufficient power to show a low and specific teratogenic risk increase. Examination of 30 induced abortions which occurred just after the accident did not disclose any gross developmental abnormalities or chromosomal aberrations (Rehder et al., 1978).

Spontaneous abortions which occurred in Cesano, Seveso, Desio, Meda and seven other cities in the area were identified by reports to the County Medical Officer and searching among admission/discharge hospital forms between July 1976 and December 1977 (Bisanti et al., 1980). Rates of spontaneous abortion (per number of pregnancies, excluding induced abortions) increased in the fourth trimester of 1976 (21.3%) in the 'most exposed' cities of Cesano and Seveso, compared with 13.9% in Desio and Meda, and 14.0% in the other seven cities ($p < 0.05$). It decreased in the following trimesters. When pregnancies were regrouped according to exposure zone, spontaneous abortion rates were always higher in Zone B than in other zones after the last trimester of 1976. [The Working Group noted that these results are hard to interpret because ascertainment bias cannot be ruled out. Inadequate details on the procedure are given to evaluate this potential problem.]

Data on births in Zone A between April 1977 (nine months after the accident) and December 1984 showed a significant excess of female births: 48 females versus 26 males ($p < 0.001$) (Mocarelli *et al.*, 1996). This ratio declined (64 females versus 60 males) in the years 1985 to 1994 and was no longer significant. Parents with an excess of female offspring were reported to have had a high 2,3,7,8-TCDD serum concentration in 1976. This observed change in the sex ratio in the years following the accident, if it is meaningful, could have several possible explanations (change in parental hormone concentrations, selective male miscarriages, mutations) in relation to high 2,3,7,8-TCDD exposure. [The Working Group noted that the number of reported births in Zone A between 1977 and 1984 (74) is much higher than the 26 births reported by Mastroiacovo *et al.* (1988) in Zone A between 1977 and 1982.]

Exposure to 2,3,7,8-TCDD occurred in eastern Missouri, after contaminated oil was sprayed for dust control in 1971. A total of 402 births (i.e., any product of conception with a gestational age of 20 weeks or longer) were identified between 1972 and 1982 among women who had potential exposure to PCDDs, based on proximity of residence to a location of known contamination (Stockbauer *et al.*, 1988); 804 unexposed births among Missouri residents were selected for comparison. Increased but not statistically significant risk ratios were observed for infant, fetal or perinatal death and low birth weight. Birth defects were not increased; however, the power of this study, as computed by the authors, for detecting a doubling in the risk of total birth defects was low at 34%.

Four ecological studies have evaluated the relationship between reproductive outcomes and the potential for environmental exposure to 2,3,7,8-TCDD. These studies have analysed correlations between annual rates of birth defects and usage of 2,4,5-T in corresponding geographical areas having different levels of aerial spraying. As in all ecological studies of this kind, it is not possible to extrapolate results to an individual level. These studies failed to show consistent patterns of birth defects or malformations (Field & Kerr, 1979; Nelson *et al.*, 1979; Thomas, 1980; Hanify *et al.*, 1981).

A summary of methods and findings of several investigations conducted in Viet Nam by Vietnamese researchers, on the reproductive effects of Agent Orange sprayings, was published by Constable and Hatch (1985) and Sterling and Arundel (1986). All these studies showed evidence of an increased risk for adverse reproductive outcomes such as abortions, stillbirths, congenital malformations (especially of the central nervous system and oral clefts) or molar pregnancies in relation to Agent Orange sprayings, both among southern Vietnamese populations and to wives of veterans from the north. Although many of the results are striking, details on the methods used are lacking and there is no reassurance that potential selection bias, reporting bias or confounding which are major problems in the type of studies presented, were avoided.

A case–control study on gestational trophoblastic disease (molar pregnancy or chorio-carcinoma) was conducted in 1990, in the Obstetrics and Gynaecology Hospital in Ho Chi Minh City (Ha *et al.*, 1996). A total of 87 cases and 87 surgical controls matched for age and area of residence (two strata: Ho Chi Minh City, province) were interviewed at the hospital. All had been married. Cumulative exposure to Agent Orange was estimated from history of residence since the sprayings and from data on spraying missions from the United States military records. There was no difference in past exposure to Agent Orange between cases and controls. Negative findings could be explained by mis-classification of exposures or by the decrease in exposure since the end of the sprayings. The 2,3,7,8-TCDD levels however remain elevated today in Vietnamese blood and tissue (Schecter *et al.*, 1995).

(iii) *Occupational studies*

A study was conducted among wives of chlorophenol production workers who were potentially exposed to PCDDs and unexposed controls (Townsend *et al.*, 1982). Information on reproductive outcomes was obtained by interview from 370 and 345 wives of exposed and unexposed workers, respectively: 737 pregnancies occurred after potential paternal exposure, whereas 2031 pregnancies were considered to be unexposed. Odds ratios were 1.1 (95% CI, 0.5–2.1) for stillbirths, 1.0 (95% CI, 0.8–1.4) for sponta-neous abortions and 0.9 (95% CI, 0.5–1.4) for congenital malformations. No specific pattern of malformations or increasing risk of unfavourable outcome with length of paternal exposure (12 months or less, more than 12 months) was seen. [The Working Group noted that this study assumed the effect of paternal exposure to PCDDs to be an irreparable event, so that every subsequent pregnancy was considered to be exposed, whatever the time since last exposure. No figures were presented according to this last variable and no detail was given on the actual level of exposure to PCDDs in the plant.]

In New Zealand, the rates of various outcomes among wives of men who sprayed 2,4,5-T at some time during the two-year period preceding birth outcome (486 pregnancies) were compared with rates among wives of agricultural contractors who did not spray pesticides during the corresponding period (401 pregnancies) (Smith *et al.*, 1982b). Relative risks were 0.9 (90% CI, 0.6–1.3) for miscarriage and 1.2 (90% CI 0.6–2.5) for congenital defect. Three stillbirths (7.0 /1000 live births) were reported in the exposed group and none in the unexposed group. The authors concluded, however, that small increases in risk, especially for individual defects, could not be ruled out. The nine pesticide applicators had been chosen because they had the longest durations of exposure to phenoxy herbicides. The average exposure of the cohort would have therefore been much lower.

Information on reproductive factors and birth defects was obtained from 189 PCDD-exposed herbicide production workers in West Virginia, USA, and 155 unexposed controls, but was not confirmed by physician or hospital records. Among 655 pre-gnancies in the exposed population and 429 in the controls, the rates of miscarriages, stillbirths or birth defects and the patterns of birth defects were similar (Suskind & Hertzberg, 1984).

4.4.2 *Experimental systems*

Developmental toxicity has been observed at lower 2,3,7,8-TCDD exposure levels than those producing male and female adult reproductive toxicity in various animals.

(a) *Developmental effects*

(i) *General embryo- and fetotoxicity*

There are numerous reviews concerning aspects of the developmental effects of PCDDs and related compounds in a range of vertebrate species (Couture *et al.*, 1990a; Birnbaum, 1991; Peterson *et al.*, 1993; Battershill, 1994; Sauer *et al.*, 1994; Birnbaum, 1995b; Brouwer *et al.*, 1995; Lindstrom *et al.*, 1995; Abbott, 1996; Birnbaum, 1996; Birnbaum & Abbott, 1997).

At dose levels below those where overt toxicity occurred in the dam, growth retardation was detected in the offspring. Thymic and splenic atrophy were also noted. Subcutaneous oedema was observed in several species and gastrointestinal haemorrhage in others. Higher levels of exposure resulted in fetal deaths and resorptions. One of the key observations has been that the dose levels associated with fetal toxicity are similar across species, regardless of the dose associated with adult lethality. For example, Han/Wistar (Kuopio) rats, that are uniquely resistant to 2,3,7,8-TCDD-induced lethality in the adult, exhibit developmental toxicity similar to that of Long-Evans (Turku) rats that are extremely susceptible to the lethal effects of 2,3,7,8-TCDD (Huuskonen *et al.*, 1994). Fetotoxicity occurs after approximately the same dose to the dam of both rats and hamsters, although the adult LD_{50} varies by over a factor of 100 (Olson *et al.*, 1990).

(ii) *Teratogenic effects*

Cleft palate and hydronephrosis

Exposure of pregnant mice to 2,3,7,8-TCDD and related compounds caused a pathognomonic syndrome of effects in the offspring at doses (e.g., a subcutaneous dose of 0.3 µg/kg/day during gestation days 6–15) that result in no overt toxicity to the mother (Couture *et al.*, 1990a). Either divided doses throughout organogenesis or a single higher dose resulted in a similar spectrum of structural malformations in the pups consisting of clefting of the secondary palate and hydronephrosis. The peak period of sensitivity for induction of palatal clefting was gestational days 11–12; exposure on gestational day 14 or later cannot induce cleft palate since fusion has already occurred. A clear window of sensitivity was not seen for hydronephrosis. The same dose (3–24 pg/kg) was associated with an identical incidence and severity of the renal lesion whenever treatment occurred during gestational days 6–12 (Couture *et al.*, 1990b). Hydronephrosis also resulted from lactational exposure only (dose 3–12 µg/kg given on gestation day 6), although this was less efficient than transplacental exposure (Couture-Haws *et al.*, 1991). Hydronephrosis was also induced at doses below those which induced palatal clefting. At low doses, mild hydronephrosis was observed, predominantly in the right kidney. At higher doses, both the incidence and severity of response increased in both kidneys. Hydronephrosis was often accompanied by hydroureter. The cause of both conditions was inappropriate proliferation of the ureteric epithelium resulting in a narrowing and blockage of the lumen (Abbott *et al.*, 1987). Urine produced by the fetal kidney was blocked from being eliminated, leading to destruction of the renal parenchyma.

Inappropriate epithelial cell proliferation also appears to play a major role in palatal clefting. 2,3,7,8-TCDD blocked fusion of the opposing palatal shelves in mice (Pratt *et al.*, 1984), although the shelves did make contact. During normal development, the medial epithelium transforms into mesenchyme (Fitchett & Hay, 1989; Shuler *et al.*, 1992). This epithelial–mesenchymal differentiation was blocked by 2,3,7,8-TCDD. The medial epithelium continued to proliferate and under the influence of 2,3,7,8-TCDD, transformed into an oral-like stratified squamous epithelium complete with desmosomes, tonofilaments and keratins (Abbott & Birnbaum, 1989a).

No species other than the mouse shows similar responses at non-toxic doses (reviewed in Couture *et al.*, 1990a). For example, cleft palate has been reported in rats exposed during organogenesis, but the dose needed to produce clefting also results in fetotoxicity, fetal wastage and maternal toxicity. Although increased incidence of hydronephrosis has been reported, in no case was the incidence statistically significant. Renal abnormalities have been seen in hamsters, but these also occurred only at doses where fetotoxicity was evident.

Although the majority of studies examining the mechanism of PCDD teratogenicity in mice have been conducted with 2,3,7,8-TCDD, there have been many investigations of the induction of cleft palate and hydronephrosis by other PCDD-like compounds (see cited reviews). Several higher chlorinated PCDDs cause the same spectrum of birth defects as 2,3,7,8-TCDD (Birnbaum, 1991).

Other developmental effects

Gastrointestinal haemorrhage has been observed in guinea-pigs and rats. Prenatal exposure of mice to either 2,3,7,8-TCDD or 2,3,4,7,8-PeCDF resulted in haemorrhage of embryonic blood into the maternal circulation because of rupture of the embryo-maternal vascular barrier (Khera, 1992).

While the majority of experimental studies with PCDDs have focused on exposure during organogenesis, treatment earlier in gestation has been noted to result in fetotoxicity (Giavini *et al.*, 1982). In addition, however, recent studies have indicated that PCDDs can accelerate differentiation of the preimplantation embryo (Blankenship *et al.*, 1993). The Ah receptor has been demonstrated to be present in the developing embryo from the eight-cell stage (Peters & Wiley, 1995).

The developing teeth also appear to be a target for PCDD-induced effects. Neonatal exposure of BALB/c mice to 150 μg/kg 2,3,7,8-TCDD by intraperitoneal injection leads to accelerated tooth eruption in mice (Madhukar *et al.*, 1984). Impaired dentin and enamel formation has been observed in the continuously growing incisors of young male Han/Wistar rats (1000 μg/kg intraperitoneal injection) (Alaluusua *et al.*, 1993) following 2,3,7,8-TCDD exposure.

The developing immune system is also a target for PCDDs (reviewed in Birnbaum, 1995a). Exposure during organogenesis results in lymphoid atrophy. Mice fail to survive because of the induction of cleft palate. To avoid this effect, mice can be treated on gestation day 14, when the palate has already fused. Under these conditions, 2,3,7,8-TCDD accelerated the differentiation of prothymocytes in the bone marrow (Fine *et al.*, 1989, 1990a,b). This suggests that thymic atrophy may be a result of altered differentiation of cells from the bone marrow. The ratio of T-lymphocyte subsets is altered in the pups as well. Holladay *et al.* (1991) also observed changes in the surface markers of lymphocytes following prenatal exposure. Exposure of rats on gestational day 15, which is developmentally slightly earlier than gestation day 14 in the mouse, leads to similar changes in T-cell subset ratios in the rat offspring (Gehrs & Smialowicz, 1994). This is associated with permanent suppression of delayed-type hypersensitivity in the rat offspring (Gehrs *et al.*, 1995), an immunological measure highly correlated with altered host resistance and increased disease sensitivity. The dose levels associated with permanent immune suppression in the developing rat are even lower than those needed in the prenatally exposed mouse. This is in contrast to the apparent resistance in adult rats to immunosuppression following exposure to PCDDs (Smialowicz *et al.*, 1994).

(iii) *Role of growth factors and hormones*

Further information on this topic is presented in Sections 4.3 and 4.6.

Alterations in proliferation and differentiation play a role in cleft palate, hydronephrosis and immunological developmental effects. While reactive oxygen species may participate in some of the teratogenic effects of 2,3,7,8-TCDD (Hassoun *et al.*, 1995), changes in various growth factors and receptors are correlated with palatal clefting. During normal development, levels of EGF decrease and TGFα increases during palatal fusion. 2,3,7,8-TCDD has little effect on EGF, but does block the increase in TGFα in the developing palate (Abbott & Birnbaum, 1990a, 1991). The EGF receptor, which is normally present in the epithelium, decreases during palatal fusion (Abbott & Birnbaum, 1989a). This decrease is blocked by 2,3,7,8-TCDD (Abbott & Birnbaum, 1989b; Abbott *et al.*, 1994b). Whether this is a compensatory increase in the receptor level due to the decrease in the presence of its ligands remains to be determined. However, these changes probably play a role in the continued proliferation of the medial epithelium resulting in cleft palate due to 2,3,7,8-TCDD. Several members of the TGFβ family also respond to 2,3,7,8-TCDD. While these growth factors frequently inhibit epithelial cell proliferation, they are often stimulatory to cells of mesenchymal origin. 2,3,7,8-TCDD causes an increase in TGFβ1 and TGFβ2 in the medial epithelium (Abbott & Birnbaum, 1990a, 1991; Abbott *et al.*, 1994b). These growth factors also increase in the underlying mesenchyme in response to 2,3,7,8-TCDD.

Cleft palate can also be induced by exposure to glucocorticoids; however, the mechanism is distinct from that of 2,3,7,8-TCDD. Glucocorticoids cause growth inhibition of the palatal shelves, resulting in small shelves which fail to make contact and thus cannot fuse (Pratt, 1985). Co-treatment of mice with hydrocortisone and 2,3,7,8-TCDD leads to a synergistic increase in the incidence of cleft palate (Birnbaum *et al.*, 1986). The size of the cleft suggests that growth inhibition plays a major role in this clefting. The changes in EGF, TGFα and β and the EGF receptor also suggest that the effects resemble those seen following exposure to hydrocortisone (Abbott, 1995). Sensitivity to glucocorticoid-induced cleft palate is related to the numbers of glucocorticoid receptors. 2,3,7,8-TCDD exposure causes an increase in the numbers of glucocorticoid receptors in the developing palate (Abbott et al., 1994c), suggesting that the synergism of hydrocortisone-induced cleft palate by 2,3,7,8-TCDD may be associated with an increase in the number of steroid receptors. However, there is an additional level of complexity in this interaction, since hydrocortisone has been shown to increase the expression of the Ah receptor in the palate (Abbott et al., 1994c). The Ah receptor is required for 2,3,7,8-TCDD induction of cleft palate, as well as for all other well studied responses (reviewed in Birnbaum, 1994a). 2,3,7,8-TCDD causes a decrease in the level of Ah receptor expression in the palate at the time of fusion (Abbott et al., 1994d). Hydrocortisone blocks this decrease, suggesting that the synergistic induction of cleft palate by 2,3,7,8-TCDD and glucocorticoids may involve interactions of multiple receptor and growth factor systems.

2,3,7,8-TCDD can also interact synergistically with retinoic acid in the induction of cleft palate (Birnbaum et al., 1989). In contrast to the interaction with hydrocortisone, the retinoid/2,3,7,8-TCDD combination results in effects on growth factors resembling those seen with 2,3,7,8-TCDD (Abbott & Birnbaum, 1989b). It is not yet known whether retinoic acid up-regulates the Ah receptor in the palate, as has been demonstrated for the glucocorticoid receptor. However, 2,3,7,8-TCDD exposure can block a retinoid-induced increase in the retinoic acid receptor (Weston et al., 1995) in cultured mouse embryonic palatal mesenchyme cells. Wanner and co-workers (1995) have also shown that retinoic acid can suppress the differentiation-induced increase in the Ah receptor in cultured keratinocytes. Thus, there appears to be potential for cross-talk between the Ah receptor and receptors in the steroid family.

While the majority of studies examining 2,3,7,8-TCDD-induced changes in growth factor and hormone receptors have concentrated on the developing palate, changes have also been observed in the developing urinary tract. An increase in EGF receptors in the ureteric epithelium in response to PCDDs is associated with the induction of hydro-nephrosis (Abbott & Birnbaum, 1990b). This is similar to that observed in the enhanced proliferation of the medial epithelium in the palate. However, while PCDDs decreased Ah receptor expression in the developing palate at the time of fusion (Abbott et al., 1994d), there were no detectable changes in the levels of Ah receptor in the developing urinary tract at the same time (Bryant et al., 1995). 2,3,7,8-TCDD exposure on gestation day 10 leads to reduced levels of EGF in the ureteric epithelial cells, while TGFα remains unchanged (Bryant et al., 1996). No other growth factors or receptors have been examined in this target tissue. However, neither retinoids nor glucocorticoids cause hydronephrosis.

(b)   Functional developmental toxicity

(i)   Male reproductive system effects

In a series of studies, Mably et al. (1992a,b,c) exposed pregnant Holtzman rats on gestational day 15 to 2,3,7,8-TCDD at oral doses ranging from 0.064 to 1.0 μg/kg. They focused on the effects upon male offspring because of the decrease in circulating androgens observed in highly exposed adult male rats (Moore *et al.*, 1985). There was no effect on anogenital distance in the PCDD-treated pups at birth and on postnatal day 4 when corrected for body weight differences with the controls. At all times when they were measured (32–120 days of age), the weights of the accessory sex organs of the prenatally exposed male offspring were decreased in a dose-related fashion and both testicular and epididymal sperm counts were permanently reduced. The decrease in epididymal sperm count was observed at the lowest maternal dose tested (0.064 µg/kg) on day 120 and at most earlier times. When these male rats were mated around 70 and 120 days of age with control females, there was no significant effect upon fertility or survival and growth of the offspring.

Male sexual behaviour was also altered. The males took longer to mount receptive females, had more difficulty in achieving intromission and took more thrusts to achieve ejaculation (Gray *et al.*, 1995a). Mably *et al.* (1992c) reported a decrease in circulating androgen levels in the male offspring at birth. However, later studies from the same laboratory were not able to replicate these findings (Roman *et al.*, 1995). Feminization of sexual behaviour was also reported. When male pups prenatally exposed to PCDDs were treated with oestrogens and progesterone following castration, they demonstrated an increased lordotic response as compared to controls. The sexually dimorphic nuclei of the preoptic area of the hypothalamus were also examined to see if there was 'demasculinization', but no change was observed (Bjerke *et al.*, 1994).

Effects due to prenatal exposure to 2,3,7,8-TCDD were investigated in another laboratory (reviewed in Gray *et al.*, 1995b) using Long-Evans rats and Syrian hamsters. Both male and female offspring were studied. Rats were dosed with 1 µg/kg bw 2,3,7,8-TCDD by gastric instillation on gestational day 8 or 15 in order to determine if certain sensitive developmental effects would have been missed by exposing only towards the end of organogenesis. Hamsters were treated on gestational day 11, which is developmentally similar to gestational day 15 in the rat (Gray & Ostby, 1995; Gray *et al.*, 1995a). Dose–response studies were also conducted in rats, with doses of 0.8, 0.2, and 0.05 µg/kg maternal weight 2,3,7,8-TCDD (Gray *et al.*, 1995b). In general, the results obtained with Long-Evans rats were similar to those with Holtzman rats described above: prenatal exposure resulted in decreased sperm counts, decreased accessory sex organ weights and altered male mating behaviour. However, there were several significant differences. The decrease in anogenital distance was associated with a decrease in body weight (Gray *et al.*, 1995a). While the decrease in testicular sperm was statistically significant, it was quite small (~ 6%) and unlikely to explain the much larger decrease in epididymal (~ 35%) and ejaculated (~ 60%) sperm counts. No feminization of sexual behaviour was seen, and there was no reduction in serum testosterone level or in ventral prostate weight.

Although the male rat pups in both of these studies appeared to become aroused as readily as controls, they had more difficulty in achieving intromission and ejaculation. Whether this was associated with subtle changes in the penis remains to be determined. However, Bjerke & Peterson (1994) have observed a decrease in the weight of the glans penis. Gray *et al.* (1995a), in confirmation of the results of Roman *et al.* (1995), failed to observed any change in androgen status, including the lack of change in the number or affinity of androgen receptors. However, the two studies contrast in that no feminization of behaviour was observed in the Long-Evans rats (Gray *et al.*, 1995b). In the male hamster, there was no effect on the weight of testes or on serum testosterone level, although there was a reduction in epididymal and ejaculated sperm (Gray *et al.*, 1995a). The delay in puberty, however, as measured by preputial separation, appears to be a consistent finding among the two strains of rats and the hamster.

A significant decrease in epididymal sperm count was seen in the Long-Evans rats at a maternal dose of 0.2 µg/kg 2,3,7,8-TCDD and the ejaculated sperm count was reduced by 25% at a 0.05 µg/kg dose (Gray *et al.*, 1995b). Few other adverse effects were observed in the male Long-Evans offspring below 0.2 µg/kg. Premature eye opening, an effect previously seen in mice (Madhukar *et al.*, 1984), was seen at 0.05 µg/kg. Prenatal exposure was more effective on gestational day 15 than on gestational day 8 in terms of male reproductive effects. This suggests that the window of sensitivity for the male effects occurs late in organogenesis. Cross-fostering studies by Bjerke and Peterson (1994), and earlier studies by Khera and Ruddick (1973), indicated that all of the male reproductive effects can be induced prenatally. The only exception is the feminization of mating behaviour, already noted as a weak, if not species- and strain-specific, response (Brouwer *et al.*,1995).

Exposure of Syrian hamsters on gestational day 11 to 2 µg/kg 2,3,7,8-TCDD (a dose over 1000 times lower than the adult LD_{50}) resulted in effects similar to those observed in rats and, in spite of a decrease in seminal vesicle weight, there were no effects on male sexual behaviour or on testis weight. Puberty was delayed, and epididymal and ejaculated sperm count were permanently decreased (Gray *et al.*, 1995a,b).

(ii)   *Female reproductive system effects*

Multiple developmental effects were observed in female rats prenatally exposed to 1 µg/kg 2,3,7,8-TCDD on gestation day 8 or gestation day 15 (Gray & Ostby, 1995) and in female hamsters prenatally exposed to 2 µg/kg 2,3,7,8-TCDD on gestation day 11 (Gray *et al.*, 1995b). Vaginal opening was delayed in both species. In rats, two structural abnormalities were seen: a persistent vaginal thread across the normal vaginal opening, and clefting of the external genitalia in the female pups. In young adult female rats, there was no change in oestrous cyclicity, suggesting a normal hormonal profile. The changes in the external genitalia occurred at a higher incidence following exposure on gestational day 15 as compared to gestational day 8. In contrast, exposure early in organogenesis was associated with premature reproductive senescence in the female pups, many of whom stopped oestrous cycling before six months of age.

Prenatal exposure of hamsters resulted in similar effects (Gray *et al.*, 1995b). In some of the hamster pups, vaginal opening could not be easily detected; it was delayed in all of the others. Clefting of the external genitalia was present in all of the female hamster pups. Fertility was also decreased in the female hamster offspring, probably due to the structural problems in the external genitalia, since no effect on cyclicity was observed.

(iii) *Central nervous system effects*

Although most of the effects of prenatal exposure to 2,3,7,8-TCDD appear to directly target the developing genitourinary system, there is some evidence for involvement of the central nervous system. Gordon *et al.* (1995, 1996) have demonstrated that prenatal 2,3,7,8-TCDD exposure permanently depresses core body temperature in both rats and hamsters. Rats were examined at 18 months of age following prenatal exposure on gestational day 15 to 1 µg/kg 2,3,7,8-TCDD and hamsters at one year of age following exposure of the dam to 2 µg/kg on gestational day 11. The set point for body temperature is in the hypothalamus. The treated animals can still respond to a cold or heat stress by raising or lowering their body temperature as required, but their body temperature is always lower than that of controls.

(iv) *Persistence of effects*

A key finding of these functional developmental toxicity studies is the permanent nature of the responses following prenatal exposure. This is in contrast to some of the biochemical responses, such as induction of hepatic cytochrome P450 content and EROD activity, which returned to control levels by 120 days of age (Mably *et al.*, 1992a).

(v) *Hormonal effects*

Many of the developmental effects of 2,3,7,8-TCDD, such as clefting of the external genitalia, resemble those seen with high doses of oestrogens (Vannier & Raynaud, 1980). Endometriosis also requires the presence of oestrogens and, while low doses of 2,3,7,8-TCDD (Cummings *et al.*, 1996) and related compounds (Johnson *et al.*, 1996) promote the growth of endometriotic lesions in rodent models, high doses which cause ovarian atrophy, and thus reduced levels of oestrogens, are less effective.

Prenatal exposure to 0.025 or 0.1 µg/kg per day 2,3,7,8-TCDD on gestational days 10 to 16 of pregnant rats results in moderately depressed plasma T4 levels at weaning (Seo *et al.*, 1995). While the pups had lowered T4 levels, no effects on thyroid status were observed in the dams. This may have been associated with an increase in peripheral T4 metabolism in the pups (Morse *et al.*, 1993).

(vi) *Neurobehavioural effects*

Hearing deficits in rats, due to an increase in the auditory threshold, can be induced by exposure to a single dose of 2,3,7,8-TCDD of 0.3, 1.3 or 10 µg/kg on gestational day 19 (Goldey *et al.*, 1995, 1996). This response can be partially blocked by the addition of exogenous thyroxine, suggesting a role for a depression in circulating thyroid hormones in this response. Late gestational and lactational exposure of rats to 2,3,7,8-TCDD can result in changes in locomotor activity and rearing behaviour (Thiel *et al.*, 1994). Prenatal and lactational exposure of rhesus monkeys to 2,3,7,8-TCDD also causes changes in object learning (Schantz & Bowman, 1989).

(c) *Reproductive effects*

Reproductive effects have been reviewed by Allen *et al.* (1979), Morrissey and Schwetz (1989) and Theobald and Peterson (1994).

Multi-generation studies have been used to assess reproductive effects in both sexes. In a three-generation study in Sprague-Dawley rats, Murray *et al.* (1979) noted that exposure to a diet providing doses of up to 0.1 μg/kg bw per day 2,3,7,8-TCDD resulted in impaired reproductive capacity in rats as indicated by reductions in fertility and litter size. While they reported a maximal no-effect level of 1 ng/kg bw per day, a different method of statistical analysis indicated a lowest observed effect level of 1 ng/kg bw per day (Nisbet & Paxton, 1982). [The Working Group noted that no sex ratio data were provided.]

(i) *Male reproductive system*

2,3,7,8-TCDD causes a loss of germ cells, degeneration of both spermatocytes and mature spermatozoa within the seminiferous tubules, and a reduction in the number of tubules with mature spermatozoa. The lowest observed effect level for decreased spermatogenesis in Sprague-Dawley rats was 1 μg/kg per day in a 13-week study (Kociba *et al.*, 1976). This dose was associated with a depression in body weight gain and food consumption, indicating that effects on spermatogenesis occur only under conditions of overt toxicity. It was suggested that these adverse effects on the male reproductive system might be due to decreases in plasma testosterone and dihydrotestosterone concentration. A single dose of 15 μg/kg 2,3,7,8-TCDD caused a significant decrease in circulating testosterone levels within one day (Moore *et al.*, 1985). The decrease in circulating androgens appears to be due to decreased testicular responsiveness to LH and enhanced sensitivity of the pituitary to feedback inhibition by androgens and oestrogens (Moore *et al.*, 1989; Bookstaff *et al.*, 1990a,b; Kleeman *et al.*, 1990; Moore *et al.*, 1991).

The Leydig cell is the primary site of steroidogenesis in the testis. At intraperitoneal 2,3,7,8-TCDD doses of 12.5–50.0 μg/kg bw, there was a dose-dependent reduction in Leydig cell volume in Harlan/Sprague-Dawley rats, due to both fewer cells and reduced size of the individual cells (Johnson *et al.*, 1992c, 1994). This could play a role in the androgenic deficiency observed. Wilker *et al.* (1995) have shown that the effects on the Leydig cells can be prevented by treatment with human chorionic gonadotropic hormone (hCG) which had been previously shown to block the decrease in circulating testosterone levels (Ruangwies *et al.*, 1991).

Under normal conditions, reduction in circulating androgens would cause an increase in plasma LH, leading to a compensatory increase in testosterone biosynthesis by the Leydig cells. In adult male rats treated with toxic doses of 2,3,7,8-TCDD (50 μg/kg bw), in which the serum levels of androgens are decreased, the pituitary feedback regulation is impaired (Moore *et al.*, 1989; Bookstaff *et al.*, 1990a,b; Kleeman *et al.*, 1990).

(ii) *Female reproductive toxicity*

Treatment of the adult female with PCDDs can lead to reduced fertility, reduced litter size (Murray *et al.*, 1979), effects on ovarian cycling and overt ovarian toxicity. In adult rats, higher levels of exposure (1 μg/kg per day for 13 weeks) led to anovulation and suppression of the oestrous cycle (Kociba *et al.*, 1976).

Several reproductive studies have also been conducted in rhesus monkeys exposed to 2,3,7,8-TCDD in the diet (Allen *et al.*, 1977, 1979; Barsotti *et al.*, 1979). Females exposed to 500 ng/kg in the diet for nine months showed overt signs of maternal toxicity, including death. Only one of eight monkeys at this dose was able to carry an infant to term. In contrast to the higher dose, no overt effect on maternal health was seen at 50 ng/kg in the diet (Allen *et al.*, 1979).

When female rhesus monkeys were exposed to 5 or 25 ng/kg of 2,3,7,8-TCDD in the diet (Bowman *et al.*, 1989a; Schantz & Bowman, 1989), reproductive performance was not impaired in the low-dose group, in which seven out of eight monkeys gave birth to live offspring. In contrast, only one of eight females gave birth to a live infant in the 25-ng/kg group. These studies suggest that fetotoxicity can occur at doses below those causing maternal toxicity. Exposure of monkeys during early pregnancy to single or divided doses of 1 µg/kg bw 2,3,7,8-TCDD resulted in only three of 16 monkeys having live offspring, with most of the fetal loss being due to abortions (McNulty, 1984, 1985).

Anovulation and suppression of the oestrous cycle indicate ovarian dysfunction, and occur in both adult rats and monkeys following high doses of 2,3,7,8-TCDD causing overt toxicity (Kociba *et al.*, 1976; Allen *et al.*, 1979; Barsotti *et al.*, 1979). Li *et al.* (1995b) demonstrated that exposure of adult female Sprague-Dawley rats to a single dose of 10 µg/kg 2,3,7,8-TCDD resulted in a decrease in the number of ova ovulated per female, a decrease in the number of females ovulating and an increase in time spent in oestrous concomitant with a decrease in pro-oestrous and dioestrous. These effects were dose-dependent (Li *et al.*, 1995c), but were statistically significant only at doses that caused a loss in body weight ($\geq$ 10 µg/kg).

Rhesus monkeys were exposed to 0, 5, or 25 ng/kg 2,3,7,8-TCDD in their diet for four years and then held for up to an additional 10 years, when laparascopic surgery was performed. Both the incidence and severity of endometriosis were increased in a dose-dependent manner (Rier *et al.*, 1993). These findings have been supported by results from surgically induced endometriosis in both rats and mice (Cummings *et al.*, 1996). In both species, treatment with 2,3,7,8-TCDD (1.3 or 10 µg/kg bw given five times over a 16-week period) led to an increase in the size of endometriotic cysts in a dose-dependent fashion. 1,3,6,8-TCDD (2 or 20 mg/kg bw) did not enhance the growth of the endometriotic cysts (Johnson *et al.*, 1996). The highest dose of 2,3,7,8-TCDD (five times 10 µg/kg) was associated with ovarian atrophy and a decrease in the endometriotic response. This is not unexpected, since promotion of endometriosis requires oestrogen (Cummings & Metcalf, 1995). Studies with rhesus monkeys demonstrated that high levels of exposure to 2,3,7,8-TCDD result in a reduction in serum 17β-oestradiol levels (Barsotti *et al.*, 1979). This could be due to increased metabolism of oestrogen due to induction of hepatic microsomal enzymes.

Thus, while oestrogen is required for PCDD-induced promotion of endometriosis, the decrease in circulating oestradiol levels suggests an antioestrogenic effect of 2,3,7,8-TCDD. However, no effects on circulating oestradiol levels were seen in pregnant rats treated with 2,3,7,8-TCDD (Shiverick & Muther, 1983) or in mice (DeVito *et al.*, 1992). Another possibility is a direct effect on gonadal tissue, as suggested more recently by Li *et al.* (1995b,c). A third possibility is an alteration in target tissue responsiveness.

4.5   Genetic and related effects (see also Appendix 3 and **Table 64** for references)

Genetic effects of 2,3,7,8-TCDD have been reviewed (Kociba, 1984; Shu *et al.*, 1987). Indirect genetic effects are discussed in Section 4.6.

4.5.1   *Humans*

In 19 women [age unspecified] exposed to 2,3,7,8-TCDD after the Seveso accident and 16 control women aged 17–37 years, abortions were induced between weeks 8 and 16 of gestation in the exposed group and between weeks 8 and 13 in the control group. Cytogenetic studies were carried out on maternal peripheral lymphocytes, placental and umbilical cord tissues and fetal tissues. Significant increases (16.8% versus 5.5% and 1.51% versus 0.96%, respectively) in the frequencies of aberrant cells and in the average number of aberrations per damaged cell were found only in the fetal tissues in the group of exposed pregnancies (Tenchini *et al.*, 1983). [The Working Group noted the absence of differences in other tissues and of data on 2,3,7,8-TCDD concentrations in the fetuses; there was no indication of the zone in which the parents lived.]

In 27 male subjects aged 54–88 years (average age, 65.3 years) who were potentially exposed to 2,3,7,8-TCDD after the BASF accident in 1953 (see Section 1.3.1(*a*)(i)) and with a current blood concentration of 2,3,7,8-TCDD on a lipid basis exceeding 40 ng/kg, and 28 controls aged 53–93 years (average age, 65.1 years) without known exposure to 2,3,7,8-TCDD and with blood concentrations of less than 10 ng/kg, no statistically significant difference was found in the frequencies of chromosomal aberrations or sister chromatid exchange in peripheral lymphocytes in 1991 (Zober *et al.*, 1993).

4.5.2   *Experimental systems*

2,7-DCDD did not induce mutations in *Salmonella typhimurium* in either the presence or absence of an exogenous metabolic system in the only reported study. 2,7-DCDD did not transform C3H 10T1/2 cells or initiate transformation in these cells subsequently treated with 12-*O*-tetradecanoylphorbol 13-acetate (TPA). Continuous exposure to 2,7-DCDD did not promote cell transformation when the same cells were initiated by treatment with *N*-methyl-*N'*-nitro-*N*-nitrosoguanidine (MNNG).

2,3,7,8-TCDD did not induce mutations in *S. typhimurium* in either the presence or absence of an exogenous metabolic system.

2,3,7,8-TCDD produced conflicting results in tests for mutation in mouse lymphoma cells.

Single treatments with 2,3,7,8-TCDD did not induce transformation of C3H 10T1/2 cells or initiate the process of transformation in cultures subsequently exposed to TPA, whereas continuous treatment with low concentrations enhanced transformation of the same cells pretreated with MNNG. Neoplastic transformation was also observed in human epidermal keratinocytes immortalized by adenovirus 12–simian virus 40 (Ad12–SV40) but not in primary human epithelial keratinocytes.

Inhibition of gap-junctional intercellular communication was observed in mouse hepatoma cells and rat hepatocytes in primary culture, but not in Chinese hamster cells or

Table 64. Genetic and related effects of PCDDs

Test system	Result[a] Without exogenous metabolic system	With exogenous metabolic system	Dose[b] (LED/HID)	Reference
2,7-Dichlorodibenzo-*para*-dioxin				
SA0, *Salmonella typhimurium* TA100, reverse mutation	–	–	128	Mortelmans et al. (1984)
SA5, *Salmonella typhimurium* TA1535, reverse mutation	–	–	128	Mortelmans et al. (1984)
SA7, *Salmonella typhimurium* TA1537, reverse mutation	–	–	128	Mortelmans et al. (1984)
SA9, *Salmonella typhimurium* TA98, reverse mutation	–	–	128	Mortelmans et al. (1984)
TCM, Cell transformation, C3H 10T1/2 mouse cells	–[f,g]	NT	5	Abernethy & Boreiko (1987)
2,3,7,8-TCDD				
SA0, *Salmonella typhimurium* TA100, reverse mutation	NT	–	10	Geiger & Neal (1981)
SA0, *Salmonella typhimurium* TA100, reverse mutation	–	–	385	Mortelmans et al. (1984)
SA5, *Salmonella typhimurium* TA1535, reverse mutation	NT	–	10	Geiger & Neal (1981)
SA5, *Salmonella typhimurium* TA1535, reverse mutation	–	–	385	Mortelmans et al. (1984)
SA7, *Salmonella typhimurium* TA1537, reverse mutation	–	–	385	Mortelmans et al. (1984)
SA7, *Salmonella typhimurium* TA1537, reverse mutation	–	–	10	Geiger & Neal (1981)
SA8, *Salmonella typhimurium* TA1538, reverse mutation	0	–	10	Geiger & Neal (1981)
SA9, *Salmonella typhimurium* TA98, reverse mutation	0	–	10	Geiger & Neal (1981)
SA9, *Salmonella typhimurium* TA98, reverse mutation	–	–	385	Mortelmans et al. (1984)

Table 64 (contd)

Test system	Result[a]		Dose[b] (LED/HID)	Reference
	Without exogenous metabolic system	With exogenous metabolic system		
2,3,7,8-TCDD (contd)				
G51, Gene mutation, mouse lymphoma L5178Y cells, methotrexate or thymidine selection	+		0.1	Rogers et al. (1982)
G51, Gene mutation, mouse lymphoma L5178Y cells, thioguanine selection	(+)		0.5	Rogers et al. (1982)
G51, Gene mutation, mouse lymphoma L5178Y cells, ouabain or AraC selection	–		0.5	Rogers et al. (1982)
G5T, Gene mutation, mouse lymphoma L5178Y cells, tk locus	–	–	1	McGregor et al. (1991)
TCM, Cell transformation, C3H 10T1/2 mouse cells	–	NT	1.6	Abernethy et al. (1985)
UIH, Unscheduled DNA synthesis, human mammary epithelial cells in vitro	–	NT	0.003	Eldridge et al. (1992)
SHL, Sister chromatid exchange, human lymphocytes in vitro	+	NT	0.0004	Nagayama et al. (1995a)
MIH, Micronucleus test, human lymphocytes in vitro	+	NT	0.0004	Nagayama et al. (1993)
TIH, Cell transformation, immortalized human keratinocytes in vitro	+	NT	0.00004	Yang et al. (1992)
TIH, Cell transformation, primary human keratinocytes in vitro	–	NT	0.001	Yang et al. (1992)
HMA, Host-mediated assay, peritoneal macrophages in mouse	+[c]		0.0004 × 1 ip	Massa et al. (1992)
DVA, DNA strand breaks, rat liver in vivo	+		0.025 × 1 po	Wahba et al. (1989)
DVA, DNA strand breaks, rat peritoneal lavage cells in vivo	+[d]		0.025 × 1 po	Alsharif et al. (1994b)
MST, Mouse spot test	–[d]		0.003 × 1 ip	Fahrig (1993)
SVA, Sister chromatid exchange, rat lymphocytes in vivo	–[c]		0.03 × 1 po	Lundgren et al. (1986)
SVA, Sister chromatid exchange, C57BL/6J and DBA/2J mouse bone marrow in vivo	–		0.15 × 1 ip	Meyne et al. (1985)
MVM, Micronucleus test, C57BL/6J and DBA/2J mouse bone marrow in vivo	–		0.15 × 1 ip	Meyne et al. (1985)

Table 64 (contd)

Test system	Result[a]		Dose[b] (LED/HID)	Reference
	Without exogenous metabolic system	With exogenous metabolic system		
2,3,7,8-TCDD (contd)				
CBA, Chromosomal aberrations, C57BL/6J and DBA/2J mouse bone marrow *in vivo*	–		0.15 × 1 ip	Meyne *et al.* (1985)
SLH, Sister chromatid exchange, human lymphocytes *in vivo*	–		NG	Zober *et al.* (1993)
CLH, Chromosomal aberrations, human lymphocytes *in vivo*	–		(Seveso)	Tenchini *et al.* (1983)
CLH, Chromosomal aberrations, human lymphocytes *in vivo*	–		NG	Zober *et al.* (1993)
CLH, Chromosomal aberrations, human lymphocytes *in vivo*	–		(Seveso)	Reggiani (1980)
CVH, Chromosomal aberrations, human placental and umbilical cord tissues *in vivo*	–		(Seveso)	Tenchini *et al.* (1983)
CVH, Chromosomal aberrations, human fetal tissues *in vivo*	?		(Seveso)	Tenchini *et al.* (1983)
BVD, Binding (covalent) to DNA, mouse liver *in vivo*	–		0.1 × 1 ip	Turteltaub *et al.* (1990)
ICR, Inhibition of intercellular communication, Chinese hamster V79 cells	–	NT	0.003	Lincoln *et al.* (1987)
ICR, Inhibition of intercellular communication, C3H 10T1/2 mouse fibroblasts *in vitro*	–	NT	0.00003	Boreiko *et al.* (1989)
ICR, Inhibition of intercellular communication, mouse hepatoma cells (Hepa1c1c7) *in vitro*	+	NT	0.00003	De Haan *et al.* (1994)
ICR, Inhibition of intercellular communication, rat hepatocytes *in vitro*	+	NT	0.000000003	Baker *et al.* (1995)
ICR, Inhibition of intercellular communication, (³H]-uridine exchange), C3H 10T1/2 mouse cells	–	NT	0.01	Boreiko *et al.* (1989)
Octachlorodibenzo-*para*-dioxin				
SA0, *Salmonella typhimurium* TA100, reverse mutation	–	–	385	Zeiger *et al.* (1988)
SA5, *Salmonella typhimurium* TA1535, reverse mutation	–	–	385	Zeiger *et al.* (1988)
SA9, *Salmonella typhimurium* TA98, reverse mutation	–	–	385	Zeiger *et al.* (1988)

Table 64 (contd)

Test system	Result[a]		Dose[b] (LED/HID)	Reference
	Without exogenous metabolic system	With exogenous metabolic system		
Octachlorodibenzo-*para*-dioxin (contd)				
SAS, *Salmonella typhimurium* TA97, reverse mutation	–	–	385	Zeiger et al. (1988)
Mixtures of PCDDs, PCDFs and PCBs				
SHL, Sister chromatid exchange, human lymphocytes *in vitro*	+	NT	0.0004	Nagayama et al. (1994)
MST, Mouse spot test	–[d]		0.128 × 1 ip	Fahrig (1993)
SLH, Sister chromatid exchange, human lymphocytes *in vivo*	–		NG	Lundgren et al. (1988)
CLH, Chromosomal aberrations, human lymphocytes *in vivo*	–		NG	Lundgren et al. (1988)
BHD, Binding (covalent) to DNA, human placenta *in vivo*	–		NG	Gallagher et al. (1994)
1,2,3,6,7,8-Hexachlorodibenzo-*para*-dioxin				
TCM, Cell transformation, C3H 10T1/2 mouse cells	–	NT	0.39	Abernethy & Boreiko (1987)
1,2,3,7,8,9-Hexachlorodibenzo-*para*-dioxin				
TCM, Cell transformation, C3H 10T1/2 mouse cells	–	NT	0.39	Abernethy & Boreiko (1987)

[a] +, positive; (+), weak positive; –, negative; NT, not tested; ?, inconclusive

[b] LED, lowest effective dose; HID, highest ineffective dose; in-vitro tests, µg/mL; in-vivo tests, mg/kg bw/day; NG, not given

[c] Administred with 12-*O*-tetradecanoyl phorbol-13-acetate

[d] Co-treatment with ethylnitrosourea enhanced ENU activity two-fold

[e] α-Naphthoflavone-induced sister chromatid exchange was enhanced in lymphocyte cultures from TCDD-treated rats compared to controls

[f] Initiated with *N*-methyl-*N'*-nitro-*N*-nitrosoguanidine

[g] Subsequently exposed to 12-*O*-tetradecanoyl phorbol-13-acetate

murine fibroblasts, as measured by a metabolic cooperation assay or dye transfer. These results are discussed in Section 4.6.

Unscheduled DNA synthesis was not induced in normal human mammary epithelial cells. Increased formation of sister chromatid exchange and micronuclei was found in human lymphocytes *in vitro* in the presence or absence of α-naphthoflavone.

In a host-mediated assay, 2,3,7,8-TCDD elicited a dose-dependent response in cell-transforming potential on peritoneal macrophages which was seven times that of the 2,3,7,8-tetrabromo analogue.

In studies *in vivo*, positive results were reported for DNA single-strand breaks in rat liver and rat peritoneal lavage cells and for sister chromatid exchange frequency in rat lymphocytes in the presence but not in the absence of α-naphthoflavone. Use of a highly sensitive accelerator mass spectrometry approach did not reveal adduct formation following very low-level exposure in mouse liver.

Mutagenic and recombinogenic effects were observed only in combination with *N*-ethyl-*N*-nitrosourea in the spot test with mice.

A method capable of detecting one DNA adduct in 10^{11} nucleotides did not show binding of 2,3,7,8-TCDD to DNA in liver of mice dosed *in vivo*.

Changes in DNA I (indigenous)-compound formation were studied in Sprague-Dawley rats treated orally by gastric instillation with 2,3,7,8-TCDD, 1,2,3,7,8-PeCDD or 1,2,4,7,8-PeCDD (1 and 5 μg/kg bw in corn oil per week for four weeks). There were significant reductions in female, but not male rat hepatic I-compound formation after treatment with the two compounds substituted in all four lateral positions, whereas 1,2,4,7,8-PeCDD was inactive in this respect. No I-compound changes were observed in renal DNA following treatment with any of the compounds (Randerath *et al.*, 1988, 1990).

1,2,3,6,7,8- and 1,2,3,7,8,9-HxCDD did not transform C3H 10T1/2 cells or initiate transformation in the same cells subsequently treated with TPA. Continuous exposure to either of these two hexachlorinated congeners promoted cell transformation when the same cells were initiated by treatment with MNNG.

OCDD was not mutagenic in *S. typhimurium* (Zeiger *et al.*, 1988).

Mutations in tumours

DNA was extracted and analysed for activating mutations in H-*ras* codon 61 arising in hepatocellular adenomas and carcinomas of male and female B6C3F1 and C57BL/6 mice treated with a single intraperitoneal dose of vinyl carbamate (0.005 μM/g bw in saline) or vehicle and then gastric instillation doses of 2,3,7,8-TCDD (2.5 μg/kg bw in corn oil) every two weeks for 52 weeks. Another group received only the vinyl carbamate treatment. Of 45 tumours from B6C3F1 mice treated with 2,3,7,8-TCDD alone, only 23 (51%) had H-*ras* codon 61 mutations and 70% of these were C→A transitions in the first base. The pattern was similar to that found in spontaneous tumours of this strain and contrasted with the combined vinyl carbamate plus 2,3,7,8-TCDD and the vinyl carbamate alone-treated groups. In these two groups, respectively, there were A→T transitions in the second base in 39/53 (74%) and 17/27 (63%) of the tumours containing activating mutations. Similar results were obtained for the C57BL/6 mouse strain. Thus, 2,3,7,8-TCDD treatment did not change the mutational spectrum arising within H-*ras* codon 61 of tumours arising either without treatment or as a result of treatment with vinyl carbamate (Watson *et al.*, 1995).

Mixture of PCDDs and/or PCDFs

Mixtures of PCDDs did not enhance mutagenic or recombinogenic effects, but in combination with *N*-ethyl-*N*-nitrosourea, positive effects were obtained in the spot test with mice.

Mixtures of PCDDs, PCDFs and coplanar PCBs increased the frequency of sister chromatid exchange formation in human lymphocytes *in vitro* in the presence or absence of α-naphthoflavone.

4.6   Mechanisms of carcinogenicity

4.6.1   *Introduction*

In lifetime bioassays for cancer in rodents, 2,3,7,8-TCDD is a multisite carcinogen in both sexes of all species tested and causes tumours at sites distant from the point of administration (see Section 3).

2,3,7,8-TCDD is the most toxic of the PCDD and PCDF congeners. PCDDs and PCDFs exhibit a similar rank order of potency across species and within different cell types for numerous biochemical and biological responses. This is consistent with a similar mechanism of action via the Ah receptor. Binding to the Ah receptor is necessary but not sufficient for the expression of toxicity for this entire class of chemicals. For this reason, 2,3,7,8-TCDD and all PCDDs/PCDFs will be considered together regarding potential mechanisms of carcinogenicity (Poland & Knutson, 1982; Goldstein & Safe, 1989).

It is likely that the dose of 2,3,7,8-TCDD determines the mechanism of toxicity and carcinogenicity. At high doses, many acute effects are seen that have not been demonstrated in chronic dosing studies utilizing lower doses more relevant to human environmental exposures. Acute and chronic dosing regimens that yield equivalent body burdens may also produce different pathologies by different mechanisms. For these reasons, only effects seen at doses well below the lethal dose will be considered here in relation to the mechanism of carcinogenesis of 2,3,7,8-TCDD (see Sections 4.3, 4.4 and 4.5).

4.6.2   *General issues regarding mechanisms of carcinogenesis*

(a)   *Carcinogenesis is a multistep process*

Fundamentally there are three ways in which a compound such as a PCDD can influence the process of carcinogenesis (Barrett, 1993):

(i)   it may induce a heritable mutation (initiation);

(ii)   it may induce a heritable epigenetic change in a critical gene(s);

(iii) it may increase the clonal expansion of a cell possessing a heritable alteration in a critical gene(s).

(b)   *Genotoxicity*

2,3,7,8-TCDD is considered a 'non-genotoxic' substance (see Section 4.5).

(c)   *Ah receptor*

It has been proposed that the broad spectrum of biological responses associated with exposure to 2,3,7,8-TCDD is due to alteration in expression of 2,3,7,8-TCDD-regulated genes mediated by the Ah receptor (Section 4.3). However, even with the same receptor and the same ligand, there are both qualitative and quantitative differences between species. Even though Ah receptor activation is likely to be required for the carcinogenicity of 2,3,7,8-TCDD, its precise role in this process remains unclear.

In analogy to the mouse, two forms of Ah receptor exhibiting about a 4–5-fold difference in binding affinity for 2,3,7,8-TCDD (K_d, ~ 0.4 nM and ~ 2 nM, respectively) have been described in humans (Ema *et al.*, 1994).

(d)   *Effects of 2,3,7,8-TCDD on gene expression*

Induction of expression of genes driven by the XRE element (recognized by the Ah receptor), e.g., CYP1A1 and CYP1A2, represents a useful marker for 2,3,7,8-TCDD effects. The broad spectrum of effects of 2,3,7,8-TCDD on hormone and growth factor systems, cytokines and other signal transduction pathways indicates that this substance is a powerful growth dysregulator (see Sections 4.3 and 4.4).

(e)   *Oxidative damage*

In a series of studies by Stohs and colleagues, single treatment of rats or mice with high doses (≥ 50 µg/kg) resulted in increased superoxide anion production by peritoneal lavage cells, lipid peroxidation and DNA single-strand breaks (Stohs *et al.*, 1990; Alsharif *et al.*, 1994b). The relevance of these high dose studies to the carcinogenicity of 2,3,7,8-TCDD is questionable.

In-vitro studies showed that the promotion of transformation of C3H mouse fibroblasts by low non-cytotoxic concentrations of 2,3,7,8-TCDD (1.5 pM) was inhibited by the antioxidants mannitol and vitamins C and A (Wölfle & Marquardt, 1996). Promotion of cellular transformation is a well documented effect of 2,3,7,8-TCDD, as discussed below, and this study provides evidence for an oxidative-stress mechanism for this effect. Another study showed an Ah receptor-dependent formation of 8-hydroxydeoxyguanine (8-OH-dG) adducts in DNA following treatment of the mouse Hepa1c1c7 cell line with 500 pM 2,3,7,8-TCDD for 48 h (Park *et al.*, 1996).

Production of oxidative damage by 2,3,7,8-TCDD is consistent across several different experimental systems, both *in vivo* and *in vitro*. The requirement in rats for ovarian hormones in the mechanism of tumour promotion by 2,3,7,8-TCDD (Lucier *et al.*, 1991) is associated with a 2–3-fold higher level of 8-OH-dG DNA adduct formation in intact compared with ovariectomized rats (Tritscher *et al.*, 1996). It has been suggested that this increase in 8-OH-dG DNA adducts is a result of a production of genotoxic metabolites via redox cycling of catechol oestrogens, although there may be alternative sources of reactive oxygen species. The role of these adducts in carcino-genicity has yet to be established.

(f)   Cell transformation

In the mouse C3H 10T1/2 embryonic fibroblast cell transformation system (which contains a functional Ah receptor (Okey *et al.*, 1983)), significant increases in foci formation in cells pre-initiated with MNNG were observed following exposure to non-cytotoxic doses of 2,3,7,8-TCDD (4–4000 pM 2,3,7,8-TCDD) in a dose-dependent pattern (Abernethy *et al.*, 1985). 2,3,7,8-TCDD also gave positive results in an in-vitro transformation assay using rat tracheal epithelial cells only after prior initiation of the cells with MNNG and at concentrations of at least 300 pM continuously for seven days (Tanaka *et al.*, 1989). These data support the observations that 2,3,7,8-TCDD acts as a tumour promoter *in vivo*.

Virally immortalized human foreskin epidermal keratinocytes treated with 100 pM 2,3,7,8-TCDD were transformed, as shown by colony formation in soft agar, foci formation, an increased maximal cell density and a 100% incidence of squamous-cell carcinomas in nude mice when injected with 1×10^7 cells compared with an incidence of zero with cells exposed to 0.1% dimethyl sulfoxide (Yang *et al.*, 1992). Maximal induction of neoplastic transformation occurred at 1 nM, whereas induction of aryl hydrocarbon hydroxylase activity was maximal at 30 nM. Neoplastic transformation of human cells occurs at a concentration similar to that needed for rodent cell trans-formation.

(g)   Cell proliferation and tumour promotion

Since 2,3,7,8-TCDD is not directly genotoxic, it either could be acting to 'promote' the development of tumours from previously initiated cells and/or may be causing mutations via an indirect mechanism.

In a rat tumour initiation–promotion protocol experiment, hepatic cell proliferation as measured by BrdU incorporation (labelling index) was decreased at a dose of 3.5 ng/kg 2,3,7,8-TCDD per day and increased an average of three-fold at 125 ng/kg 2,3,7,8-TCDD per day, after 30 weeks of 2,3,7,8-TCDD treatment (Maronpot *et al.*, 1993). Significant interindividual variation was observed in labelling index, with approximately half of the animals exhibiting significantly higher labelling indices than similarly treated animals. Preneoplastic GSTP-positive foci were elevated only at 125 ng/kg per day. Cell proliferation was significantly stronger in initiated than in non-initiated rats. In another study by Stinchcombe *et al.* (1995), 2,3,7,8-TCDD only marginally affected DNA synthesis in GSTP-positive liver foci after treatment with a dose 100 ng/kg 2,3,7,8-TCDD per day for 115 days. However, in this study, apoptosis in foci was markedly reduced.

(h)   Suppression of immune surveillance

Effects on the immune system can have significant effects on the disease process and the manifestation of toxicity in other organ systems. This is particularly relevant to cancer, where a primary effect of 2,3,7,8-TCDD on immune function could secondarily aid in the progression and development of malignancy by allowing genetically altered cells to escape immune surveillance. There is a wealth of information concerning immune suppression in laboratory animals, but results on immune function in human studies are inconsistent (see Sections 4.2.1 and 4.2.2(*b*)).

4.6.3 *Tissue-specific mechanisms of carcinogenicity of 2,3,7,8-TCDD*

(*a*) *Liver*

(i) *Sex differences in carcinogenicity in the liver*

Female rats appear to be more sensitive than male rats to the hepatocarcinogenic effects of 2,3,7,8-TCDD. This sex difference has not been observed in mice. Furthermore, sex differences in carcinogenic responsiveness were not observed in either rats or mice given a mixture of 1,2,3,6,7,8-HxCDD and 1,2,3,7,8,9-HxCDD (see Section 3).

(ii) *Possible role of ovarian hormones in tumorigenesis*

Sex-dependent cell proliferation and altered hepatic foci formation were observed in the livers of intact but not ovariectomized rats in a 2,3,7,8-TCDD tumour promotion study, an effect which was not attributable to differences in liver concentrations. This suggests a possible role of ovarian hormones, presumably oestrogens. On the basis of these results, an indirect genotoxic mechanism of tumour promotion by TCDD was suggested. This involves induction of cytochromes P450 which metabolize 17β-oestradiol to catechols (Lucier *et al.*, 1991). These catechols (e.g., 2-hydroxyoestradiol and 4-hydroxyoestradiol) can be converted to semiquinone intermediates, possibly forming reactive singlet oxygen species (Liehr & Roy, 1990), subsequently leading to an increase in oxidative stress or DNA damage (Liehr, 1990; Yager & Liehr, 1996).

Another hypothesis for the role of ovarian hormones in the mechanism of liver tumour development is an alteration in the signal transduction pathway for oestrogens. Hepatic oestrogen receptor complex level and binding capacity are down-regulated in rats after in-vivo exposure to 2,3,7,8-TCDD (Romkes *et al.*, 1987; Romkes & Safe, 1988; Harris *et al.*, 1990; Clark *et al.*, 1991a; Zacharewski *et al.*, 1991, 1992, 1994).

(iii) *Effects on epidermal growth factor receptor*

2,3,7,8-TCDD decreases the amount of detectable plasma membrane EGF receptor in liver *in vivo* and keratinocytes *in vitro* (Madhukar *et al.*, 1984; Hudson *et al.*, 1985; Astroff *et al.*, 1990; Choi *et al.*, 1991; Lin *et al.*, 1991a; Sewall *et al.*, 1993, 1995). In one study, however, changes in cell proliferation occurred in populations of hepatocytes different from those in which there was induction of CYP1A1/CYP1A2 (Fox *et al.*, 1993), while down-regulation of the EGF receptor occurs throughout the liver (Sewall *et al.*, 1993).

In a tumour initiation–promotion protocol, there was no effect of 2,3,7,8-TCDD on the EGF receptor in ovariectomized rats paralleling the tumour incidence data, even though CYP1A1 and CYP1A2 induction profiles were similar. The maximal decrease in EGF receptor binding was three-fold at a dose of 125 ng/kg per day and an ED_{50} of 10 ng/kg per day (1.5 μg 2,3,7,8-TCDD/kg liver fat). EGF receptor effects occur at lower doses than induction of cell proliferation or foci, consistent with this effect being a contributing factor in the hepatocarcinogenic action of TCDD. Decreased EGF receptor binding may be indicative of increased EGF expression and thus a mechanistically plausible predictor of increased cell proliferation (Clark *et al.*, 1991a; Lucier *et al.*, 1991; Sewall *et al.*, 1993).

(iv) *Cellular localization*

Induction of CYP1A1 and CYP1A2 protein following chronic exposure to 2,3,7,8-TCDD exhibited a dose-dependent increase in acinar zones 2 and 3 (Tritscher *et al.*, 1992). In contrast, changes in cell proliferation following 2,3,7,8-TCDD exposure do not show an acinar-dependent pattern and in one study occurred in different populations of hepatocytes than induction of CYP1A1/CYP1A2 (Fox *et al.*, 1993). In addition, down-regulation of the EGF receptor (Sewall *et al.*, 1993) and expression of the Ah receptor are observed throughout the liver. This may imply that there is a differential sensitivity of hepatocytes to 2,3,7,8-TCDD induction.

(v) *Alterations in gap-junctional communication by 2,3,7,8-TCDD*

Whether inhibition of gap-junctional intercellular communication (GJIC) has a causal role in the mechanism of carcinogenesis for 2,3,7,8-TCDD, or is a response that occurs as a result of other events during tumour promotion is unknown.

Alterations in connexin (Cx) expression and alterations in GJIC have been observed following exposure to 2,3,7,8-TCDD *in vitro* and *in vivo* in rodents. Treatment of Fischer 344 rats (that had been initiated orally with 10 mg/kg NDEA) with 100 ng/kg 2,3,7,8-TCDD per day for eight months resulted in a significant increase in altered hepatic foci. In these foci, there was decreased expression of Cx32, increased Cx26 expression, and a complete absence of Cx43 expression (Neveu *et al.*, 1994). 2,3,7,8-TCDD inhibited GJIC in rat hepatocytes grown in primary culture in a time-, dose- and Ah receptor-dependent manner at doses of 2,3,7,8-TCDD from 10^{-12} to 10^{-8} M, indicating that inhibition of GJIC is a highly sensitive response to 2,3,7,8-TCDD (Baker *et al.*, 1995). Cx32 expression was decreased, while Cx26 was unaffected.

Alteration of GJIC has also been seen with other PCDDs and PCDFs. Inhibition of GJIC by PCDD and PCDFs correlated well with their potency to induce CYP1A1 (as measured by EROD activity in Hepa1c1c7 cells (De Haan *et al.*, 1996). The concentration required for half-maximal response (EC_{50}) for both responses for all congeners was ≤ 1 nM and the dose–response curves were parallel. These same authors previously demonstrated that this effect was Ah receptor-dependent (De Haan *et al.*, 1994). 2,3,7,8-TCDD had no effect on GJIC in mouse V79 or C3H 10T1/2 cells (Lincoln *et al.*, 1987; Boreiko *et al.*, 1989).

(vi) *Cytotoxicity as mechanism for hepatic lesions*

Hepatocellular toxicity has been observed in rat carcinogenicity experiments (see Section 3) and might play a role in carcinogenesis.

(*b*)   *Other target tissues*

2,3,7,8-TCDD-induced carcinogenesis has been reported in a number of other tissues including lung, nasal ethnoturbinates, thyroid, lymphoid tissues, skin and tongue (see Section 3). Ah receptor expression and receptor-dependent responses have been observed in many of these tissues (see Section 4.3) and may play a role in carcinogenesis. A study in congenic strains of mice and using a number of isomers has indicated a role for the Ah receptor in PCDD-induced skin papilloma (Poland *et al.*, 1982).

In the case of thyroid carcinogenesis, an indirect mechanism has been proposed involving enhanced metabolism of thyroid hormones in the liver (see Section 4.3) (Hill *et al.*, 1989; Kohn *et al.*, 1996).

4.6.4   *Mechanisms for reduced cancer incidence following 2,3,7,8-TCDD exposure*

Two mechanisms have been proposed to explain negative trends in cancer incidence. Firstly, reductions in tumour incidence could be due to alterations in body weight (known since Tannenbaum, 1940) as a result of 2,3,7,8-TCDD exposure. Secondly, 2,3,7,8-TCDD disrupts the endocrine homeostasis, and may thereby reduce the incidence of hormone-dependent cancers such as mammary and uterine cancers.

5.   Summary of Data Reported and Evaluation

5.1   Exposure data

Polychlorinated dibenzo-*para*-dioxins (PCDDs) are formed as inadvertent by-products, sometimes in combination with polychlorinated dibenzofurans (PCDFs), during the production of chlorophenols and chlorophenoxy herbicides, and have been detected as contaminants in these products. PCDDs and PCDFs also may be produced in thermal processes such as incineration and metal-processing and in the bleaching of paper pulp with free chlorine. The relative amounts of PCDD and PCDF congeners produced depend on the production or incineration process and vary widely.

PCDDs are ubiquitous in soil, sediments and air. Excluding occupational or accidental exposures, most human exposure to PCDDs occurs as a result of eating meat, milk, eggs, fish and related products, as PCDDs are persistent in the environment and accumulate in animal fat. Occupational exposures to PCDDs at higher levels have occurred since the 1940s as a result of production and use of chlorophenols and chloro-phenoxy herbicides. Even higher exposures have occurred sporadically in relation to accidents in these industries.

Mean background levels of 2,3,7,8-tetrachlorodibenzo-*para*-dioxin (2,3,7,8-TCDD) in human tissues today are in the range of 2–3 ng/kg fat. Available data suggest that these levels have decreased by a factor of 3 to 5 since the late 1970s, when the development of gas chromatography/mass spectrometry methodology first permitted these extremely low levels of PCDDs in tissues and the environment to be measured accurately. Similarly, since the mid-1980s, mean tissue levels of total PCDDs and PCDFs (measured as international toxic equivalents (I-TEQs)) in the general population have decreased by two- to three-fold. Human exposures related to occupation or accidents have led to tissue levels of 2,3,7,8-TCDD up to several orders of magnitude higher than background levels.

5.2   Human carcinogenicity data

In the evaluation of the evidence of carcinogenicity of 2,3,7,8-TCDD, more weight has been given to studies with direct 2,3,7,8-TCDD measurements and to studies involving heavy exposure to herbicides likely to be contaminated with 2,3,7,8-TCDD. The effects of 2,3,7,8-TCDD and those of the products in which it was found cannot be separated in most of the epidemiological studies; however, the focus here is on the contaminant.

The most important studies for the evaluation of the carcinogenicity of 2,3,7,8-TCDD are four cohort studies of herbicide producers (one each in the United States and the Netherlands, two in Germany), and one cohort of residents in a contaminated area from Seveso, Italy. These studies involve the highest exposures to 2,3,7,8-TCDD among all epidemiological studies, although the exposures at Seveso were lower and the follow-up shorter than those in the industrial settings. In addition, the multi-country cohort study from IARC is of special interest because it includes three of four high-exposure cohorts and other industrial cohorts, many of them not reported in separate publications, as well as some professional applicators. Most of the four industrial cohorts include analyses of sub-cohorts considered to have the highest exposure and/or longest latency. These cohorts, and their respective high-exposure sub-cohorts, are the focus of the summary here. Additional studies of herbicide applicators, both cohort and case–control studies, who have considerably lower exposures to 2,3,7,8-TCDD, are not considered critical for the evaluation.

An increased risk for all cancers combined is seen in the cohort studies cited above. The magnitude of the increase is generally low; it is higher in sub-cohorts considered to have the heaviest 2,3,7,8-TCDD exposure within the cohorts listed above. Furthermore, statistically significant positive dose–response trends for all cancers combined were present in the largest and most heavily exposed German cohort. A positive trend ($p = 0.05$) was also seen in the smaller German cohort where an accident occurred with release of large amounts of 2,3,7,8-TCDD; the positive trend in this cohort was limited to smokers. Cumulative dose in both these trend analyses was estimated by combining data from blood 2,3,7,8-TCDD levels and knowledge of job categories, work processes and calendar time of exposure. Increased risks for all cancers combined were also seen in the longer-duration longer-latency sub-cohort of the United States study. These positive trends with increased exposure tend to reinforce the overall positive association between all cancers combined and exposure, making it less likely that the increase is explained by confounding, either by smoking or by other carcinogenic exposures in the industrial setting.

An increased risk for lung cancer is also present in the most informative cohort studies, again especially in the more highly exposed sub-cohorts. The relative risk for lung cancer in the combined highly exposed sub-cohorts was estimated to be 1.4 (statistically significant). It is possible that lung cancer relative risks of this order could result from confounding by smoking, but only if there were a pronounced difference in smoking habits between the exposed population and the referent populations, a difference which seems unlikely. It therefore seems unlikely that confounding by smoking can explain all the excess lung cancer risk, although it could explain part of it. It is also possible that other occupational carcinogens, many of which would affect the lung, are causing some confounding.

An excess risk for soft-tissue sarcoma, based on a small number of deaths, has been reported. Incidence data for soft-tissue sarcoma were generally not available. A case–control study nested in the IARC international cohort found a dose–response relationship with estimated 2,3,7,8-TCDD exposure; however, strong positive trends were also found with estimated exposure to 2,4-dichlorophenoxyacetic acid (2,4-D) and 2,4,5-trichloro-phenoxyacetic acid (2,4,5-T). A similar increase in soft-tissue sarcoma was present in the Seveso population, but only in the zone which overall had the lowest exposure. No such increase is present in the German or Dutch cohort studies. Soft-tissue sarcomas are subject to serious misclassification on death certificates; although it is unlikely that this occurs differentially in the exposed and the referent populations, reclassification of a few cases would have important consequences on results based on small numbers.

An increased risk for non-Hodgkin lymphoma was found in most of the populations studied in the four industrial cohort studies and in the Seveso population, although the relative risks were mostly nonsignificant and below 2. A case–control study nested in the IARC international cohort provided weak evidence of a dose–response relationship with estimated 2,3,7,8-TCDD exposure. Although it is plausible that other chemicals cause non-Hodgkin lymphoma, strong potential confounding factors are not known. The lack of complete consistency among the studies and the weak effect detected in most of the positive ones, however, caution against a causal interpretation of the findings.

Increased risks for several other malignant neoplasms have been sporadically reported among workers exposed to 2,3,7,8-TCDD, and at Seveso, perhaps most notable being for digestive system cancers and multiple myeloma. The available results are not fully consistent, and several studies have not reported the results for each individual cancer site.

Overall, the strongest evidence for the carcinogenicity of 2,3,7,8-TCDD is for all cancers combined, rather than for any specific site. The relative risk for all cancers combined in the most highly exposed and longer-latency sub-cohorts is 1.4. While this relative risk does not appear likely to be explained by confounding, this possibility cannot be excluded. There are few examples of agents which cause an increase in cancers at many sites; examples are smoking and ionizing radiation in the atomic bombing survivors (for which, however, there are clearly elevated risks for certain specific cancer sites). This lack of precedent for a multi-site carcinogen without particular sites predominating means that the epidemiological findings must be treated with caution; on the other hand, the lack of precedent cannot preclude the possiblity that in fact 2,3,7,8-TCDD, at high doses, does act as a multi-site carcinogen. It should be borne in mind that the general population is exposed to levels far lower than those experienced by the industrial populations.

5.3   Animal carcinogenicity data

2,3,7,8-TCDD was tested for carcinogenicity by oral administration in three experiments in mice and in three experiments in rats. It was also tested by exposure of immature mice and by intraperitoneal or subcutaneous injection in one study in hamsters, and by skin application in mice.

In three experiments in two strains of mice, administration of 2,3,7,8-TCDD orally by gastric instillation increased the incidence of hepatocellular adenomas and carcinomas in both males and females. In one of these three experiments, 2,3,7,8-TCDD increased the incidence of follicular-cell adenomas of the thyroid, lymphomas and subcutaneous fibrosarcomas in female mice; a trend for an increased incidence of alveolar/bronchiolar adenomas or carcinomas in male mice was also observed.

Oral administration of 2,3,7,8-TCDD by gastric instillation or in the diet to rats increased the incidence of benign hepatocellular neoplasms (identified as adenomas, neoplastic nodules and hyperplastic nodules) in females in two strains and the incidence of hepatocellular carcinomas in one strain. An increased incidence of follicular-cell adenomas of the thyroid in male and female rats in the study with administration by gastric instillation was reported. In the feeding study, 2,3,7,8-TCDD increased the incidence of squamous-cell carcinomas of the tongue, hard palate, nasal turbinates and lung in both sexes of rats. In the feeding study, a high incidence of endocrine-related tumours (pituitary adenomas, phaeochromocytomas and pancreatic islet-cell tumours) was observed in control female rats. The incidence of these tumours was lower after treatment with 2,3,7,8-TCDD, associated with decreased body weight.

In one experiment involving oral administration to immature mice of two strains, 2,3,7,8-TCDD increased the incidence of hepatocellular adenomas and carcinomas in males and that of hepatocellular adenomas in females of one strain. Treatment of immature mice increased the incidence of thymic lymphomas in male and female mice of both strains.

Application of 2,3,7,8-TCDD to the skin increased the incidence of dermal fibrosarcomas in female mice. Intraperitoneal or subcutaneous administration of 2,3,7,8-TCDD to small groups of hamsters increased the incidence of squamous-cell carcinomas of the skin.

In several studies in mice, administration of 2,3,7,8-TCDD following administration with known carcinogens enhanced the incidences of skin papillomas, lung adenomas, liver adenomas and hepatoblastomas. 2,3,7,8-TCDD enhanced the incidence of focal hepatic lesions in several strains of female rats following administration of various N-nitrosamines. In one study, 2,3,7,8-TCDD enhanced the incidence of lung carcinomas in ovariectomized compared with intact female rats following administration of N-nitrosodiethylamine.

In summary, 2,3,7,8-TCDD administered at low doses by different routes to rats and mice causes tumours at multiple sites. It also causes tumours in hamsters.

Dibenzo-*para*-dioxin was tested for carcinogenicity by oral administration in one experiment in mice and in one experiment in rats. No increased incidence of tumours at any site was observed in mice or rats of either sex.

2,7-Dichlorodibenzo-*para*-dioxin (2,7-DCDD) was tested for carcinogenicity by oral administration in one experiment in mice and in one experiment in rats. No increased incidence of tumours was seen at any site in rats of either sex. In male but not in female mice, an increased incidence of hepatocellular adenomas was observed, but the impurity of the chemical confounds an evaluation of its carcinogenicity. In one study, 2,7-DCDD did not enhance the incidence of skin papillomas in mice treated with *N*-methyl-*N'*-nitro-*N*-nitrosoguanidine.

A mixture of 1,2,3,6,7,8- and 1,2,3,7,8,9-hexachlorodibenzo-*para*-dioxins was tested for carcinogenicity by oral administration in mice and in rats, and by administration to the skin in mice. The incidence of hepatocellular adenomas was increased in male and female mice and in female rats following oral administration. Impurities in the mixture were unlikely to have been responsible for the observed response. No significant increase in tumours at any site was observed following application to the skin in mice.

In other studies, administration of either 1,2,3,7,8-pentachlorodibenzo-*para*-dioxin or 1,2,3,4,6,7,8-heptachlorodibenzo-*para*-dioxin led to an increased incidence of hepatic focal lesions in female rats following treatment with nitrosamines.

Administration of a defined mixture of 49 PCDDs increased the incidence of hepatic focal lesions in female rats following treatment with *N*-nitrosomorpholine.

5.4   Other relevant data

5.4.1   *Kinetics*

In most vertebrate species, the 2,3,7,8-substituted PCDDs are the congeners which are predominantly retained. If chlorine atoms are present on all 2,3,7,8 positions, the biotransformation rate of PCDDs is strongly reduced, resulting in significant bioaccumulation. In most species the liver and adipose tissue are the major storage sites.

As Ah receptor-mediated effects are caused primarily by the parent compound, biotransformation to more polar metabolites should be considered to be a detoxification process. Although kinetics influence the biological and toxic effects, genetic factors seem to play a dominant role.

5.4.2   *Toxic effects*

Human exposure to 2,3,7,8-TCDD or other PCDD congeners due to industrial or accidental exposure has been associated with chloracne and alterations in liver enzyme levels in both children and adults. Changes in the immune system and glucose metabolism have also been observed in adults. Infants exposed to PCDDs and PCDFs through breast milk exhibit alterations in thyroid hormone levels and possible neurobehavioural and neurological deficits.

The extraordinary potency of 2,3,7,8-TCDD and related 2,3,7,8-substituted PCDDs has been demonstrated in many animal species. The lethal dose of 2,3,7,8-TCDD, however, varies more than 5000-fold between the guinea-pig, the most sensitive, and the hamster, the least sensitive species. In all mammalian species tested so far, lethal doses of 2,3,7,8-TCDD result in delayed death preceded by excessive body weight loss ('wasting').

Other signs of 2,3,7,8-TCDD intoxication include thymic atrophy, hypertrophy/-hyperplasia of hepatic, gastrointestinal, urogenital and cutaneous epithelia, atrophy of the gonads, subcutaneous oedema and systemic haemorrhage.

In tissue culture, 2,3,7,8-TCDD affects growth and differentiation of keratinocytes, hepatocytes and cells derived from other target organs. Toxicity of 2,3,7,8-TCDD segregates with the Ah receptor, and relative toxicity of other PCDD congeners is associated with their ability to bind to this receptor.

PCDDs cause suppression of both cell-mediated and humoral immunity in several species at low doses.

PCDDs have the potential to suppress resistance to bacterial, viral and parasitic challenges in mice.

5.4.3   Effects on reproduction

Most studies on reproductive effects of PCDDs in humans concerned paternal exposure, usually long after high exposure had occurred. Most studies have a limited power to detect elevations in specific birth defects. The studies also showed discordant results concerning an increase in the risk of spontaneous abortions. Some studies have shown alterations in hormone levels and sperm characteristics after PCDD exposure.

2,3,7,8-TCDD is both a developmental and reproductive toxicant in experimental animals. The developing embryo/fetus appears to display enhanced sensitivity to the adverse effects of PCDDs. Perturbations of the reproductive system in adult animals require overtly toxic doses. In contrast, effects on the developing organism occur at doses > 100 times lower that those required in the mother. Sensitive targets include the developing reproductive, nervous and immune systems. Perturbation of multiple hormonal systems and their metabolism due to PCDD exposure may play a role in these events.

5.4.4   Genetic effects

In human studies after in-vivo exposure, there have been no unequivocal reports of effects of 2,3,7,8-TCDD or other PCDD congeners upon the frequencies of chromosomal aberrations.

In animal studies *in vivo* and in cultured human and animal cells *in vitro*, 2,3,7,8-TCDD gave conflicting results with regard to several genetic endpoints, such as DNA damage, gene mutations, sister chromatid exchange and cell transformation.

Experimental data indicate that 2,3,7,8-TCDD and probably other PCDDs and PCDFs are not direct-acting genotoxic agents.

5.4.5 *Mechanistic considerations*

The administration of 2,3,7,8-TCDD in rodent bioassays significantly increased the incidence of benign and/or malignant tumours in various tissues (liver, lung, lymphatic system, soft tissue, nasal turbinates, hard palate, thyroid and tongue) in both sexes. The number of tumours per animal (multiplicity) was small. Prior exposure to a known carcinogen and subsequent exposure to 2,3,7,8-TCDD enhanced (promoted) tumour incidence and/or multiplicity and resulted in the appearance of tumours at earlier times. While 2,3,7,8-TCDD has been demonstrated to increase tumour incidence at different sites, the pattern of tumour sites is a function of species, sex and study.

2,3,7,8-TCDD is not directly genotoxic. A number of hypotheses addressing the mechanisms of 2,3,7,8-TCDD-mediated tumour promotion have been presented. These hypotheses include Ah receptor-mediated alteration in expression of networks of genes involved in cell growth and differentiation, DNA damage mediated by cytochrome P450-catalysed metabolic activation pathways, expansion of preneoplastic cell populations via inhibition of apoptosis, positive modulation of intra- or extracellular growth stimuli, or suppression of immune surveillance. For thyroid tumour induction, an indirect mechanism of 2,3,7,8-TCDD-induced carcinogenesis has also been proposed. In rodents, the induction of hepatic uridine diphosphate-glucuronosyl transferase resulted in enhanced elimination of thyroid hormones as glucuronides from the circulation, and subsequent enhanced stimulation of the thyroid gland via elevated levels of circulating thyroid-stimulating hormone.

(a) *Ah receptor*

The Ah receptor is a ubiquitous transcription factor found in both rodents and humans. PCDDs bind to human and rodent Ah receptors with very similar structure–activity relationships; 2,3,7,8-TCDD has the highest affinity of the PCDDs for both rodent and human receptors.

Both in humans and in mice, two forms of Ah receptor have been identified which exhibit a 5–10-fold difference in binding affinity for 2,3,7,8-TCDD. In humans, one form of the Ah receptor exhibits a K_d (a measure of binding affinity) for 2,3,7,8-TCDD of 0.4 nM, whereas the other form binds 2,3,7,8-TCDD with a K_d of about 2 nM.

In congenic mouse strains, expression of the lower or higher affinity forms of receptor has been extensively demonstrated to result in proportional differences in sensitivity to 2,3,7,8-TCDD with regard to biochemical changes and toxic effects. Thus, congenic mice expressing the lower-affinity form of receptor require higher doses of 2,3,7,8-TCDD to elicit these effects than strains expressing higher-affinity forms. A similar difference in sensitivity to PCDDs has also been demonstrated in tumour promotion studies in skin of congenic mouse strains. In these studies, PCDDs show the same rank order of potency in Ah receptor binding *in vitro* and tumour induction *in vivo*. Taken together, these data strongly support a receptor-mediated mechanism of mouse skin carcinogenesis.

(b)   Gene expression

The best studied 2,3,7,8-TCDD-dependent gene expression response is the induction of *CYP1A1* and *CYP1A2*. In both rodent and human cells, this response is mediated by the Ah receptor. In rodent and human cells, PCDDs show very similar potencies in inducing *CYP1A1* and *CYP1A2* expression in rodent and human cells. The role, if any, of the induction of these genes in carcinogenesis by 2,3,7,8-TCDD is unclear. 2,3,7,8-TCDD-induced gene regulatory responses and biochemical effects documented in rodent tissues and/or cells have also been observed in human tissues or cells.

(c)   Comparison of tissue concentrations in humans and animals

Four epidemiological studies of high-exposure industrial cohorts in Germany, the Netherlands and the United States found an increase in overall cancer mortality.

In these cohorts, the blood lipid 2,3,7,8-TCDD levels estimated to the last time of exposure were 2000 ng/kg (mean) (up to 32 000 ng/kg) in the United States cohort, 1434 ng/kg geometric mean (range, 301–3683 ng/kg) among accident workers in the Dutch cohort, 1008 ng/kg geometric mean in the group of workers with severe chloracne in the BASF accident cohort in Germany and measurements up to 2252 ng/kg in the Boehringer cohort in Germany. These calculated blood 2,3,7,8-TCDD levels in workers at time of exposure were in the same range as the estimated blood levels in a two-year rat carcino-genicity study. In rats exposed to 100 ng/kg bw 2,3,7,8-TCDD per day, hepatocellular carcinomas and squamous-cell carcinomas of the lung were observed. Estimated blood levels were 5000–10 000 ng/kg 2,3,7,8-TCDD. In the same study, in rats exposed to 10 ng/kg bw 2,3,7,8-TCDD per day, hepatocellular nodules and focal alveolar hyperplasia were observed. Estimated blood levels were 1500–2000 ng/kg 2,3,7,8-TCDD. These results indicate parallel tumorigenic responses to high exposure to 2,3,7,8-TCDD in both humans and rats.

In view of the results mentioned above, it should be noted that the present background levels of 2,3,7,8-TCDD in human populations (2–3 ng/kg) are 100 to 1000 times lower than those observed in this rat carcinogenicity study. Evaluation of the relationship between the magnitude of the exposure in experimental systems and the magnitude of the response (i.e., dose–response relationships) do not permit conclusions to be drawn on the human health risks from background exposures to 2,3,7,8-TCDD.

5.5   Evaluation[1]

There is *limited evidence* in humans for the carcinogenicity of 2,3,7,8-tetrachloro-dibenzo-*para*-dioxin.

There is *sufficient evidence* in experimental animals for the carcinogenicity of 2,3,7,8-tetrachlorodibenzo-*para*-dioxin.

There is *evidence suggesting lack of carcinogenicity* in experimental animals for dibenzo-*para*-dioxin.

---

[1] For definition of the italicized terms, see Preamble, pp. 26–27.

There is *limited evidence* in experimental animals for the carcinogenicity of a mixture of 1,2,3,6,7,8- and 1,2,3,7,8,9-hexachlorodibenzo-*para*-dioxins.

There is *inadequate evidence* in experimental animals for the carcinogenicity of 2,7-dichlorodibenzo-*para*-dioxin.

There is *inadequate evidence* in experimental animals for the carcinogenicity of 1,2,3,7,8-pentachlorodibenzo-*para*-dioxin.

There is *inadequate evidence* in experimental animals for the carcinogenicity of 1,2,3,4,6,7,8-heptachlorodibenzo-*para*-dioxin.

Overall evaluation

2,3,7,8-Tetrachlorodibenzo-*para*-dioxin is *carcinogenic to humans (Group 1)*.

In making the overall evaluation, the Working Group took into consideration the following supporting evidence:

(i) 2,3,7,8-TCDD is a multi-site carcinogen in experimental animals that has been shown by several lines of evidence to act through a mechanism involving the Ah receptor;

(ii) this receptor is highly conserved in an evolutionary sense and functions the same way in humans as in experimental animals;

(iii) tissue concentrations are similar both in heavily exposed human populations in which an increased overall cancer risk was observed and in rats exposed to carcinogenic dosage regimens in bioassays.

Other polychlorinated dibenzo-*para*-dioxins are *not classifiable as to their carcinogenicity to humans (Group 3)*.

Dibenzo-*para*-dioxin is *not classifiable as to its carcinogenicity to humans (Group 3)*.

POLYCHLORINATED DIBENZOFURANS

1. Exposure Data

1.1 Chemical and physical data

1.1.1 *Nomenclature and molecular formulae and weights*

Chemical Abstracts Service (CAS) names and synonyms, CAS Registry numbers, molecular formulae and molecular weights for selected polychlorinated dibenzofurans (PCDFs) are presented in **Table 1**. The tetra-, penta-, hexa- and hepta-chlorinated compounds are referred to here as TCDFs, PeCDFs, HxCDFs and HpCDFs, or collectively as, for example, Cl_4–Cl_7 PCDFs or hepta/octa-CDFs.

Table 1. Nomenclature, molecular formulae and molecular weights of selected polychlorinated dibenzofurans

CAS Registry No.	CAS name and synonyms[a]	Molecular formula	Molecular weight
51207-31-9	**2,3,7,8-Tetrachlorodibenzofuran**; F83; TCDF; 2,3,7,8-TCDF; 2,3,7,8-tetra-CDF	$C_{12}H_4Cl_4O$	305.98
57117-41-6	**1,2,3,7,8-Pentachlorodibenzofuran**; F94; 1,2,3,7,8-PeCDF; 1,2,3,7,8-penta-CDF	$C_{12}H_3Cl_5O$	340.42
57117-31-4	**2,3,4,7,8-Pentachlorodibenzofuran**; F114; 2,3,4,7,8-PeCDF; 2,3,4,7,8-PnCDF; 2,3,4,7,8-penta-CDF	$C_{12}H_3Cl_5O$	340.42
70648-26-9	**1,2,3,4,7,8-Hexachlorodibenzofuran**; F118; 1,2,3,4,7,8-HxCDF; 1,2,3,4,7,8-hexa-CDF	$C_{12}H_2Cl_6O$	374.87
57117-44-9	**1,2,3,6,7,8-Hexachlorodibenzofuran**; F121; 1,2,3,6,7,8-HxCDF; 2,3,4,7,8,9-hexachlorodibenzofuran; 1,2,3,6,7,8-hexa-CDF	$C_{12}H_2Cl_6O$	374.87
72918-21-9	**1,2,3,7,8,9-Hexachlorodibenzofuran**; F124; 1,2,3,7,8,9-HxCDF; 1,2,3,7,8,9-hexa-CDF	$C_{12}H_2Cl_6O$	374.87
60851-34-5	**2,3,4,6,7,8-Hexachlorodibenzofuran**; F130; 2,3,4,6,7,8-HxCDF; 2,3,4,6,7,8-hexa-CDF	$C_{12}H_2Cl_6O$	374.87
67562-39-4	**1,2,3,4,6,7,8-Heptachlorodibenzofuran**; F131; 1,2,3,4,6,7,8-HpCDF; 1,2,3,4,6,7,8-hepta-CDF	$C_{12}HCl_7O$	409.31
55673-89-7	**1,2,3,4,7,8,9-Heptachlorodibenzofuran**; F134; 1,2,3,4,7,8,9-HpCDF; 1,2,3,4,7,8,9-hepta-CDF	$C_{12}HCl_7O$	409.31
39001-02-0	**Octachlorodibenzofuran**; F135; OCDF; octa-CDF; perchlorodibenzofuran	$C_{12}Cl_8O$	444.76

[a] Names in bold letters are the Chemical Abstracts Service (CAS) names

1.1.2 *Structural formulae*

The general structure of the PCDFs is shown in **Table 2**. Any or all of the eight hydrogen atoms on dibenzofuran can be replaced with chlorine, giving rise to 135 possible chlorinated dibenzofuran structures. All of the 135 are referred to as congeners (members of a like group) of one another, and congeners having the same number of chlorines are isomers (Clement, 1991).

Table 2. Dibenzofuran structural formula and numbers of chlorinated isomers

Formula

No. of chlorines $(x + y)$	No. of isomers
1	4
2	16
3	28
4	38
5	28
6	16
7	4
8	1
Total	135

1.1.3 *Chemical and physical properties*

Knowledge of basic chemical and physical properties is essential to understanding and modelling environmental transport and fate as well as pharmacokinetic and toxico-logical behaviour. The most important parameters for the PCDFs appear to be water solubility, vapour pressure, and octanol/water partition coefficient (K_{ow}). The ratio of vapour pressure to water solubility yields the Henry's Law constant for dilute solutions of organic compounds, an index of partitioning for a compound between the vapour and aqueous solution phases (Mackay *et al.*, 1991). Chemical and physical properties of selected PCDFs are presented in **Table 3**.

Limited research has been carried out to determine physical and chemical properties of PCDFs. As with the polychlorinated dibenzo-*para*-dioxins (PCDDs), the tetra- to octa-chloro congeners with 2,3,7,8-chlorination have received the most attention. Of the large number of possible congeners, only the 2,3,7,8-chlorinated compounds and a few others are available commercially, and preparation and synthesis can be both time-consuming and difficult. Some of the PCDF congeners have not yet been prepared in pure form. Like the PCDDs, the PCDFs are intentionally prepared only for research purposes.

Table 3. Chemical and physical properties of selected PCDFs[a]

Chemical	Melting point (°C)	Water solubility (mg/L)	Vapour pressure (Pa) at 25 °C	Henry's Law constant (Pa × m³/mol)[b]	log K_{ow}
2,3,7,8-TCDF	227–228	4.19×10^{-4} at 22.7 °C	2×10^{-6}	1.5	6.53
1,2,3,7,8-PeCDF	225–227		2.3×10^{-7}		6.79
2,3,4,7,8-PeCDF	196–196.5	2.36×10^{-4} at 22.7 °C	3.5×10^{-7}	[0.5]	6.92
1,2,3,4,7,8-HxCDF	225.5–226.5	8.25×10^{-6} at 22.7 °C	3.2×10^{-8}	[1.43]	
1,2,3,6,7,8-HxCDF	232–234	1.77×10^{-5} at 22.7 °C	2.9×10^{-8}	[0.6]	
1,2,3,7,8,9-HxCDF	246–249		2.4×10^{-8}		
2,3,4,6,7,8-HxCDF	239–240		2.6×10^{-8}		
1,2,3,4,6,7,8-HpCDF	236–237	1.35×10^{-6} at 22.7 °C	4.7×10^{-9}	[1.4]	7.92
1,2,3,4,7,8,9-HpCDF	221–223		6.2×10^{-9}		
OCDF	258–260	1.16×10^{-6} at 25 °C	5×10^{-10}	[0.2]	8.78

[a] From Burkhard & Kuehl (1986); Rordorf (1989); Sijm *et al.* (1989); Friesen *et al.* (1990); Mackay *et al.* (1991)
[b] Values in brackets have been calculated by the Working Group.

The concept of toxic equivalency factors (TEFs) was developed by several agencies and national and international organizations (Ahlborg, 1989; Safe, 1990; Ahlborg *et al.*, 1992; Birnbaum & De Vito, 1995) to aid in the interpretation of the complex database and in the evaluation of the risk of exposure to mixtures of structurally related PCDDs and PCDFs. TEF values are derived by evaluating the potency of each PCDD and PCDF isomer relative to that of tetrachlorodibenzo-*para*-dioxin (2,3,7,8-TCDD). TEFs are order-of-magnitude estimates that are based on the evaluation of all available infor-mation, including binding to the Ah receptor (see Section 4) and other in-vitro responses as well as in-vivo effects ranging from enzyme induction to tumour formation (Ahlborg *et al.*, 1992; Birnbaum & De Vito, 1995).

The levels of all the individual PCDDs and PCDFs in a mixture may be converted into one value of toxic equivalents (TEQs), as follows:

$$\text{TEQ} = \Sigma \ (\text{TEF} \times \text{concentration})$$

Assignment of relative potencies in a quantitative sense imposes appreciable demands on the experimental data. All congeners must exhibit parallel dose–response curves for the effects studied to be treated as additive. Additivity is an implicit assumption of the TEF concept. Many in-vitro and in-vivo studies have supported the hypothesis that the toxic effects of combinations of PCDDs and PCDFs are additive and have supported the applicability of the TEF concept in practice (Ahlborg *et al.*, 1992a).

Toxicologists have widely adopted the set of TEFs shown in **Table 4** (I-TEFs, also adopted by NATO (North Atlantic Treaty Organization)). Other sets of TEFs have been used in the past (e.g. BGA (German), Nordic, Swiss, Eadon (american)), but TEQs calculated with these TEFs normally do not differ from those based on I-TEFs by more than a factor of 2 (Ahlborg *et al.*, 1988; Rappe *et al.*, 1993).

Table 4. I-TEFs for 2,3,7,8-substituted PCDFs[a]

Congener	I-TEF
2,3,7,8-TCDF	0.1
1,2,3,7,8-PeCDF	0.05
2,3,4,7,8-PeCDF	0.5
1,2,3,4,7,8-HxCDF	0.1
1,2,3,6,7,8-HxCDF	0.1
1,2,3,7,8,9-HxCDF	0.1
2,3,4,6,7,8-HxCDF	0.1
1,2,3,4,6,7,8-HpCDF	0.01
1,2,3,4,7,8,9-HpCDF	0.01
OCDF	0.001
All other PCDFs	0

[a] From Ahlborg *et al.* (1992a);
Rappe *et al.* (1993)
I-TEF, international toxic equivalency factor

1.1.4   *Methods of analysis*

Analysis for PCDFs in the environmental and biological matrices uses essentially the same methods as those developed for PCDDs. In fact, analyses for PCDFs and PCDDs are very frequently performed concurrently. Thus, methods of analysis for both classes of compounds are discussed in the monograph on PCDDs, and the designations A-W used here are those given in Table 5 of the PCDD monograph on page 39.

1.2   **Formation and destruction**

PCDFs can be formed by a number of different reactions including synthetic chemical, thermal, photochemical and biochemical; analogous pathways can be used for their destruction. PCDFs already present in reservoir sources such as sediments, soil and sewage sludge are significant contributors to current environmental levels.

1.2.1   *Formation of PCDFs*

(a)   *Chemical reactions*

(i)   *Polychlorinated biphenyls (PCBs)*

Mixtures of PCBs (see IARC, 1987d) have been widely used since the 1930s as dielectric fluids in electrical equipment such as cables, transformers and capacitors. They have also been used as non-flammable heat-exchange liquids and as additives to plastics and in cutting oil. The total world production is estimated to exceed 500 000 tonnes

(Rappe *et al.*, 1979a). Primarily due to environmental problems, use of PCBs has now been phased out in most European countries and in many others.

Vos *et al.* (1970) identified PCDFs (tetra- and penta-CDFs) in samples of European PCBs (Phenoclor DP-6 and Clophen A60) but not in a sample of American Aroclor 1260. The toxic effects of these PCBs were found to parallel the levels of PCDFs present. Bowes *et al.* (1975) examined a series of Aroclors as well as the same samples of Aroclor 1260, Phenoclor DP-6 and Clophen A60 previously analysed by Vos *et al.* (1970). They used packed column gas chromatography (GC) with low-resolution mass spectrometry and very few standard compounds and reported that the most abundant PCDFs were PeCDFs (**Table 5**). Using a complete set of PCDF standards and high-resolution GC, Rappe *et al.* (1985a) determined the levels of 2,3,7,8-substituted PCDFs in commercial PCB products (see **Table 6**).

Table 5. Concentrations of PCDFs in PCBs (mg/kg)

PCB[a]	TCDFs	PeCDFs	HxCDFs	Total
Aroclor 1248 (1969)	0.5	1.2	0.3	2.0
Aroclor 1254 (1969)	0.1	0.2	1.4	1.7
Aroclor 1254 (1970)	0.2	0.4	0.9	1.5
Aroclor 1260 (1969)	0.1	0.4	0.5	1.0
Aroclor 1260 (lot AK3)	0.2	0.3	0.3	0.8
Aroclor 1016 (1972)	ND	ND	ND	
Clophen A 60	1.4	5.0	2.2	8.4
Phenoclor DP-6	0.7	10.0	2.9	13.6

From Bowes *et al.* (1975)
ND, not detected at 0.001 mg/kg
[a] Production year in parentheses

(ii) *Chlorophenols*

Chlorophenols (see IARC, 1986b; 1987c) have been used extensively since the 1950s as insecticides, fungicides, mould inhibitors, antiseptics and disinfectants. In 1978, the annual world production was estimated to be approximately 150 000 tonnes (Rappe *et al.*, 1979a). Due to occupational and environmental risks, the use of chlorophenols has now been phased out in most European countries and in a few countries outside Europe. The most important use of 2,4,6-tri-, 2,3,4,6-tetra- and pentachlorophenol (PCP) and their salts is for wood preservation. PCP is also used as a fungicide for slime control in the manufacture of paper pulp and for a variety of other purposes such as in cutting oils and fluids, for tanning leather and in paint, glues and outdoor textiles. **Table 7** summarizes a number of relevant analyses of the levels of PCDFs in commercial chlorophenol formulations (Rappe *et al.*, 1978b).

Buser and Bosshardt (1976) reported the results of a survey of the PCDF and PCDD content of PCP and its sodium salt from commercial sources in Switzerland (analytical method AC). On the basis of the results, the samples could be divided into two groups:

Table 6. Concentrations of PCDFs in commercial PCBs (µg/kg)

PCB type	Tri-CDF	TCDFs		PeCDFs			HxCDFs					HpCDFs
	Total	2378-	Total	12348-/12378-	23478-	Total	123479-/123478	123678-	123789-	234678-	Total	Total
Pyralene	700	53	630	10	T	35	ND	ND	ND	ND	ND	ND
Aroclor 1254	63	19	1 400	690	490	4 000	2 500	2 100	190	130	10 000	960
Aroclor 1260	10	13	110	48	56	260	500	120	190	27	1 500	1 300
Aroclor 30	500	35	573	14	28	160	50	59	ND	ND	220	T
Aroclor 40	1 300	180	2 600	96	8	1 700	79	68	ND	T	310	ND
Aroclor 50	7 400	3 300	20 000	760	1 100	8 000	700	360	18	98	3 100	75
Clophen A60	770	840	6 900	1 100	990	8 100	1 600	330	170	330	6 800	2 000
Clophen T64	47	23	360	97	122	840	520	390	58	41	2 600	220
Clophen	710	54	1 200	34	30	270	ND	T	ND	ND	T	ND

T, traces; ND, not detected
From Rappe et al. (1985a)

a first series with generally low levels (HxCDD, < 1 mg/kg) and a second series with much higher levels (HxCDD, > 1 mg/kg) of PCDDs. Samples with high PCDD levels also had high levels of PCDFs. The ranges of the combined levels of PCDFs were 1–26 mg/kg for the first series of samples and 85–570 mg/kg for the second series of samples. The levels of OCDF were as high as 300 mg/kg and this congener dominated the PCDF content of the samples.

Table 7. Levels of PCDFs in commercial chlorophenols (mg/kg)

	2,4,6-Tri-chlorophenol	2,3,4,6-Tetra-chlorophenol	Pentachlorophenol	
			Sample A	Sample B
TCDFs	1.5	0.5	0.9	≤ 0.4
PeCDFs	17.5	10	4	40
HxCDFs	36	70	32	90
HpCDFs	4.8	70	120	400
OCDF	< 1	10	130	260

From Rappe *et al.* (1978b); Rappe & Buser (1981)

(iii) *Pulp bleaching*

During the 1950s, free chlorine gas was introduced for the bleaching of pulp in pulp and paper mills. In 1986–87, it was first reported that bleaching pulp using free chlorine gas produced 2,3,7,8-TCDF (Rappe *et al.*, 1987a). A survey performed in 1987 in the United States showed that the concentrations of 2,3,7,8-TCDF in bleached pulp ranged from undetectable (at a detection limit of 1.2 ng/kg) up to 330 ng/kg, with a median concentration of 50 ng/kg and a mean of 93 ng/kg (Gillespie & Gellman, 1989).

New technology has been developed for pulp bleaching using chlorine dioxide (ECF, elemental chlorine free) or non-chlorinated reagents (TCF, total chlorine free). 2,3,7,8-TCDF at a level of about 0.2 ng/kg was found in ECF- and TCF-bleached pulp (Rappe & Wågman, 1995).

(iv) *Production of chlorine*

Chlorine is produced primarily by the electrolysis of brine. The annual world production in 1995 was estimated to be 40 million tonnes (Fauvarque, 1996). Rappe *et al.* (1991) reported that residues from the production of chlorine using the chloralkali process were highly contaminated with PCDFs. The problem is particularly associated with the use of graphite electrodes in the process. The graphite electrode process was for a long time the dominant technology and is still very widespread. Chlorine butter, a by-product from this process, was already identified as a chloracnegen 100 years ago. Only a few samples from chloralkali plants have been analysed, primarily from landfills. Total PCDF concentrations of 0.6–0.7 mg/kg have been found. The pattern of PCDFs is dominated by the 2,3,7,8-substituted tetra- to hepta-CDFs, resulting in a nordic TEQ value of 10–30 µg/kg (see **Table 8**).

Table 8. Levels of PCDFs (ng/kg) in three samples of electrode sludge from chloralkali plants

	Sample 1	Sample 2	Sample 3
2,3,7,8-TCDF	26 000	56 000	57 000
Total TCDFs	64 000	150 000	140 000
1,2,3,4,8-/1,2,3,7,8-PeCDF	25 000	55 000	56 000
2,3,7,8-PeCDF	12 000	25 000	24 000
Total PeCDFs	75 000	240 000	240 000
1,2,3,4,7,9-/1,2,3,7,8-HxCDF	32 000	71 000	73 000
1,2,3,6,7,8-HxCDF	7 000	16 000	15 000
Total HxCDFs	68 000	140 000	140 000
1,2,3,4,6,7,8-HpCDF	9 100	19 000	19 000
1,2,3,4,7,8,9-HpCDF	8 100	19 000	20 000
Total HpCDFs	24 000	53 000	54 000
OCDF	31 000	76 000	71 000
TEQ (nordic)	13 000	28 000	28 000

From Rappe *et al.* (1991)

(v)   *Production of vinyl chloride*

Stringer *et al.* (1995) reported the analyses of three samples of residues from the production of vinyl chloride (see IARC, 1987e), an intermediate in the production of polyvinyl chloride (PVC) (analytical method ACS). In all samples, the concentrations of PCDFs were much higher than those of PCDDs and the higher chlorinated 2,3,7,8-substituted congeners constituted a substantial proportion (see **Table 9**).

(b)   *Thermal reactions*

(i)   *Incineration of municipal waste*

Olie *et al.* (1977) reported the occurrence of PCDDs and PCDFs in fly ash from three municipal incinerators in the Netherlands. Their results indicated only the presence of PCDFs, without isomer identification or quantification. Buser *et al.* (1978a) quantified PCDDs and PCDFs in fly ash from a municipal incinerator and an industrial heating facility in Switzerland. In the former, the level of total PCDFs was 0.1 mg/kg. In the industrial incinerator fly ash, the level was 0.3 mg/kg.

In 1986, a working group of experts convened by the World Health Organization Regional Office for Europe (WHO/EURO, 1987) reviewed the available data on emissions of PCDDs from municipal solid-waste incinerators. They concluded that, because of their high thermal stability, PCDFs were destroyed only after adequate residence times (> 2 s) at temperatures above 800 °C. Total emissions of PCDFs from tests on municipal solid-waste incinerators were reported to range between a few and several thousand ng/m^3 dry gas at 10% carbon dioxide. The WHO working group prepared a table giving a range of estimated isomer-specific emissions for those isomers of major concern with respect to municipal solid-waste incinerators operating under various conditions (**Table 10**).

Table 9. Concentrations of PCDFs in still bottoms and residues from vinyl chloride production (µg/kg)

	Sample 1[a]	Sample 2[b]	Sample 3[c]
2,3,7,8-TCDF	0.91	680	0.44
Total TCDF	15	20 600	6
1,2,3,7,8-PeCDF	9.5	975	1.8
2,3,4,7,8-PeCDF	1.6	1 050	0.58
Total PeCDFs	65	45 300	11
1,2,3,4,7,8-HxCDF	110	10 100	11
1,2,3,6,7,8-HxCDF	24	9 760	2.4
1,2,3,7,8,9-HxCDF	9.5	21 800	1.3
2,3,4,6,7,8-HxCDF	3.1	930	0.89
Total HxCDFs	300	63 700	27
1,2,3,4,6,7,8-HpCDF	250	13 400	38
1,2,3,4,7,8,9-HpCDF	51	1 340	6
Total HpDFs	450	16 600	58
OCDF	390	43 500	650
I-TEQ	20	6 370	3.9

From Stringer *et al.* (1995)
[a] Sample 1 is a process waste including, but not limited to, distillation residues, heavy ends, tars and reactor clean-out wastes, from the production of certain chlorinated aliphatic hydrocarbons by free radical catalysed processes.
[b] Sample 2 is a waste from heavy ends from the distillation of ethylene in ethylene dichloride production.
[c] Sample 3 is a waste from heavy ends from the distillation of vinyl chloride in vinyl chloride monomer production.

The emissions tabulated in column 1 are those which the working group considered to be achievable in modern, highly controlled and carefully operated plants in use in 1986. The results given in column 1 are not representative of emissions that might be expected from such plants during start-up or during occasional abnormal conditions. Emission levels listed in column 2 were considered by the working group to be indicative of the upper limit of emissions from modern municipal solid-waste incinerators. These plants might experience such emissions during start-up or during occasional abnormal conditions, although some of the data reviewed have shown that the figures in column 2 should not be considered to be an absolute maximum. However, most plants existing in 1986, if carefully operated, will have had PCDF emissions in the range between columns 1 and 2. The highest values for municipal solid-waste incinerators (column 3) were obtained by multiplying the values in column 2 by a factor of 5. Emission data that were reported to the working group from all tests and under all circumstances were no greater than these values. Generally, these emission levels are associated with irregular or unstable operating conditions, high moisture content of the municipal solid waste or low combustion or afterburner temperatures. Of special importance is the observation that the major contributor to the TEQ was 2,3,4,7,8-PeCDF.

Table 10. Estimated range of emissions of PCDFs from municipal solid-waste (MSW) and municipal sewage sludge (MSS) incinerators

| | Emissions from MSW combustion (ng/m³) | | | | Emissions from MSS combustion (ng/m³) |
| | Achievable with modern plants with no gas cleaning | Maximum from average operation | High emissions[a] | Achievable with modern plants with gas cleaning[b] | Most probably highest emissions |
	(1)	(2)	(3)	(4)	(5)
2,3,7,8-TCDF	0.9	10	50	0.1	0.9
1,2,3,7,8-/1,2,3,4,8-PeCDF	2.3	52	260	0.2	2.3
2,3,4,7,8-PeCDF	2.0	40	200	0.2	2.0
1,2,3,4,7,8-/1,2,3,4,7,9-HxCDF	1.1	48	240	0.1	1.1
1,2,3,6,7,8-HxCDF	1.3	40	200	0.1	1.3
1,2,3,7,8,9-HxCDF	0.06	52	260	–	0.06
2,3,4,6,7,8-HxCDF	2.0	36	180	0.2	2.0

From WHO/EURO (1987) excepted when noted
[a] Values obtained by multiplying values in column 2 by a factor of 5
[b] Adapted from ECETOC (1992)

During the second half of the 1980s and 1990, regulatory agencies in several countries, such as Germany, the Netherlands and Sweden, announced strict regulations for municipal solid-waste incinerators. The European Union value is 0.1 ng TEQ/m^3 (European Union, 1994) (see column 4, **Table 10**). This directive has resulted in the introduction of modern air pollution control devices and, together with improved burning conditions, has led to a decrease in PCDF emissions from municipal solid-waste incinerators, which had been considered to be major sources.

(ii) *Incineration of sewage sludge*

Sludge from municipal waste-water treatment plants may be incinerated after being dehydrated. The WHO working group in 1986 reviewed the available data from municipal sewage sludge incinerators and found that PCDD and PCDF emissions from this type of plant were generally lower than emissions from municipal solid-waste incinerators (see Table 10, column 5) (WHO/EURO, 1987).

(iii) *Incineration of hospital waste*

Doyle *et al.* (1985) claimed that the incomplete combustion of certain hospital wastes containing halogenated compounds could produce high emissions of PCDFs. They found the mean levels of total PCDFs to be 156 ng/m^3, but no isomer-specific data were available. Data cited by the United States Environmental Protection Agency indicate that flue gas emissions from hospital waste incinerators are in the range of 10–100 ng I-TEQ/m^3, higher than the levels achievable with modern municipal solid-waste incinerators (United States Environmental Protection Agency, 1994; Thomas & Spiro, 1995). [The Working Group noted that, due to smaller emission volumes, the overall emissions from hospital waste incinerators are generally lower than those from the municipal solid-waste incinerators.]

(iv) *Incineration of polyvinyl chloride (PVC)*

The extent to which PCDFs are formed during the combustion of PVC is a controversial issue. However, the incineration conditions appear to be quite important. On the basis of laboratory experiments, Christmann *et al.* (1989a) considered PVC to be an important source of PCDFs. However, experiments performed in incinerators showed the effect of PVC on the formation of PCDFs to be minimal (Frankenhaeuser *et al.*, 1993; Wikström *et al.*, 1996).

(v) *Combustion of wood*

Schatowitz *et al.* (1994) studied PCDD/PCDF emissions from small-scale laboratory studies of combustion of wood and household waste (analytical method ABS). The results (in ng I-TEQ/m^3) are summarized in **Table 11**. Data on PCDDs and PCDFs are not separated.

(vi) *Automobile emissions*

Hagenmaier *et al.* (1990) reported on the emissions of PCDFs and the lower chlorinated congeners and brominated analogues in automobile emissions from four representative experiments using leaded gasoline, unleaded gasoline with or without catalytic converters and diesel fuel (analytical method ABS). The results are summarized in **Table 12**.

Table 11. PCDD/PCDF emissions from wood and household waste combustion

Fuel	Furnace	PCDD/PCDFs (ng I-TEQ/m^3)
Beech wood sticks	Fireplace	0.064
Beech wood sticks	Stick wood boiler	0.019–0.034
Wood chips	Automatic chip furnace	0.066–0.214
Uncoated chipboard	Automatic chip furnace	0.024–0.076
Waste wood chips	Automatic chip furnace	2.70–14.42
Household waste	Household stove, closed	114.4

From Schatowitz *et al.* (1994)

Table 12. PCDFs from automobile emissions (pg/m^3)

	Leaded gasoline	Unleaded gasoline	Unleaded gasoline with catalytic converter	Diesel engine
TCDFs	6 628	110	6.8	3.9
2,3,7,8-TCDF	201.4	8.5	0.55	1.04
PeCDFs	1 514	180	6.9	2.0
1,2,3,7,8-PeCDF	141.2	8.6	0.43	< 0.26
2,3,4,7,8-PeCDF	58.4	4.0	0.31	0.36
HxCDFs	824	73	4.3	1.3
1,2,3,4,7,8-HxCDF	111.8	8.1	0.62	0.33
1,2,3,6,7,8-HxCDF	111.8	4.1	0.81	0.34
1,2,3,7,8,9-HxCDF	< 10.0	7.3	0.02	< 0.26
2,3,4,6,7,8-HxCDF	35.7	10.5	0.59	< 0.26
HpCDFs	737	92	3.5	4.1
1,2,3,4,6,7,8-HpCDF	529.2	5.4	2.11	2.07
1,2,3,4,7,8,9-HpCDF	< 10.0	3.2	< 0.02	0.43
OCDF	30	23	3.6	4.8
Total tetra- to octaCDFs	**9 733**	**478**	**25.1**	**16.1**
I-TEQ pg/m^3	141.5	9.8	0.93	1.20
I-TEQ pg/L fuel	1 083.3	50.7	7.20	23.60

From Hagenmaier *et al.* (1990)

(vii) *Metal production*

Steel mills and the manufacturing of iron and steel are considered to be major sources of PCDDs and PCDFs in the environment. The concentrations of PCDFs are much higher than the concentrations of PCDDs in these samples (Rappe, 1994). Jager (1993) reported on the contamination of scrap samples and I-TEQ levels in flue gas emissions from German steel mills (see **Table 13**) (analytical method ABS).

Table 13. PCDD/PCDF contamination of flue gas, clean gas and flue dust from a steel mill

Proportion of non-metals in scrap added	Flue gas (ng I-TEQ/m^3)	Clean gas (ng I-TEQ/m^3)	Flue dust (ng I-TEQ/g)
Low	0.9	0.02	4.8
Average	1.7	0.04	5.1
High	2.7	0.06	6.0

From Jager (1993)

(viii) *Accidents with electrical equipment containing PCBs*

Buser *et al.* (1978b) reported that pyrolysis of PCBs could cause formation of PCDFs and they issued a warning for this risk. Such an accident occurred in 1981 in the State Office building in Binghamton, NY (United States), when a transformer in the basement exploded and contaminated soot was spread throughout the building (O'Keefe *et al.*, 1985; Schecter, 1986). In the 1980s, following similar accidents involving both transformers and capacitors, people were evacuated from houses and workplaces in the United States, Canada, Sweden, Finland and France (Rappe *et al.*, 1985b; Hryhorczuk *et al.*, 1986; Rappe *et al.*, 1986b). In many cases, analyses showed elevated concentrations of PCDFs in the soot (as high as 2168 mg/kg; the major constituents being 2,3,6,7-/2,3,7,8-TCDFs, 2,3,4,7,8-PeCDF and 1,2,3,4,7,8-/1,2,3,6,7,8-HxCDFs) (Rappe *et al.*, 1985b).

(c) *Photochemical reactions*

The photochemical dechlorination of OCDF on soil has been studied by Tysklind *et al.* (1992). Dechlorination occurs preferentially in the lateral (2,3,7,8) positions. Consequently, no 2,3,7,8-substituted PCDFs could be identified in the dechlorination products. Similar results were obtained by Friesen *et al.* (1996) for the photochemical degradation of 2,3,4,7,8-PeCDF, where no 2,3,7,8-TCDF was found.

(d) *Biochemical reactions*

Öberg *et al.* (1990) showed that chlorinated phenols could be transformed *in vitro* to PCDFs by peroxidase-catalysed oxidation.

1.2.2 *Destruction of PCDFs*

Although PCDFs are considered to be very stable, they can undergo a series of chemical degradation reactions. Peterson and Milicic (1992) and Oku *et al.* (1995) reported the degradation of a series of PCDFs using a mixture of potassium hydroxide in polyethylene glycol or sodium or potassium hydroxide in 1,3-dimethyl-2-imidazolidinone.

Vollmuth and Niessner (1995) reported no significant degradation of PCDFs by ultra-violet radiation, ozone or a combination of the two.

Thermal degradation of PCDFs occurs at temperatures above 800 °C and at residence times of longer than 2 s (WHO/EURO, 1987), but the conditions required for thermal degradation are matrix-dependent.

Adriaens et al. (1995) reported on the biologically mediated reductive dechlorination of 2,3,4,7,8-PeCDF in sediments using inocula derived from contaminated environments.

1.3 Occurrence

All tissue concentrations reported in this section are lipid-based (as ng/kg fat), unless otherwise stated.

1.3.1 Occupational and accidental exposures to PCDFs

(a) Occupational exposures

(i) Exposure during production of PCBs

Although several cohorts of PCB workers have been studied, no study has taken PCDFs into account.

(ii) Exposure during production of TCP and 2,4,5-T

In the Boehringer-Ingelheim plant in Hamburg manufacturing a range of herbicides, Flesch-Janys et al. (1996a) studied 48 workers (45 men and 3 women) (see also monograph on PCDD, p. 55). The blood concentrations of PCDFs in these workers are given in **Table 14**.

Table 14. Concentrations of PCDFs (ng/kg fat) in blood of workers at a German herbicide plant (Boehringer-Ingelheim plant)

	No.[a]	First blood sample[b]		Last blood sample[c]	
		Median	Range	Median	Range
2,3,4,7,8-PeCDF	5	105.9	76.4–406.7	71.3	47.9–108
1,2,3,4,7,8-HxCDF	42	116.7	37.5–1035	61.5	21.9–489.4
1,2,3,6,7,8-HxCDF	31	50.4	28.5–374	30.2	13.6–205.9
2,3,4,6,7,8-HxCDF	6	16.3	10.1–38	8.8	6.1–14.8
1,2,3,4,6,7,8-HpCDF	22	123.1	47.3–1028	45.8	24.7–243
1,2,3,4,7,8,9-HpCDF	6	14.8	3.6–26	3	1.6–5.4

From Flesch-Janys et al. (1996a)
[a] Number of persons whose levels exceeded upper background concentrations at all points in time
[b] Mean, 5.4 years after end of employment
[c] Mean, 5.6 years after the first blood sample

(iii) *Exposure during handling and spraying of 2,4,5-T*

Professional pesticide applicators involved in ground-level spraying of 2,4,5-T in New Zealand are claimed to be the group most heavily exposed to agricultural use of 2,4,5-T in the world (Smith *et al.*, 1992a). Many of the applicators sprayed for more than six months per year and some were spraying for more than 20 years. Measurements of PCDFs in blood serum of nine of these workers are given in **Table 15** (see also monograph on PCDDs, p. 57).

Table 15. Levels of PCDFs in serum of nine 2,4,5-T applicators and nine matched control subjects in New Zealand

Congener	Average level (ng/kg fat ± SE)[a]		Ratio[b]
	Applicator	Matched control	
2,3,7,8-TCDF	1.6 ± 0.3	1.7 ± 0.3	0.9
1,2,3,7,8-PeCDF	< 2.1 ± 0.2	< 2.0 ± 0.2	1.1
2,3,4,7,8-PeCDF	8.0 ± 0.9	7.4 ± 0.8	1.1
1,2,3,4,7,8-HxCDF	5.4 ± 0.3	5.1 ± 0.5	1.1
1,2,3,6,7,8-HxCDF	5.5 ± 0.4	5.6 ± 0.6	1.0
1,2,3,7,8,9-HxCDF	< 0.8 ± 0.1	< 0.8 ± 0.1	1.0
2,3,4,6,7,8-HxCDF[c]	< 1.1 ± 0.4	< 1.7 ± 0.2	1.1
1,2,3,4,6,7,8-HpCDF	14.2 ± 0.7	16.0 ± 2.3	0.9
1,2,3,4,7,8,9-HpCDF[c]	< 1.6 ± 0.1	< 1.9 ± 0.3	0.8

From Smith *et al.* (1992a)
[a] Values are adjusted for total lipids in serum.
[b] Ratio, average for applicators/average for matched control subjects
[c] A number of positive signals were below the limit of quantification.

Military personnel in Viet Nam: Nygren *et al.* (1988) analysed adipose tissue and blood samples collected 15–20 years after military service from 27 men, 10 of whom were heavily exposed during their service in Viet Nam, 10 of whom had marginal exposure during service and served as Viet Nam controls and seven veterans who did not serve in Viet Nam and were used as 'era' controls. The results for PCDFs levels are summarized in **Table 16** (see also Section 1.3.1(*a*)(ii) of the monograph on PCDDs).

(iv) *Exposure at incinerators*

Studies of workers at incinerators have not found elevated tissue levels of PCDFs. Rappe *et al.* (1992), Päpke *et al.* (1993a) and Böske *et al.* (1995) found only elevated tissue levels of PCDDs.

(v) *Metal production and recycling*

Triebig *et al.* (1996) analysed the concentrations of PCDFs in the blood of 76 workers in a non-iron recycling plant in the south-western part of Germany. The results were compared with those from a group of 102 controls. Elevated concentrations of PCDFs

Table 16. Concentrations of PCDFs in blood plasma of exposed and unexposed groups of United States Army veterans (ng/kg fat)

Isomers	Arithmetic means								Geometric means		
	Exposed Viet Nam veterans		Viet Nam controls		Era controls[a]				Exposed Viet Nam veterans	Viet Nam controls	Era controls
	Mean	SEM[b]	Mean	SEM	Mean	SEM			Mean	Mean	Mean
2,3,7,8-TCDF	4.0	2.1	3.6	0.9	3.4	1.7			2.3	2.1	1.0
2,3,4,7,8-PeCDF	14.0	2.5	15.2	2.4	19.2	5.9			11.9	13.4	15.2
1,2,3,4,7,8-HxCDF[c]	13.5	1.5	9.3	1.7	11.5	3.0			12.8	7.6	9.2
1,2,3,6,7,8-HxCDF	9.1	1.3	5.4	1.3	7.5	2.6			8.2	3.7	5.7
2,3,4,6,7,8-HxCDF	2.9	0.7	1.9	0.4	1.7	1.7			2.3	1.7	1.5
1,2,3,4,6,7,8-HpCDF	27.2	4.4	20.5	3.6	19.6	2.6			24.6	13.3	16.6

From Nygren et al. (1988)

[a] Era controls are veterans who served outside Viet Nam during the period of the Viet Nam conflict.

[b] SEM, standard error of mean

[c] 1,2,3,4,7,8-/1,2,3,4,7,9-HxCDF

were found in the exposed group (up to 1138 ng/kg), around six times above the maximal blood concentrations in controls. Elevated levels were found particularly for 2,3,4,7,8-PeCDF and for HxCDFs (analytical method ACS). In another study, Bergschicker et al. (1994) found elevated concentrations of the same PCDFs in a group of 34 workers employed in a primary and secondary copper smelter (analytical method ACS).

Menzel et al. (1996) reported elevated blood concentrations of PCDDs/PCDFs in a group of 14 workers employed in welding and cutting of metals (welders: median, 29.9; burners: median, 46.7; referents, 28.3 ng I-TEQ/kg).

Hansson et al. (1995) reported a significant increase in Cl_5–Cl_8 PCDFs in the blood of nine workers from a magnesium plant in Norway. They analysed blood samples from workers employed at the plant for 10–36 years and from a control group of nine non-production workers. OCDF was the congener with the highest exposure levels (see **Table 17**).

Table 17. Mean concentrations of PCDFs (expressed in ng/kg fat) in blood plasma from metal workers and controls

PCDF	Controls ($n = 9$)		Workers ($n = 9$)		p value[a]
	Mean	Range	Mean	Range	
2,3,7,8-TCDF	2.9	1.2–4.7	3.5	1.5–6.1	0.5
1,2,3,7,8-PeCDF	2.2	< 1–3	5.4	< 1–11	0.06
2,3,4,7,8-PeCDF	20	14–29	51	19–170	0.02
1,2,3,4,7,8-HxCDF	22	5.9–94	59	23–150	0.01
1,2,3,6,7,8-HxCDF	12	5.7–31	59	19–190	0.002
2,3,4,6,7,8-HxCDF	3.4	< 1–6.8	5.4	2–9.6	0.09
1,2,3,4,6,7,8-HpCDF	14	4.7–32	85	21–150	0.0007
1,2,3,4,7,8,9-HpCDF	< 2		6.9	< 2–16	0.0005
OCDF	7.5	< 3–18	216	17–560	0.0005
I-TEQ	25	17–42	60	27–190	0.007

From Hansson et al. (1995)
[a] Mann-Whitney U test for comparison between groups (two-tailed)

(vi) Exposure during production of chlorine gas

Svensson et al. (1993) reported that in a small cohort of workers at a chloralkali plant in Sweden, handling sludge from graphite electrodes had caused exposure to 2,3,7,8-substituted PCDFs (2,3,4,7,8-PeCDF and HxCDFs). However, exposure to contaminated soil did not result in elevated concentrations of PCDFs (analytical method ACS).

(vii) Exposure in bleached pulp mills

Rosenberg et al. (1995) analysed 34 blood samples from workers at a pulp mill and 14 controls. They found no statistically significant differences in lipid-adjusted concentrations of PCDFs between the two groups.

(viii) *Exposure during production of PVC*

Hansson *et al.* (1997) reported a weak correlation between length of employment in production of PVC (or vinyl chloride monomer) and concentrations of PCDFs in the blood, especially 1,2,3,4,7,8- and 1,2,3,6,7,8-HxCDFs and 1,2,3,4,6,7,8-HpCDF.

(b)   Accidental exposure

Repeated heating of PCBs in the presence of oxygen can result in formation of PCDFs, polychlorinated quaterphenyls (PCQs) and other compounds. In Japan and Taiwan, the use of PCBs as heat exchangers during the deodorizing of cooking oil resulted in contamination of cooking oil, presumably when the processing machines leaked. These incidents caused thousands of cases of PCB/PCDF poisoning when the contaminated oil was distributed and consumed.

(i)   Yusho *incident, Japan, 1968*

A mass poisoning, called the *yusho* ('oil disease') incident, occurred in western Japan in 1968. The disease was caused by ingestion of a specific brand of rice oil that was contaminated not only with PCBs but also with PCDFs, PCQs and other substances. About 2000 affected individuals (Chen *et al.*, 1985a) were identified (1870 had been registered by 31 May 1990), primarily in the Fukuoka and Nagasaki prefectures on the island of Kyushu (Ikeda & Yoshimura, 1996). Although *yusho* patients had ingested more than 40 different PCDF congeners, Rappe *et al.* (1979b) found that only a few congeners had been retained by the patients. Most of the retained congeners were found to have the 2, 3, 7 and 8 positions chlorinated. The missing congeners, apparently metabolized and excreted, were those with two vicinal hydrogenated carbon atoms in at least one of the rings. Masuda (1994) determined concentrations of the major PCDF congeners identified in tissues and blood at different sampling times (**see Table 18**). The highest concentrations were found for 2,3,4,7,8-PeCDF and 1,2,3,4,7,8-/1,2,3,6,7,8-HxCDFs. Five years after exposure ended, the mean concentrations of PCBs in the adipose tissue, liver and blood of *yusho* cases were 1.9 mg/kg (ppm), 0.08 mg/kg and 6.7 µg/kg, respectively (Masuda *et al.*, 1985), which were about twice the levels in the control group. Levels of PCDFs in adipose tissue ranged from 6 to 13 µg/kg (Masuda *et al.*, 1985). Sixteen years after exposure, the mean level of PCQs in adipose tissue of *yusho* cases was 207 µg/kg, approximately 100 times the level in Japanese controls (Kashimoto *et al.*, 1985).

(ii)   Yucheng *incident, Taiwan, 1979*

In 1979, 11 years after the Japanese *yusho* incident, a similar incident occurred in central Taiwan. About 2000 persons were identified as *yucheng* patients, primarily from Taichung and Changhwa counties (Chen & Hites, 1983; Chen *et al.*, 1985a). Oil samples were found to be contaminated with PCBs, PCDFs and PCQs, like the *yusho* oil. However, the average chlorination level seemed to be higher in the Taiwanese oil than in

Table 18. Concentrations of PCDF congeners in tissues of *yusho* patients

Year of sampling	Tissue	PCBs (mg/kg)	PCDFs (µg/kg wet weight)			
			2,3,7,8-TCDF	2,3,4,7,8-PeCDF	1,2,3,4,7,8-/1,2,3,6,7,8-HxCDF	1,2,3,4,6,7,8-HpCDF
1969	Liver	1.4	0.3	6.9	2.6	
1969	Liver	0.2	0.02	1.2	0.3	
	Adipose	2.8	0.3	5.7	1.7	
1972	Liver	0.03	< 0.01	0.3	0.03	
	Adipose	4.3	ND	0.8	0.2	
1975	Adipose	0.2	ND	0.1	0.5	
1977	Liver	0.06	ND	1.49	5.31	1.39
	Adipose	3.0	0.002	1.45	1.99	0.22
	Lung	0.016	0.002	0.365	0.41	0.05
1985	Uterus	0.005	ND	0.026	0.031	ND
1982	Comedo	0.2	ND	0.36	0.39	0.1
1986	Adipose[a]	2.2	0.003	1.4	0.51	
1986	Adipose[b]	2.3	0.028	0.77	0.66	0.036
	Blood[b]	0.0085	0.0025	0.0025	0.0004	
	Control subject					
1986	Adipose[c]	1.1	0.007	0.02	0.02	0.0009
	Blood[c]	0.0033	0.00007	0.00006	0.0009	

From Masuda (1994)

[a] Average of seven patients

[b] Average of six patients

[c] Average of three controls

the Japanese oil. The major PCDF was 1,2,3,4,7,8-HxCDF. Chen & Hites (1983) analysed tissue samples from a deceased patient (see **Table 19**). PCDFs in the blood of 10 patients were analysed by GC with negative chemical ionization–mass spectrometry. The blood samples were collected 9–27 months after the onset of poisoning. The total PCDFs in the blood of 10 patients ranged from 0.02 to 0.20 µg/kg, the major components being 1,2,3,4,7,8-HxCDF and 2,3,4,7,8-PeCDF. Minor amounts of 1,2,3,4,6,7,8-HpCDF and 1,2,4,7,8-PeCDF were also found (Chen *et al.*, 1985b). In *yucheng* patients, within the first year of exposure, mean serum PCB, PCDF and PCQ levels for 15 cases were 60 mg/kg (range, 4–188 mg/kg, 0.14 µg/kg (range, < 0.005–0.27 µg/kg) and 19.3 µg/kg (range, 0.9–63.8 µg/kg), respectively (Kashimoto *et al.*, 1985). Analysis of PCB levels in 1980–81 in 165 cases (mean, 38 µg/kg; range, 10–720 µg/kg) (Rogan, 1989) and in 1985 in 32 cases (mean, 15.4 µg/kg; range, 0.6–86.8 µg/kg) (Lundgren *et al.*, 1988) suggested that some PCBs were being eliminated. [The Working Group noted that it was not clear from the reports if the samples were drawn from distinctly different individuals or included some of the same individuals.]

Table 19. Concentrations of PCDF congeners in the tissues of a deceased patient with *yucheng* in Taiwan

Tissue	Level of PCDF congener (μg/kg)		
	1,2,4,7,8-PeCDF	2,3,4,7,8-PeCDF	1,2,3,4,7,8-HxCDF
Liver	3.4	6.3	25.4
Intestinal fat	0.9	4.0	7.8
Bronchus	0.4	1.8	3.2
Large intestine	0.3	1.2	2.3
Heart	0.2	0.8	1.4
Stomach	0.05	0.23	0.4
Small intestine	0.05	0.21	0.34
Kidney	0.04	0.18	0.32
Lung	0.01	0.06	0.15
Brain	0.01	0.06	0.15
Spleen	0.01	0.08	0.1

From Chen & Hites (1983)

(iii) *PCB explosions and fires*

After the accident at Binghamton, NY (United States), in 1981 (see Section 1.2.1(*b*)(viii), 74.7 ng/kg 2,3,4,7,8-PeCDF, 149 ng/kg 1,2,3,4,7,8-HxCDF, 39.3 ng/kg 1,2,3,4,6,7,8-HpCDF and 25.9 ng/kg 1,2,3,4,7,8,9-HpCDF were found in the adipose tissue of an exposed person (Schecter *et al.*, 1985a). After an accident in Reims, France, in 1985, < 4 ng/kg 2,3,4,7,8-PeCDF, < 2 ng/kg 1,2,3,4,7,8-HxCDF, < 14 ng/kg total HpCDFs as well as < 12 ng/kg total HpCDDs and < 23 ng/kg OCDD were found in the blood of 6 exposed persons (Rappe *et al.*, 1986b).

1.3.2 *Environmental occurrence* (see also Appendix 2)

Most of the analytical data on environmental levels of PCDFs are from studies measuring PCDDs and PCDFs, often reported as a total I-TEQ (see the monograph on PCDDs as well as Appendix 1). However, in some studies, separate data on PCDFs were reported.

(a) *Air* (see Appendix 2, Table 1)

In a baseline study on PCDDs and PCDFs in ambient air (Eitzer & Hites, 1989), 55 samples were taken between 1985 and 1987 at three sites in Bloomington, IN (United States). A set of samples was also taken in the Trout Lake, WI, area, a much more rural area than Bloomington. There was consistency in the isomer pattern within a group of isomers, but overall levels of the various groups had somewhat more variation. Some of this variation was related to the atmospheric temperature; for example, more of the lower chlorinated PCDFs were found in the vapour phase at higher temperatures. The TCDF distribution between vapour and particulate phases at various temperatures (with a detection limit of 1 fg/m^3 (femtogram = 10^{-15} g)) was as follows: at 3 °C, 50% vapour phase and 50% particulate phase; at 12 °C, 80% vapour phase and 20% particulate phase; and at 26 °C, > 95% vapour phase and < 5% particulate phase.

Airborne concentrations of PCDDs and PCDFs in office buildings and in ambient outdoor air in Boston, MA (United States), were measured by Kominsky and Kwoka (1989). Twelve of the 16 samples were collected inside the buildings and four samples were collected at the ambient air intake plenums of the buildings. PCDFs were generally not detected, except for three samples that showed detectable concentrations of TCDFs and PeCDFs. Two of these samples (one inside and one ambient air) contained 2,3,7,8-TCDF. The I-TEQs for the two samples containing 2,3,7,8-TCDF were 0.34 and 0.20 pg/m^3, respectively.

(b)   Water (see Appendix 2, Table 2)

Muir et al. (1995) analysed water and other matrices downstream from a bleached kraft pulp mill on the Athabasca River (Alberta, Canada) in 1992. The 'dissolved phase' and the suspended particulates from centrifuged samples were analysed for 41 PCDDs/-PCDFs ranging from mono- to octa-chlorinated congeners. Most PCDD congeners (including 2,3,7,8-TCDD) were undetectable (< 0.1 pg/L) in the centrifugate; however, concentrations of 2,3,7,8-TCDF were above the detection limits at the 1 km site (Weldwood; 0.1 pg/L) and at 48 km (Emerson Lake; 0.09 pg/L). In 1993, 2,3,7,8-TCDF was not detected in the dissolved phase (< 0.1 pg/L) either 1 or 19 km downstream.

In a survey conducted in 1986 for PCDDs/PCDFs and other pollutants in finished water systems throughout New York State (United States), two TCDFs were found at concentrations of 1 pg/L in one finished drinking-water (Meyer et al., 1989). Except for a trace of OCDF detected in one location, no other PCDD or PCDF was detected in any of the 19 other community water systems surveyed.

(c)   Soil (see Appendix 2, Table 3; also Appendix 1, Tables 4, 5 and 8)

Topsoil samples were collected at six typical locations in Flanders, Belgium, including potential PCDD/PCDF source areas, and analysed [but not reported] isomer-specifically for PCDDs and PCDFs (Van Cleuvenbergen et al., 1993). Concentrations in the 0–3-cm soil fraction, averaged per location, ranged between 2.1 ng/kg at a rural location and 8.9 ng/kg (both as I-TEQ) in an industrialized area. Generally, PCDFs made up 70 ± 6% of the I-TEQ, whereas they accounted for 34 ± 6% of the sum of the concentrations of the seventeen 2,3,7,8-substituted congeners.

At the end of 1990, high levels of PCDFs and PCDDs (10–100 μg I-TEQ/kg) were detected in the surface gravel of playgrounds and sports fields in Germany during routine monitoring. The source of this contamination was identified as a fine-grained copper slag which originated from a former copper smelter at Marsberg, Germany. This material had been used as a cover layer due to its red colour (Kieselrot), its reduced dust formation compared to other gravels and its quick drying after rain. The PCDDs/PCDFs in the copper slag were formed as by-products of a chlorinating roasting process when up to 8% sodium chloride and coal were added to a copper slag from an old mining process.

About 800 000 tonnes of red copper slag was produced by this process, and a large quantity was used. *Kieselrot* contains a large number of highly chlorinated aromatic compounds as its main organic components. It shows an unusual congener profile for PCDDs and PCDFs. The total amount of PCDFs was about one order of magnitude higher than that of PCDDs. Furthermore, the concentrations increased from TCDFs to OCDF by at least one order of magnitude. The levels of OCDF exceeded those of OCDD by more than a factor of 10. These concentration ratios are typical for metallurgical processes and have been found in the emissions from magnesium production. Typical OCDF and I-TEQ values in *Kieselrot* were 6311 and 64.5 µg/kg, respectively (Döring *et al.*, 1992; Theisen *et al.*, 1993).

In connection with analyses of highly contaminated samples related to the production and use of chlorine (e.g., chloralkali electrolysis sludge and chromate sludge) in Sweden, Rappe *et al.* (1991b) also found high PCDF levels in surface soil samples in the vicinity of the production plant. A typical PCDF congener pattern, called the 'chloralkali pattern', was identified in these soil samples.

(d)   Food (see Appendix 2, Table 4)

All of the relevant data on PCDFs in foods derive from studies of both PCDFs and PCDDs. The monograph on PCDDs in this volume should be consulted for general remarks. The data included have been selected to meet a number of criteria, including: relevance to dietary intake rather than environmental monitoring, appropriate detection limits and appropriate analytical methodology. Some exceptions have, however, been made and some data that are available only as summed TEQs have been included where they seem to be of value. Additionally, the results included either were available on a lipid basis or could be so converted using either reported fat contents or reasonable assumptions. Some further results omitted from the tables are discussed in the text below. Certain entries in the Appendix 1 tables (for PCDDs) do not appear in Appendix 2, since PCDFs were either not determined, or not reported separately from the summed TEQ.

Summed TEQ concentrations are included in Tables 9–18 in Appendix 1 and these have, in most cases, been recalculated using I-TEF values and assuming that congeners that were not detected were present at the full value of the detection limit, unless limits of detection were not reported (indicated as 'ND').

Ryan *et al.* (1990) found an average concentration of 73.3 ng/kg 2,3,7,8-TCDF in cow's milk, much higher than in other reports (see Appendix 2, Table 4), and in a subsequent study showed this to be due to migration into milk from bleached paperboard containers (Ryan *et al.*, 1991). In Germany, Beck *et al.* (1990a) also found elevated levels of 2,3,7,8-TCDF in milk from cardboard containers, in the range 1.6–28 ng/kg (mean, 9.6 ng/kg), contrasting with a range of < 0.1–1.4 ng/kg (mean, 0.7 ng/kg) in other milk. The non-toxic 1,2,7,8-TCDF isomer also migrates. This congener is not normally present in milk but was found at a mean concentration of 4.9 ng/kg in milk from cardboard packages (Beck *et al.*, 1990a) and by Ryan *et al.* (1991) at a mean concentration of 80 ng/kg. Similar increases in 2,3,7,8-TCDF levels were found in studies in New Zealand (Buckland *et al.*, 1990b), the United Kingdom (Startin *et al.*, 1990) and the United States (Glidden *et al.*, 1990) and elsewhere. However, in Sweden, Rappe *et al.* (1990b) found little or no such migration in cardboard-packaged milk from four out of five towns (5 ng/kg in one). Since 1990, the concentrations of PCDFs in pulp products have been substantially reduced. Thus, in samples from the United Kingdom Total Diet Study (Wright & Startin, 1995), a relatively high 2,3,7,8-TCDF level of 6.6 ng/kg was found in milk collected in 1982, together with 1,2,7,8-TCDF clearly indicating chlorine bleaching as the source, while neither congener was detected in milk collected in 1992.

If Ryan's atypical data are excluded, the samples of milk and dairy products from various locations, which are dominated by European samples from the late 1980s and early 1990s, have mean concentrations of individual PCDFs between about 0.2 and 2.8 ng/kg (Appendix 2, Table 4). The ratios between the lowest and highest measurements for different PCDF congeners vary from around 30 to several hundred. [The Working Group noted that data for OCDF should be treated with particular caution; at these concentrations, this congener is especially difficult to determine accurately and the range of reported concentrations is wide.] Apart from OCDF, 2,3,4,7,8-PeCDF tends to have the highest concentration in most European samples, but not in the single analysis presented of milk from the United States (Eitzer, 1995).

Milk produced close to sites associated with contamination from incineration and similar processes can contain relatively high concentrations of PCDFs (**Table 20**).

Analyses of meats and meat products indicate mean concentrations for most 2,3,7,8-chlorinated congeners of between 1 and 4 ng/kg, with 1,2,3,7,8,9-HxCDF and 1,2,3,4,7,8,9-HpCDF generally at lower concentrations. As with PCDDs, samples of animal liver show considerably higher concentrations.

The rather limited data on poultry meat and eggs suggest that concentrations are usually of the same order of magnitude as those seen in other animal products.

In fish, the pattern of concentrations of different congeners tends to be more extreme and more variable. It is unusual for 1,2,3,7,8,9-HxCDF to be detectable, while most of the tetra- and pentachlorinated congeners are present at higher concentrations than in terrestrial animal products. The predominant congener in fatty fish from the Baltic Sea is 2,3,4,7,8-PeCDF (Svensson *et al.*, 1991). 2,3,7,8-TCDF has been reported in retail samples of marine fish species at concentrations around 100 ng/kg (Beck *et al.*, 1989a; Liem *et al.*, 1991a).

1.4   Human tissue measurements (see **Table 21**)

Most of the analytical data on biological monitoring of PCDFs have been reported in studies in which both PCDDs and PCDFs were measured (see the monograph on PCDDs in this volume; Section 1.4 and Tables 24, 25 and 27).

In some studies, individual data on PCDFs are reported. All concentrations reported in this section are lipid-based (as ng/kg fat), unless otherwise stated.

Table 20. Concentrations of PCDFs in cow's milk from contaminated areas

Reference	Origin	Sample year	No.	PCDF concentration (ng/kg fat)									
				TCDF	PeCDF		HxCDF				HpCDF		OCDF
				2378	12378	23478	123478	123678	123789	234678	1234678	1234789	
Riss et al. (1990)	Austria, Brixlegg (metal reclamation)	1988	1	7.4	6.3	29.5	26.5	17.1	–	18.8	–	–	–
			1	9	6.5	57.6	26.8	17.8	–	9.4	–	–	–
Rappe et al. (1987b)	Switzerland,	–											
	Hunzenschwil (MSWI)			[< 0.49]	[< 0.45]	[9.62]	[2.91]	[4.25]	ND	[6.26]	[11.0]	ND	[< 3.58]
	Rheinfelden (Cl compound manuf.)			[< 0.80]	[< 0.92]	[6.59]	[2.41]	[1.69]	ND	[1.40]	[< 5.16]	ND	[< 14.9]
	Suhr (MSWI)			[< 1.01]	[< 1.14]	[6.94]	[1.89]	[3.00]	ND	[3.79]	[8.83]	ND	[< 6.62]
Startin et al. (1990)	UK, incinerator	1989	1	[0.25]	[0.075]	[1.775]	[1.05]	[0.75]	[< 0.525]	[0.65]	[0.575]	[< 0.5]	[< 3.825]
			1	[0.275]	[< 0.6]	[2.625]	[1.25]	[1.025]	[< 0.55]	[0.925]	[< 1.8]	[< 0.85]	[< 3.05]
	UK, urban/industrial	1989	1	[0.525]	[0.3]	[6.1]	[1.375]	[0.9]	[< 0.425]	[0.725]	[0.425]	[< 0.25]	[< 1.95]
			1	[0.45]	[0.35]	[3.875]	[0.875]	[0.55]	[< 0.25]	[0.375]	[< 0.5]	[< 0.5]	[< 4]
Harrison et al. (1996)	UK, Derbyshire (Cl compd. Manuf.) (Farm A) (4% fat assumed)	1990	1	[0.5]	[0.5]	[7.75]	[2.75]	[3]	[< 0.25]	[3.25]	[1.5]	[0.25]	[0.75]
Eitzer (1995)	USA, Connecticut, (incineration) (4% fat assumed)	1993	12	[0.325]	[0.0325]	[0.0825]	[0.1725]	[0.0975]	[0.06675]	[0.1725]	[0.8]	[0.185]	[8.5]

Summed I-TEQs are given in the PCDD monograph in this volume.

–, not reported; ND, not detected and limit of detection not reported; [ ], calculated by the Working Group; MSWI, municipal solid-waste incinerator.

Table 21. Concentrations of PCDFs in human samples

Reference	Origin; sample description (and no.)	Coll. period	Anal. meth.	PCDF concentration (ng/kg, lipid-based)									
				TCDF	PeCDF	HxCDF				HpCDF			OCDF
				2378	12378	23478	123478	123678	123789	234678	1234678	1234789	1234789
Austria													
Riss *et al.* (1990)	Brixlegg; (1) blood from farmer (1)	88	CSN	<14 <10	7.5 1.8	839 119	116 27.2	113 30	— —	15 3.2	— —	— —	— —
Canada													
Ryan *et al.* (1985b)	Kingston/Ottawa[a]; adipose (8)	79–81	BSIW	2.9 ± 1.9 (6 pos.)	—	16.9 ± 21.4 (6 pos.)	—	—	—	—	—	—	—
Ryan *et al.* (1985c)	Adipose Québec (5)	72	BSIW			20.5 (4 pos.)		17.0 (1 pos.)			28.9		
	(10)	76				21.7		2.8 (8 pos.)			23.5 (9 pos.)		
	British Columbia (5)	72				30.8		59.7			55.1		
	(10)	76				18.3		21.8			38.3		
	Maritimes (10)	76				16.3					25.1		
	Ontario (6)	76				10.4		12.7			28.0		
	Prairies (10)	76				14.8		22.4 (6 pos.)			48.9 (8 pos.)		
	E. Ontario[a] (10)	80				18.4 ± 6.3		17.3 ± 6.9			39.4 ± 19.6		
LeBel *et al.* (1990)	Adipose Ontario (76)	84	BSO	2.4 ± 2.6 (ND–10.8)		31.3 ± 19.1 (3.4–113)		35.6 ± 20.6 (6.1–107.6)		3.7 ± 3.1 (ND–15.2)	25.2 ± 15.0 (8.1–113)		4.7 ± 5.2 (ND–27.9)
	Kingston[a] (13)	79–81		3.5		39.0		47.5		5.9	44.2		16.7
	Ottawa[a] (10)	79–81		3.1		27.6		35.0		4.4	29.9		7.3
Teschke *et al.* (1992)	British Columbia; adipose, residents of forest industry region (41)	90–91	CSO	2.2 (0.46–7.5)	1.9 (0.22–13)	10 (2.6–27)	11 (1.2–27)	10 (2.9–26)	3.3 (1.4–9.6)	0.80 (0.06–4.2)	19 (7.6–61)	0.60 (0.33–0.89)	3.7 (1.4–7.0)
China													
Ryan *et al.* (1987)	Shanghai; adipose[b] LC, 58% (1)	84	BSOW	9.7		12			<2		<2		—
	LC, 50% (1)			7.4		5.8			<2		<2		—
	LC, 73% (1)			6.4		15			<2		<2		—
	LC, 70% (1)			2.7		12			16		<2		—
	LC, 73% (1)			<2.8		14			25		<2		—
	LC, 72% (1)			<2		9.9			18		<2		—
	LC, 76% (1)			<1.8		14			14		<2		—

Table 21 (contd)

Reference	Origin; sample description (and no.)	Coll. period	Anal. meth.	PCDF concentration (ng/kg, lipid-based)									
				TCDF	PeCDF		HxCDF				HpCDF		OCDF
				2378	12378	23478	123478	123678	123789	234678	1234678	1234789	
China (contd)													
Schecter (1994)	Blood, general population; 15–19 years (50)	92	BSOW	<4.2	<1.6	2.7	3.4	2.1	<1.0	1.9	5.1	<1.2	<5.0
	>40 years (50)			2.7	<1.0	2.7	4.7	3.0	<1.0	2.7	7.7	<2.3	<5.0
Finland													
Rosenberg et al. (1995)	Plasma, general population; age, 28–60 years (14)	89–90	BSIW	1.9 (0.4–5.3)	1.2 (0.3–2.7)	29 (7.8–60)	10 (3.8–17)	9.5 (4.4–18)	1.6 (1.4–1.8)	4.8 (2.6–10)	64 (14–136)	<0.2	–
France													
Huteau et al. (1990a)	Paris; adipose; 6 patients, age, 54–82 years (8)	<90	BSO	5.7 (7 pos.) (2.4–12)	18.3 (3 pos.) (1–35.4)	104 (8 pos.) (19.3–242)	12.7 (4 pos.) (9.8–16.0)	11.5 (3 pos.) (9.8–14.4)	6 (1 pos.)	–	59.7 (2 pos.) (16.2–103)	–	–
Germany													
Beck et al. (1989b)	Hamburg residents; adipose (20)	86	BSIW	2.5 (0.7–6.0)	0.4 (0.1–1.6)	40 (10–101)	15 (4.8–39)	16 (4.7–47)	–	4.7 (2.1–10)	20 (7.2–35)	–	0.4 (0.1–0.8)
Thoma et al. (1990)	Munich residents	<89	BSO										
	Adipose (28)			2.5 (0.7–12.8)		35.2 (7.6–93.3)		41.4 (15.8–146.0)			14.2 (3.8–45.6)		4.0 (1.2–13.5)
	Liver (28)			5.5 (0.9–45.3)		173.7 (36.7–643)		398.5 (40.8–1801)			218.9 (12.2–757)		29.7 (4.3–65.8)
	Infants; adipose (8)			2.1 (1.0–4.6)		16.1 (5.3–38.7)		10.4 (3.9–23.6)			4.2 (1.9–7.3)		4.8 (2.5–9.1)
Päpke et al. (1992)	General population; blood (102)	89–90	BSOW	2.3 (0.5–6.7)	2.0 (0.5–7.1)	37 (6.3–99)	15.4 (3.6–49.0)	13.3 (2.7–53.0)	1.7 (0.5–9.4)	4.3 (0.5–14.0)	23.4 (4.8–55.0)	1.5 (0.5–4.0)	4.2 (1.0–15.0)
Kieselrot-studie (1991)	General population; blood (56)	91	BSOW	4.2 (ND–12)	1.4 (ND–4.4)	34.5 (11–91)	13.9 (4.0–34)	15.9 (6.6–33)	0.5 (ND–4.7)	4.5 (ND–7.9)	22.4 (10–66)	0.4 (ND–4.2)	3.5 (ND–71)
Päpke et al. (1993b)	General population; blood (44)	92	BSOW	1.2 (1.2–3.8)	0.4 (ND–2.5)	18.8 (6.8–48.2)	10.9 (4.4–24.5)	7.8 (3.1–20.7)	ND (ND–1.2)	2.9 (ND–9.9)	19.0 (8.5–38.4)	0.4 (ND–2.4)	0.4 (ND–2.4)

Table 21 (contd)

Germany (contd)

Reference	Origin; sample description (and no.)	Coll. period	Anal. meth.	PCDF concentration (ng/kg, lipid-based)									
				TCDF 2378	PeCDF 12378	23478	HxCDF 123478	123678	123789	234678	HpCDF 1234678	1234789	OCDF
Schrey et al. (1992)	General population; blood (95)	91	BSOW	1.37 (0.16–5.9)	0.64 (0.30–1.1)	34.3 (6.7–110)	11.5 (3.9–29)	16.5 (5.3–42)	–	3.67 (62–7.9)	15.4 (6.8–45)	0.48 (0.28–1.1)	1.10 (0.24–3.3)
Päpke et al. (1994b)	General population; blood (70)	93	BSOW	2.2 (0.5–5.4)	0.7 (0.5–2.8)	15.3 (5.0–42.1)	8.8 (3.9–22.0)	6.5 (2.4–18.8)	ND	2.8 (1.0–5.6)	12.5 (5.1–36.3)	0.9 (0.5–3.1)	3.5 (1.9–6.1)
Päpke et al. (1996)	General population; blood (134)	94	BSOW	1.9 (0.9–4.3)	0.5 (ND–1.8)	12.8 (3.2–41.3)	7.9 (2.5–19.4)	5.8 (1.8–16.3)	ND	2.6 (1.0–6.9)	11.4 (4.0–27.4)	0.6 (ND–2.0)	2.6 (ND–2.0)
	General population; blood	96	BSOW										
	18–71 years (139)			1.2 (ND–2.0)	0.6 (ND–1.0)	10.9 (3.2–29.7)	6.5 (2.6–14.5)	4.7 (2.0–8.9)	ND	2.4 (0.5–4.8)	8.1 (4.1–18.3)	0.9 (0.5–0.9)	2.4 (1.5–3.2)
	18–30 years (47)			1.2 (0.5–1.9)	0.6 (0.5–1.9)	8.2 (3.2–14.3)	5.8 (2.6–11.6)	4.1 (2.2–8.5)	ND	2.4 (1.4–4.1)	9.2 (4.2–18.3)	1.0 (0.7–1.6)	2.5 (1.8–2.5)
	31–42 years (48)			1.3 (0.5–1.8)	0.6 (0.5–1.0)	10.9 (4.8–20.1)	6.4 (2.8–14.5)	4.8 (2.0–8.4)	ND	2.4 (0.5–4.4)	7.8 (4.7–16)	1.0 (0.8–1.8)	2.4 (1.6–3.1)
	43–71 years (44)			1.2 (0.5–2.0)	0.5 (ND–1.0)	13.8 (5.2–29.7)	6.9 (3.0–13.3)	5.3 (2.2–8.9)	ND	2.5 (1.0–4.8)	7.1 (4.1–15.1)	0.8 (0.5–1.0)	2.4 (1.5–3.2)
Wittsiepe et al. (1993)	Marberg, near copper smelter; blood (56)	91	BSOW	4.9 (ND–12)	1.8 (ND–10)	41.6 (13–240)	24.4 (5.1–120)	35.1 (6.5–280)	1.1 (ND–8.0)	5.6 (0.7–20)	42.1 (7.4–180)	0.5 (ND–3.2)	5.8 (ND–57)
Körner et al. (1994)	Mammary tumour tissue (7)		BSO	3.2 (1.1–7.0)	1.3 (<2–4.1)	39.3 (19.5–73.8)			33.5 (16.8–52.3)		14.4 (6.1–23.8)	–	8.1 (2.9–13.8)
Wuthe et al. (1990)	Near metal reclamation plant; blood (22)	89	BSOW	4.9 (1.4–9.8)		72.9 (28–228)			108.6 (43.7–411)		48.3 (16–190)		4.3 (1.2–8.8)
Wuthe et al. (1993)	One woman (1)	92	BSOW										
	Blood			1.8		9.7			19.1		15.4		<4.4
	Milk			1.0		13.3			16.3		5.7		0.5
Ewers et al. (1994)	Allotment gardeners; blood (21)	92	BSOW	1.1 (0.5–4.1)		32 (23–76)			27 (16–54)		12 (0.6–30)		2.7 (1.3–6.7)

Table 21 (contd)

Reference	Origin; sample description (and no.)	Coll. period	Anal. meth.	TCDF 2378	PeCDF 12378	23478	HxCDF 123478	123678	123789	234678	HpCDF 1234678	1234789	OCDF
Germany (contd)													
Beck et al. (1994)	Infants, 3–23 months	< 93	BSOW										
	Adipose (8)			1.1 (< 0.5–3.1)	< 0.5	8.7 (1.6–33)	4.4 (1.0–12)	2.8 (0.7–9.3)	–	1.0 (< 0.5–3.0)	5.2 (1.0–12)	–	< 0.5 (< 0.5–1.2)
	Liver (8)			–	–	23 (3.3–82)	27 (< 2–107)	30 (2.9–85)	–	5.6 (< 1–14)	50 (< 4–169)	–	9.1 (4.5–15)
	Spleen (8)			2.1 (< 1–< 10)	2.1 (< 1–< 10)	15 (< 5–68)	7.0 (1.4–28)	5.0 (1.3–16)	–	4.6 (1.0–20)	10 (1.9–31)	–	1.6 (< 1–< 5)
	Thymus (8)			5.6 (3.2–7.5)	3.4 (< 1–7.5)	14 (6.1–37)	5.1 (2.2–< 15)	5.6 (3.5–< 15)	–	5.0 (2.1–< 15)	8.3 (2.6–19)	–	4.2 (< 1–< 15)
Jödicke et al. (1992)	Infant, 3 months	91	BSO										
	Stool (1)			< 2	< 2	11.0		12.7	–	< 5	30.7	–	< 5
	Mother's milk (2)			< 0.5–< 0.7	0.4–< 0.7	13.5–17.5		7.1–7.3	–	1.3–1.6	3.8–4.3	–	< 1–< 2
Welge et al. (1993)	Blood	92	BSOW										
	Vegetarians (24)			0.94 (0.16–2.3)	0.64 (0.42–0.89)	25.8 (11–50)	8.1 (4.2–13)	11.8 (5.3–18)	–	3.16 (0.8–5.0)	14.2 (5.6–72)	0.40 (0.3–0.5)	2.0 (0.2–6.7)
	Non-vegetarians (24)			1.3 (0.36–2.1)	0.66 (0.36–1.1)	25.5 (9.9–80)	9.1 (4.2–20)	12.9 (5.3–33)	–	3.16 (0.66–7.9)	14.6 (8.5–22)	0.38 (0.4–0.77)	1.4 (0.66–3.6)
Abraham et al. (1995a)		93–94	BSOW										
	Mother's blood (3)			[< 2.2]	[< 1.0]	[8.5]	[4.7]	[3.2]	–	[1.0]	[4.8]	–	[< 2.4]
	Placenta (3)			[< 2.4]	[< 1.0]	[8.0]	[2.5]	[1.7]	–	[< 1.0]	[2.2]	–	[< 3.0]
	Umbilical cord (3)			[< 2.0]	[< 1.0]	[4.3]	[2.7]	[1.7]	–	[< 1.0]	[4.3]	–	[< 5.0]
	Meconium (1)			[< 2.8]	[< 1.0]	[4.3]	[2.2]	[1.8]	–	[1.0]	[4.3]	–	[< 5.0]
Guam													
Schecter et al. (1992)	Whole blood (10)	89	BSOW	3.9	0.5	9.3	6.3	5.4	0.5	1.2	34.1	0.9	6.4
Japan													
Miyata et al. (1977)	Omentum (5)	75	CRO	< 5	ND–45.4				< 5.0		–	–	–
	Liver (4)			< 5	ND–17.2				< 5.0		–	–	–
	Mamma (1)			< 5	19.7				< 5.0		–	–	–

Table 21 (contd)

Reference	Origin; sample description (and no.)	Coll. period	Anal. meth.	TCDF	PeCDF	HxCDF					HpCDF		OCDF
				2378	12378	23478	123478	123678	123789	234678	1234678	1234789	
Japan (contd)													
Ryan (1986)	Adipose	84	BSIW										
	Age 21; LC, 43% (1)			–		17			20				–
	Age 33; LC, 37% (1)			–		51			ND				–
	Age 46; LC, 67% (1)			–		31			64				–
	Age 55; LC, 80% (1)			–		29			41				–
	Age 64; LC, 71% (1)			–		31			49				–
	Age 70; LC, 56% (1)			–		36			168				–
	Mean; LC, 59% (1)			–		33			68				–
Ono et al. (1986)	Cancer patients; adipose[a] (13)	85	CSI	9 (3–12)	–	25 (4–71)	15 (4–24)	14 (3–28)	–	8 (4–16)	–	–	–
Okagi et al. (1987)	Big city: adipose (1)	85	CRI	6	–	29	14	–	–	–	–	2	8
Hirakawa et al. (1991)	Controls; adipose (8)	<91	BSI	3 (1–7)	–	21 (8–30)	7 (3–13)	9 (3–20)	–	–	5 (2.8)	–	–
Masuda (1996)	Control; serum	91–92	BSIW	4.7	11.4	0.8	11.9	8.3	–	3.4	0.9	–	–
Netherlands													
van Wijnen et al. (1990)	Liver	<90	BSIW										
	Fetus (4)			–	–	0.12	0.12	0.10	–	–	0.10	–	–
	Infant not nursed (1)			–	–	0.12	0.04	0.04	–	–	0.09	–	–
	Infant nursed (1)			–	–	2.47	2.09	2.74	–	–	5.39	–	–
	Fat												
	Infant not nursed (1)			–	–	5.20	ND	ND	–	–	1.80	–	–
	Infant nursed (1)			–	–	14.66	2.61	2.05	–	–	4.43	–	–
	Placenta (1)			–	–	1.01	0.17	0.12	–	–	0.18	–	–
New Zealand													
Smith et al. (1992a)	Control group for 2,4,5-T applicators; serum	88	BSIW	1.7 ± 0.3	<2.0 ± 0.2	7.4 ± 0.8	5.1 ± 0.5	5.6 ± 0.6	<0.8 ± 0.1	<1.7 ± 0.2	16.0 ± 2.3	1.9 ± 0.3	–

PCDF concentration (ng/kg, lipid-based)

Table 21 (contd)

Reference	Origin; sample description (and no.)	Coll. period	Anal. meth.	TCDF 2378	PeCDF 12378	PeCDF 23478	HxCDF 123478	HxCDF 123678	HxCDF 123789	HxCDF 234678	HpCDF 1234678	HpCDF 1234789	OCDF
Norway													
Johansen et al. (1996)	Blood	93	BSO										
	Controls (10)			2.8 (0.6–5.0)	1.8 (ND–10.9)	17.1 (4.9–34)	8.7 (1.9–21)	9.7 (2.3–22)	0.9 (ND–1)	4.3 (1.6–6.7)	18 (2.5–53)	1.0 (ND–0.9)	8.6 (1.3–30)
	Moderate crab intake (15)			5.1	7.2	54.0	55	45	3.6	8.9	44	4.8	13.4
	High crab intake (9)			7.2 (1.7–16.5)	13.4 (1.3–35)	102 (52–148)	130 (34–233)	103 (27–217)	2.3 (ND–5.4)	14.3 (3.2–29)	93 (27–201)	26 (ND–5.3)	5.4 (2.1–8.8)
Russian Federation													
Schecter et al. (1992)	Whole blood	88–89	BSOW										
	Baikalsk (8)			3.0	<1.8	15	13	6.8	<1.6	2.1	4.6	<1.0	<8
	St Petersburg (pool) (60)			2.3	<1.0	9.2	8.1	3.9	<1.0	1.2	6.3	<2.2	–
Spain													
Jiménez et al. (1995)	Madrid, unexposed; serum (11)	93	BSO	4.7 ± 3.8 (9 pos.) (0.8–11.5)	1.4 ± 1.0 (9 pos.) (0.5–3.4)	7.0 ± 2.1 (10 pos.) (2.5–9.6)	5.8 ± 1.1 (10 pos.) (4.8–8.2)	5.1 ± 0.8 (10 pos.) (3.9–6.5)	1.8 ± 1.7 (5 pos.) (0.1–4.9)	2.6 ± 1.2 (9 pos.) (1.2–5.0)	12.8 ± 3.3 (11 pos.) (7.5–18.0)	5.0 ± 4.2 (9 pos.) (0.9–13)	20.6 ± 11.1 (9 pos.) (0.9–38.6)
Gonzáles et al. (1997)	Mataró; blood, 10 pools (198)	95	BSOW	1.2		6.2			10.6			7.1	2.4
Sweden													
Rappe (1984b)	Background; adipose [a] (6)	82	CS	3		40			22			50	3
Nygren et al. (1986)	Adipose [b]	84	BSIW										
	Unexposed (18)			4.2 (0.3–11)	–	32 (9–54)	5 (1–6)	4 (1–5)	–	2 (1–4)	10 (1–18)	–	–
	Cancer patients (17)			3.4 (0.3–7.2)	–	45 (9–87)	6 (1–15)	5 (1–13)	–	2 (1–7)	13 (1–49)	–	–
	Non-cancer patients (14)			4.6 (0–11)	–	33 (11–65)	5 (2–7)	4 (2–7)	–	2 (1–4)	10 (5–16)	–	–

PCDF concentration (ng/kg, lipid-based)

Table 21 (contd)

Reference	Origin; sample description (and no.)	Coll. period	Anal. meth.	TCDF	PeCDF		HxCDF					HpCDF		OCDF
				2378	12378	23478	123478	123678	123789	234678	1234678	1234789	
Sweden (contd)													
Rappe (1992)	Blood	90	BSIW										
	No fish consumption			1.5	0.15	12	5.4	4.4	–	2.1	10	–	1.0
	Normal fish consumption			1.8	0.5	20	7.1	5.4	–	2.2	14	–	1.0
	High fish consumption			3.0	1.3	79	8.3	11	–	2.8	10	–	1.0
Svensson et al. (1995a)	Blood; pool[a]	95	BSI										
	South of Bothnia Fishermen			4.8	ND	198	ND	ND	ND	5.0	16	–	ND
	Controls			ND	ND	40	5.9	6.8	ND	ND	19	–	ND
	Baltic Proper Fishermen			ND	ND	110	9.7	12	ND	4.0	16	–	ND
	Controls			ND	ND	41	7.0	7.0	ND	2.6	15	–	3.2
	Baltic South Fishermen			4.8	ND	163	19	23	ND	7.3	31	–	ND
	Controls			2.6	ND	59	10	10	ND	ND	20	–	6.8
	West Coast Fishermen (100)			ND	ND	47	8.0	8.0	ND	3.0	14	–	2.9
	Controls (98)			ND	ND	42	8.9	9.6	ND	4.8	18	–	3.2
Hardell et al. (1995)	Blood		BSI										
	Cancer patients (7)	> 86		3.3 (0.7–7.2)	1.0 (0.3–1.9)	59 (22–200)	8.6 (3.9–17)	7.9 (2.7–15)	2.0 (1–3)	2.7 (0.5–7)	16 (3–49)	0.8 (0.3–1)	< 3
	Non-cancer patients (12)	> 86		5.0 (2.4–11.4)	< 1.0	35 (11–65)	5.3 (3–7)	3.8 (2–6)	–	2.1 (1–4)	9.9 (5–16)	< 1.0	–
Switzerland													
Wacker et al. (1990)	Background		CSO										
	Adipose[a] (21)			0.8	3.3	48.5	8.3	7.4	–	8.0	1.2	–	0.4
	Liver[a] (21)			0.2	2.3	7.3	3.7	4.7	–	1.8	1.6	–	0.2
Taiwan													
Ryan et al. (1994)	Control children; serum	91	BSW	< 5	–	19			25		34	–	–

Table 21 (contd)

Reference	Origin; sample description (and no.)	Coll. period	Anal. meth.	PCDF concentration (ng/kg, lipid-based)									
				TCDF	PeCDF		HxCDF				HpCDF		OCDF
				2378	12378	23478	123478	123678	123789	234678	1234678	1234789	
United Kingdom													
Duarte-Davidson et al. (1993)	Wales, 5 pools; adipose (5)	90/91	CSO	<10	13	24 (20–27)	26 (18–42)	15 (9–27)	–	–	34 (24–49)	–	46 (36–62)
United States													
Ryan et al. (1985c)	NY State: adipose (6)	83/84	CSOW	–	–	14.7 ± 2.5 (10.9–17.0)	28.7 ± 7.2 (15.1–52.8)	–	–	–	16.4 ± 4.0 (12.5 ± 23.8)	–	–
Ryan et al. (1986)	NY State	<83	BSIW										
	Adipose (mean LC, 67%) (3)			–	–	13.9 (6.5–17)	32.4 (ND–52)	–	–	–	12.1 (ND–24)	–	–
	Liver (mean LC, 24%) (3)			–	–	4.1 (ND–6.9)	9.9 (4.2–17)	–	–	–	3.3 (ND–7.7)	–	–
	Adrenal (LC, 28 and 25%) (2)			–	–	4.9–5.5	8.5–11	–	–	–	3.5–4.5	–	–
	Bone marrow (LC, 26%) (1)			–	–	4.4	9.4	–	–	–	2.7	–	–
	Muscle (mean LC, 11%) (3)			–	–	1.1 (ND–2.3)	2.4 (1.7–3.4)	–	–	–	ND	–	–
	Kidney (LC, 3.0 and 4.0%) (2)			–	–	ND	ND	–	–	–	ND–1.7	–	–
Ryan (1986)	NY State, one man, 22 years old	85	BSIW										
	Adipose (LC, 83%) (1)					4.2							–
	Liver (LC, 4.4%) (1)					2.6							–
Schecter et al. (1986a)	Binghamton; adipose[a]	83–84	CRO										
	(1)			<2	–	12.5	11.4	5.6	–	–	16.3	ND	<20
	(1)			4.1	–	10.9	9.3	5.8	–	–	13.7	ND	<20
	(1)			<2	–	17.0	13	8.8	–	–	12.5	19.6	1.2
	(1)			<2	–	16.5	22.9	15.4	–	–	23.8	20.6	1.5

Table 21 (contd)

Reference	Origin; sample description (and no.)		Coll. period	Anal. meth.	PCDF concentration (ng/kg, lipid-based)									
					TCDF	PeCDF		HxCDF				HpCDF		OCDF
					2378	12378	23478	123478	123678	123789	234678	1234678	1234789	OCDF
United States (contd)														
Schecter et al. (1986a) (contd)	Adipose; LC, 70.6% (46%-88%)	(8)	<85	BNW	–	–	14.3 (3.1-19.7)	–	31.3 (15.1-46.9)	–	–	16.5 (12.5-23.8)	–	–
Stanley et al. (1986)	US general population; adipose	(46)	82	BSO	9.1 ± 9.6 (<2-32)	–	27 ± 16 (<1.8-77)	–	18 ± 8.3 (2.9-55)	–	–	18 ± 12 (<10-55)	–	60 ± 110 (<2-360)
Nygren et al. (1988)	Era control; serum	(1)	<88	BSIW	<18	–	10	3.1	2.2	–	<4	13.6	–	–
		(1)			<0.1	–	16.4	17.6	12.6	–	<3	23	–	–
		(1)			2.6	–	27	26	19	–	4.8	51	–	–
		(1)			10.4	–	51	10.4	3.6	–	<1.5	12.6	–	–
		(1)			<0.4	–	5.3	4.4	2.8	–	<2	10	–	–
		(1)			0.6	–	10.9	8.5	5.4	–	1.4	10.7	–	–
		(1)			<2.0	–	14.1	10.3	6.5	–	<2.5	16.4	–	–
Schecter et al. (1989b)	One person		<89	N										
	Fat[a]	(1)			–	–	17	–	52	–	–	15	–	–
	Abdomen	(1)			–	–	17	–	22	–	–	12	–	–
	Subcutaneous	(1)			–	–	4.9	–	8.5	–	–	3.5	–	–
	Adrenal[a]	(1)			–	–	4.4	–	9.4	–	–	2.7	–	–
	Bone marrow[a]	(1)			–	–	ND	–	4.2	–	–	2.1	–	–
	Liver[a]	(1)			–	–	1.1	–	2.1	–	–	ND	–	–
	Muscle[a]	(1)			–	–	ND	–	2.1	–	–	ND	–	–
	Kidney[a]	(1)			–	–	ND	–	ND	–	–	ND	–	–
	Lung[a]	(1)			–	–	–	–	–	–	–	–	–	–
Schecter et al. (1990b; 1991a)	Plasma	(20)	<90	BSOW	1.3	–	6.1	6.9	5.4	–	1.2	25.1	–	<3
	Adipose	(20)	<90		1.6	–	6.8	5.6	3.7	–	1.5	16.4	–	<1
	Whole blood	(4)	88/89		3.0	–	70.5	22.7	23.5	–	8.2	29	–	–
	Adipose	(4)	88/89		3.9	–	70.8	14.5	17.8	–	5.3	23.3	–	4.2
Kang et al. (1991)	Adipose Viet Nam veterans	(36)	78	N	2.9	1.7	23.1	21.5	10.7	1.5	3.8	37.4	2.2	3.6
	Non-Viet Nam veterans	(79)			2.4	1.1	22.2	19.3	9.9	0.9	3.2	32.9	1.9	4.5
	Civilians	(80)			3.3	1.9	23.3	23.2	12.0	0.9	3.6	39.1	2.2	3.4

Table 21 (contd)

Reference	Origin; sample description (and no.)	Coll. period	Anal. meth.	PCDF concentration (ng/kg, lipid-based)									
				TCDF	PeCDF		HxCDF				HpCDF		OCDF
				2378	12378	23478	123478	123678	123789	234678	1234678	1234789	
United States (contd)													
Paccitelli et al. (1992)	Referents; serum (79)	87/88	BSIW	1.2	–	11 (3.3–28)	11 (4.2–28)	8.5 (3.7–18)	–	1.5	20 (2 pos.) (8.7–46)	0.8	1.1
Patterson et al. (1994)	General population; adipose (4)	84/86	BSIW	1.1 (0.7–1.8)	–	3.7 (3.3–4.3)	3.7 (3.2–4.1)	5.8 (4.0–8.3)	–	–	12.0 (8.9–15)	–	–
Schecter et al. (1994b)	Placenta; pool (14)	<94	BSOW	1.9	<1.0	3.6	4.0	2.0	1.7	<1.0	6.3	<1	<5
	Placenta (1)	<94		0.5	0.5	6.8	8.6	1.8	0.8	<0.2	4.6	<0.6	4
	Blood, pool (50)	<94		2.3	1.2	8.8	10.6	6.9	2.8	2.8	19.6	3.1	9.3
	Fetal tissue, 8–14 weeks, pool (10)	94		1.3	<0.2	1.1	2.2	1.0	–	1.5	3.1	<0.9	<3.2
Schecter et al. (1996c)	Adipose (5)	96	BSNW	0.59	0.45	2.6	4.3	2.3	0.12	1.2	6.5	0.3	0.8
	Blood, before nursing (5)	96	BSNW	0.87	0.52	3.0	5.9	3.4	ND	1.7	8.9	ND	1.9
	Placenta (5)	96	BSNW	0.61	0.58	4.0	3.3	1.8	ND	0.53	2.7	0.52	2.2
	Cord blood (5)	96	BSNW	<1.2	<0.7	0.87	1.5	1.5	ND	1.4	3.5	ND	<5
	Mother's milk (5)	96	BSNW	0.49	0.37	2.8	3.9	2.4	ND	1.4	5.4	0.53	<2.9
Schecter et al. (1996d)	Blood pool (100)	96	BSIW	<2.0	<1.4	11.1	14.1	7.9	3.5	<3.7	12.0	<4	<5
	Serum pool (100)	96	BSIW	<2.0	<1.9	9.3	14.0	7.9	4.0	<4.1	13.9	4.9	<5
Viet Nam													
Schecter et al. (1986b)	N. Viet Nam; adipose (LC, 50%) (7)	84	BSOW	–	–	9.7		9.3	–	–	4.2	–	–
	S. Viet Nam; adipose (LC, 60%) (13)			–	–	13.0		31.7	–	–	17.0	–	–
Schecter et al. (1986c)	N. Viet Nam; adipose (LC, 56%) (9)	84	BSOW	–	–	14.7 (ND–29.4)			13.3 (ND–20)		7 (ND–10.7)	–	–
	S. Viet Nam; adipose (LC, 62%) (15)			–	–	21.0 (4.3–45.5)			58.3 (13.6–166.7)		28.9 (4.2–74.9)	–	–
Schecter et al. (1989c)	S. Viet Nam; adipose (27)	84–88	ABN	7 (ND–17)	–	–	–	–	–	–	–	–	–

Table 21 (contd)

Reference	Origin; sample description	(and no.)	Coll. period	Anal. meth.	PCDF concentration (ng/kg, lipid-based)									
					TCDF	PeCDF		HxCDF				HpCDF		OCDF
					2378	12378	23478	123478	123678	123789	234678	1234678	1234789	1234789
Viet Nam (contd)														
Nguyen et al. (1989)	Ho Chi Minh City; adipose* (mean LC, 76%)	(9)	84/85	BSNW	–		13 (4.3–23)			49 (14–93)			29 (7.8–72)	–
Huteau et al. (1990b)	S. Viet Nam; Adipose	(27)	< 90	BSO	1.9 (20 pos.) (0.8–3.9)	4.1 (10 pos.) (1.0–16.8)	25 (21 pos.) (6.5–67.8)	26.2 (22 pos.) (1.4–121)	26.2 (22 pos.) (1.4–121)	8.9 (14 pos.) (2.0–38.9)	9.2 (2 pos.) (8.6–9.8)	47.3 (17 pos.) (9.5–238)	–	–
Schecter et al. (1990c)	Adipose N. Viet Nam	(10)	80s	BSO	1.4	0.6	9.1	4.6	4.0	1.7	ND	8.0	0.3	2.2
	S. Viet Nam	(13)			0.8	0.7	7.4	6.4	5.1	0.8	–	13.2	0.2	1.6
Schecter et al. (1990d)	Liver, stillborn	(1)	< 89	BSOW	0.5	0.8	2.4	5.6	2.6	<0.2	0.6	3.9	<0.2	<0.3
	infants	(1)			1.2	2.3	2.6	5.7	3.8	<0.4	0.8	6.6	<0.5	<0.7
		(1)			0.9	0.6	2.2	2.5	1.5	<0.3	0.3	2.8	<0.3	<0.5
Schecter et al. (1992)	Blood N. Viet Nam; pool	(82)	< 91	BSOW	4.6	1.7	7.6	20.6	11.1	0.5	2.2	46.7	1.9	4.2
	S. Viet Nam; pool	(383)			2.4	2.0	9.3	23.9	14.7	0.8	2.6	42.7	3.8	4.4
Schecter et al. (1995)	Blood S. Viet Nam; pool	(433)	91/92	BSOW	2.1	1.8	8.3	21.1	13	0.7	2.3	37.6	3.4	3.9
	Centr. Viet Nam; pool	(183)			2.9	2.2	14.9	67.4	40.0	0.9	3.0	75.7	1.9	5.1

Data presented are means and, if available, ± standard deviation, with range in parentheses, unless otherwise indicated. Levels of congeners not detected at a known detection limit (for example, 4.2 ng/kg) are presented as < 4.2 when detection limit is given.

Explanation for analytical methods: All analyses use high-resolution gas chromatography: B, HRMS; C, LRMS; I, isomer-specific; O, others; N, no information; S, sophisticated clean-up; R, reduced clean-up; W, WHO-accepted laboratory; –, not reported; ND, not detected; LC, lipid content; pos., positive; S, south; N, north; Centr, central; [ ] Calculated by the Working Group

Summed TEQ values for PCDDs/PCDFs in these studies are given in Table 25 of the monograph on PCDDs in this volume.

*Overlap between these studies

*Concentrations on wet weight-basis

*Contained also 5.5 and 4.7 ng/kg 1,2,7,8-TCDF, respectively

*150 fishermen and 150 controls between all groups

1.4.1   *Blood and tissue samples*

   (a) *Austria*

Samples of milk from cows grazing in the vicinity of a metal reclamation plant showed significantly higher PCDD/PCDF levels than control samples. In the blood of two farmers, an increase in levels of certain PCDD and PCDF isomers was found. The highest PCDF value in one sample was 2,3,4,7,8-PeCDF at 839 ng/kg (Riss *et al.*, 1990).

   (b) *Canada*

Ryan *et al.* (1985b) reported that some samples of adipose tissue from older subjects (> 60 years old) who had died in Ontario hospitals in 1979–81 contained small (mean, 3 ng/kg) amounts of 2,3,7,8-TCDF and larger amounts of 2,3,4,7,8-PeCDF (mean, 17 ng/kg).

   (c) *China*

Human adipose tissue from seven patients (four men, three women; mean age, 54 years) undergoing general surgery in Shanghai was analysed by Ryan *et al.* (1987). Compared with data from other countries, the values for most congeners were low. [The presence of 1,2,7,8-TCDF suggests that sample contamination (from paper/pulp products) may explain, in part, the relatively high levels of 2,3,7,8-TCDF.]

   (d) *Finland*

In conjunction with a study of possible effects of PCDDs and PCDFs on pulp and paper mill workers in Finland (Rosenberg *et al.*, 1995) (see also Section 1.3.1(*a*)(vii)), measurements were made in a comparison group with no known exposure (*n* = 14; mean age, 41 years). The mean I-TEQ level in blood plasma was 49 ng/kg (range, 20–99 ng/kg) (see monograph on PCDDs in this volume, Section 1.4.1). 2,3,4,7,8-PeCDF represented about one-third of the TEQ.

   (e) *France*

Measurements of PCDDs and PCDFs in adipose tissue from eight persons living in Paris were reported by Huteau *et al.* (1990a). Most of the 2,3,7,8-substituted isomers were found, in some cases at unexpectedly high values (2,3,7,8-TCDF, 1,2,3,7,8-PeCDF and 2,3,4,7,8-PeCDF). Surprisingly, non-2,3,7,8-substituted isomers were also reported at relatively high values (TCDFs, TCDDs, HpCDFs). [Sample contamination cannot be excluded.]

   (f) *Germany*

Age-related increases in blood levels of 2,3,4,7,8-PeCDF and the HxCDFs as well as I-TEQ have been reported (Schrey *et al.*, 1992; Sagunski *et al.*, 1993; Päpke *et al.*, 1996). No or very little age-dependence was observed for 2,3,7,8-TCDF, 1,2,3,7,8-PeCDF, HpCDF or OCDF.

The Kieselrotstudie (Wittsiepe *et al.*, 1993) was designed to assess the degree of exposure to PCDDs and PCDFs in 56 persons living in the vicinity of a former copper smelter located in Marsberg (see Section 1.3.2(c)). The median I-TEQ values of the Marsberg subjects (43.2 ng/kg) and a reference group from Steinfurt (43.0 ng/kg) were similar, whereas the mean of the Marsberg group (52.7 ng/kg) was higher than that of the control group (44.4 ng/kg). The individuals of the Marsberg group had significantly higher levels of PeCDFs, HxCDFs and HpCDFs on average than the individuals of the reference group.

Near a metal reclamation plant in Rastatt, Baden-Württemberg, PCDD/PCDF contamination of soil, dust from homes, indoor air and vegetables was investigated in 1987. Blood samples from 22 volunteers living in the vicinity of the plant were analysed for PCDDs/PCDFs. Levels of certain Pe-, Hx- and HpCDF isomers were increased, in a similar pattern to the contamination throughout the area. The increase in PCDD/PCDF levels was attributed to occupational exposure in the case of workers and to food intake in the other cases. For children (four samples), soil and/or dust ingestion may be a pathway of special importance (Wuthe et al., 1990).

No correlation was seen between adipose tissue or liver concentrations and age or sex in 28 subjects aged between 26 and 80 years (Thoma et al., 1989, 1990). Large differences in the concentrations of PCDDs and PCDFs between adipose and liver were demonstrated for most of the isomers. Thoma et al. (1990) also reported concentrations of PCDDs and PCDFs in adipose tissue from eight infants (age, 2–12 months). The levels were lower than in adults for nearly all isomers (see **Table 22**).

Table 22. Concentrations of PCDF isomers in adipose and liver tissues from German adults and adipose tissues of infants

Compound	Adult; ratio liver : adipose	Adipose tissue; ratio infant : adult
TCDF	2.20	0.75
PeCDF	4.93	0.36
HxCDF	9.38	0.22
HpCDF	15.43	0.23
OCDF	7.43	1.02

From Thoma et al. (1989, 1990)

Background data on PCDDs and PCDFs in human blood from Germany published by Päpke et al. (1989b) have been updated since 1991 by various authors (see Table 27 of the monograph on PCDDs in this volume). The results suggest a decrease in PCDD/PCDF blood levels in Germany over the past decade.

(g)   *Japan*

The first reports of PCDDs/PCDFs in human tissue from the general population were presented by Miyata et al. (1977) in connection with the *yusho* poisoning in Japan. Levels of PCDFs (isomers not separated) in the range of 17–45 ng/kg were reported in four of six fat and in one of four liver biopsy/autopsy samples taken from the general Japanese population. At that time, no TCDFs or HxCDFs were detected.

Kashimoto *et al.* (1985) detected PCBs and PCQs in blood of *yusho* and *yucheng* patients. PCDFs were found only in *yucheng* patients. In 60 unexposed individuals, PCDFs were not detected at a detection limit of 10 ng/kg (in whole blood).

Thirteen samples of human adipose tissue from cancer patients were analysed for tetra- to octa-CDDs and -CDFs (Ono *et al.*, 1986). These compounds were identified in all of the analysed samples. Total PCDF concentrations were in the range of 7–120 ng/kg on a wet weight basis, and 2,3,4,7,8-PeCDF levels ranged from 4 to 71 ng/kg.

(h) Taiwan

In connection with the determination of blood serum levels of PCDFs (and PCBs) in *yucheng* children perinatally exposed to contaminated rice oil, Ryan *et al.* (1994) analysed a matched control population. The total PCDD/PCDF profile for the two pooled control sera from the matched children were very similar. The mean of two measurements was given, with an I-TEQ of 12.6 ng/kg for PCDFs. The characteristic '*yucheng* isomers', 2,3,4,7,8-PeCDF and 1,2,3,4,7,8-HxCDF, showed levels 10–15 times and 15–25 times, respectively, higher in the exposed children than in the matched controls.

(i) United Kingdom

PCDD/PCDF background data were measured in pooled human adipose tissue samples from five areas in Wales (Duarte-Davidson *et al.*, 1993). With the exception of OCDF, which was found at unexpectedly high values in all pooled samples (36–62 ng/kg), the concentrations were similar to those in other industrialized countries. 2,3,7,8-TCDD and 2,3,7,8-TCDF were not detected at detection limits of 10 ng/kg.

(j) United States

Six samples from both biopsy and autopsy fat taken in 1983–84 from New York State residents were analysed (Ryan *et al.*, 1985c). PCDDs and PCDFs were found in all samples with total (Cl_4–Cl_8) PCDD levels about an order of magnitude higher than total (Cl_5–Cl_7) PCDFs. Only the penta-, hexa- and hepta-PCDF congeners were detected, at levels that were of the same order of magnitude (15–29 ng/kg). TCDF and OCDF were absent.

The tissue distribution of PCDDs and PCDFs was studied in three autopsy subjects from the general population of New York State (Ryan, 1986; Ryan *et al.*, 1986). These were the first reports to show that several 2,3,7,8-chlorine substituted PCDDs/PCDFs are present not only in adipose tissues from the general population, but also in all other tissues assayed. The ratios of the PCDD/PCDF congeners to each other were similar in each tissue, with overall levels on a wet weight basis decreasing in the order fat, adrenal, bone marrow, liver, muscle, spleen, kidney and lung. If the levels are expressed on a lipid basis rather than on a wet weight basis, liver had the highest value and the variation between tissues showed only a two- to four-fold difference.

Analysis for Cl_4–Cl_8 PCDDs/PCDFs was performed for 46 adipose tissue samples prepared from the United States Environmental Protection Agency National Human

Adipose Tissue Survey (NHATS) as composites from over 900 specimens to represent the nine United States census divisions and three age groups (0–14, 15–44 and ≥ 45 years) (Stanley *et al.*, 1986). The results demonstrate that PCDDs/PCDFs are prevalent in the general United States population and that differences exist with age. Only means and ranges of all data were reported.

A comparison of PCDD/PCDF levels in whole blood, plasma and adipose tissue was performed by Schecter *et al.* (1994b). There were few differences in PCDD/PCDF levels between blood, plasma and adipose tissue and also between whole blood and adipose tissue when reported on lipid basis. Total PCDDs/PCDFs appeared higher in plasma than in adipose tissue, if reported by actual measurement. Comparing whole blood with adipose tissue, values were more similar.

PCDDs and PCDFs in adipose tissue of United States Viet Nam veterans and controls were determined by Kang *et al.* (1991). The samples were collected in 1978. The geometric mean (± SD) 2,3,7,8-TCDF levels in adipose tissue for Viet Nam veterans, non-Viet Nam veterans and civilian controls were 2.9, 2.4 and 3.3 ng/kg, respectively. The mean levels for all isomers for these groups were not significantly different from each other.

In a study by Schecter *et al.* (1994b), levels of PCDDs and PCDFs in placenta, blood and fetal tissue were measured. The highest I-TEQ values (lipid-based) were found in blood, followed by placenta. The fetal tissue contained approximately one third of the I-TEQ of the adult values.

In a further study of partitioning of PCDDs/PCDFs in human maternal tissues, including blood, milk, adipose tissue and placenta, Schecter *et al.* (1996c) collected samples from five American women (mean age, 21.6 years; range, 21–34 years) residing in upstate New York and undergoing caesarean section deliveries between September 1995 and January 1996. Blood, placenta and fat were collected at the time of delivery. The milk and second blood were collected about four to eight weeks later. The lowest concentrations were found in the cord blood, at about one half of the maternal adipose and blood levels. A reduction in PCDD/PCDF levels was observed in the 'second' blood samples after a breast-feeding period of between four and eight weeks.

PCDD/PCDF levels in two pools of whole blood and serum (*n* = 100) collected in 1996 were compared with older blood data; a decrease was not clearly shown. Mean age of the blood donors was not specified (Schecter *et al.*, 1996d).

(k) Viet Nam

Adipose tissue samples from south Viet Nam were compared with those from north Viet Nam (where there was no exposure to Agent Orange) (Schecter *et al.*, 1986b). 2,3,7,8-TCDF was not detectable. Most of the other chlorinated PCDFs were found at higher values in samples from south Viet Nam. A further 27 individual and 10 pooled human adipose tissue specimens, collected from persons in south and north Viet Nam, respectively, were analysed for 2,3,7,8-TCDD and 2,3,7,8-TCDF (Schecter *et al.*, 1989c). The mean values were 19 ng/kg 2,3,7,8-TCDD and 7 ng/kg 2,3,7,8-TCDF in the samples from persons in the south; no 2,3,7,8-TCDD or 2,3,7,8-TCDF was detected in samples from persons in the north.

PCDD/PCDF levels in 27 adipose tissue samples from south Viet Nam were reported by Huteau *et al.* (1990b). Besides the usual 2,3,7,8-substituted isomers, they found non-2,3,7,8-substituted isomers in many samples. [Sample contamination cannot be excluded.]

In connection with analysis of blood samples from various geographical locations for PCDDs/PCDFs, Schecter *et al.* (1992) reported results for pooled samples from north Viet Nam (two analyses with a total of 82 persons) and south Viet Nam (nine analyses totalling 383 persons). The I-TEQ values for samples from north and south Viet Nam were 15 and 36 ng/kg, respectively.

1.4.2   *Human milk*

There have been a large number of studies of PCDD/PCDF concentrations in human milk. Many of the available results are shown in **Table 23** and summarized in **Table 24**. In terms of the I-TEQ concentrations, PCDFs account for between 17 and 78% of the total in human milk. The discussion in Section 1.4.2 of the monograph on PCDDs in this volume is equally applicable to PCDFs.

1.5   Regulations and guidelines

In Germany, an occupational technical exposure limit value of 50 pg I-TEQ/m^3 in air has been established for PCDDs and PCDFs (Deutsche Forschungsgemeinschaft, 1996).

At present, the regulatory requirements for incinerator emissions vary widely among the countries of the European Union. The European Union (1994) published a 'Council Directive on the incineration of hazardous waste' which would require that "the emission of PCDDs and PCDFs shall be minimized by the most progressive techniques" and which defines 0.1 ng/m^3 as a guide value which should not be exceeded by all average values measured over the sample period of 6–16 h.

Germany and the Netherlands have set daily average limit values of 0.1 ng I-TEQ/m^3 of exhaust gases for PCDDs/PCDFs from industrial waste incinerators, Sweden 0.1–0.5 ng TEQ/m^3, and the United Kingdom 1 ng I-TEQ/m^3 with a goal to reduce PCDD/-PCDF emissions from industrial and municipal waste incinerators to 0.1 ng/m^3 (ECETOC, 1992; Liem & van Zorge, 1995).

In Germany, sewage sludge used as a fertilizer for farmland is not allowed to contain more than 100 ng I-TEQ/kg dry matter (Ordinance on Sewage Sludge, 1992; Liem & van Zorge, 1995).

The Canadian Government has proposed a tolerable daily intake (TDI) value of 10 pg I-TEQ/kg bw per day for PCDDs and PCDFs (Government of Canada, 1993).

In Japan, a limit of 0.5 ng I-TEQ/m^3 2,3,7,8-PCDD/PCDF is recommended for municipal waste incinerators (Liem & van Zorge, 1995).

For milk and milk products, a maximal tolerable concentration for PCDDs/PCDFs of 17.5 ng I-TEQ/kg fat has been set in the United Kingdom. In Germany, PCDDs/PCDFs

Table 23. Concentrations of PCDFs in human milk

Reference	Origin	No.	Coll. period	Mean PCDF concentration (ng/kg fat)									
				TCDF	PeCDF		HxCDF				HpCDF		OCDF
				2378	12378	23478	123478	123678	123789	234678	1234678	1234789	
Albania													
WHO (1996)	Librazhd; unpolluted area (WHO criteria)	10	92–93	0.3	0.2	3.7	1.4	1.2	<0.1	0.8	2.7	0.1	0.3
	Tirana; polluted area (WHO criteria)	10	92–93	0.4	0.3	4.7	1.7	1.5	<0.1	0.8	1.3	0.1	0.1
Austria													
WHO (1996)	Brixlegg; industrial area (WHO criteria)	13	92–93	0.9	0.3	13.5	3.5	2.6	<0.1	1.3	4.6	0.1	2
Yrjänheikki (1989)	Tulln (WHO criteria)	51	86–88	3.9	1.3	16.9	5.3	4.8	ND	2.3	8.7	–	15.4
WHO (1996)	Tulln; rural area (WHO criteria)	21	92–93	0.6	0.2	8.5	3.4	2.3	<0.1	1.2	2.6	0.1	2
Yrjänheikki (1989)	Vienna (WHO criteria)	54	86–88	4.4	1	16.2	4.8	3.6	ND	1.8	6.5	–	18.2
WHO (1996)	Vienna; urban area (WHO criteria)	13	92–93	0.7	0.2	9.2	3.3	2.1	<0.1	1	4.9	0.1	5.9
Belgium													
Yrjänheikki (1989)	Industrial (WHO criteria)	–	86–88	6.2	2.9	32	14	6.5	1.4	6.6	7.3	–	0.3
	Rural (WHO criteria)	–	86–88	3.3	1.4	35	16	7.6	–	7	12	–	–
	Urban (WHO criteria)	–	86–88	4	1.3	32	13	6.1	3.3	–	2.2	–	5
WHO (1996)	Brabant Wallou (WHO criteria)	8	93	0.5	0.3	20.1	5.2	4.7	<0.1	2.2	3.2	0.1	0.3
	Brussels (WHO criteria)	6	93	0.6	0.3	22	5.4	4.8	<0.1	2.4	4.1	0.2	1.2
	Liege (WHO criteria)	20	93	0.7	0.3	26.7	5.8	5.3	0.1	2.1	3.8	0.1	0.3
Cambodia													
Schecter et al. (1991b)	Phnom Penh	8		0.52	0.32	1.6	0.74	0.79	<0.5	0.41	2.2	<0.5	2.4

Table 23 (contd)

Reference	Origin	No.	Coll. period	Mean PCDF concentration (ng/kg fat)									
				TCDF	PeCDF		HxCDF				HpCDF		OCDF
				2378	12378	23478	123478	123678	123789	234678	1234678	1234789	
Canada													
WHO 1996	All provinces (WHO criteria)	200	81	4.2	<1	13	17		<1	4.3	15	<1	<2
	All provinces (WHO criteria)	100	92	1.4	<1	6.2	8.1		<1	2.3	9.2	<1	<2
Yrjänheikki 1989	British Columbia	23	86–88	2.4	<1	10.3	5.2	4.3	<1	2.2	7.6	–	<2
	Maritimes	19	86–88	8	<1	6.7	3.5	2.2	<1	<1	5.6	–	<2
	Ontario N & E	32	86–88	2.9	<1	7.4	3	2.7	<1	1.5	3.8	–	<2
	Ontario SW	44	86–88	1.8	<1	9.1	3.6	2.8	<1	1.5	5	–	<2
	Prairies	31	86–88	5.7	<1	5.6	4.8	4.2	<1	2	6	–	<2
	Québec	34	86–88	4	1.7	7.1	4.2	3.5	<1	1.3	6.2	–	<2
Dewailly et al. (1991)	Québec (rural area)	16	86–88	6.1	–	5.2	3.3	2.3	–	1.1	4.5	–	–
Croatia (Yugoslavia)													
Yrjänheikki (1989)	Krk (WHO criteria)	14	86–88	<3.1	0.9	11.3	2.6	3	–	1.3	2.1	–	–
	Zagreb (WHO criteria)	41	86–88	<2	<0.9	9.7	3.2	2.9	–	1.6	1.9	–	–
WHO (1996)	Krk (WHO criteria)	10	93	0.4	0.2	7.9	2.5	2	<0.1	0.8	1.7	0.1	0.3
	Zagreb (WHO criteria)	13	93	0.9	0.6	13.5	4	3.5	<0.1	1.7	2.8	0.1	0.3
Czech Republic													
WHO (1996)	Kladno (WHO criteria)	11	93	0.9	0.4	16.3	5.7	3.8	<0.1	1.1	3.4	0.1	0.2
	Uherske Hradiste (WHO criteria)	11	93	1.1	0.4	25.5	7.3	4.7	<0.1	1.8	2.9	0.1	0.2

Table 23 (contd)

Reference	Origin	No.	Coll. period	Mean PCDF concentration (ng/kg fat)									
				TCDF	PeCDF		HxCDF				HpCDF		OCDF
				2378	12378	23478	123478	123678	123789	234678	1234678	1234789	
Denmark													
Yrjänheikki (1989)	WHO criteria	10	86–88	1.2	–	12.8	7	5	–	1.5	8.5	–	–
	Pool	42	86~	1.2	–	12	5.6	4.4	–	1.5	8.8	–	–
WHO (1996)	7 cities (WHO criteria)	48	93	0.5	0.2	11.1	3.5	3	0.1	1.2	6.1	0.1	0.4
Abraham et al. (1995b)	Faeroe Islands	1	94~	<0.5	<0.5	7	3	2.4	–	<0.5	2.4	–	<2
		1	94~	1.6	<0.5	6.2	5.4	3.5	–	2.2	5.3	–	<2
		1	94~	1	<0.5	6	6	4.5	–	<0.5	6.2	–	2.8
		1	94~	<3	<3	5.3	<3	<3	–	<3	9.4	–	9.2
	pool	9	94~	0.7	<0.2	4.2	2.5	1.9	–	0.9	1.6	–	<0.5
Estonia													
Mussalo-Rauhamaa & Lindström (1995)	Tallinn (primipara)	6	91	0.7	0.2	12.8	4.7	2.5	<0.1	0.4	1.9	<0.1	0.9
	Tarto (primipara)	6	91	1.3	0.2	23.8	3.6	2.6	<0.1	0.8	3.9	<0.1	1.2
Finland													
Yrjänheikki (1989)	Helsinki (WHO criteria)	38	86–88	0.3	0.2	15	2.6	1	<0.5	2	8.8	–	1.6
WHO (1996)	Helsinki (WHO criteria)	10	93	1.1	0.5	19	4.5	3.5	0.1	1.5	9.9	0.1	1.9
Yrjänheikki (1989)	Kuopio (WHO criteria)	31	86–88	0.3	0.3	14	2.9	1.3	<0.5	2.3	12	–	1.9
WHO 1996	Kuopio (WHO criteria)	24	93	0.6	0.3	9.6	2.6	2.1	<0.1	0.9	6.9	0.1	0.3
France													
González et al. (1996)	Paris	15	90	1.8	0.5	16.5			20.4			45	19

Table 23 (contd)

Reference	Origin	No.	Coll. period	Mean PCDF concentration (ng/kg fat)									
				TCDF	PeCDF		HxCDF				HpCDF		OCDF
				2378	12378	23478	123478	123678	123789	234678	1234678	1234789	
Germany													
Beck et al. (1992a)	Mother having 1, 2 or 3 children	728	82–92	ND	ND	28.3	ND	ND	ND	ND	ND	ND	ND
	1 child	34	NR	2.1	1	13	5.1	5.7	–	2.7	5.9	–	0.3
	2 children	23	NR	2.9	1	24	8.6	8.9	–	3.6	9.9	–	1.8
	3 children	34	NR	2.9	1	18	7.4	7.2	–	2.9	7.6	–	0.9
Frommberger (1990)	Baden-Württemberg	490	88–89	4.2	0.3	38	7.9	5.9	–	2.9	6.8	–	1
Beck et al. (1987)	Berlin	30		2.5	<1	20	8.7	7.8	–	3	8.5	–	<3.1
Beck et al. (1989c)	Berlin	35		2.8	1	21	8.6	7.9	–	3.2	8.6	–	3
Yrjänheikki (1989)	Berlin (WHO criteria)	40	86–88	1.4	0.7	22	8.7	7.7	–	2.7	13	–	0.9
WHO (1996)	Berlin (WHO criteria)	10	93	<0.4	<0.4	11.9	5.5	4.4	<0.4	1	3.3	<0.1	<0.1
Beck et al. (1989c)	Flensburg (Baltic coast)	6		1.6	0.6	25	8.7	8.4	–	2.6	9.3	–	0.3
Fürst et al. (1992b)	North-Rhine Westphalia	526	84–91	1.7	0.5	26.7	7.8	6.5	–	3.4	5.5	–	1.4
Yrjänheikki (1989)	North-Rhine Westphalia (WHO criteria)	79	86–88	2.3	0.6	30	8.2	6.7	<0.5	3.8	5.3	–	7.2
Yrjänheikki (1989)	Oldenburg (WHO criteria)	35	86–88	2.4	0.9	23.7	15.2	15	ND	6.2	12.8	–	6.7
Beck et al. (1989c)	Recklinghausen; industrial area	10		1.4	0.7	22	7.7	9.2	–	3.1	13	–	4
Yrjänheikki (1989)	Recklinghausen (WHO criteria)	23	86–88	1.4	0.9	26	8.5	8	ND	3	8.4	–	1.3
Beck et al. (1989c)	Rheinfelden (rural area/PCP manuf.)	9		5.8	1.3	24	11	9.7	ND	3.9	12	ND	1.5
Beck et al. (1989c)	Weiden; rural area	14		3.3	1.1	22	7.4	7.5	–	3.3	8.7	–	0.7

Table 23 (contd)

Reference	Origin	No.	Coll. period	Mean PCDF concentration (ng/kg fat)									
				TCDF	PeCDF		HxCDF				HpCDF		OCDF
				2378	12378	23478	123478	123678	123789	234678	1234678	1234789	
Hungary													
Yrjänheikki (1989)	Budapest (WHO criteria)	100	86–88	0.5	<0.5	5.7	<2	<2	–	0.5	3.3	–	6.5
WHO (1996)	Budapest (WHO criteria)	20	93	0.3	0.2	5.9	2.6	2.1	<0.1	0.8	2.8	0.1	0.2
Yrjänheikki (1989)	Szentes (WHO criteria)	50	86–88	0.7	<0.5	7.6	<2	<2	–	0.4	<2	ND	7.6
WHO (1996)	Szentes (WHO criteria)	10	93	0.4	0.3	5.6	2.5	2	<0.1	1	2.7	0.1	0.3
Japan													
Schecter et al. (1989d)/Yrjänheikki (1989)	Fukuoka	6	86	3	1.3	26	4.5	3	<1	2	4	–	<2
Hirakawa et al. (1995)	Fukuoka (primipara)	7	94	2.3	0.6	11.4	4.3	4.5	1.9	2	2	0.2	2.7
Hirakawa et al. (1995)	Fukuoka (multipara)	8	94	2	0.6	7.8	3.3	3.2	1.6	1.5	2.1	0.7	3
Hashimoto et al. (1995b)	Various locations	26	93–94	1.7	1.6	38	6.5	6.8	1.2	4	4.2	5.9	3.6
Jordan													
Alawi et al. (1996b)	Amman; pool	4–6	94	<3.2	<3.2	<3.2	<3.2	<3.2	<3.2	<3.2	9.6	<3.2	<32
	Amman; pool		94	<6.3	<6.3	<6.3	<6.3	<6.3	<6.3	<6.3	<6.3	<6.3	<31
	Aqaba; pool		94	<4.5	4.5	10.1	17.9	<4.5	<4.5	<4.5	<4.5	<4.5	<22
	Irbid; pool		94	8.3	11.1	75.9	161	104	7.4	54.6	391	106	189
	Madaba; pool		94	<11	16.8	84.1	112	96.1	<11	<11	<11	<11	<22
	Zarka; pool		94	<2.6	2.6	4.4	5.2	4.4	<2.6	<2.6	<2.6	<2.6	<17
Kazakhstan													
Petreas et al. (1996)	WHO criteria	40	96	1.1	0.77	5.3	2.3	1.9	0.75	1.2	2.4	1	3

Table 23 (contd)

Reference	Origin	No.	Coll. period	Mean PCDF concentration (ng/kg fat)									
				TCDF	PeCDF	HxCDF					HpCDF		OCDF
				2378	12378	23478	123478	123678	123789	234678	1234678	1234789	
Lithuania													
WHO (1996)	Anykshchiai; rural area (WHO criteria)	12	93	0.8	0.4	10.3	3.8	2.7	<0.4	1.3	3.4	0.2	0.6
	Palanga; coastal area (WHO criteria)	12	93	1.1	0.4	16.4	4.1	3.2	<0.2	1.6	1.8	0.1	0.2
	Vilnius; urban area (WHO criteria)	12	93	1.3	0.9	9.1	4	3	<0.5	1.8	3.8	0.5	0.8
Netherlands													
Liem et al. (1995)	Primipara	103	93	0.4	0.2	18	5.2	4.4	–	2.4	6	0.1	0.3
Yrjänheikki (1989)	Rural area (WHO criteria)	13	86–88	3.1	0.8	24	7	6.3	ND	2.6	16	–	0.8
	Urban area (WHO criteria)	13	86–88	2.8	0.7	23	7.1	7.1	ND	ND	ND	–	2.4
WHO (1996)	WHO criteria	17	93	0.3	0.3	17.2	5.1	4.4	<0.5	2.6	6	<0.5	0.3
Norway													
Clench-Aas et al. (1992)	Hamar; rural area (WHO criteria)	10	85–86	4.1	0.8	11.4	4.6	2.7	0.7	1	5.5	–	1.2
WHO (1996)	Hamar; rural area (WHO criteria)	10	93	1.1	0.4	7.5	2	1.9	<0.5	1.1	4.3	<0.6	1.5
Clench-Aas et al. (1992)	Skien-Porsgrunn; Mg production (WHO criteria)	10	85–86	4.9	1.3	17.7	7.8	5.3	0.7	1.7	5.6	–	2.5
WHO (1996)	Skien-Porsgrunn; industrial area (WHO criteria)	10	93	1.2	0.5	10.9	4.5	3.7	<0.5	1.4	5.2	<0.6	1.3

Table 23 (contd)

Reference	Origin	No.	Coll. period	Mean PCDF concentration (ng/kg fat)									
				TCDF 2378	PeCDF 12378	23478	HxCDF 123478	123678	123789	234678	HpCDF 1234678	1234789	OCDF
Norway (contd)													
Clench-Aas et al. (1992)	Tromsø; coastal area (WHO criteria)	11	85–86	4.3	0.8	12.9	3.6	2.6	0.7	0.9	6.2	–	1.1
WHO (1996)	Tromsø (WHO criteria)	10	93	1.8	0.3	7.6	1.9	1.7	<0.3	1.4	18.7	<0.5	3.3
New Zealand													
Buckland et al. (1990a)	Auckland (WHO criteria)	11	90~	0.8	0.35	4.9		5.9	<0.6	0.71	6.2	<0.5	<6
	Christchurch (WHO criteria)	9	90~	0.74	0.23	5.8		7.7	<0.9	0.84	7.4	<0.8	<6
	N. Canterbury (WHO criteria)	8	90~	0.78	0.2	6.6		8.8	<0.6	0.91	7.8	<0.7	<6
	Northland (WHO criteria)	9	90~	1.1	0.22	4.7		8.6	<0.7	1.1	7.5	<0.7	<8
Pakistan													
Schecter et al. (1990e)	Pool	7		1.2	<4.3	6.5		5.8	<3.9	1.5	4.3	<3.5	<6.6
WHO (1996)	Lahore (WHO criteria)	14	93	<0.02	<0.01	2.9	1.3	1.1	<0.1	0.5	3.9	<0.02	13.8
Poland													
Yrjänheikki (1989)	WHO criteria	5	86–88	1.7	4.3	15.4	18.6	10	–	5.9	35.1	–	–
Russian Federation													
WHO (1996)	Arkhangelsk	1	93	1.5	0.5	12.9	3.2	2.3	0.1	1	1.9	0.1	0.2
Schecter et al. (1990f)	Baikalsk; pool	5	88–89	2.7	1.3	9.6	8.2	3.2	<0.5	0.6	1.4	<0.5	0.4
	Irkutsk; pool	4	88–89	6.3	2.3	19	15	5	<0.5	1.8	2.6	<0.5	2
	Kachug; pool	4	88–89	2.8	1	7.4	5.7	2.2	<0.5	0.7	0.6	<0.5	0.5
WHO (1996)	Karhopol	1	93	0.7	0.2	5	1.4	0.9	<0.1	0.3	0.8	0.1	0.1
Schecter et al. (1990f)	Moscow	1	88–89	1.9	0.4	11	4	2.5	<0.5	1.1	1.5	<0.5	0.8
	Novosibirsk; pool	10	88–89	1.7	0.8	8.4	5.4	2.4	<0.5	0.8	0.7	<0.5	1.5

Table 23 (contd)

Reference	Origin	No.	Coll. period	TCDF	PeCDF		HxCDF				HpCDF		OCDF
				2378	12378	23478	123478	123678	123789	234678	1234678	1234789	
Slovakia													
WHO (1996)	Michalovce (WHO criteria)	10	93	1.1	0.4	21	5.8	3.5	<0.1	1.1	5.5	0.1	0.2
	Nitra (WHO criteria)	10	93	0.8	0.5	14.5	5.4	4	0.1	1.4	2.7	0.1	0.3
South Africa													
Schecter et al. (1990e)	Pool												
	Black	6		0.8	0.3	2	2.4	1.8	0.6	0.6	5.2	0.6	6.1
	White	18		1.5	0.4	5.5	3.4	3.1	ND	1.3	4.7	0.4	2.8
Spain													
WHO (1996)	Bizkaia (WHO criteria)	19	93	0.9	0.4	16.9	5	4	0.1	1.5	3	0.2	0.5
	Gipuzkoa (WHO criteria)	10	93	0.7	0.4	20.9	6	4.7	0.1	2.2	3.1	0.1	0.2
González et al. (1996)	Madrid	13	90	1	0.7	0.9			30			7.2	18
Sweden													
Yrjänheikki (1989); Clench-Aas et al. (1992)	Borlänge; rural area	10	85–86	3.6	0.8	17	7	3.7	<1.5	1.3	5.7	–	<2.5
	Gothenburg; city (WHO criteria)	10	85–86	4.1	–	17.4	5.2	3.7	<1.5	2.6	11.4	–	<2.5
	Sundsvall; industrial (WHO criteria)	10	85–86	3.8	–	19.6	4	3.3	<1.5	2	6.7	–	<2.5
	Uppsala (MSWI) (WHO criteria)	10	85–86	3.7	–	17.1	5.3	4.4	<1.5	2.4	12.1	–	<2.5
Thailand													
Schecter et al. (1991b)	Bangkok	10		1.8	0.7	2.6	1.2	0.9	<0.5	0.6	0.9	<0.5	0.6

Table 23 (contd)

Reference	Origin	No.	Coll. period	Mean PCDF concentration (ng/kg fat)									
				TCDF	PeCDF		HxCDF				HpCDF		OCDF
				2378	12378	23478	123478	123678	123789	234678	1234678	1234789	
United Kingdom													
Wearne et al. (1996)	Cambridge (WHO criteria)	20	93–94	0.82	0.47	16	4.4	4	0.09	2.5	4	0.19	0.57
Startin et al. (1989)	Glasgow (WHO criteria)	50	87~	0.9	0.3	19	7.2	5	ND	2.3	7.1	–	6.9
Wearne et al. (1996)	Glasgow (WHO criteria)	20	93–94	0.78	0.3	15	4.2	3.6	< 0.1	2.2	4	0.15	0.81
Startin et al. (1989)	Sutton Coldfield (WHO criteria)	50	87~	1.4	0.5	25	8.3	7.8	ND	3.6	9.5	–	6.8
Wearne et al. (1996)	Birmingham (WHO criteria)	20	93–94	1	0.29	14	4.2	3.6	< 0.1	2	2.9	0.13	0.72
Ukraine													
WHO (1996)	Kiev (WHO criteria)												
	Area 1	5	93	0.8	0.6	9.5	7.1	4.4	0.2	1.3	5.7	0.8	1.9
	Area 2	5	93	0.8	0.5	9.9	7.1	4.6	0.2	1.3	4.6	0.7	1
United States													
Schecter et al. (1989d; 1994b; 1996a,b)	United States	43	88	2.85	0.45	7.3	5.6	3.2	< 0.75	1.9	4.1	< 1	4.1
Schecter et al. (1990e)	Tennessee; pool	9	–	1	< 1.5	4.1	7.8		< 1.4	1.2	8.1	< 2.7	< 5.8

Table 23 (contd)

Reference	Origin	No.	Coll. period	Mean PCDF concentration (ng/kg fat)									
				TCDF	PeCDF		HxCDF				HpCDF		OCDF
				2378	12378	23478	123478	123678	123789	234678	1234678	1234789	
Viet Nam													
Schecter et al. (1990e)	Binh Long; pool	4		1	1.3	7.1	8.8	6.7	< 1.3	2	13.2	< 3.5	< 7
Schecter et al. (1991b); Schecter (1994)	Da Nang	11	85–90	2.2	4.1	17	34	18	< 0.5	10	40	< 0.5	7.4
	Dong Nai	11	85–90	1.6	1	13	19	11	< 0.5	2.1	6.2	< 0.5	0.9
	Hanoi	30	85–90	2	1	6.1	4.2	3.1	< 0.5	1.4	3.4	< 0.5	2.1
Schecter et al. (1989d); Schechter (1994)	Ho Chi Minh	38	85–90	2.8	1.4	8.1	5.7	3.6	< 0.5	1.6	8	ND	2.6
	Song Be	12	85–90	2	2	8.7	12	7.8	< 0.5	2.7	10	ND	1.8
Schecter et al. (1990e)	Tay Ninh; pool	4		1.1	2	10.9		16.3	< 2.4	3.1	14.9	< 5.9	< 14
	Vung Tau	5		2	1.4	9.3	9.5	5.4	0.7	1.6	11.8	< 4.9	< 7

ND, not detected and detection limit not reported; –, not reported

WHO criteria are described in Section 1.4.2 of the monograph on PCDDs in this volume.

Summed TEQ values for PCDDs/PCDFs in these studies are given in Table 29 of the monograph on PCDDs in this volume.

Table 24. Summary of concentrations (ng/kg fat) of PCDFs in human milk (as reported in Table 23)

	TCDF	PeCDF		HxCDF				HpCDF		OCDF
	2378	12378	23478	123478	123678	123789	234678	1234678	1234789	
Mean	2.0	1.1	15	8.4	6.6	1.1	2.6	9.9	3.2	5.7
Minimum	0.3	0.2	0.9	0.74	0.79	0.09	0.3	0.6	0.1	0.1
5th percentile	0.4	0.2	4.2	1.6	1.3	0.1	0.58	1.5	0.1	0.2
25th percentile	0.8	0.3	7.3	3.5	2.7	0.1	1.1	3.3	0.1	0.4
Median	1.4	0.6	12	5.2	4.1	0.5	1.6	5.6	0.1	1.5
75th percentile	2.8	1	19	7.3	6.6	1.4	2.4	8.5	0.4	3.4
95th percentile	5.7	3.9	31	17	16	3.3	6.3	15	5.9	17
Maximum	8.3	17	84	161	104	7.4	55	391	106	189

must not exceed 5 ng I-TEQ/kg milk fat and, in the Netherlands, they must not exceed 6 ng I-TEQ/kg milk and milk product fat (Liem & van Zorge, 1995).

2. Studies of Cancer in Humans

Human beings have not been documented to have been exposed to toxicologically significant amounts of PCDFs alone. There have been two food poisonings in Asia in which PCBs contaminated by PCDFs were the etiological agent. The blood levels of PCBs of the victims in these incidents were higher than those of the general population but lower than are seen in highly exposed workers. [The Working Group noted that several cohorts with occupational exposure to PCBs have been followed; there is some evidence of increased incidence of liver and biliary cancer combined but not increased primary liver cancer (Brown, 1987).] The morbidity experienced by the poisoning victims was greater than is usually seen in PCB workers, and this difference in toxicity is usually attributed to the admixed PCDFs. Strictly, though, inferences about the toxicity of PCDFs, PCBs, or any component of the oil are not justified, since all the victims were exposed to all components. There has also been exposure to PCDFs in accidents, such as the Binghamton, NY, fire (see Section 1.2.1(b)(viii)), but they have been in situations in which there was also documented exposure to 2,3,7,8-TCDD, other PCDDs, PCBs, and other compounds.

The most toxic PCDFs are estimated to have a potency within one or two orders of magnitude of that of 2,3,7,8-TCDD. Thus, for some groups with environmental exposures, such as consumers of Baltic Sea fish, PCDFs may make up the major part of their potentially toxic exposures as estimated by total TEQs.

2.1 Rice oil contamination incidents

The poisoning incidents in Japan and Taiwan involving consumption of contaminated rice oil are described in Section 1.3.1(b)(i).

2.1.1 Japan

In 1968, in Fukuoka and Nagasaki, Japan, there was an outbreak of an illness consisting of severe cystic acne, hyperpigmentation and conjunctivitis. Clinical and epidemiological investigation showed a strong association with the consumption of specific lots of rice bran cooking oil (Kuratsune *et al.*, 1972). The illness was termed '*yusho*', Japanese for 'oil disease'. Initially, chemical analysis could show only that there was a large amount of chlorine in the oil; the contaminant was later shown to be PCBs and related compounds.

Eventually about 2000 cases were registered with Japanese health authorities. The reasons for registration included not only epidemiological surveillance but also clinical care and in some cases eligibility for compensation. [The Working Group noted that some people who were genuine cases may have avoided registration, and some with minimal exposure may be included, but the combination of general publicity and the linking of registration to care probably means that most of those eligible were registered.]

The Japanese oil contained of the order of 1000 mg/kg PCBs and 5 mg/kg PCDFs. Estimates of intake are based on a study of 141 cases (Masuda, 1994). These patients consumed about 500 mL oil before becoming symptomatic, and about another 200 mL before the cause of the illness was determined and oil consumption ceased. Thus, they ingested about 500 mg PCBs and 2.5 mg PCDFs before becoming symptomatic, and about 600 mg PCBs and 3.5 mg PCDFs in total. This occurred over a period of weeks.

Ikeda and Yoshimura (1996) followed 1815 *yusho* patients identified from the registry from the Japanese Ministry of Health and Welfare to the end of March 1990. They then contacted the local health departments and obtained a copy of the death certificate for each of those who had died. The causes of death, standardized mortality ratios (SMRs) and confidence intervals (CIs) are presented in **Table 25**. The overall analysis used Japanese national data for its comparison group, but regional data were used for specific cancer sites in order to see whether regional variations explained observed excesses in mortality. The SMR for total mortality was 1.1 [95% CI, 0.9–1.2]; for total cancer in men, it was 1.6 [95% CI, 1.2–2.1]; and, for liver cancer in men, it was 3.4 [95% CI, 1.8–6.0]. Women had decreased total cancer mortality but a nonsignificant increase in liver cancer mortality (SMR, 2.3; [95% CI, 0.5–6.7]) based on three deaths. There was no excess mortality from cancer in women. Both sexes showed a nonsignificant excess mortality from non-malignant liver disease.

2.1.2 Taiwan

Although the rice oil processing machines were banned in Japan, at least one found its way to Taiwan. In 1979, an extraordinary replication of the Japanese incident occurred there (Hsu *et al.*, 1985), called '*yucheng*', meaning 'oil disease' in Chinese, again involving about 2000 persons.

The Taiwanese oil contained about 100 mg/kg PCBs and 0.4 mg/kg PCDFs. Estimates are based on a study of 99 cases. Patients consumed about 300 mg PCBs and 1.3 mg PCDFs during latency and about 1 g PCBs and 3.8 mg PCDFs in total (Hsu *et al.*, 1994). Some persons consumed the oil for six months before becoming symptomatic. The ratio of PCBs to PCDFs was similar in the *yusho* and *yucheng* episodes, and the dose of PCBs and PCDFs causing symptoms was roughly similar, although the Taiwanese consumed more oil that was less contaminated.

Yu *et al.* (1996) reported that a total of 2061 subjects were included in the *yucheng* registry by 1983; no cases were added nor active follow-up carried out after that year. They acquired the registry and traced cohort members through 31 December 1991. For the deceased cases, they acquired a copy of the death certificate from the local household registration offices and abstracted information on date, place and cause of death. The overall and cause-specific mortality of the exposed group was compared with that of the Taiwan general population using 1 January 1979 as the date of the incident and, as the end of follow-up, 31 December 1991, the date of death or the last date a subject was known to be living. Of the 2061 subjects in the 1983 *yucheng* registry, 70 were actually offspring of the exposed subjects who were born after 30 June 1978 and were excluded. Of the remaining 1991 *yucheng* subjects, 154 did not have valid addresses and thus could not be traced; therefore, a total of 1837 *yucheng* subjects were included. Vital status was determined for 99.5%; 83 of the subjects had died during the follow-up period. The SMR for total mortality was 0.8 (95% CI, 0.7–1.0). There were 10 cancer deaths (SMR, 1.2; 95% CI, 0.6–2.3) including three from liver cancer (SMR, 0.8; 95% CI, 0.2–2.4). There was a 2.7-fold (1.3–4.9) excess of cirrhosis and non-malignant liver disease, based on 10 deaths. Hsieh *et al.* (1996) independently studied the Taiwanese cohort during the same time period and came to similar conclusions.

Table 25. Follow-up studies of mortality in the Asian PCB/PCDF poisonings

	Yusho (Japan)		*Yucheng* (Taiwan)			
	Ikeda & Yoshimura (1996)		Yu *et al.* (1996)		Hsieh *et al.* (1996)	
Number	1815		1837		1940	
Male	816		851		929	
Female	899		986		1011	
Years of follow-up	1968–90		1979–91		1979–91	
Median age at exposure	[~ 25 years]		[~ 22 years] (46% were < 20 years old)		[~ 22 years]	
Deaths	No.	SMR (95% CI)	No.	SMR (95% CI)	No.	SMR (95% CI)
Total deaths	200	1.1 [0.9–1.2]	83	0.8 (0.7–1.0)	102	1.1 (0.9–1.3)
Male	127	1.2 [1.0–1.4]	47	0.8 (0.6–1.1)	55	1.0 (0.8–1.3)
Female	73	0.9 [0.7–1.1]	36	0.9 (0.6–1.2)	47	1.3 (1.0–1.8)
Cancer deaths	58	1.2 [0.9–1.6]	10	1.2 (0.6–2.3)	11	0.6 (0.3–1.0)
Male	45	1.6 [1.2–2.1]	8	1.6 (0.7–3.2)	8	0.7 (0.3–1.4)
Female	13	0.7 [0.3–1.0]	2	0.6 (0.1–2.3)	3	0.4 (0.1–1.2)
Liver cancer deaths	15	3.1 [1.7–5.1]	3	0.8 (0.2–2.4)	2	0.7 (0.1–2.5)
Male	12	3.4 [1.8–6.0]	2	0.7 (0.1–2.5)	1	0.3 (0.0–1.6)
Female	3	2.3 [0.5–6.7]	1	1.3 (0.02–7.1)	1	1.1 (0.0–6.0)
Liver disease deaths	9	1.8 [0.8–3.5]	10	2.7 (1.3–4.9)	15	3.2 [1.8–5.3]
Male	6	1.7 [0.6–3.6]	7	2.5 (1.0–5.1)	9	2.5 [1.2–4.8]
Female	3	2.3 [0.5–6.7]	3	3.4 (0.7–9.8)	6	5.2 [1.9–11.4]

[ ] Calculated by the Working Group

2.1.3 *Comparison of Japan and Taiwan*

The cancer findings in the 12-year follow-up data from Taiwan are not consistent with the 22-year follow-up data from Japan. There was a clear excess of liver cancer mortality in males in Japan that was not seen in Taiwan. The excess of liver cancer was even greater in the Japanese data at 15 years of follow-up (Ikeda *et al.*, 1986) (SMR, 5.6) than it was at 22 years (SMR, 3.4). Both cohorts showed an excess of non-malignant liver disease. The exposures to the heat-degraded PCBs appear to have been similar. Masuda (1994) showed that the differences in blood levels of PCBs and PCDFs reported between *yusho* and *yucheng* were a function of the time after the incident that the samples were drawn, rather than due to differences in exposure. The methods of cohort selection and follow-up do not appear to favour ascertainment of those with cancer in Japan compared with those in Taiwan. The belief among physicians that the status of being a *yusho* (or *yucheng*) case increases cancer risk, leading to a more frequent diagnosis, cannot be ruled out. However, such a diagnostic bias would have to be specific to Japan and to liver cancer to produce the observed effect. Liver disease and liver cancer are common in both countries, and the recognition and management of them is a regular part of clinical training. It is unlikely that liver cancer is being under-diagnosed among the Taiwanese.

Chronic hepatitis B infection confers a relative risk of as high as 100 for liver cancer. In the 1970s and 1980s, Japan as a whole probably had about a 2% seroprevalence for antibody to hepatitis B surface antigen, while Taiwan had about 15% (IARC, 1994a). It is therefore unlikely to be a confounder.

Hepatitis C virus is probably more prevalent in Japan than in Taiwan (IARC, 1994b). Ito *et al.* (1991), in a community-based survey of Japanese over the age of 40 years, showed a prevalence of 2.3% using a (relatively non-specific) first-generation ELISA assay. In Taiwan, Lin *et al.* (1991) showed a prevalence of 0.6% in pregnant women using a second-generation recombinant immunoblot assay. Thus, Japan has a four-fold higher rate, but the prevalences are low. Hepatitis C appears to be as carcinogenic as hepatitis B but, unless there is a different chemical interaction with the two viruses (for which there is no evidence), the difference in prevalence cannot account for the liver cancer excess in *yusho* patients in Japan.

Hepatitis B and possibly C infection increases dramatically at lower latitudes, and the prefectures of Japan involved, Nagasaki and Fukuoka, are southern ones. Relatively minor differences in the prevalence of hepatitis virus infection could readily produce a relative risk of 3 for liver cancer, since the national rates are dominated by the population centres further north. Ikeda and Yoshimura (1996), however, considered this possibility and found that, when the liver cancer rates among *yusho* patients were compared with the Nagasaki and Fukuoka rates, the relative risk declined from 3.4 to 2.3 in men but remained statistically significant. This may be too conservative, since only about half of the cases actually lived in Nagasaki and Fukuoka.

2.2 Fish consumption

Swedish investigators have studied mortality and cancer incidence in Swedish fishermen and their wives (Rylander & Hagmar, 1995) from the Baltic coast, who prefer salmon, herring and other fatty fish, and compared them both with the rates in the Swedish population (Hagmar *et al.*, 1992) and those of fishing families from the Atlantic coast, who prefer less fatty cod and flat fish (Svensson *et al.*, 1995a). Swedish fishermen were believed to eat about twice as much fish as the general population, and this was confirmed by dietary interviews in a sample of the wives. Baltic fish are contaminated by organochlorine compounds, and the concentration of these substances in human body fat relates to the amount of fish consumed. The predominant exposure in terms of PCDDs and PCDFs from fatty fish from the Baltic Sea is to 2,3,4,7,8-PeCDF (Svensson *et al.*, 1991) [although even heavy fish consumers probably have body fat concentrations about three orders of magnitude lower than those of the victims of the Asian poisonings]. These fish also contain PCBs and other persistent chlorinated compounds.

The fishermen (> 99% of the cohort members were men) cohorts were formed from the records of the local fishermen's organizations. For the Atlantic coast, 8493 persons (16 women) had ever been members of the organization and, for the Baltic coast, 2907 persons (24 women). The cohorts consisted of 8477 Atlantic coast and 2896 Baltic coast fishermen observed from 1965 for the Atlantic and from 1968 for the Baltic. After the fishermen were identified, the wives were sought through linkage to the national Swedish population registry and also records in local parishes. For the Atlantic coast, 7166 women were identified who either were or had been married to one of the fishermen. For the Baltic coast, there were 2175 women. Information was updated for everyone to 31 December 1988, including a subset of the Baltic coast men who had been reported on previously (Hagmar *et al.*, 1992). Data on death came from Statistics Sweden and those on cancer occurrence from the Swedish Cancer Registry (Svensson *et al.*, 1995b).

Stomach cancer occurred more frequently in the Baltic coast fishermen. Compared with the regional population, the standardized incidence ratio (SIR) was 1.6 (95% CI, 1.0–2.4) and, compared with Atlantic coast fishermen, the incidence rate ratio (IRR) was 2.2 (1.3–3.5). Squamous-cell cancer of the skin was diagnosed more frequently in the Baltic coast fishermen (SIR, 2.3; 1.5–3.5) compared with the regional population and (IRR, 1.9; 1.2–3.1) compared with the Atlantic coast fishermen. Both cohorts of fishermen had higher mortality from multiple myeloma compared with the general population, with SMRs of 3.1 on the Baltic coast and 1.3 on the Atlantic coast. Ischaemic heart disease was decreased among the Baltic coast fishermen but not among those from the Atlantic coast, consistent with their reported differences in diet and the possible protective role of *n*-3 polyunsaturated fatty acids found in the fatty fish preferred by the former population (Svensson *et al.*, 1995b). Compared to the Swedish rates, the Baltic coast wives had a slightly higher and the Atlantic coast wives a slightly lower incidence of breast cancer, but comparisons with neither the population nor the other group were significant (Rylander & Hagmar, 1995).

2.3   Industrial cohorts

[The Working Group noted that exposure to PCDFs may have occurred among workers in the phenoxy herbicides/chlorophenols industrial production cohorts which have been reviewed in the monograph on PCDDs. Exposure to PCDFs, however, is inadequately characterized in these cohorts. Furthermore, the Working Group considered that confounding by concomitant exposure to PCDDs seriously complicates any interpretation of these data regarding cancer risk in relation to PCDF exposure.]

3.   Studies of Cancer in Experimental Animals

3.1   Administration with known carcinogens

Studies on PCDFs in combination with known carcinogens are summarized in **Table 26**.

3.1.1   *Mouse skin*

2,3,7,8-Tetrachlorodibenzofuran

Groups of 20 female HRS/J hairless (*hr/hr*) mice, eight weeks of age, were given skin applications of 0 or 5 µmol/animal *N*-methyl-*N'*-nitro-*N*-nitrosoguanidine (MNNG) in 50 µL acetone followed by 1 µg/animal 2,3,7,8-TCDF in 50 µL acetone twice weekly for 20 weeks. Skin papillomas developed in 19/19 mice (4.9 tumours/mouse) in mice treated with MNNG plus 2,3,7,8-TCDF compared with 1/20 (0.05 tumours/mouse) in mice treated with 2,3,7,8-TCDF alone and 0/23 with MNNG alone (Poland *et al.*, 1982).

2,3,4,7,8-Pentachlorodibenzofuran

Three groups of 20 female HRS/J hairless (*hr/hr*) mice, five to eight weeks of age, were treated with single skin applications of 5 µmol/animal MNNG in 50 µL acetone. Starting seven days later, the mice were treated with 25, 50 or 100 ng/animal 2,3,4,7,8-PeCDF in 25 µL acetone twice weekly for 20 weeks. A control group of 20 mice received acetone followed by 100 ng/animal 2,3,4,7,8-PeCDF. The numbers of surviving mice with papillomas of the skin were 9/19, 11/18 and 8/18 in mice treated with MNNG and 25, 50 or 100 ng/animal 2,3,4,7,8-PeCDF compared with 0/20 in mice treated with 2,3,4,7,8-PeCDF alone and 1/19 in mice treated with MNNG alone. Skin carcinomas were found in 1/19 mice treated with MNNG + 25 ng 2,3,4,7,8-PeCDF, 1/19 mice treated with MNNG + 100 ng 2,3,4,7,8-PeCDF and in 1/19 mice treated with MNNG alone (Hébert *et al.*, 1990a).

1,2,3,4,7,8-Hexachlorodibenzofuran

Three groups of 20 female HRS/J hairless (*hr/hr*) mice, five to eight weeks of age, were treated with single skin applications of 5 µmol/animal MNNG in 50 µL acetone. Starting seven days later, the mice were treated with 250, 500 or 1000 ng/animal 1,2,3,4,7,8-HxCDF in 25 µL acetone twice weekly for 20 weeks. A control group of 20 mice received acetone followed by 1000 ng/animal 1,2,3,4,7,8-HxCDF. The numbers of surviving mice with papillomas of the skin were 15/19, 7/14 and 3/17 in mice treated with MNNG and 250, 500 or 1000 ng/animal 1,2,3,4,7,8-HxCDF compared with 1/17 in mice treated with 1,2,3,4,7,8-HxCDF alone. Skin carcinomas occurred in 1/19 mice treated with MNNG + 250 ng 1,2,3,4,7,8-HxCDF, 2/17 mice treated with MNNG + 1000 ng 1,2,3,4,7,8-HxCDF and 1/19 mice treated with MNNG alone (Hébert *et al.*, 1990a).

Table 26. Enhancement of tumorigenesis in animals by administration of PCDFs in combination with known carcinogens

Strain/species (sex)	Known carcinogen	Route of administration	Interval	Dose and frequency	Route of administration	Enhancement	Reference
Skin							
HRS/J hairless mice (hr/hr) (F)	5 µmol MNNG	Skin		1 µg 2,3,7,8-TCDF/2 per wk/20 wk	Skin	+	Poland et al. (1982)
HRS/J hairless mice (hr/hr) (F)	5 µmol MNNG	Skin	7 days	25 ng 2,3,4,7,8-PeCDF/2 per wk/20 wk	Skin	+	Hébert et al. (1990a)
		Skin	7 days	50 ng 2,3,4,7,8-PeCDF/2 per wk/20 wk	Skin	+	
		Skin	7 days	100 ng 2,3,4,7,8-PeCDF/2 per wk/20 wk	Skin	+	
		Skin	7 days	250 ng 1,2,3,4,7,8-HxCDF/2 per wk/20 wk	Skin	+	
		Skin	7 days	500 ng 1,2,3,4,7,8-HxCDF/2 per wk/20 wk	Skin	+	
		Skin	7 days	1000 ng 1,2,3,4,7,8-HxCDF/2 per wk/20 wk	Skin	+	
Liver							
Wistar rats (M)	50 mg/L NDEA in drinking-water for 4 weeks	Oral	None	10 µg/kg bw 2,3,4,7,8-PeCDF per wk/16, 20 wk	s.c.	−	Nishizumi & Masuda (1986)
		Oral	None	10 µg/kg bw 2,3,4,7,8-PeCDF per wk/24 wk	s.c.	+	
		Oral	None	100 µg/kg bw 2,3,4,7,8-PeCDF per wk/16, 20, 24 wk	s.c.	+	
		Oral	None	10 µg/kg bw 1,2,3,4,7,8-HxCDF per wk/24 wk	s.c.	−	
		Oral	None	100 µg/kg bw 1,2,3,4,7,8-HxCDF per wk/24 wk	s.c.	+	
SD rat (F)	PH/30 mg/kg bw NDEA	i.p.	35 days	0.8 then 0.16 µg/kg bw 2,3,4,7,8-PeCDF per wk/20 wk	s.c.	−	Waern et al. (1991)
		i.p.	35 days	3.2 then 0.64 µg/kg bw 2,3,4,7,8-PeCDF per wk/20 wk	s.c.	+	
		i.p.	35 days	13 then 2.6 µg/kg bw 2,3,4,7,8-PeCDF per wk/20 wk	s.c.	+	

MNNG, N-methyl-N′-nitro-N-nitrosoguanidine; NDEA, N-nitrosodiethylnitrosamine; i.p., intraperitoneal injection; PH, partial hepatectomy; F; female; M, male

3.1.2 *Rat liver*

2,3,4,7,8-Pentachlorodibenzofuran

Groups of 12 male Wistar rats, five weeks of age, were given 50 mg/L (ppm) *N*-nitrosodiethylamine (NDEA) in the drinking-water for four weeks. The rats were then given weekly subcutaneous injections of olive oil or 10 or 100 μg/kg bw 2,3,4,7,8-PeCDF for 16, 20 or 24 weeks. At the end of treatment, the animals were killed (four per treatment per time point) and the number and size of liver tumours (hepatocellular carcinomas and hyperplastic nodules) were assessed. The numbers of liver tumours per rat were significantly greater in the 2,3,4,7,8-PeCDF-NDEA animals (at 24 weeks, 10 μg 2,3,4,7,8-PeCDF + NDEA, 17/rat; 100 μg 2,3,4,7,8-PeCDF + NDEA, 24.3/rat) than in the rats treated with NDEA alone (at 24 weeks, 3/rat). The number of hepatocellular neoplasms was increased at the 16-week observation period in the 100 μg/kg 2,3,4,7,8-PeCDF/NDEA rats (3.3/rat) compared with those treated with NDEA alone (0.3/rat). The lesions were also larger in animals receiving the 2,3,4,7,8-PeCDF/NDEA combination treatment than in those treated with NDEA alone (Nishizumi & Masuda, 1986). [The Working Group noted that the number of animals with tumours was not given.]

Groups of 10 female Sprague-Dawley rats [age unspecified] were subjected to a 70% partial hepatectomy followed by administration of 30 mg/kg bw NDEA by intraperitoneal injection and treatment with corn oil vehicle or 2,3,4,7,8-PeCDF by subcutaneous injection starting five weeks later for 14 or 20 weeks. The 2,3,4,7,8-PeCDF was given as an initial loading dose (5 × maintenance dose) followed by weekly maintenance doses of 0.16, 0.64 and 2.6 μg/kg bw 2,3,4,7,8-PeCDF for 19 weeks. The rats were killed after 20 weeks of treatment with vehicle or 2,3,4,7,8-PeCDF and analysed for the presence of γ-glutamyltransferase-positive focal hepatic lesions. A significant increase in the percentage of liver occupied by these lesions was observed for all doses (approximately: low-dose, 0.25%; mid-dose, 0.5%; high-dose, 0.5%) compared with NDEA alone (0.15%). A significant increase in the number of foci per liver was also seen at the two highest doses (approximately: low-dose, 2500; mid-dose, 3500; high-dose, 4500) as compared to NDEA alone (2000) (Waern *et al.*, 1991).

1,2,3,4,7,8-Hexachlorodibenzofuran

Groups of 12 male Wistar rats, five weeks of age, were given 50 mg/L (ppm) NDEA in the drinking-water for four weeks. The rats were then given weekly subcutaneous injections of olive oil or 10 or 100 μg/kg bw 1,2,3,4,7,8-HxCDF for 16, 20 or 24 weeks. At the end of treatment, the animals were killed (four per treatment per time point) and the number and size of hepatocellular carcinomas and hyperplastic nodules were assessed. At 24 weeks, the highest dose of 1,2,3,4,7,8-HxCDF increased the number of liver tumours per rat (12/rat) as compared to NDEA alone (3/rat). No effect was seen at the low dose (2.3 tumours/rat) (Nishizumi & Masuda, 1986). [The Working Group noted that the number of animals with tumours was not given.]

4. Other Data Relevant to an Evaluation of Carcinogenicity and its Mechanisms

4.1 Absorption, distribution, metabolism and excretion

4.1.1 *Humans*

Kinetic data on PCDFs have been reviewed (Olson, 1994).

In an individual exposed accidentally to PCDFs during a fire in Binghamton, NY, United States (see page 364), elimination half-lives of 2,3,4,7,8-PeCDF, 1,2,3,4,7,8-HxCDF, 1,2,3,6,7,8-HxCDF and 1,2,3,4,6,7,8-HpCDF were found to be 4–7 years (Schecter *et al.*, 1990a). Flesch-Janys *et al.* (1996a) investigated 48 workers who had been exposed to PCDDs and PCDFs in a herbicide-producing plant and calculated median half-lives that ranged from 3.0 years for 1,2,3,4,5,6,7,8-HpCDF to 19.6 years for 2,3,4,7,8-PCDF. In *yucheng* patients who had ingested PCB-contaminated rice oil in 1979 (see pages 362–363), half-lives of 2–3 years were found for 2,3,4,7,8-PeCDF, 1,2,3,4,7,8-HxCDF and 1,2,3,4,6,7,8-HpCDF during the period 1–12 years after the incident. *Yusho* patients were contaminated in 1968 and were examined 15–25 years after the incident showed considerably longer half-lives of 8–13 years (Ryan *et al.*, 1993; Masuda, 1996). These data suggest an increase in half-lives at lower dose levels. This behaviour is reflected in the kinetic model of Carrier *et al.* (1995b).

Half-lives of 1.3 years for 2,3,7,8-TCDF and 6.3 years for 2,3,4,7,8-PeCDF were calculated (Schlatter, 1991) using a method that compares daily intakes and body burdens of PCDFs of the normal population with those of 2,3,7,8-TCDD.

Concentrations of 2,3,4,7,8-PeCDF and 1,2,3,4,7,8- and 1,2,3,6,7,8-HxCDFs were 3–5-fold higher in adipose tissue than in liver (wet weight basis) in deceased *yusho* patients but considerably lower in adipose tissue than in liver in *yucheng* patients (Olafsson *et al.*, 1988). In the normal population, the concentration ratios of liver : fat (on a wet weight basis) were 0.2 for 2,3,4,7,8-PeCDF, 0.5 for OCDF and 1.1 for 1,2,3,4,6,7,8-HpCDF (Thoma *et al.*, 1990; Wacker *et al.*, 1990).

During one year of breast-feeding, PCDD and PCDF levels in human milk fell by 50–70% and those in the milk of mothers nursing their second child were 20–30% lower than those in the milk of mothers nursing their first child (Fürst *et al.*, 1989). These results are concordant with predictions of kinetic models (Carrier *et al.*, 1995b; Van der Molen *et al.*, 1996).

4.1.2 *Experimental systems*

(a) Absorption

The efficiency of absorption of 2,3,7,8-TCDF and 2,3,4,7,8-PeCDF has been studied in rats, hamsters and guinea-pigs after oral uptake using oily vehicles. For both compounds, 70–90% absorption from the gastrointestinal tract was observed (Birnbaum *et al.*, 1980; Yoshimura *et al.*, 1986; Brewster & Birnbaum, 1987; Kamimura *et al.*,

1988). In the guinea-pig, gastrointestinal uptake of 2,3,7,8-TCDF was more efficient than that of 2,3,7,8-TCDD and this was attributed to higher solubility of the former compound (Nolan *et al.*, 1979; Decad *et al.*, 1981a). As with PCDDs, gastrointestinal absorption of PCDFs depends on the vehicle, molecular size and solubility of the congener. The latter two properties appear to be the more significant in decreasing absorption of the hepta- and octa-CDFs (McLachlan *et al.*, 1990). As for 2,3,7,8-TCDD, it was shown that enterohepatic circulation was not significant for 1,2,3,7,8-PeCDF or its metabolites in rats (Brewster & Birnbaum, 1988).

Percutaneous absorption of 2,3,4,7,8-PeCDF in rats was age-dependent, with much more effective uptake in younger animals (Banks *et al.*, 1990). The dermal absorption of 2,3,7,8-TCDF and 1,2,3,7,8- and 2,3,4,7,8-PeCDFs in rats was also found to be dose- and structure-dependent, with 2,3,7,8-TCDF absorbed most efficiently (Brewster *et al.*, 1989). Compared with oral uptake, skin permeation is much slower. After dermal application of 1,2,3,7,8-PeCDF to the skin of a rhesus monkey, 99% of the dose was still present at the application site after 6 h (Brewster *et al.*, 1988). The uptake of seven compounds from a dermal application site showed a good inverse correlation with the octanol–water partition coefficients (Jackson *et al.*, 1993).

As with PCDDs, the adsorption of PCDFs on environmental matrices such as soil and combustion particles can strongly reduce the bioavailability of these compounds. The oral bioavailability factor which has been suggested for PCDDs (25–50% for Cl_4- and Cl_6-congeners) can also be considered applicable to PCDFs (Van den Berg *et al.*, 1994).

(b) Distribution

The PCDFs have a similar tissue distribution to that of the PCDDs in both rodents and non-human primates, the liver, adipose tissue and skin being the major storage sites. The 2,3,7,8-substituted PCDFs are the major congeners retained in most mammalian tissues and fluids. In this respect, the guinea-pig forms a distinct exception, as it also retains in the liver PCDFs with a 2,3,(4),6,7-chlorine substitution pattern, which apparently cannot be effectively metabolized by the cytochrome P450 system of the guinea-pig (Van den Berg *et al.*, 1986c; Ahlborg *et al.*, 1990). In other rodent species, the retention of these 'pseudolateral' PCDFs (for example, 2,3,4,6,7-PeCDF) is rarely observed (Van den Berg *et al.*, 1994). Some tissue retention of non-2,3,7,8-substituted PCDFs has been found in rats and marmosets (Abraham *et al.*, 1989; Neubert *et al.*, 1990a), but the concentrations observed are not considered to be toxicologically relevant when compared with the predominance of 2,3,7,8-substituted congeners. An increasing binding affinity to plasma proteins is found for the higher-chlorinated PCDFs and binding to plasma proteins and lipoproteins appears to be the major mode of transport in the blood (Patterson *et al.*, 1989; Schecter *et al.*, 1990e).

Studies with 2,3,7,8-TCDF and -TCDD have shown these compounds to have similar tissue distribution in the rat (Birnbaum *et al.*, 1980). A number of higher-chlorinated PCDFs, especially 2,3,4,7,8-PeCDF, have a much higher liver affinity in rodents than 2,3,7,8-TCDD. For these PCDFs, liver retention of 75–90% of the administered dose has been reported (Van den Berg *et al.*, 1994). Studies with mixtures of both PCDDs and PCDFs showed that tissue distribution in rats and hamsters was not significantly different between the hepta- and octa-CDFs and -CDDs (Van den Berg *et al.*, 1986c, 1987). In rhesus monkeys, the liver retention of 2,3,4,7,8-PeCDF, which is unusually high in rodents, is lower and not much different from that of 2,3,7,8-TCDD in rhesus monkeys (Kuroki *et al.*, 1980; Brewster *et al.*, 1988). In contrast, marmosets more closely resemble rats in tissue distribution of PCDFs as well as PCDDs (Abraham *et al.*, 1989). As with 2,3,7,8-TCDD, dose-dependent hepatic retention of PCDFs has been observed in a number of rodent studies, but some other studies have not found this dose-dependence (Van den Berg *et al.*, 1994). With respect to the occurrence of inducible hepatic binding sites in rodent liver (Poland *et al.*, 1989a), it should be noted that 2,3,4,7,8-PeCDF is a strongly binding substrate as well as an inducer of CYP1A2 (Yoshimura *et al.*, 1984; Kuroki *et al.*, 1986; Yoshimura *et al.*, 1987).

(c)   Metabolism

As with the PCDDs, the oxidation of PCDFs occurs preferentially on the 2, 3, 7 or 8 positions, yielding a higher number of hydroxylated metabolites than with the PCDDs due to the asymmetric structure of the dibenzofuran molecule (Veerkamp *et al.*, 1981; Poiger *et al.*, 1989). Based on studies with rats and 2,3,7,8-TCDF, it appears that the preferred site of metabolism of 2,3,7,8-TCDF is near the furan oxygen, with oxygenation at C4 predominating over oxygenation at C3 (Burka *et al.*, 1990). In rats, the CYP1A1 protein is directly involved in phase I metabolism of 2,3,7,8-TCDF (Olson *et al.*, 1994) and not the CYP1A2 protein (Tai *et al.*, 1993). Sulfur-containing metabolites have also been observed as minor metabolites, with S substitution preferentially at the 4 position (Kuroki *et al.*, 1989, 1990). In contrast to the PCDDs, the 4-4a positions in the dibenzofuran molecule are more susceptible to metabolic mixed function oxidase attack (Plüss *et al.*, 1987; Burka *et al.*, 1990). As a result, the biotransformation of 2,3,7,8-TCDF and 1,2,3,7,8-PeCDF is much more rapid than that of their dioxin analogues. If chlorine atoms on the 4 or 6 position are present in a 2,3,7,8-substituted PCDF, metabolism is strongly decreased, leading to an extremely low rate of elimination from the body (Brewster & Birnbaum, 1987, 1988; Van den Berg *et al.*, 1989a,b). Further chlorination of 2,3,7,8-substituted PCDFs results in a decrease in the number of metabolites and elimination rate (Veerkamp *et al.*, 1981; Poiger *et al.*, 1989). Virtually no information is available on differences between species in PCDF metabolism. In **Figure 1**, a generalized scheme for metabolic pathways of PCDFs is given, which is based on mammalian studies *in vivo* (Van den Berg *et al.*, 1994).

(d)   Excretion

The elimination of PCDFs, like that of the PCDDs, depends strongly on the position of the chlorine atoms. Those congeners with a 2,3,7,8-chlorine substitution pattern exhibit the slowest elimination rates in all laboratory species studied. As PCDFs are stored primarily in the liver and adipose tissue, the whole-body half-life of these compounds is governed mainly by the elimination from these two body compartments. Although kinetic information for PCDFs is more limited, elimination rates and half-lives

Figure 1. A generalized scheme of pathways for the biotransformation of PCDFs based on the information from in-vivo mammalian studies

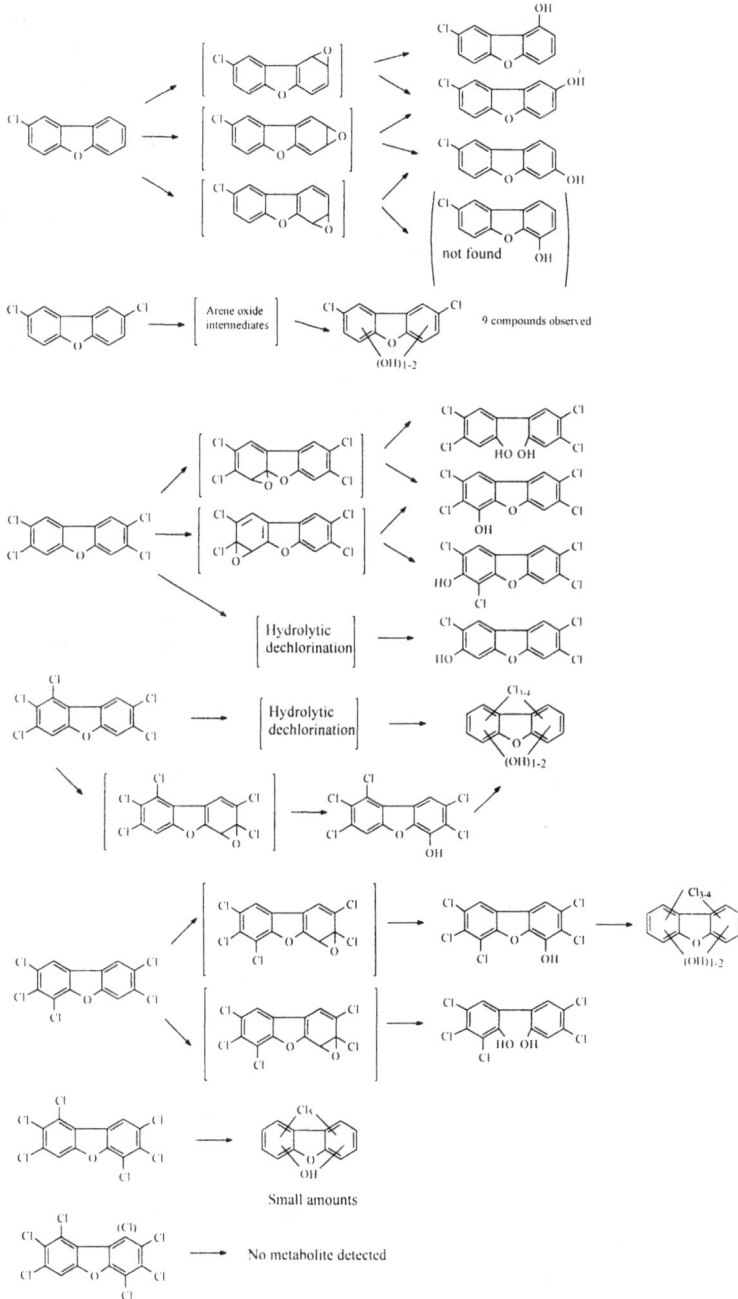

From Van den Berg *et al.* (1994)

appear to be similar to those of the PCDDs (Van den Berg *et al.*, 1994). Exceptions are seen with 2,3,7,8-TCDF and 1,2,3,7,8-PeCDF, for which elimination in rodents is much faster than for the other 2,3,7,8-substituted PCDFs. This rapid elimination can be directly attributed to the higher susceptibility of the C-4 position to metabolic attack in the dibenzofuran molecule. The presence of a chlorine atom on the C-4 position dramatically decreases the rate of elimination (Birnbaum *et al.*, 1981; Brewster & Birnbaum, 1988; Brewster *et al.*, 1988; Van den Berg *et al.*, 1989a,b; Ahlborg *et al.*, 1990). As a result, the half-life in the liver of the rat increases from several days for 1,2,3,7,8-PeCDF to more than 100 days for 2,3,4,7,8-PeCDF (Brewster & Birnbaum, 1988; Van den Berg *et al.*, 1989b). This importance of chlorine substitution on the 4/6 position is also seen in the short half-life of 1,2,3,7,8,9-HxCDF of less than 10 days in rats, compared with those of 2,3,4,6,7,8-HxCDF, 1,2,3,6,7,8-HxCDF and 1,2,3,4,7,8-HxCDF (Ahlborg *et al.*, 1990). Guinea-pigs eliminate 2,3,7,8-TCDF less efficiently than mice, the half-life in guinea-pigs being 20 days, compared with 4 days in DBA/2J mice and just 2 days in C57BL/6J mice (Decad *et al.*, 1981a,b; Ioannou *et al.*, 1983). The fact that the acute toxicities of 2,3,7,8-TCDD and -TCDF in the guinea-pig are in the same range has been attributed to the limited ability of this species to metabolize and eliminate the latter congener (Van den Berg *et al.*, 1994).

As in rodents, the elimination rates of 2,3,7,8-TCDF and 1,2,3,7,8-PeCDF in primates are faster than those of the other 2,3,7,8-substituted congeners. The half-lives for both compounds in rhesus monkeys and marmosets have been estimated to be approximately one week or less (Birnbaum *et al.*, 1981; Neubert *et al.*, 1990a,b). As for PCDDs, the elimination of PCDFs from most body compartments can be described as a one-compartment open model, but models with two- or three-phase eliminations for 2,3,7,8-TCDF in rodents and monkeys have been reported. In view of the non-linear distribution of PCDDs in many experimental systems, the use of physiologically based pharmaco-kinetic models has been successfully applied (Carrier *et al.*, 1995a,b).

4.2 Toxic effects

4.2.1 *Humans*

The results in this section are not lipid-based.

[The Working Group noted that in the *yusho* and *yucheng* incidents, exposures were to PCDFs and planar and non-planar PCBs and that one cannot unequivocally attribute the effects to one class of chemicals or the other.]

(a) *Non-cancer effects of ingestion of rice oil contaminated with polychlori-nated dibenzofurans, quaterphenyls and biphenyls in Japan* (yusho) *and Taiwan* (yucheng)

In both groups, the most notable acute effects were dermatological and neurological signs and symptoms of fatigue, headaches and gastrointestinal distress (nausea, vomiting, abdominal pain) (Kuratsune, 1989; Rogan, 1989).

Yusho

The initial recognition of *yusho* occurred in 1968. About 2000 individuals were identified as part of the *yusho* population (Masuda *et al.*, 1985). Tissue concentrations of PCDFs in these people are given in **Table 18**.

Effects observed shortly after exposure included elevated triglyceride levels and effects on female reproductive hormones manifest as changes in menstrual and basal body temperature patterns and lowered excretion of oestrogens and pregnanediol in exposed women (Kuratsune, 1989). However, fertility and other measures of reproductive function were not evaluated. Evidence of chronic bronchitis and respiratory infections still remained 14 years after exposure ended (Nakanishi *et al.*, 1985). However, more than 10 years after exposure, PCB levels were not related to serum levels of triiodothyronine, thyroxine and thyroxine-binding globulin (Murai *et al.*, 1987). Although the liver is the suspected target organ for halogenated hydrocarbons and marked proliferation of the endoplasmic reticulum was observed in that organ, clinical evidence of liver damage, such as alterations in liver enzymes or liver disease, was not observed (Kuratsune, 1989).

Dermatological effects were the most evident signs, characterized by hyperpigmentation of the nails, gingivae and face and by nail deformities, horny plugs, comedones, acneform eruptions, cysts and other abnormal keratotic changes. Acneform eruptions were observed on the face, cheeks, auricles, retroauricular areas, inguinal regions and external genitalia (Urabe & Asahi, 1985). More than 80% of *yusho* cases experienced one or more dermatological effects (Kuratsune, 1989), which diminished in severity over time (Urabe & Asahi, 1985).

Ophthalmological effects were characterized by swelling and hypersecretion of the meibomian glands and pigmentary changes of the conjunctiva (Kuratsune *et al.*, 1972). More than 80% of *yusho* cases exhibited ocular changes, which, in some cases, appeared to persist 15 years after exposure ended (Kuratsune, 1989).

Thirty per cent of the cases reported having at least one symptom consistent with neurological involvement, such as limb paraesthesia and spasms, weakness, headaches and fatigue (Kuratsune, 1972). As summarized by Kuratsune (1989), Kuriowa *et al.* (1969) found mostly sensory deficits, identified through slowed nerve conduction velocities in 23 cases. Follow-up of these cases indicated that the neurological symptoms disappeared over time; however, conduction velocity measurements were not repeated.

A number of studies examined the immune status of *yusho* cases (Kuratsune, 1989). Significant decreases in mean IgA and IgM and increases in IgG were noted in 28 cases tested in 1970 ($p < 0.05$). Within two years, means levels of all three immunoglobulins returned to normal. Small increases in the percentage of CD4$^+$ cells, small decreases in the percentage of CD8$^+$ cells and enhanced lymphocyte stimulation were also noted in *yusho* cases (Nakanishi *et al.*, 1985).

Mortality in the *yusho* population was assessed among 1761 patients registered by the end of 1983. Among 887 men and 874 women, there were 79 and 41 deaths, respectively (Masuda, 1994). Mortality from chronic liver disease and cirrhosis was elevated in men only (6 deaths; SMR, 2.7).

Studies of offspring of *yusho* cases have been limited to descriptions of effects on newborns exposed *in utero*. An early description of 13 children born to exposed mothers noted two stillborn infants, one of whom was diffusely and deeply hyperpigmented (Rogan, 1982). Neonates described in other reports were darkly pigmented and had marked secretions of the conjunctival palpebra, gingival hyperplasia, hyperkeratosis, calcification of the skull, low birth weight and natal teeth (Yamashita & Hayashi, 1985). The abnormal pigmentation disappeared after 2–5 months. No other physical abnormalities (neurological, cardiovascular or malformations) were identified.

Yucheng

The initial recognition of *yucheng* occurred in 1979. As of 1983, approximately 2000 individuals were found to have been exposed to the contaminated rice oil. Serum concentrations of PCDFs in these people are given in **Table 19**.

The ophthalmological and dermatological changes observed in *yucheng* cases were very similar in character and anatomical distribution to those noted in *yusho* cases (Lü & Wu, 1985). In 89 cases followed for up to 17 months, dermatological conditions of 38% of the cases improved, 54% remained the same and 7% showed deterioration of their condition (Lü & Wong, 1984).

Like *yusho* cases, *yucheng* cases examined within two years of exposure for nerve function exhibited slowing of sensory nerve conduction. They also exhibited motor nerve slowing and mixed deficits (Chen *et al.*, 1981, 1983; Chia & Chu, 1984; Chen *et al.*, 1985a). Of a population of 27 individuals, 20% also had abnormal electroencephalograms (EEGs) (Chia & Chu, 1984). However, the authors suggested that any correlation between PCB exposure and the abnormal EEGs might be spurious due to low PCB levels in the cerebrospinal fluid (0.5–2.3 µg/kg, measured in four subjects), despite much higher blood PCB levels of 48–64 µg/kg. A sample of 28 individuals with peripheral neuropathy in 1980 was re-examined in 1982 and was found to have normal EEGs and some recovery of sensory and motor nerve conduction velocity (Chia & Chu, 1985).

In 1981, immunological function was assessed on several subsets of *yucheng* cases and summarized by Lü and Wong (1984). In 30 cases compared with unexposed controls, both IgA and IgM were significantly decreased, while IgG did not differ from controls. In this same group, percentages of active T cells and T cells (E-rosette lymphocytes) were significantly decreased ($p < 0.05$), while total lymphocyte count and percentage of B cells were unchanged. Significant decreases in helper T cells (T4) but not suppressor T cells (T8) were also observed. In another group of cases, response to lymphocyte-stimulating mitogens was mixed and the findings were unclear. In 143 cases, reaction to streptococci antigen appeared to be significantly ($p < 0.05$) depressed relative to controls.

Alterations in porphyrin levels and liver enzymes have been identified as acute reactions to exposure to halogenated polycyclic hydrocarbons, including PCBs. Porphyrin levels were measured in two exposed groups (Chang *et al.*, 1980; Gladen *et al.*, 1988). In 1980, statistically significant elevations in 24-h urinary excretion of uroporphyrin (exposed, 41.23 µg ± 24.56; unexposed, 13.57 µg ± 11.76; $p < 0.01$) and α-aminolaevulinic acid (exposed, 1.002 mg ± 0.600; unexposed, 0.715 mg ± 0.337; $p < 0.05$) were noted among 69 poisoned and 20 normal subjects (Chang et al., 1980). Coproporphyrin and porphobilinogen levels were increased (but not significantly) in the exposed group. The second study group was composed of 75 children born between June 1978 and March 1985 to mothers who ingested contaminated rice oil (Gladen et al., 1988). Spot urines were collected in 1985. Mean total porphyrin (exposed, 95.2 µg/L; unexposed, 80.7 µg/L) and coproporphyrin (exposed, 72.4 µg/L; unexposed, 59.8 µg/L) excretion was elevated in the exposed, possibly due to extremely high levels (> 200 µg/L) in eight exposed children and two controls (Rogan et al., 1988). However, no porphyria cutanea tarda, a severe form of porphyria, was observed in either group of children. Moderate, but statistically significant, increases were observed in aspartate transaminase and alanine transaminase levels in 23 cases tested one year after exposure (Lü & Wong, 1984). Lactate dehydrogenase and bilirubin levels were not significantly elevated. As in yusho cases, triglyceride levels were significantly increased to approximately twice the level in unexposed controls.

Effects observed in offspring of yucheng cases are described in Section 4.4.1.

4.2.2 Experimental studies

(a) Species comparisons of toxic effects

(i) General effects

Thirteen-week dietary studies of Sprague-Dawley rats given 1,2,3,4,8-PeCDF, 1,2,3,7,8-PeCDF, 2,3,4,7,8-PeCDF or 1,2,3,6,7,8-HxCDF revealed that both toxicity, including body weight loss and thymic atrophy, and depletion of hepatic vitamin A followed the rank order of the compounds to bind to the Ah receptor and to induce CYP1A activity (Plüss et al., 1988a,b; Håkansson et al., 1990). When these PCDFs were administered as a mixture, it was observed that the individual PCDF toxicity was additive (Plüss et al., 1988b). Toxicity of 1,2,3,7,8-PeCDF was significantly lower than that of 2,3,4,7,8-PeCDF and this was attributed to rapid detoxification by biotransformation (see Section 4.1.2(c)) (Brewster & Birnbaum, 1988; Plüss et al., 1988a).

In male Sprague-Dawley rats fed 10 mg 2,3,7,8-TCDF per kg of diet, thymus, ventral prostate and seminal vesicle weights were significantly decreased (Oishi et al., 1978), and haemoglobin and haematocrit values were reduced.

Guinea-pigs given a single oral dose of 1–15 µg/kg 2,3,7,8-TCDF or 2,3,4,7,8-PeCDF showed a reduction in body weight gain. All animals that received 10 µg/kg or 15 µg/kg 2,3,7,8-TCDF or 2,3,4,7,8-PeCDF died 9–20 days after dosing. In mice, 22 daily oral doses of 30–300 µg/kg bw/day 2,3,7,8-TCDF did not induce clinical signs of toxicity (Moore et al., 1979). In contrast with other rodents, 2,3,7,8-TCDF was highly toxic to guinea-pigs, the acute toxicity being similar to that of 2,3,7,8-TCDD in this species (Ioannou et al., 1983; Moore et al., 1979). The high sensitivity of the guinea-pig was attributed to the low biotransformation rate in this species (see Section 4.1.2(b)) (Van den Berg et al., 1994).

A single dose of 1500 µg/kg 2,3,7,8-TCDF was lethal to 2/2 rhesus monkeys (Moore et al., 1979). Those animals which survived a dose of 1000 µg/kg (2/4) developed facial oedema and loss of eyelashes, fingernails and toenails. Most animals accumulated a white, wax-like exudate in the ear canal and showed a dry, leathery texture of the skin. Blood analysis 28 days after dosing revealed mild anaemia, relative lymphopenia and marked relative and absolute neutrophilia. Serum cholesterol was decreased by 33–50%. Major microscopic lesions were hyperkeratosis of the epidermis, squamous metaplasia of the meibomian and ceruminous glands (eyelid and ear canal, respectively) and a dilatation of hair follicles filled with keratinaceous debris in the facial area. The thymus showed extensive reduction of the cortex and necrotic debris in the medulla. Furthermore, the bile duct mucosa was found to be extremely hyperplastic with cystic dilatation and inflammation. Mild skin lesions were also found in the two rhesus monkeys that had received 500 μg/kg.

Packed blood cell volume and serum triglyceride and bile acid concentrations were significantly increased in rhesus monkeys after a single intravenous dose of 34 μg/kg 2,3,4,7,8-PeCDF (Brewster et al., 1988). Serum cholesterol, protein, albumin, triiodothyronine and thyroxine concentrations were decreased. After 28–58 days, the animals exhibited alopecia, hyperkeratinization of the toe- and finger-nails, facial chloracne-like lesions and loss of body weight. Two out of three animals subsequently died. Pathological findings indicated hyperplastic and metaplastic changes in the gastric mucosa, the meibomian glands of the eyelid and the ceruminous glands of the ear.

In cynomolgus monkeys (Macaca fascicularis), PCB mixtures similar to those ingested by yusho patients but without PCDFs caused immunosuppression and enlargement and histopathological changes of the liver (interstitial inflammation, proliferation of bile-duct epithelial cells). Treatment with a PCDF-containing PCB mixture, however, led to more pronounced decreases in body weight, immunosuppression, fatty liver and histopathological changes. In addition, the PCDF-containing mixture caused hair loss, acneform skin eruptions, oedema of the eyelid, congestions and abscesses of the meibomian gland and cornification of the skin (Hori et al., 1982).

(ii) Skin

In haired and hairless newborn and adult mice, dermal application of 2,3,4,7,8-PeCDF or 1,2,3,4,7,8-HxCDF caused involution of sebaceous glands (Puhvel & Sakamoto, 1988). Epidermal hyperplasia and hyperkeratinization, however, were induced in the hairless mice only. The density of inflammatory cell infiltrates in the dermis was not reduced by topical treatment with anti-inflammatory agents. The distinct pattern of chloracne observable in hairless mice (Puhvel et al., 1982) did not include hyperkeratinization of the sebaceous follicles typical of human chloracne. Histopathological changes observed with all acnegenic compounds were epidermal hyperkeratosis and hyperplasia, loss of sebaceous glands, keratinization of intradermal pilar cysts and diffuse lymphohistiocytic infiltration of the dermis. Atrophy or complete absence of the hair follicles were evident in severe lesions (Hébert et al., 1990a). In these cases, the epidermis was hypoplastic with increased keratin on the surface. The data for dermal toxicity and changes in body weight and organ weights indicated that 2,3,4,7,8-PeCDF was 0.2–0.4 times, and 1,2,3,4,7,8- HxCDF 0.08–0.16 times, as toxic as 2,3,7,8-TCDD following repeated dermal exposure.

The ability of several PCDFs to induce a flat, cobblestone-like morphology in cell cultures was studied in a nonkeratinizing derivative (XBF) of the keratinizing XB mouse epithelial cell line cocultured with irradiated 3T3 feeder cells. The minimum concentrations required to produce these changes from the normal spindle-shape cells, over a 14-day exposure period, were > 2.38 µg/kg for 2,6-DCDF, 0.032 µg/kg for 2,3,7,8-TCDF, 0.378 µg/kg for 2,3,4,6,7,8-HxCDF and 4.48 µg/kg for OCDF (Gierthy & Crane, 1985).

Osborne and Greenlee (1985) reported that 2,3,7,8-TCDF decreased DNA synthesis, proliferation and epidermal growth factor (EGF) binding, and induced differentiation in several lines of human keratinocytes.

(iii) *Liver*

While no histopathological signs of liver damage were observed in guinea-pigs treated with 15 µg/kg 2,3,7,8-TCDF or 20 µg/kg 2,3,4,7,8-PeCDF, Sprague-Dawley rats showed liver cell vacuolization, necrosis of single hepatocytes and Kupffer cell hypoplasia after treatment with 1,2,3,6,7,8-HxCDF (200 µg/kg in the diet). These alterations were less pronounced with 1,2,3,7,8-PeCDF (200 µg/kg in the diet) and 1,2,3,6,7,8-HxCDF (20 µg/kg in the diet). No liver lesions were observed after administration of 1,2,3,4,8-PeCDF (6000 µg/kg in diet) (Plüss *et al.*, 1988a).

C57BL/6fh(J67) mice receiving 22 daily oral doses of 300 µg/kg 2,3,7,8-TCDF showed a 17% increase in liver weight and a 25% increase in liver/body weight ratio; fluorescence indicative of porphyria was not observed. Guinea-pigs receiving single oral doses of up to 15 µg/kg 2,3,7,8-TCDF did not develop liver pathology. In rhesus monkeys, single oral doses of 2,3,7,8-TCDF up to 1500 µg/kg resulted in inconsistently increased liver weight but no histopathological liver lesion (Moore *et al.*, 1979). Brewster *et al.* (1988) did not report histopathological liver changes except for deposits of haemosiderin in Kupffer cells after administration of a single intravenous dose of 34 µg/kg 2,3,4,7,8-PeCDF to rhesus monkeys.

(b) *Immunological responses*

Only five out of 135 PCDF congeners have been studied for their effects on the mammalian immune system (Holsapple, 1995).

Kerkvliet *et al.* (1985) studied the humoral immunosuppressive effect of a single oral dose of 1,2,3,4,6,7,8-HpCDF in C57BL/6 mice, two days before sheep red blood cell (SRBC) challenge. Splenic IgM antibody response was measured five days later ('HAIR-assay'). The 50% immunosuppressive dose (ID_{50}) was calculated as 208 µg/kg, while the ID_{50} for 1,2,3,4,5,6,7,8-HpCDD was 85 µg/kg. [For comparison, the ID_{50} for 2,3,7,8-TCDD was 0.74 µg/kg (Kerkvliet & Brauner, 1990)].

Davis and Safe (1991) compared the effects of a series of congeners with respect to their suppression of the in-vitro plaque-forming anti-SRBC response using cells from either C57BL/6 or DBA/2 mice. The immunosuppressive potencies of 2,3,4,7,8-PeCDF, 2,3,7,8-TCDF, 1,2,3,7,9-PeCDF and 1,3,6,8-TCDF in this in-vitro assay were similar to each other and to that of 2,3,7,8-TCDD, using spleen cell cultures from both mouse strains, although *in vivo* their immunotoxic potentials differ by up to 14 900-fold in C57BL/6 mice (Davis & Safe, 1988).

Harper *et al.* (1993) studied the effects of a single intraperitoneal injection of 2,3,7,8-TCDD, 2,3,4,7,8-PeCDF, 1,2,3,7,9-PeCDF or 1,3,6,8-TCDF on the splenic plaque-forming cell (PFC) response to the T-cell-independent antigen TNP-LPS in C57BL/6 and DBA/2 mice. The effective doses (μg/kg) required to decrease by 50% (ED_{50}) the end-point 'PFCs/10^6 viable cells' were:

Congener	C57BL/6 mice	DBA/2 mice
2,3,7,8-TCDD	1.5	9.7
2,3,4,7,8-PeCDF	2.0	2.6
1,2,3,7,9-PeCDF	391	4 690
1,3,6,8-TCDF	1 484	17 167

Similarly designed experiments were performed with B6C3F1 mice. The effects induced by the same four congeners after intraperitoneal injection were compared with those observed after in-vitro exposure of mouse splenocytes. The ED_{50} of the PFC response to 2,3,7,8-TCDD, 2,3,4,7,8-PeCDF and 1,2,3,7,8-PeCDF and 1,3,6,8-TCDF was 14.1, 5.5, 1695 and 34 800 nmol/kg, respectively. Corresponding values derived from in-vitro studies were 7.0, 10.6, 149 and 2325 nM, respectively (Harper *et al.*, 1995).

Vecchi *et al.* (1983) studied the suppressive effects of a single intraperitoneal injection of 180 μg/kg bw 2,3,7,8-TCDF on antibody production in C57BL/6 mice and in DBA/2 mice. A pronounced decrease in the number of PFC as a response to the injection of SRBCs was observed in C57BL/6 mice only.

A single dose of 20 ng/kg 2,3,4,7,8-PeCDF had no effect on the proportions of sub-populations of lymphocytes in peripheral blood of marmosets, studied by flow cytometry. In contrast, 10 μg/kg bw 2,3,7,8-TCDD induced a decrease in the number of $CD20^+$ cells and the number of $CD4^+$ $CDW29^+$ cells (Neubert *et al.*, 1993b).

(c)   Biochemical responses

There appear to have been few studies of the biochemical responses attributable to PCDF exposure, other than those on induction of CYP1A1 and CYP1A2 expression (see Section 4.3).

EGF receptor autophosphorylation was decreased in placenta after in-utero exposure to PCBs and PCDFs ingested from contaminated rice oil in the *yucheng* incident (Sunahara *et al.*, 1987). In contrast, EGF receptor expression was increased in mouse embryonic palatal medial epithelial cells (Abbott & Birnbaum, 1989b). Support for the role of the Ah receptor in mediating downregulation of the EGF receptor was supported by structure–activity studies in mice (Ryan *et al.*, 1989b) and the differential responsiveness of congenic mice differing only at the Ah locus (Lin *et al.*, 1991a).

4.3   Interaction with Ah receptor and its early molecular consequences and other biochemical responses

Laterally substituted PCDF congeners bind to the Ah receptor and produce the same biological and toxic effects as the PCDDs. Among these PCDFs, the congeners with the 2,3,7,8-chlorine substitution pattern are the most potent ones (Poland & Knutson, 1982; Safe, 1990). The binding affinities of 2,3,7,8-TCDF, 1,2,3,7,8- and 2,3,4,7,8-PeCDFs to the Ah receptor are of the same order of magnitude as that of 2,3,7,8-TCDD (see Section 4.3 in the monograph on PCCDs in this volume). The Ah receptor binding affinity for the class of congeners is dependent upon the extent and pattern of chlorination (Whitlock, 1986; Okey, 1990; Safe, 1990).

In general, induction of *CYP1A1* gene expression by PCDFs tends to follow the same rank order of potency as receptor binding *in vitro*. Like many planar aromatic substances, including 2,3,7,8-TCDD, the 2,3,7,8-substituted PCDFs also induce CYP1A2 and bind strongly to this protein (Yoshimura *et al.*, 1984; Kuroki *et al.*, 1986; Poland *et al.*, 1989b). Ah receptor-regulated genes encoding phase-two metabolizing enzymes (e.g., UDP-glucuronosyl transferase and DT diaphorase) are also induced following PCDF exposure, but information is limited (Safe, 1990; Van den Berg *et al.*, 1994).

Although the binding of some 2,3,7,8-substituted PCDFs to the Ah receptor and associated *CYP1A1* induction *in vitro* is similar to that of 2,3,7,8-TCDD, the general toxicity of some of these congeners is significantly lower due to faster biotransformation in several rodent species. This is especially the case for 2,3,7,8-TCDF and 1,2,3,7,8-PeCDF (Van den Berg *et al.*, 1994).

Enzyme induction has been observed in both pre- and postnatally exposed rats; the endocrine implications of these effects are unclear (Waalkens-Berendsen *et al.*, 1996).

Numerous PCDF congeners have been shown to produce Ah receptor-mediated responses such as thymic atrophy, immunotoxicity and teratogenicity in many mammalian species (reviewed by Safe, 1990).

Like the 2,3,7,8-substituted PCDDs (see Section 4.3 in the monograph on PCDDs), PCDFs negatively modulate some 17β-oestradiol-induced biological responses in certain target tissues. The above effects can be of the same order of magnitude as those produced by 2,3,7,8-TCDD (Safe *et al.*, 1991).

The binding of these compounds to the Ah receptor and associated biological responses depend on the cell type, species, sex, age and assay used (Poland & Knutson, 1982; Safe, 1986; Whitlock, 1986; Okey, 1990; Safe, 1990).

Four PCDFs have been shown to increase levels of both hepatic and urinary porphyrins following subchronic exposure in mice, as observed with 2,3,7,8-TCDD and 1,2,3,7,8-PeCDD (van Birgelen *et al.*, 1996b).

4.4   Reproductive and developmental effects

4.4.1   *Humans*

Fetal PCB syndrome, as described among babies in Japan born to mothers who consumed contaminated oil, is characterized at birth by brown pigmentation ('cola-coloured babies') on the skin and the mucous membrane, gingival hyperplasia, very early postnatal eruption of the teeth or natal teeth, calcification of the skull and low birth weight (Yamashita & Hayashi, 1985). In addition, among *yucheng* babies born between 1979 and 1983, a high perinatal mortality rate was observed (eight of 39) (Hsu *et al.*, 1985). Retrospective ascertainment of neonatal dermatological findings among 128 children exposed transplacentally and born in Taiwan between 1979 and 1985, indicated increased rates of hyperpigmentation, eyelid swelling and discharge, deformed nails, acne, natal teeth and swollen gums, compared with 115 control children (Rogan *et al.*, 1988; Gladen *et al.*, 1990). In neither Japan nor Taiwan was there a clear relationship between symptoms or fetopathy and PCB dose (Yu *et al.*, 1991).

Many follow-up studies were initiated among *yucheng* children to assess metabolic impairment or anomalies in physical or cognitive development. In 1985, a cohort was constructed to include all children born between June 1978 and March 1985 who had been exposed prenatally. The exposed cohort consisted of 132 children, living in 1985, from 159 pregnancies occurring among 74 women (Rogan *et al.*, 1988). In April 1985, 117 exposed children aged one month to six years (average, 32 months) and 108 control children (average age, 31 months) were examined. Exposed children were smaller (93% of control weight and 97% of control height) than controls of the same age and sex. Medical histories since birth indicated a higher rate of bronchitis among exposed children. Clinical examination showed a higher frequency of hyperpigmentation and nail deformities, differences in eyebrow flare, hypertelorism and clinodactyly, and an increased prevalence of clinically detectable developmental delay (10% exposed versus 3% controls).

One hundred and fifteen exposed children from the original cohort and 115 highly matched controls were tested for cognitive development annually from 1985 through 1990. The exposed children scored approximately five points lower on age-appropriate tests of intelligence from the age of two to the age of seven. Children born later were as affected as children born shortly after the outbreak (Yu *et al.*, 1991; Chen *et al.*, 1992; Lai *et al.*, 1994).

A behavioural survey was performed on the same groups (Chen *et al.*, 1994). At each year of follow-up and at each age, exposed children scored higher on tests for hyperactivity and conduct disorders.

At school-age, there was evidence of higher prevalence of congenital lack of permanent teeth among some exposed *yucheng* children (five of 18) compared with controls (one of 44) matched for sex, age, father's occupation, family economic status and area of residence (Lan *et al.*, 1989). [Selection of exposed children is not clearly described, and control children had a low participation rate of 61%.]

In a series of 55 *yucheng* children (out of 132 identified during the same period of 1978–85) and 55 controls matched for age and sex, there was evidence in 1991 of decreased height and decreased muscular development (as indicated by total lean mass) among exposed children (Guo *et al.*, 1994).

Seven to nine years after the poisoning, there was no difference in any immunological or haematological parameters investigated between 19 exposed children and 32 matched controls (Lan *et al.*, 1990).

In an examination conducted in 1993 of 104 exposed children, *yucheng* girls were significantly shorter (2.5 cm) than controls, and the penile length of *yucheng* boys, aged 11–14 years, was shorter than that of controls. Neither effect was related to sexual development by the Tanner scale (Guo *et al.*, 1993). In a separate examination, 22% of tympanic membranes in 110 *yucheng* children were abnormal versus 17% of controls ($p < 0.01$) (Chao & Hsu, 1994).

Analysis of physical and cognitive development began in October 1991 of 104 children whose mothers were exposed and 109 children whose fathers but not mothers were exposed and of three matched controls born after 1985 (Guo *et al.*, 1993; Chen *et al.*, 1992). Like children born before 1985, the later-born children were shorter in stature and lower in weight than controls, although the differences were no longer statistically significant. *Yucheng* children were reported to have higher activity levels but no physical temperament, habit or other behavioural problems. Overall, scores on all tests among paternally exposed children were similar to those of the controls. However, maternally exposed children scored lower on the Stanford-Binet IQ test Wechsler and on all subscales of the Wechsler Intelligence Scale for Children. In a follow-up study based on a random sample of the above children, the exposed children had significantly lower verbal and full-scale IQs and auditory event related potential. No neurophysiological changes were observed, including pattern visual evoked potentials and short-latency somatosensory evoked potentials.

In summary, there is evidence that babies born after the *yusho* incident or after the *yucheng* incident (for which more data are available) present signs of intra-uterine growth retardation and congenital anomalies at birth. Some authors have proposed that these findings were consistent with a generalized disorder of ectodermal tissue (Rogan *et al.*, 1988). Sunahara *et al.* (1987) showed that *yucheng* babies with low birth-weight had depressed autophosphorylation capacity of the EGF receptor in the placenta, induced by exposure to PCBs and PCDFs during gestation. There is evidence of deficits on cognitive development scores among *yucheng* children up to seven years of age.

4.4.2 *Experimental systems*

PCDFs are teratogenic in mice, causing the same spectrum of birth defects and developmental toxicity as 2,3,7,8-TCDD (Birnbaum, 1991). Whether administered orally to the dam as a single dose during the middle of organogenesis or in divided doses on gestation days 10–13, 2,3,7,8-TCDF, 1,2,3,7,8-PeCDF, 2,3,4,7,8-PeCDF and 1,2,3,4,7,8-HxCDF cause cleft palate and hydronephrosis at doses which are not maternally or fetally toxic (Weber & Birnbaum, 1985; Birnbaum *et al.*, 1987a,b). The dose–response curves for these four PCDFs are parallel to each other and to that of 2,3,7,8-TCDD. The ED_{50} values and the relative potency values for induction of cleft palate are as follows: 2,3,7,8-TCDD 3.4 µg/kg, 1.0; 2,3,7,8-TCDF 70.1 µg/kg, 0.05; 1,2,3,7,8-PeCDF 132.9 µg/kg, 0.025; 2,3,4,7,8-PeCDF 35.9 µg/kg, 0.1; and 1,2,3,4,7,8-HxCDF 344.8 µg/kg, 0.01. The ED_{50} for hydronephrosis was about five times lower than that for cleft palate. Mixtures of these chemicals demonstrate strict additivity for induction of cleft palate.

Prenatal exposure of mice to 2,3,4,7,8-PeCDF results in haemorrhage of embryonic blood into the maternal circulation because of rupture of the embryo–maternal vascular barrier (Khera, 1992). Exposure of pregnant rats on gestation day 1 to 43 nmol/kg (15 µg/kg) 2,3,4,7,8-PeCDF resulted in a decrease in sperm count in the male offspring and a delay or lack of vaginal opening in the females (Waalkens-Berensen et al., 1996).

Oral treatment of adult mice with 100 µg/kg 2,3,4,7,8-PeCDF five times over a 16-week period led to an increase in the growth of surgically induced endometriosis (Johnson et al., 1996).

4.5   Genetic and related effects (see also Appendix 3 and **Table 27**)

4.5.1   *Humans*

Peripheral lymphocytes from 35 Taiwanese women exposed in the *yucheng* incident (Lundgren et al., 1988) that occurred in 1979 and those from 24 matched controls were assessed for the levels of sister chromatid exchange in the presence or absence of α-naphthoflavone and for chromosomal aberrations in 1985. Serum levels of PCBs were measured for 32 individuals and those of PCDFs were measured for only 12 exposed women. Blood concentrations of total PCBs in the exposed population and in controls averaged approximately 15 and 0.34 µg/kg, respectively. PCDFs detected were primarily 1,2,3,4,7,8-HxCDF (10.8 ng/kg) and 2,3,4,7,8-PeCDF (2.7 ng/kg). Sister chromatid exchange frequencies in the absence of α-naphthoflavone and chromosomal aberrations were similar in control and exposed populations. Differences in the level of α-naphtho-flavone-induced sister chromatid exchange between the two groups were highly signi-ficant. These findings indicate that exposure to PCBs or PCDFs *in vivo* results in an enhanced sensitivity of lymphocytes to the sister chromatid exchange-inducing effects of α-naphthoflavone.

Placentas from nonsmoking Taiwanese women (38–35 years of age) from the *yucheng* cohort were obtained in 1983 and 1984. The formation of DNA adducts in pla-cental DNA was investigated using ^{32}P-postlabelling, but none was detected (Gallagher et al., 1994).

4.5.2   *Experimental systems* (see **Table 27**)

3-Chlorodibenzofuran induced reverse mutation in *Salmonella typhimurium*. Elevated frequencies of sister chromatid exchange and micronucleus formation were induced by 2,3,4,7,8-PeCDF in human lymphocytes *in vitro* in the presence or absence of α-naphthoflavone.

Table 27. Genetic and related effects of PCDFs

Test system	Result[a]		Dose[b] (LED/HID)	Reference
	Without exogenous metabolic system	With exogenous metabolic system		
3-Chlorodibenzofuran				
SAO, *Salmonella typhimurium* TA100, reverse mutation	+	+	100	Matsumoto & Ando (1991)
SA9, *Salmonella typhimurium* TA98, reverse mutation	+	+	40	Matsumoto & Ando (1991)
2,3,4,7,8-Pentachlorodibenzofuran				
SHL, Sister chromatid exchange, human lymphocytes *in vitro*	+	NT	0.0008	Nagayama *et al.* (1995a)
MIH, Micronucleus test, human lymphocytes *in vitro*	+	NT	0.005	Nagayama *et al.* (1993)
BVD, Binding (covalent) to DNA, rat liver *in vivo* (^{32}P-postlabelling)	–		0.1 p.o. × 4	Randerath *et al.* (1993)
1,2,3,7,8-Pentachlorodibenzofuran				
BVD, Binding (covalent) to DNA, rat liver *in vivo* (^{32}P-postlabelling)	–		0.1 p.o. × 4	Randerath *et al.* (1993)
1,2,4,7,8-Pentachlorodibenzofuran				
BVD, Binding (covalent) to DNA, rat liver *in vivo* (^{32}P-postlabelling)	–		0.1 p.o. × 4	Randerath *et al.* (1993)
2,3,4,6,7,8-Hexachlorodibenzofuran				
BVD, Binding (covalent) to DNA, rat liver *in vivo* (^{32}P-postlabelling)	–		0.1 p.o. × 4	Randerath *et al.* (1993)
Mixed PCDFs and PCBs				
BVD, Binding (covalent) to DNA, human placenta *in vivo* (^{32}P-postlabelling)	–		NG	Gallagher *et al.* (1994)

[a] +, positive; (+), weak positive; –, negative; NT, not tested; ?, inconclusive
[b] LED, lowest effective dose; HID, highest ineffective dose; in-vitro tests, μg/mL; in-vivo tests, mg/kg bw/day; p.o., oral; NG, not given

Changes in DNA I (indigenous)-compound formation were studied in female Sprague-Dawley rats treated by gastric instillation with 1,2,3,7,8-PeCDF, 1,2,4,7,8-PeCDF, 2,3,4,7,8-PeCDF or 2,3,4,6,7,8-HxCDF (100 µg/kg bw in corn oil per week for four weeks). No test compound–DNA adducts were detected, but there were significant, structure-dependent reductions in hepatic I-compound formation. Potencies increased in the order: control (100%, 122 modifications in 10^9 DNA nucleotides) = 1,2,4,7,8-PeCDF (104%) < 1,2,3,7,8-PeCDF (80%) < 2,3,4,7,8-PeCDF (61%) = 2,3,4,6,7,8-HxCDF. These activities parallel the reported Ah receptor-binding activities (Randerath et al., 1993).

5. Summary of Data Reported and Evaluation

5.1 Exposure data

Polychlorinated dibenzofurans (PCDFs) are formed as inadvertent by-products in the production and use of polychlorinated biphenyls (PCBs) and, in combination with polychlorinated dibenzo-para-dioxins (PCDDs), in the production of chlorophenols and have been detected as contaminants in these products. PCDFs and PCDDs also may be produced in thermal processes such as incineration and metal processing and in the bleaching of paper pulp with free chlorine. PCDFs are also found in residual waste from the production of vinyl chloride and the chloralkali process for chlorine production. The relative amounts of PCDF and PCDD congeners produced depend on the production or incineration process and vary widely.

Like PCDDs, PCDFs are ubiquitous in soil, sediments and air. Excluding occupational or accidental exposures, most background human exposure to PCDFs occurs as a result of eating meat, milk, eggs, fish and related products, as PCDFs are persistent in the environment and accumulate in animal fat. High exposures have occurred in relation to incidents in Japan (yusho) and Taiwan (yucheng) involving contamination of rice oil and in accidents involving electrical equipment containing PCBs. Occupational exposures also may occur in metal production and recycling, and in the production and use of chlorophenols and PCBs.

Based on limited data, the sum of the mean background levels of the penta- and hexachlorinated PCDF congeners commonly found in human tissues is generally in the range of 10–100 ng/kg fat, and the PCDF contribution to tissue international toxic equivalent (I-TEQ) values is typically of the same order of magnitude as that of the PCDDs. Since the mid-1980s, mean tissue levels of total PCDFs and PCDDs (measured as I-TEQ) in the general population have decreased by two- to three-fold. Five-fold higher tissue levels have been found in subpopulations consuming large amounts of PCDF-contaminated fish. Accidental exposures to PCDFs have led to tissue levels one or more orders of magnitude higher than background levels.

5.2   Human carcinogenicity data

In the *yusho* and *yucheng* incidents, each involving about 2000 cases, people were exposed to sufficient PCBs and PCDFs to produce symptoms. Fatal liver disease is 2–3 times more frequent than national rates in both cohorts. In Japan, at 22 years of follow-up, there is a three-fold excess of liver cancer mortality in men, which was already detectable and even higher at 15 years of follow-up. In Taiwan, at 12 years of follow-up, there is no excess of liver cancer mortality. This difference does not appear to be the result of study design, differences in diagnostic habits, exposure or age at exposure, but may be related to differences in the time of follow-up.

5.3   Animal carcinogenicity data

There are no long-term carcinogenicity studies on PCDFs.

2,3,7,8-Tetrachlorodibenzofuran (2,3,7,8-TCDF) treatment following a single dose of *N*-methyl-*N′*-nitro-*N*-nitrosoguanidine (MNNG) resulted in an increased incidence of mouse skin papillomas.

2,3,4,7,8-Pentachlorodibenzofuran (2,3,4,7,8-PeCDF) treatment following a single dose of MNNG resulted in an increased incidence of mouse skin papillomas. 2,3,4,7,8-PeCDF treatment following four weeks' treatment with *N*-nitrosodiethylamine (NDEA) resulted in an increased incidence of hepatocellular carcinomas and hyperplastic nodules in male rats. Treatment with the same compound after a single dose of NDEA increased the incidence of focal hepatic lesions in female rats.

1,2,3,4,7,8-Hexachlorodibenzofuran (1,2,3,4,7,8-HxCDF) treatment following a single dose of MNNG resulted in an increased incidence of mouse skin papillomas. 1,2,3,4,7,8-HxCDF treatment following four weeks' treatment with NDEA resulted in an increased incidence of hepatocellular carcinomas and hyperplastic nodules in male rats. Treatment with the same compound after a single dose of NDEA increased the incidence of focal hepatic lesions in female rats.

5.4   Other relevant data

Kinetics

The half-lives of PCDFs in humans are much longer than those in experimental animals.

In most vertebrate species, the 2,3,7,8-substituted PCDFs are the congeners which are preferentially retained in tissues. Oxidation by cytochrome P450 primarily occurs at the 4 and 6 positions in the molecule and the presence of chlorine atoms at these positions reduces metabolism more than substitution at the 1 and 9 positions. Consequently, chlorine substitution on these positions strongly hinders elimination. In rodents, some PCDFs, e.g. 2,3,4,7,8-PeCDF, show an extremely high affinity for liver tissue, which has been attributed to binding to the CYP1A2 protein. As Ah-receptor-mediated effects are primarily caused by the parent compound, biotransformation should be considered as a detoxification process.

Toxic effects

In animal experiments, 2,3,7,8-substituted PCDFs exhibit the same pattern of toxicity as those documented for PCDDs.

Studies of adults in Japan (*yusho*) and Taiwan (*yucheng*) who ingested rice oil contaminated with PCBs, PCDFs and other by-products of PCB thermal degradation have observed effects in multiple systems. In both situations the poisonings were characterized by chloracne, elevated triglyceride levels, abnormal neurological symptoms, ophthalmic changes and alterations in immune parameters. In *yucheng*, porphyrin levels were also elevated.

Biochemical responses and mechanism of action

2,3,7,8-Substituted PCDFs bind to the Ah receptor and, as documented for PCDDs, induce *CYP1A1* and *CYP1A2* gene expression. Ah-receptor-binding affinities of 2,3,7,8-TCDF, 1,2,3,7,8- and 2,3,4,7,8-PeCDF are of the same order of magnitude as that observed for 2,3,7,8-TCDD. With increasing chlorination, receptor binding affinity decreases. The enzyme induction follows the same structure–activity relationship.

Reproductive and developmental effects

In the *yucheng* population, eight of 39 children exposed *in utero* died before birth. Surviving children showed signs of intra-uterine growth retardation and congenital anomalies at birth, a deficit of cognitive development up to seven years of age, and defects in musculoskeletal development and pigmentation.

Several PCDFs have been shown to be teratogenic in mice, causing cleft palate and hydronephrosis. 2,3,4,7,8-PeCDF leads to persistent reproductive effects (reduced sperm count, structural alterations of the female genital tract) following prenatal exposure. It also promotes the growth of surgically induced endometriosis in mice. All of these effects are also observed with 2,3,7,8-TCDD.

Genetic and related effects

2,3,4,7,8-PeCDF increased the frequencies of sister chromatid exchange and micronucleus formation in human lymphocytes *in vitro*.

5.5   Evaluation[1]

There is *inadequate evidence* in humans for the carcinogenicity of polychlorinated dibenzofurans.

There is *inadequate evidence* in experimental animals for the carcinogenicity of 2,3,7,8-tetrachlorodibenzofuran.

There is *limited evidence* in experimental animals for the carcinogenicity of 2,3,4,7,8-pentachlorodibenzofuran.

---

[1] For definition of the italicized terms, see Preamble, pp. 26–27.

There is *limited evidence* in experimental animals for the carcinogenicity of 1,2,3,4,7,8-hexachlorodibenzofuran.

Overall evaluation

Polychlorinated dibenzofurans *are not classifiable as to their carcinogenicity to humans (Group 3).*

APPENDIX 1

TABLES ON OCCURRENCE (PCDDs)

Table 1. Concentrations of PCDDs in air

Reference	Origin; sample description (and no.)	Coll. period	Samp. meth. / Anal. meth.	PCDD concentration (pg/m^3) TCDD 2378	PeCDD 12378	HxCDD 123478	123678	123789	HpCDD 1234678	OCDD	I-TEQ PCDD/PCDF
Australia											
Taucher et al. (1992)	Sydney; ambient air (8)	10/90	G/P/X BSI				No information				0.016–0.062
Austria											
Moche & Thanner (1996a)	Mostly urban Ambient, winter (41) Ambient, summer (43)	92/93	G/P BN				No information				0.050–0.222 0.022–0.041
Moche & Thanner (1996b)	Graz; ambient air, winter (20) Linz; ambient air, winter (15)	93/94 94/95	G/P BN				No information				0.07–0.42 <0.01–0.180
Christmann et al. (1989b)	Brixlegg; ~280 m from Cu reclamation plant (1) (1) (1) (1)	2/88 5/88 6/88 7/88	G/P CSI	0.1 0.07 0.03 ND	0.4 0.4 0.2 0.2	ND ND 0.04 ND	ND 0.2 0.08 ND	ND ND 0.05 ND	2.1 1.2 0.4 0.5	2.7 2.1 0.5 1.0	2.3[a] 1.9[a] 1.2[a] 1.5[a]
Belgium											
Wevers et al. (1992)	Antwerp Tunnel air (1) (3) Ambient air (4)	91	G/P BSN	0.017	0.0126	0.0025	0.0042 No information No information	0.0030	0.0047	0.0022	0.080 (0.030–0.116) 0.035 (0.021–0.055)
Wevers et al. (1993)	Near emission sources (20)	92	G/P BSN				No information				0.165 (0.018–0.379)

Table 1 (contd)

Reference	Origin; sample description (and no.)	Coll. period	Samp. meth. / Anal. meth.	TCDD 2378	PeCDD 12378	HxCDD 123478	123678	123789	HpCDD 1234678	OCDD	I-TEQ PCDD/PCDF
Canada											
Reiner et al. (1995)	Close to cement kiln; ambient air (6)	6/89	G/P B/ CSO				No information				0.015–0.035
	Toronto Island; ambient air (6)	9/88–7/89					No information				0.063
Steer et al. (1990a)	SW Ontario; burning tyre dump	2/90	G/P CSO								
	1 km downwind (5)						I-TEQ (PCDD only), 0.01–0.34				0.02–2.5
	3 km downwind (4)						I-TEQ (PCDD only), 0.014–0.039				0.046–0.27
Germany											
Bruckmann & Hackhe (1987)	Hamburg; dump site	2/85	G/P/Si BSI								
	Dump site, oil (1)	4/85		< 0.02	< 0.03	< 0.02	< 0.02	ND	ND	0.27	0[a]
	Residential, west of dump (1)	4/85		< 0.1	–	–	–	–	1.1	1.0	0.038[a]
	(2)	3/86		< 0.1–0.02	0.06	0.05	0.22	0.09	1.5	1.2–4.2	0.032–0.072[a]
	Residential, highway, dump, industrial (5)	85–87		< 0.02–0.11	< 0.01–0.60	0.06–1.0	0.08–2.2	0.07–5.2	2.15–15.4	1.1–40	0.164–2.186[a]
	Close to copper industry (2)	1&2/87		< 0.01	0.04	0.03–0.04	0.06–0.12	0.06–0.09	2.15–3.69	0.65–0.7	0.093–0.206[a]
	Industry, highway (2)	1&10/86		0.02–0.20	0.04–0.22	0.19–0.26	0.60–0.71	< 0.17–0.36	4.8–5.3	7.4–9.4	0.525–0.612[a]
	Industry, 2 MWI (2)	85–86		< 0.01–0.085	0.1–0.052	< 0.09–0.19	< 0.09–0.90	< 0.09–0.38	1.5–7.7	3.7–7.7	0.156–1.081[a]
	Highway tunnel (2)	1/86		< 0.01–0.06	0.28–0.31	< 0.17–0.37	0.66–1.19	< 0.17–0.44	3.4	6.3–6.4	0.457–0.569[a]
	Suburb, highway (1)	9/86		< 0.02	< 0.04	0.06	0.09	< 0.04	2.31	2.9	0.085[a]
	Suburb (North) (1)	8/86		< 0.02	< 0.03	< 0.03	0.07	0.06	1.23	1.0	0.032[a]
	Suburb (13 km SE) (1)	4/86		0.02	< 0.02	< 0.08	0.23	< 0.08	0.60	0.37	0.084[a]
	Forest (20 km N) (1)	4/86		< 0.02	< 0.03	< 0.03	< 0.03	< 0.03	0.28	0.37	0.001[a]

PCDD concentration (pg/m³)

Table 1 (contd)

Reference	Origin; sample description (and no.)	Coll. period	Samp. meth. / Anal. meth.	PCDD concentration (pg/m^3)							I-TEQ PCDD/PCDF
				TCDD 2378	PeCDD 12378	HxCDD 123478	123678	123789	HpCDD 1234678	OCDD	
Kirschmer (1987)	Rhine-Ruhr; Mean of 11 sites/wide range of uses (33)	85–86	G/P CSI	ND	0.02	0.03	0.06	0.03	1.14	0.98	0.1 (0.02–0.4)[a]
Christmann et al. (1989b)	Ambient air; Berlin-Dahlem (10)	1/87	G/P CSI	ND	ND	ND	ND	ND	6.6	8.5	0.1
	Bad-Kreuzberg (1)	2/88		ND	ND	ND	ND	ND	1.3	2.2	0.07[a]
	Gelsenkirchen (5)	87/88		ND	ND	ND	ND	ND	3.2	8.5	0.1 (0.03–0.3)[a]
	Recklinghausen (3)	5–9/87		ND	ND–0.5	ND	ND	ND	ND–1.7	6.1	0.2 (0.1–0.3)[a]
	Indoor air; PCP application (1)			ND	ND	ND	6.2	ND	63.3	103	2.6[a]
Päpke et al. (1989a)	Indoor air; PCP application (kindergartens) (1)	86	G/P BSI	ND	ND	0.04	0.92	0.11	77.0	131.5	2.46[a]
	(15)						No information				0.696 (0.018–2.46)[a]
König et al. (1993)	Hessen; ambient air	90	G/P BSI								
	Rural (21)			0.002	0.009	0.013	0.026	0.024	0.267	3.18	0.048
	Rural/industry (21)			0.004	0.020	0.025	0.052	0.044	0.629	6.44	0.087
	Rural industry (21)			0.003	0.021	0.019	0.048	0.036	0.527	5.80	0.079
	Industry (21)			0.005	0.029	0.034	0.071	0.061	0.570	8.77	0.146
	Industry (21)			0.004	0.022	0.024	0.053	0.044	0.603	6.77	0.110
	Traffic (21)			0.002	0.018	0.017	0.042	0.036	0.435	5.14	0.078

Table 1 (contd)

Reference	Origin; sample description (and no.)	Coll. period	Samp. meth. / Anal. meth.	PCDD concentration (pg/m³)							I-TEQ PCDD/PCDF
				TCDD 2378	PeCDD 12378	HxCDD 123478	123678	123789	HpCDD 1234678	OCDD	
Wallenhorst et al. (1995)	Baden-Württemberg; ambient air	92	G/P BSI								
	Rural					No information					0.021 (0.008–0.054)
	Rural with special exposure					No information					0.018 (0.005–0.049)
	Suburban					No information					0.056 (0.009–0.098)
	Urban					No information					0.083 (0.021–0.217)
	Multitype					No information					0.062 (0.014–0.130)
Hiester et al. (1995)	Ambient air; Essen, mostly residential	93–94	G/P CSI			No information					0.076
	Duisburg, industrial					No information					0.124
	Dortmund, downtown					No information					0.120
	Cologne, mostly residential					No information					0.040
Hippelein et al. (1996)	Augsburg; ambient air (means)		G/X BSI								
	March–April (6)	92		<0.0035	0.0086	<0.013	0.021	0.021	0.270	0.720	0.040
	April–May (6)	92		<0.0017	0.0039	<0.0049	<0.0081	<0.0074	0.087	0.280	0.019
	June–July (6)	92		<0.0012	0.0024	<0.0043	<0.0058	<0.0046	0.089	0.320	0.014
	July–September (6)	92		<0.0014	<0.0022	<0.0061	<0.0078	<0.0062	0.120	0.430	0.015
	Sept.–October (6)	92		<0.0030	<0.0076	<0.015	<0.021	0.021	0.310	0.750	0.042
	Oct.–November (6)	92		0.0037	0.012	<0.019	0.030	0.030	0.510	1.300	0.060
	Nov.–January (6)	92–93		0.0069	0.027	0.034	0.063	0.063	0.830	2.000	0.120
	Jan.–February (6)	93		<0.0036	0.018	0.027	0.045	0.044	0.530	1.200	0.087
	Mean of mean (48)	92–93		0.0031	0.010	0.015	0.030	0.024	0.340	0.870	0.049

Table 1 (contd)

Reference	Origin; sample description (and no.)		Coll. period	Samp. meth. / Anal. meth.	PCDD concentration (pg/m³)							I-TEQ PCDD/PCDF
					TCDD 2378	PeCDD 12378	HxCDD 123478	123678	123789	HpCDD 1234678	OCDD	
Rabl et al. (1996)	Bavaria; ambient air			G/P BSI								
	1.3 km E of MWI	(1)	96					No information				0.034
	2.0 km NE of MWI	(2)	95–96					No information				0.055–0.064
	3.3 km NNE of MWI	(2)	95–96					No information				0.034–0.062
Päpke et al. (1994a)	Workplace air		93	G/P/Ps BSI								
	Plant 1	(4)						No information				0.70–3.79
	Plant 2	(3)						No information				0.06–0.18
	Plant 3	(5)						No information				0.06–0.60
	Plant 1	(3)		G/P BSI				No information				0.15–1.90
	Plant 2	(5)						No information				0.08–0.15
	Plant 3	(5)						No information				0.07–0.54
Menzel et al. (1996)	Workplace air;		95	G/P/Ps N								
	Welding, MWI1 boiler pipes	(1)			Total 2,3,7,8-isomers, 541							56
	Welding, MWI2 waste chute	(2)			Total 2,3,7,8-isomers, 204–1058							11–44
	Milling, MWI1 boiler pipes	(1)			Total 2,3,7,8-isomers, 975							87
	Fitting, MWI1 waste chute	(2)			Total 2,3,7,8-isomers, 20 038–21 678							1830–2430
	Fitting, MWI2 waste chute	(2)			Total 2,3,7,8-isomers, 794–2680							30–140
	Air burning, MWI2 waste chute	(2)			Total 2,3,7,8-isomers, 354–6911							20–80
	Cutting/welding, wood chip dryer	(1)			Total 2,3,7,8-isomers, 61							2

Table 1 (contd)

Reference	Origin; sample description (and no.)	Coll. period	Samp. meth. / Anal. meth.	PCDD concentration (pg/m³)							I-TEQ PCDD/PCDF
				TCDD 2378	PeCDD 12378	HxCDD 123478	123678	123789	HpCDD 1234678	OCDD	
Menzel *et al.* (1996) (contd)	Open-air burning, power plant demol. (2)			Total 2,3,7,8-isomers, 20–39							358–459
	Open-air burning, metal reclamation 1 (2)			Total 2,3,7,8-isomers, 227–1266							98–858
	Open-air burning, metal reclamation 2 (2)			Total 2,3,7,8-isomers, 95–300							348–1183
Japan											
Sugita *et al.* (1993)	Urban area	92	GP / BSI								
	Ambient air, mean summer (2)			0.007	0.087	0.180	0.274	0.191	2.375	4.624	0.469–1.427[a]
	Ambient air, mean winter (2)			0.040	0.193	0.376	0.683	0.555	4.213	10.358	0.294–2.990[a]
Kurokawa *et al.* (1994)	Site A	< 94	GP / BSO								
	Ambient air, particle phase			No information						Summer	0.025
										Winter	0.291
	Ambient air, vapour phase			No information						Summer	0.035
										Winter	0.012
	Site B										
	Ambient air, particle phase			No information						Summer	0.184
										Winter	0.310
	Ambient air, vapour phase			No information						Summer	0.407
										Winter	0.046
	Site C										
	Ambient air, particle phase			No information						Summer	0.273
										Winter	0.614
	Ambient air, vapour phase			No information						Summer	0.218
										Winter	0.072

Table 1 (contd)

Reference	Origin; sample description (and no.)	Coll. period	Samp. meth. / Anal. meth.	PCDD concentration (pg/m³)							I-TEQ PCDD/PCDF
				TCDD 2378	PeCDD 12378	HxCDD 123478	123678	123789	HpCDD 1234678	OCDD	
Norway											
Oehme et al. (1991)	Tunnel air; Northbound	89	G/P / CSI								
	Inlet, weekday (1)			0.02	0.021	0.028	0.049	0.041	0.29	1.5	0.097[c]
	Outlet, weekday (1)			0.04	0.20	0.084	0.34	0.29	1.7	1.6	0.98[c]
	Inlet, weekend (1)			<0.01	0.018	0.018	0.091	0.029	0.36	2.3	0.089[c]
	Outlet, weekend (1)			0.03	0.054	0.050	0.12	0.09	0.52	2.8	0.55[c]
	Southbound										
	Inlet, weekday (1)			0.01	0.042	0.013	0.066	0.037	0.32	1.9	0.131[c]
	Outlet, weekday (1)			0.02	0.015	0.022	0.092	0.028	0.38	2.2	0.230[c]
	Inlet, weekend (1)			<0.01	0.021	0.086	0.063	0.024	0.18	1.1	0.101[c]
	Outlet, weekend (1)			0.01	0.031	–	0.048	0.028	0.24	1.7	0.134[c]
	Central Oslo; ambient air			No information							0.040[c]
Schlabach et al. (1996)	Spitbergen, arctic; ambient air	5/95 8/95	G/P / BSI	0.0002	0.0005	0.0009	0.0013	0.0002	–	–	0.0023
	(1)			0.0001	0.0002	0.0001	0.0003	0.0002	0.0016	0.0044	0.0011
Poland											
Grochowalski et al. (1995)	Cracow centre; market square (1)	3/95	G/C / CSI	0.15	0.18	0.21	0.2	0.16	2.7	10.4	0.95
	Mateczny crossroad (1)			1	1.15	2.15	3	1.05	55	280	11.95
Russian Federation											
Kruglov et al. (1996)	Oil fire; residential area	96	BSO								
	100 m downwind (1)			0.56	0.85	0.32	1.84	0.52	7.77	62.45	1.72
	100 m upwind (1)			0.17	0.12	0.09	0.12	0.08	4.26	39.3	0.5

Table 1 (contd)

Reference	Origin; sample description (and no.)	Coll. period	Samp. meth. / Anal. meth.	PCDD concentration (pg/m³)							I-TEQ PCDD/PCDF
				TCDD 2378	PeCDD 12378	HxCDD 123478	123678	123789	HpCDD 1234678	OCDD	
Slovakia											
Holoubek et al. (1991)	Ambient air	90	P N								
	Urban/industrial						No information				ND–6.3
	Rural						No information				0.0002–4.9
	Rural/industrial						No information				3.0–6.0
	Suburban						No information				0.0035–2.9
	Resid./industrial						No information				0.23–5.5
	Urban/industrial						No information				2.0–3.0
Spain											
Abad et al. (1996)	Catalonia (ambient air); urban, traffic (8)	93–95	G/P BSI	*0.026	0.031	0.029	0.064	0.076	0.385	1.110	0.28 (0.05–0.62)
	Rural, near MWI (12)			0.006	0.009	0.008	0.023	0.031	0.218	1.286	0.05 (0.01–0.5)
	Urban (3)			0.003	0.010	0.013	0.027	0.043	0.277	0.803	0.13 (0.11–0.15)
	Urban (3)			0.007	0.014	0.013	0.020	0.033	0.223	1.237	0.20 (0.07–0.43)
	MWI influence (2)			0.010	0.050	0.060	0.155	0.210	1.720	5.695	0.55 (0.15–0.95)
	Industrial, MWI influence, traffic (3)			0.007	0.020	0.040	0.103	0.150	0.867	2.313	0.28 (0.20–0.36)
	MWI (2)			0.005	0.010	0.010	0.015	0.020	0.135	0.770	0.08 (0.01–0.05)
	Heavy industry (2)			0.040	0.045	0.100	0.150	0.140	1.035	2.920	0.52 (0.16–0.88)

Table 1 (contd)

Reference	Origin; sample description (and no.)	Coll. period	Samp. meth. / Anal. meth.	PCDD concentration (pg/m³)							I-TEQ PCDD/PCDF
				TCDD 2378	PeCDD 12378	HxCDD 123478	123678	123789	HpCDD 1234678	OCDD	
Sweden											
Rappe *et al.* (1989a)	Rörvik; ambient air		G / BSI								
	Wind WSW (1)	9/85		<0.001	0.003	<0.001	<0.001	<0.001	0.057[f]	0.050	
	Wind W, N & E (1)	1/86		<0.001	0.005	<0.001	0.004	0.005	0.140[f]	0.064	
	Wind E & N (1)	1/86		0.002	0.009	0.002	0.005	0.006	0.210[f]	0.160	
	Wind SE (1)	1/86		0.005	0.035	0.007	0.014	0.032	1.00[f]	0.540	
	Wind NE (1)	2/86		<0.001	0.004	<0.001	0.002	0.004	0.110[f]	–	
	(1)	2/86		<0.001	0.007	0.003	0.005	0.006	0.270[f]	0.160	
	Gothenburg; ambient air										
	Wind W, N & E (1)	1/86		0.003	0.017	0.003	0.011	0.006	0.380[f]	0.290	
	Wind E & N (1)	1/86		0.009	0.066	0.019	0.046	0.092	2.900[f]	1.900	
	Wind SE (1)	2/86		<0.001	0.006	0.002	0.004	0.007	0.230[f]	1.040	
Antonsson *et al.* (1989)	Workplace air (steelmills); close to furnace	88	G/X / BSI	No information							0.80–6.4[c]
	Overhead crane			No information							1.8–14[c]
	Crane cabin			No information							2.8–5.6[c]
United Kingdom											
Clayton *et al.* (1993)	Ambient air		N / B								
	Cardiff (42)	1/91–9/92		Mean (range) total 2,3,7,8-isomers, 2.3 (ND–66)							0.100 (ND–0.86)
	Manchester (43)	3/91–9/92		Mean (range) total 2,3,7,8-isomers, 2.1 (ND–46)							0.102 (0.001–1.81)
	London (43)	1/91–11/92		Mean (range) total 2,3,7,8-isomers, 2.2 (ND–17)							0.06 (ND–0.65)
	Stevenage (43)	1/91–4/92		Mean (range) total 2,3,7,8-isomers, 1.7 (ND–9)							0.039 (ND–0.80)

Table 1 (contd)

Reference	Origin; sample description (and no.)	Coll. period	Samp. meth. / Anal. meth.	PCDD concentration (pg/m³)							I-TEQ PCDD/PCDF
				TCDD 2378	PeCDD 12378	HxCDD 123478	123678	123789	HpCDD 1234678	OCDD	
Dyke & Coleman (1995)	Ambient air	11/94	GP / CSI								
	Before bonfire (1)					No information					0.12–0.15
	During bonfire (1)					No information					0.62–0.65
	After bonfire (1)					No information					0.14–0.17
United States											
Eitzer & Hites (1989)	Bloomington; ambient, municipal (55)	85–87	GP / CSN			No further isomers reported				0.89	
	Trout Lake; ambient, rural (2)					No further isomers reported				0.16	
Smith et al. (1989)	Niagara Falls; ambient air		GP / CSI								
	Downwind from industry (1)	11/86		ND	ND	0.05	0.06	0.11	0.55	1.59	
	(1)	11/86		ND	0.49	0.64	1.06	ND	5.43	8.88	
	(1)	1/86		ND	ND	0.04	0.05	0.07	ND	1.83	
	Upwind from industry (1)	11/86		ND	ND	ND	ND	ND	0.34	1.40	
	(1)	1/87		ND	ND	ND	ND	0.03	0.37	1.36	
	(1)	2/87		ND	ND	ND	ND	ND	0.51	5.79	
Edgerton et al. (1989)	Akron; 2 km from MWI	87	GP / BSN	< 0.20	< 0.27	0.035	0.052	0.050	0.52	1.00	
				< 0.16	< 0.11	0.055	0.053	0.026	0.53	1.20	
				< 0.01	< 0.03	0.032	0.053	0.017	0.57	1.20	
	Columbus;										
	3/4 km from RDF			< 0.82	< 0.06	< 0.028	< 0.028	< 0.028	0.26	0.51	
	1/4 km from SSI			< 0.24	< 0.05	< 0.039	0.078	0.064	0.52	1.10	
	Highway			< 0.15	< 0.08	< 0.032	< 0.032	< 0.032	0.32	0.96	
	Waldo; Background			< 0.06	< 0.03	0.031	0.025	0.025	0.24	0.50	

Table 1 (contd)

Reference	Origin; sample description (and no.)	Coll. period	Samp. meth. / Anal. meth.	PCDD concentration (pg/m³)							I-TEQ PCDD/PCDF
				TCDD 2378	PeCDD 12378	HxCDD 123478	123678	123789	HpCDD 1234678	OCDD	
Hahn et al. (1989)	Workplace air; bottom ash conveyor	1/88	G/P/X / N	ND	ND	ND	ND	ND	0.431	2.141	
	Feed table floor			ND	ND	ND	ND	0.039	1.012	9.494	
Tierman et al. (1989)	Dayton, OH; ambient air, near MWI	88	N	ND	0.57	0.63	1.19	0.91	6.02	8.26	
Kominsky & Kwoka (1989)	Boston Office building (12) / Ambient air (4)	9/86	G/Si / CN	<0.3–<1.4 / <0.4–<0.6	<0.2–<1.1 / <0.5–<1.6		<0.25–<0.95 / <0.27–<0.51		<0.66–2.0 / <1.2–1.6	3.2–7.6 / 3.5–5.6	
Harless et al. (1990)	Green Bay, WI; ambient air (4)	89	G/P / BSI	<0.01–<0.04	<0.02–<0.08	<0.01–<0.01	0.01–0.03	<0.01–0.02	0.1–0.2	0.3–0.4	
Hunt & Maisel (1990)	Bridgeport, CT; ambient air (29)	87–88	G/P / BSI	0.012	0.024	0.030	0.043	0.075	0.477	2.10	
Maisel (1990)	Bridgeport MWI; ambient air preoperational (22)	87–88	G/P / BSI	<0.010	0.021	0.030	0.046	0.080	0.47		
Maisel & Hunt (1990)	Los Angeles, CA; ambient air (1)	W/87	G/P / BSI	<0.010	<0.039	<0.076	<0.083	<0.086	0.25	1.9	

Table 1 (contd)

Reference	Origin; sample description (and no.)		Coll. period	Samp. meth. / Anal. meth.	PCDD concentration (pg/m³)							I-TEQ PCDD/PCDF
					TCDD 2378	PeCDD 12378	HxCDD 123478	123678	123789	HpCDD 1234678	OCDD	
Hunt & Maisel (1992)	S. California;			G/P / BSI								
	Session I	(6)	12/87		<0.020	<0.136	<0.196	<0.410	<0.392	2.02	2.46	
	Session II	(2)	12/87		<0.006	<0.014	<0.010	<0.008	<0.010	0.230	1.25	
	Session III	(5)	7/88		<0.026	<0.060	<0.086	<0.082	<0.104	<1.796	3.18	
	Session IV	(6)	7/88		<0.034	<0.056	<0.082	<0.076	<0.150	<3.52	5.26	
	Session V	(7)	9/88		<0.024	<0.026	<0.032	<0.050	<0.028	0.377	1.13	
	Session VI	(1)	11/88		<0.012	<0.022	<0.036	<0.054	<0.050	0.227	0.437	
	Session VII	(6)	3/89		<0.024	<0.186	<0.026	<0.026	<0.030	0.248	2.05	
	Mean, all sessions	(33)			<0.024	<0.088	<0.076	<0.118	<0.128	<2.02	<5.60	
Schecter & Charles (1991)	Binghamton;			N								
	transformer incident site		81–82					No information				352'
			89–90					No information				74'
	Upper floors		81–82					No information				202'
			89–90					No information				2.9'
Lorber et al. (1996a)	Columbus, OH;			N								
	running MWI	(6)	3/94					No information				0.067
		(6)	4/94					No information				0.118
	Shut down MWI	(7)	6/95					No information				0.049
	Columbus high; running MWI	(2)	94					No information				0.26
	Shut down MWI	(2)	95					No information				0.09
	Columbus low; running MWI	(2)	94					No information				0.03
	Shut down MWI	NG	95					No information				0.02

Table 1 (contd)

Reference	Origin; sample description (and no.)		Coll. period	Samp. meth. / Anal. meth.	PCDD concentration (pg/m³)								I-TEQ PCDD/PCDF
					TCDD 2378	PeCDD 12378	HxCDD 123478	123678	123789	HpCDD 1234678	OCDD		
Riggs et al. (1996)	Edgemont, OH; 2.4 km N of MWI	(6)	9/95	G/P CSO				No information					0.206
	Kettering; 1.6 km N of MWI	(6)						No information					0.057
	Site 8; 0.5 km SW of MWI	(6)						No information					0.045
	Miami Villa; 1.4 km SW of MWI	(6)						No information					0.016
	Background; 15 km N of Dayton	(1)						No information					0.006

Analytical methods: All analyses use high-resolution gas chromatography; B, high-resolution mass spectrometry; C, low-resolution mass spectrometry; I, isomer-specific; O, others; N, no information; S, sophisticated clean-up; R, reduced clean-up; W, WHO-accepted laboratory

Sampling methods: G, glass fibre filter; P, polyurethane foam; X, XAD; C, carbon; Si, silica; Ps, personal sampling

ND, not detected; HWI, hospital waste incinerator; MWI, municipal waste incinerator; SSI, sewage sludge incinerator; RDF, refuse-derived fuel incinerator; W, winter

Data presented are means. Figures in parentheses are ranges. Levels of congeners not detected at known detection limits (for examples, 0.02 pg/m³) are presented as < 0.02

[a] German TEQ
[b] Including PCBs contribution
[c] Nordic TEQ
[d] Contains non-toxic isomers
[e] Eadon-TEQ

Table 2. Concentrations of PCDDs in water

Reference	Origin; sample description (and no.)		Coll. period	Anal. meth.	PCDD concentration (pg/L; ppt)							I-TEQ PCDD/PCDF
					TCDD 2378	PeCDD 12378	HxCDD 123478	123678	123789	HpCDD 1234678	OCDD	
Canada												
Jobb et al. (1990)	Ontario; Amherstburg, drinking water, raw	5	85–86	AB/CS	–	–	–	–	–	–	20–115	
	Cayuga; drinking water, raw	1	87		–	–	–	–	–	–	42	
	Lambton Area; drinking water, raw	2	86		–	–	–	–	–	–	13–38	
	Mitchell's Bay; drinking water, raw	4	85–86		–	–	–	–	–	–	24–140	
	South Peel Area; drinking water, raw	1	83		–	–	–	–	–	–	30	
	St. Catharines; drinking water, raw	3	83–86		–	–	–	–	–	–	39–90	
	Stoney Point; drinking water, raw	4	85–86		–	–	–	–	–	–	24–120	
	Wallaceburg; drinking water, raw	2	85–86		–	–	–	–	–	–	12–175	
	Wallaceburg; drinking water, treated	1	86		–	–	–	–	–	–	19	

Table 2 (contd)

Reference	Origin; sample description (and no.)		Coll. period	Anal. meth.	PCDD concentration (pg/L; ppt)							I-TEQ PCDD/PCDF
					TCDD 2378	PeCDD 12378	HxCDD 123478	123678	123789	HpCDD 1234678	OCDD	
Canada (contd)												
Jobb et al. (1990) (contd)	Walpole Island; drinking water, treated	2	86	AB/CS	–	–	–	–	–	–	28–41	
	Walpole Island; drinking water, raw	2	86		–	–	–	–	–	–	9–35	
	Welland river; drinking water, raw	1	86		–	–	–	–	–	–	25	
	Windsor; drinking water, raw	8	85–86		–	–	–	–	–	–	22–63	
	Windsor; drinking water, treated	1	86		–	–	–	–	–	–	46	
Germany												
Götz et al.(1994)	River Elbe;			ABSIW								
	Bunthaus d and PB		8/90		0.220	0.409	0.732	1.120	1.936	15.065	64.6	3.15
	Blankenese d and PB		8/90		0.090	0.107	0.322	0.351	0.814	3.209	12.8	1.21
Japan												
Hashimoto et al. (1995a)	Matsuyama		8/90	ACIS								
	Coastal seawater, d	1a			ND	ND	ND	ND	ND	ND	ND	
	Coastal sea-water, PB	1b			ND	ND	ND	ND	ND	0.068	2.5	

Table 2 (contd)

Reference	Origin; sample description (and no.)		Coll. period	Anal. meth.	PCDD concentration (pg/L; ppt)							I-TEQ PCDD/PCDF
					TCDD 2378	PeCDD 12378	HxCDD 123478	123678	123789	HpCDD 1234678	OCDD	
Japan (contd)												
Hashimoto et al. (1995a) (contd)	Misaki											
	Coastal seawater, d	1a	8/90	ACIS	ND	ND	ND	ND	ND	ND	0.10	
	Coastal seawater, PB	1b			ND	ND	ND	ND	ND	ND	1.1	
Matsumara et al. (1994)	Coastal seawater	1	NG	ABIS	0.020	0.014	0.040	0.070	0.088	0.250	0.340	
Miyata et al. (1992, 93)	Nagahama		10–11/91	ABIS								
	Wellwater, S	1a			ND	ND	ND	ND	ND	ND	0.19	
	Wellwater, PB	1b			ND	ND	ND	ND	ND	0.62	11.73	
	Home tap water, S	1a			ND	ND	ND	ND	ND	ND	0.29	
	Home tap water, PB	1b			ND	ND	ND	ND	ND	ND	0.24	
	Hirakata		10–11/91									
	Home tap water, S	2a			ND	ND	ND	ND	ND	ND	0.72–0.88	
	Home tap water, PB	2b			ND	ND	ND	ND	ND	ND	0.51–0.79	
	Osaka		10–11/91									
	Home tap water, S	2a			ND	ND	ND	ND	ND	0.09–0.14	0.85–1.33	
	Home tap water, PB	2b			ND	ND	ND	ND	ND	ND	0.58–0.86	
Russian Federation												
Fedorov (1993)	Ufa, north; drinking water		4/92	N	27.5							
	Ufa, south; drinking water		4/92		48.8							

Table 2 (contd)

Reference	Origin; sample description (and no.)	Coll. period	Anal. meth.	PCDD concentration (pg/L; ppt)							
				TCDD 2378	PeCDD 12378	HxCDD 123478	123678	123789	HpCDD 1234678	OCDD	I-TEQ PCDD/PCDF
Russian Federation (contd)											
Fedorov (1993) (contd)	Ufa, Iziak; drinking water	4/92		167.0							
	Ufa; Dem; drinking water	4/92	N	83.5							
	Chapaevsk; Artesian drinking water	6–9/92		20.3	31.3		18.0	16.7	235	55.7	
	Ufa, Chapaevsk; river water	3–6/90							25 000	760 000	
Khamitov & Maystrenko (1995)	Ufa; drinking water	90	N	No isomer-specific information							0.5–1.0
	Belaja river; river water	90		No isomer-specific information							2.3–5.7
	Belaja river/Ufa; river water	90		No isomer-specific information							1.7–6.0
	Ufa river/w.i.; river water	90		No isomer-specific information							0.6–1.0
	Inzer river; river water	90		No isomer-specific information							1.8
	Ziliim river; river water	90		No isomer-specific information							0.2
Sweden											
Rappe et al. (1989b)	Bälinge, Uppsala; MWTP, in 1	87	ABIS	<1.2	<3.6	<7	<5	<5	62	730	
	MWTP, out 1	87		<0.26	<0.77	<2	<1.5	<1.5	2.8	14	
	Henriksdal, Stockholm; MWTP, in 1	87		<1.6	<4.8	<9	<14	<20	70	620	
	MWTP, out 1	87		<0.28	<0.70	<2	<3	<4	<6.1	39	

Table 2 (contd)

Reference	Origin; sample description (and no.)	Coll. period	Anal. meth.	PCDD concentration (pg/L; ppt)							I-TEQ PCDD/PCDF
				TCDD 2378	PeCDD 12378	HxCDD 123478	123678	123789	HpCDD 1234678	OCDD	
Sweden (contd)											
Rappe et al. (1989b) (contd)	Järnsjön; Eman river	1	87	ABIS	<0.024	<0.039	0.054	0.120	0.075	0.300	2.000	
	Fliseryd; Eman river	1	87		<0.020	<0.025	<0.014	<0.013	<0.015	0.150	0.790	
	Filtered water; Eman river	1	87		<0.023	<0.019	<0.027	<0.024	<0.029	0.057	0.170	
	Blank; Laboratory	1	87		<0.039	<0.034	<0.045	<0.040	<0.049	<0.083	0.180	
Rappe et al. (1990a)	Ringhals, in; sea cooling water	1	89	ABIS	<0.005	<0.003	0.011	0.0047	0.0054	0.110	0.620	0.0083
	Ringhals, out; sea cooling water	1	89		<0.005	<0.003	<0.006	0.0067	<0.005	0.070	0.240	0.0075
	Ringhals, in; sea cooling water	1	89		0.0019	0.0009	0.0011	0.0015	<0.002	0.030	0.185	0.0057
	Ringhals, out; sea cooling water	1	89		0.0026	0.0004	<0.002	0.0023	0.0012	0.031	0.154	0.0063
	River Ljusnan	3	89		0.001–0.0021	0.0037–0.0048	0.0018–0.0022	0.018–0.021	0.0093–0.017	0.059–0.110	0.140–0.170	0.013–0.017
	River Ljungan	1	89		0.0031	<0.0004	<0.0006	0.0046	0.0027	0.036	0.140	0.014
	Drinking water	1	89		0.0005	<0.0005	<0.0008	0.001	<0.0009	0.0044	0.017	0.0029
United States											
Meyer et al. (1989)	Lockport; Finished water, S	1	8/86	AC/BOS	<1.0	<1.8		<0.9		<0.9	5.0	
	Finished water, PB	1			<0.7	<1.6		<0.6		<0.5	3.6	

Table 2 (contd)

Reference	Origin; sample description (and no.)		Coll. period	Anal. meth.	PCDD concentration (pg/L; ppt)							I-TEQ PCDD/PCDF
					TCDD 2378	PeCDD 12378	HxCDD 123478	123678	123789	HpCDD 1234678	OCDD	
United States (contd)												
Meyer et al. (1989) (contd)	Blank; Distilled water, soluble	1	9/86		<1.1	<3.9		<1.2		<1.4	6.5	
	Distilled water; PB	1			<1.0	<3.9		<0.9		<0.8	2.3	
	Lockport; Finished water, S	1	2/88		<3.8	<4.9		<6.3		<12	<23	
	Finished water, PB	1			<4.0	<4.8		<6.0		<9.4	<19	
	Lockport; Finished water, S	1	8/88		<3.4	<3.9		<4.7		<6.8	31	
	Finished water, PB	1			<2.6	<3.8		<4.4		<5.4	15	
	19 other locations; Finished water, S	19	86–87		ND (0.4–2.6)	ND (1.2–7.4)		ND (0.4–3.6)		ND (0.4–6.1)	ND (0.9–15)	
	Finished water, PB	19			ND (0.3–2.0)	ND (1.0–8.9)		ND (0.5–4.1)		ND (0.4–15.4)	ND (0.9–69)	

Analytical methods: A, high-resolution gas chromatography; B, high-resolution mass spectrometry; C, low-resolution mass spectrometry; I, isomer-specific; N, no information; S, sophisticated clean-up; R, reduced clean-up; W, WHO-accepted laboratory

ND, not detected; w.i., water intake; NG, not given

Data presented are means. Figures in parentheses are ranges. Levels of congeners not detected at known detection limits (for examples, 0.02 pg/m^3) are presented as <0.02

S, soluble; PB, particle bound; d, water dissolved; MWTP, municipal water treatment plant

Table 3. Concentrations of PCDDs in soil

Reference	Origin; sample description (and no.)	Coll. period	Anal. meth.	PCDD concentration (ng/kg; ppt)							I-TEQ PCDD/PCDF
				TCDD 2378	PeCDD 12378	HxCDD 123478 / 123678 / 123789			HpCDD 1234678	OCDD	
Australia											
Sund et al. (1993)	Melbourne;		ABSN								
	Park; urban area	1	90	ND	No further isomer-specific information					1200	2.1
	Near Tullamarine tip; industrial area	1	90	ND	No further isomer-specific information					1200	2.1
	Near Maid-road; industrial area	1	90	ND	No further isomer-specific information					190	0.47
	Near incinerator; industrial area	1	90	ND	No further isomer-specific information					230	0.09
	Park; urban area	1	90	ND	No further isomer-specific information					2900	1.8
	Gardens; urban area	1	90	ND	No further isomer-specific information					11 000	8.2
	Near incinerator; industrial area	1	90	ND	No further isomer-specific information					1 000	1.0
	Werribee farm; land filtration paddock	1	90	34	No isomer-specific information					75 000	520
Buckland et al. (1994)	300 m fr. road; burnt area	1	94	ABSI	No isomer-specific information						2.2
	100 m fr. road; unburnt area	1	94		No isomer-specific information						3.1
	300 m fr. road; burnt area	1	94		No isomer-specific information						35.1/38.5
	5 m fr. road; unburnt area	1	94		No isomer-specific information						8.7
	1 km fr. highway; burnt area	1	94		No isomer-specific information						3.0
	5 m fr. highway; unburnt area	1	94		No isomer-specific information						10.0
	High traffic; unburnt area, Sydney	1	94		No isomer-specific information						42.6
Austria											
Weiss et al. (1993, 1994)	Linz area; grassland; depth, 0–5 cm	13	< 93	ABSI	No further isomer-specific information						[1.6–14.4]

Table 3 (contd)

Reference	Origin; sample description (and no.)		Coll. period	Anal. meth.	PCDD concentration (ng/kg; ppt)						OCDD	I-TEQ PCDD/PCDF
					TCDD	PeCDD	HxCDD			HpCDD		
					2378	12378	123478	123678	123789	1234678		
Austria (contd)												
Riss et al. (1990)	Brixlegg (Tyrol)											
	200m downwind	NG	87		No isomer-specific information							420*
	400 m downwind	NG	87		No isomer-specific information							170*
	700 m downwind	NG	87		No isomer-specific information							46*
Boos et al. (1992)	Salzburg:			ACSI								
	Meadow; urban emission	1	90/91		ND	ND	ND	ND	ND	7.3	19.4	2.3
	Park; urban emission	1	90/91		ND	ND	ND	ND	ND	10.5	65.0	1.8
	Traffic island; heavy traffic	1	90/91		ND	4.6	3.2	5.6	1.6	64.3	305	8.3
	Meadow; urban emission	1	90/91		ND	ND	1.5	3.3	3.0	57.7	892	5.2
		1	90/91		ND	ND	ND	1.1	ND	45.5	328	1.8
		1	90/91		ND	1.1	ND	2.4	ND	38.9	270	3.9
		1	90/91		ND	ND	2.0	3.9	4.6	121.8	1022	4.5
	Park; urban emission	1	90/91		ND	ND	ND	ND	ND	10.6	40.8	2.2
	Meadow; cable proc. plant	1	90/91		ND	ND	ND	ND	ND	17.2	48.5	4.0
		1	90/91		ND	ND	0.8	1.8	1.6	13.8	29.4	6.9
		1	90/91		ND	ND	ND	1.8	1.6	16.2	57.2	3.5
	Meadow; diffuse emission	1	90/91		ND	ND	1.1	1.1	ND	10.8	19.2	3.0
	Diffuse emission, highway 100m	1	90/91		ND	ND	ND	ND	ND	3.7	10.1	0.8
		1	90/91		ND	ND	ND	ND	ND	3.9	13.2	0.6
	Diffuse emission, highway 200m	1	90/91		ND	ND	ND	ND	ND	3.5	7.5	0.9
	Steel foundry	1	90/91		ND	ND	ND	ND	ND	6.3	17.9	1.0
	Steel foundry	1	90/91		ND	ND	0.4	0.9	1.1	5.9	17.7	1.8
	Industry	1	90/91		ND	1.9	ND	2.3	2.5	13.6	28.7	3.7

Table 3 (contd)

Reference	Origin; sample description (and no.)	Coll. period	Anal. meth.	PCDD concentration (ng/kg; ppt)								I-TEQ PCDD/PCDF
				TCDD 2378	PeCDD 12378	HxCDD 123478	123678	123789	HpCDD 1234678	OCDD		
Austria (contd)												
Boos et al. (1992) (contd)	Meadow; Alpine background	1	90/91	ND	ND	ND	ND	ND	1.8	3.6		0.1
	Urban outsk.; 2ndary Al Smelter	1	90/91	ND	ND	1.1	1.2	1.6	6.6	24.2		2.8
	2ndary Al Smelter	1	90/91	ND	ND	2.0	2.3	1.5	7.0	23.5		5.3
	Diffuse emission	1	90/91	ND	ND	0.6	1.5	1.2	11.4	26.0		3.6
	Meadow; highway 0.5 m	1	90/91	ND	ND	0.7	1.9	2.1	24.6	89.1		3.1
	Industrial area; metal smelter	1	90/91	ND	ND	ND	ND	ND	92.0	241		11.5
Belgium												
Van Cleuven- bergen et al. (1993)	Mol; rural	92	ABSI	No isomer-specific information								2.14
	Moerkerke; rural	92		No isomer-specific information								2.27
	Berendrecht; harbour Antwerp	92		No isomer-specific information								3.81
	Zelzate; industry, highway	92		No isomer-specific information								8.94
	Ham; industry, highway	92		No isomer-specific information								2.72
	Vilvoorde; industry, power plant	92		No isomer-specific information								5.76
Brazil												
Krauss et al. (1995)	Amazone basin; rural	< 95	ABSI	No isomer-specific information								0.02–0.4
	Rio de Janeiro; industrial region	< 95		No isomer-specific information								3–654
	Rio de Janeiro; recreation areas	< 95		No isomer-specific information								0.03–1.8
	Cubatao; heavy industry	< 95		No isomer-specific information								11–341

Table 3 (contd)

Reference	Origin; sample description (and no.)	Coll. period	Anal. meth.	PCDD concentration (ng/kg; ppt)							I-TEQ PCDD/PCDF
				TCDD 2378	PeCDD 12378	HxCDD 123478	123678	123789	HpCDD 1234678	OCDD	
Canada											
McLaughlin et al. (1989)	Hamilton, Ontario; vicinity incinerator	14	7/83	ACSO	No further isomer-specific information					50–3 500	
Pearson et al. (1990)	Hamilton; vicinity incinerator	11	83		No further isomer-specific information					663 [ND–3 500]	
	Scarborough; vicinity incinerator	12	87		No further isomer-specific information					570 [ND–1 500]	
	Ontario; rural soils	1	83		No further isomer-specific information					810	
	Rural soils	26	87		No further isomer-specific information					30 [ND–100]	
	Rural soils	15	88		No further isomer-specific information					3 [ND–45]	
	Rural soils	1	88		No further isomer-specific information					ND	
	Urban soils	2	83		No further isomer-specific information					2 070 [940–3 200]	
	Urban soils	11	87		No further isomer-specific information					1 461 [ND–11 000]	
	Urban soils	15	88		No further isomer-specific information					3 402 [ND–1 600]	
	Urban soils	1	88		No further isomer-specific information					220	
China											
Wu et al. (1995)	Ya-Er lake area; 1	1	91–94	ACSI	ND	ND	ND	ND	ND	0.49	14.6	0.11
	Ya-Er lake area; 2	1	91–94	ACSI	ND	ND	ND	ND	ND	6.78	24.4	0.15
Czech Republic											
Zemek & Kocan (1991)	TCP prod. plant[a];			ACSI								
	East	5	86		10–400	No further isomer-specific information						
	North, interm.[a]	10	86		20–10 800	No further isomer-specific information						
	North, extern.[b]	13	86		20–2 200	No further isomer-specific information						
	West[a]	18	86		ND–11 800	No further isomer-specific information						
	South[a]	14	86		ND–1 300	No further isomer-specific information						
	Drum dump[a]	33	86		ND–29 800	No further isomer-specific information						
Finland											
Sandell & Tuominen (1993)	0–20 cm; Sawmill soil	14	NG	ABSI	No isomer-specific information						1 700–85 000[c]
	20–50 cm; Sawmill soil	14	NG		No isomer-specific information						100–9 800[c]

Table 3 (contd)

Reference	Origin; sample description (and no.)	Coll. period	Anal. meth.	PCDD concentration (ng/kg; ppt) TCDD 2378	PeCDD 12378	HxCDD 123478	123678	123789	HpCDD 1234678	OCDD	I-TEQ PCDD/PCDF
Finland (contd)											
Assmuth & Vartiainen (1995)	Sawmill soil; depth 0–50 cm (10)	NG	ABSI	84–240	ND	ND	130–8 700	ND–290	110–20 000	370–21 000	
Germany											
Rotard et al. (1987)	Soil waste; oil contamination	NG	N	ND	–	ND	ND	ND	300–1 200	ND	
Schlesing (1989)	Herbicide plant;		ANSI								
	Typical										
	Depth, 1 m (1)	<89		6300	PnCDD-HpCDD, only totals reported					2 129 000	
	Depth, 2 m (1)	<89		5300	PnCDD-HpCDD, only totals reported					36 800	
	Depth, 3 m (1)	<89		12 700	PnCDD-HpCDD, only totals reported					29 000	
	Depth, 4 m (1)	<89		400	PnCDD-HpCDD, only totals reported					10 300	
	Contaminated										
	Depth, 1 m (1)	<89		166 000	PnCDD-HpCDD, only totals reported					349 000	
	Depth, 2 m (1)	<89		698 000	PnCDD-HpCDD, only totals reported					202 000	
	Depth, 3 m (1)	<89		54 900	PnCDD-HpCDD, only totals reported					164 000	
	Depth, 4 m (1)	<89		200	PnCDD-HpCDD, only totals reported					700	
	Depth, 5 m (1)	<89		400	PnCDD-HpCDD, only totals reported					2 500	
	Depth, 6 m (1)	<89		500	PnCDD-HpCDD, only totals reported					3 900	
	Depth, 7 m (1)	<89		98 200	PnCDD-HpCDD, only totals reported					931 000	
	Depth, 8 m (1)	<89		300	PnCDD-HpCDD, only totals reported					1 500	
	Depth, 9 m (1)	<89		400	PnCDD-HpCDD, only totals reported					300	
Hagenmaier et al. (1992)	Rastatt; Cu smelter		ABSI								
	Site 1 (1)	87		2	4	3	8	8	62	400	30
	(1)	89		1	2	5	9	5	49	280	26
	Site 2 (1)	87		90	470	590	1 040	580	6 760	8 000	5 900
	(1)	89		90	540	550	950	540	6 770	6 600	5 110
	Site 3 (1)	87		10	60	60	100	60	760	1 600	600
	(1)	89		10	60	50	100	80	700	1 000	600
	Site 4 (1)	87		10	40	40	80	80	650	1 300	400
	(1)	89		10	50	70	110	70	820	1 100	510
She & Hagenmaier (1996)	Rastatt; all samples[a] (77)	87	ABSI	7 [1–130]	27 [2–1970]	35 [1–2080]	61 [4–3 680]	48 [4–3 430]	420 [31–22 400]	800 [40–20 800]	300 [12–14 500]

Table 3 (contd)

Reference	Origin; sample description (and no.)		Coll. period	Anal. meth.	PCDD concentration (ng/kg; ppt)							I-TEQ PCDD/PCDF
					TCDD 2378	PeCDD 13378	HxCDD 123478	123678	123789	HpCDD 1234678	OCDD	
Germany (contd)												
Deister & Pommer (1991)	Schwabach			N								
	750 m from MSWI	5	<91									0.2–4.3*
	750 m from MSWI	2	<91									3.7–14.5*
	550 m from MSWI	5	<91									0.2–4.1*
	350 m from MSWI	5	<91									0.6–4.4*
	350 m from MSWI	1	<91									20.7*
Unger & Prinz (1991)	B5 road, 43 000*; 0.1 m from road		<91	NNSN	No isomer-specific information							23.0
	B3 road, 15 000*; 1.0 m from road		<91		No isomer-specific information							2.6
	B5 road, 43 000*; 1.0 m from road		<91		No isomer-specific information							9.7
	B31 road, 50 000*, 1.0 m from road		<91		No isomer-specific information							44.8
	B5 road, 43 000*; 2.5 m from road		<91		No isomer-specific information							20.0
	B5 road, 43 000*; 5.0 m from road		<91		No isomer-specific information							2.6
	B3 road, 15 000*, 10 m from road		<91		No isomer-specific information							0.6
	B5 road, 43 000*; 10 m from road		<91		No isomer-specific information							1.0
	B31 road, 50 000T, 10 m from road		<91		No isomer-specific information							2.5
	B5 road, 43 000*; 25 m from road		<91		No isomer-specific information							0.4
	B5 road, 43 000*; 50 m from road		<91		No isomer-specific information							0.4
Theisen et al. (1993)	Kieselrot, Cu slag		92	ABSI	1800	8000	3800	4200	3900	78 300	530 000	64 500
	Near Kieselrot, sports ground; garden soil		92		4	26	8	14	11	439	3 450	154
	Corresponding standard soil		92		<0.5	1.4	0.7	2	2	26.8	170	3.8

Table 3 (contd)

Reference	Origin; sample description (and no.)		Coll. period	Anal. meth.	PCDD concentration (ng/kg; ppt)							I-TEQ PCDD/PCDF
					TCDD 2378	PeCDD 12378	HxCDD 123478	123678	123789	HpCDD 1234678	OCDD	
Germany (contd)												
McLachlan &	Bavaria;			ACSI								
Reissinger (1990)	Field 1; no sludge	1	89		0.04	0.14	0.12	0.28	0.21	3.3	9.4	0.84*
	Field 2: sludge for 10 y	1	89		0.05	0.47	0.76	5.0	2.7	44	100	3.7*
	Field 3: sludge for 30 y	1	89		0.16	1.1	2.1	17.0	8.2	130	250	9.4*
	Meadow; Sludge for 30 y	1	89		0.24	1.9	3.9	25	13	200	360	15*
	Sewage sludge	1	89		1.1	4.9	4.9	31	20	910	4 400	42*
Rotard et al. (1994)	Ploughland	14	<94	ACSI	ND	ND	1.2 [0.8–1.4]	1.5 [1.1–1.8]	2.0 [1.6–2.4]	9.1 [4.1–21.9]	32 [7.4–88]	1.7 [0.3–3.7]
	Grassland	7	<94		ND	0.4 [0.4–0.4]	ND [ND]	1.9 [1.4–2.9]	1.7 [1.7–1.7]	14.6 [7.1–35]	44 [26–87]	2.3 [0.4–4.8]
	Deciduous forest	9	<94		1.4 [0.5–3.0]	8.3 [1.1–29]	6.5 [1.5–20.9]	12.4 [3.1–49]	19.1 [3.6–82]	121 [23–399]	283 [60–759]	38 [5.9–102]
	Coniferous forest	11	<94		1.3 [ND–4.0]	5.1 [ND–8.9]	5.8 [2.1–14]	11.1 [3.7–29]	16.2 [5.3–54]	109 [36–272]	320 [100–692]	37 [11.1–112]
Kujawa et al. (1995)	Brandenburg; Rural	49	<94	ACSN	No isomer-specific information							1–54
Italy												
di Domenico et al. (1993b)	Sea level	10	91	ACSI	0.025+	0.045	0.068	0.11	0.23	2.2	15	
	Alt. 800–1300 m	11	91		0.036+	0.084	0.074	0.18	0.32	3.6	29	
	Caves	6	91		0.025+	0.030+	0.038+	0.038+	0.038+	0.11	2.5	
Japan												
Nakamura et al. (1994)	Agricultural field	1	NG	ABSI	No isomer-specific information							271
	Agricultural field	1	NG		No isomer-specific information							49.6
	Urban field	1	NG		No isomer-specific information							42.4

Table 3 (contd)

Reference	Origin; sample description (and no.)	No.	Coll. period	Anal. meth.	TCDD 2378	PeCDD 12378	HxCDD 123478	123678	123789	HpCDD 1234678	OCDD	I-TEQ PCDD/PCDF
								PCDD concentration (ng/kg; ppt)				
Jordan												
Alawi et al. (1996a)	Landfill Amman			ACSI								
	Sample 1	1	95		<10	343	536	733	567	3 960	3250	1 470*
	Sample 2	1	95		<10	87	85	132	98	1390	3 510	323*
	Sample 3	1	95		<10	37	48	86	56	453	474	122*
	Sample 4	1	95		<10	36	31	50	34	210	202	192*
	Sample 5	1	95		<10	30	16	35	22	428	544	111*
	Sample 6	1	95		<10	<10	<10	<10	<10	66	154	8.2*
The Netherlands												
van Wijnen et al. (1992)	Scrap car dealer	4	6/88	ACSI	ND	ND–110	ND–12	30–80	24–88	290–820	790–3 600	60–160
	Cable burning	3	6/88		ND–1100	67–2 000	0–2 100	91–6 800	130–3 400	550–25000	860–17 000	380–16 000
	Scrap metal dealer, cable burning	1	6/88		170	590	72	460	280	21000	89 000	1600
		2	6/88		ND	ND	ND	ND	ND	950–14 000	4 600–5 000	230–800
	Scrap car and open air cable burning	4	6/88		130–840	350–2 200	ND–1 200	360–3400	320–2 800	900–14 000	1 100–10 000	1 200–9 900
		3	6/88		2100–3400	6 800–8 800	8 100–14 000	30 000–33 000	20 000–28 000	150 000–200 000	140 000–370 000	72 000–98 000
		3	6/88		190–240	100–930	610–1 900	1 900–4 800	1 300–3 400	13 000–37 000	8 500–730 000	4 100–12 000
Russian Federation												
Pervunina et al. (1992)	Bashkiriya; Chlorophenol, 2,4-D production site	3	NG	ACSI	900–40 000	No further isomer-specific information						
	Moscow region; TCP production site	2	NG		1 000–4 800	No further isomer-specific information						
	Samara region; PCP production site	1	NG		18 700	No further isomer-specific information						
Fedorov (1993)	Chapaevsk			N								
	Soil, near sect. 23	1	10/90		18 700	Only total reported					–	
	Street dust	1	6/91		0.2	Only total reported				660	2 000	
	Farming area	1	6/91		–	Only total reported				34	120	
	Farming area	1	7/92		–	Only total reported					9 600	
	Potato field	1	7/92		68	Only total reported					13 300	

Table 3 (contd)

Reference	Origin; sample description (and no.)	No.	Coll. period	Anal. meth.	PCDD concentration (ng/kg; ppt)							I-TEQ PCDD/PCDF
					TCDD 2378	PeCDD 12378	HxCDD 123478	123678	123789	HpCDD 1234678	OCDD	
Russian Federation (contd)												
Fedorov (1993) (contd)	Chapaevsk; rest zone	1	7/92		56	Only total reported				76	256	
	Incinerator Ufa											
	Near sect. N 15		10/90		8 000	1 230			1 900	56 000	18 100	
	Near sect. N 11		10/90		40 000	9 000			4 300	10 200	29 000	
Fedorov et al. (1993)	Chapaevsk; CFP on site	3	92–93	ACNN	20–3 000						30 000–134 000	100–46 200
	1.5 km from CFP	2	92–93		<1–7.5	Only total reported					3 900–64 000	50–298
	2 km from CFP	1	92–93		1.5	Only total reported					13 000	40
	3 km from CFP	1	92–93		<1	Only total reported					4 800	30
	6 km from CFP	1	92–93		<1	Only total reported					4 310	14
	7 km from CFP	1	92–93		<1	Only total reported					960	10
	8 km from CFP	1	92–93		<1	Only total reported					200	4
	12 km from CFP	1	92–93		<1	Only total reported					<5	<4
Spain												
Jiménez et al. (1996a)	Madrid;			ABSO								
	SW, 400 m fr. CWI	1	93		0.98	0.23	–	0.23	–	1.60	6.52	2.28
	SE, 1200 m fr. CWI	1	93		1.51	0.53	0.42	1.18	1.53	26.24	136.7	4.11
	NE, 600 m fr. CWI	1	93		ND	0.31	0.15	0.36	ND	4.28	20.4	1.85
	NW, 1200 m fr. CWI	1	93		–	0.36	–	–	–	1.73	6.84	1.36
	W, 2000 m fr. CWI	1	93		0.89	ND	ND	ND	ND	2.07	8.76	1.99
	SW, 2000 m fr. CWI	1	93		2.62	1.04	1.27	2.92	4.05	34.6	171.3	11.4
	N, 2000 m fr. CWI	1	93		ND	0.14	0.13	0.21	0.29	1.75	9.42	0.69
	S, 1200 m fr. CWI	1	93		–	–	0.15	0.30	0.61	1.74	7.43	2.03
	NE, 2600 m fr. CWI	1	93		0.13	0.24	0.21	0.32	0.39	2.93	15.7	1.23
	NE, 2600 m fr. CWI	1	93		1.03	0.37	0.27	0.43	0.57	3.64	24.9	2.59
	NE, 2600 m fr. CWI	1	93		0.10	0.30	0.18	0.40	0.52	3.66	21.9	1.83
	NE, 3000 m fr. CWI	1	93		ND	0.26	0.15	0.32	0.46	3.75	17.5	1.52
	NE, 3000 m fr. CWI	1	93		0.13	0.20	0.08	0.20	0.25	2.54	23.01	0.82
	NE, 3000 m fr. CWI	1	93		ND	0.16	0.10	0.21	0.25	1.58	7.01	0.82
	Control; NW, 4500 m fr. CWI	1	93		ND	ND	0.13	0.32	0.48	1.36	5.93	0.71

Table 3 (contd)

Reference	Origin; sample description (and no.)		Coll. period	Anal. meth.	PCDD concentration (ng/kg; ppt)							I-TEQ PCDD/PCDF
					TCDD 2378	PeCDD 12378	HxCDD 123478	123678	123789	HpCDD 1234678	OCDD	
Spain (contd)												
Jiménez et al. (1996a) (contd)	Madrid, control; NE, 4500 m fr. CWI	1	93	ABSO	0.07	0.16	0.06	0.16	0.32	1.52	8.85	0.69
Schuhmacher et al. (1996)	Tarragona;			ABSO								
	250 m fr. MSWI	6	< 96		ND	0.10	0.05	0.09	0.17	2.12	234.1	0.48
	500 m fr. MSWI	6	< 96		0.03	0.06	0.12	0.22	0.15	3.39	23.1	0.36
	750 m fr. MSWI	6	< 96		0.01	0.11	0.18	0.26	0.35	6.67	54.8	0.84
	1000 m fr. MSWI	6	< 96		0.02	0.09	0.08	0.14	0.21	1.72	7.62	0.53
	NE fr. MSWI	8	< 96		0.03	0.06	0.07	0.08	0.11	0.69	2.27	0.23
	SE fr. MSWI	8	< 96		0.04	0.08	0.23	0.45	0.23	8.11	60.0	0.63
	SE fr. MSWI	8	< 96		–	0.05	0.07	0.13	0.12	1.37	7.06	0.23
Sweden												
Rappe et al. (1991b)	Plant B; soil I	1	90	ABSI	< 10	< 11	< 2.8	< 13	< 2.4	33	160	11 000[a]
	Plant B; soil II	1	90		< 7	< 11	< 3.3	< 6.9	< 2.2	69	400	870[a]
	Outside plant B	1	90		< 0.1	< 0.1	0.2	0.3	0.3	4.1	25	5.3[a]
	Grassfield; soil III											
	Plant B; soil IV	1	90		< 0.1	< 0.1	< 0.2	3.6	2	81	820	440[a]
	Plant B; soil V	1	90		< 0.4	< 0.4	< 0.8	< 0.7	< 0.8	1.5	30	96[a]
	Plant B; Cl$_2$ prod.; soil VI	1	90		< 0.5	< 0.5	< 1.2	21	9.9	6.8	49	1 400[a]
Taiwan												
Huang et al. (1992)	Electric wire	1	89	ABSI	17	64	25	81	20	607	37	
	incinerator site	1	89		2	249	242	289	242	2162	5	
	Mainly magnetic card	1	89		ND	ND	1	–	–	8	1	
	incinerator site	1	89		ND	ND	ND	ND	ND	ND	ND	
		1	89		8	4	–	2	2	9	–	
					ND	ND	ND	ND	ND	1	–	
Soong & Ling (1996)	PCP production plant	1	< 96	ACSO	19	69	192	794	375	39530	433 900	2 150
	site	1	< 96		2646	28850	50 770	1 337 000	130 600	23 670 000	206 900 000	1 357 000

Columns under HpCDD: 1234678; HxCDD sub-columns: 123478, 123678, 123789.

Table 3 (contd)

Reference	Origin; sample description (and no.)	Coll. period	Anal. meth.	PCDD concentration (ng/kg; ppt) TCDD 2378	PeCDD 12378	HxCDD 123478	123678	123789	HpCDD 1234678	OCDD	I-TEQ PCDD/PCDF
United Kingdom											
Kjeller et al. (1991)	Rothamsted (semi-rural); 1	1846	ABSI	0.048	0.13	0.18	0.31	0.28	2.8	13	13
	Archived samples (0–23 cm depth) 1	1856		0.033	0.09	0.13	0.12	0.14	1.2	7.8	
	1	1893		0.029	0.09	0.12	0.1	0.13	1.5	11	
	1	1914		0.040	0.11	0.16	0.23	0.18	2.0	11	
	1	1944		0.043	0.18	0.21	0.20	0.17	1.8	12	
	1	1956		0.049	0.18	0.26	0.46	0.34	3.5	13	
	1	1966		0.060	0.22	0.29	0.52	0.51	5.3	32	
	1	1980		0.079	0.20	0.30	0.67	0.41	4.6	20	
	1	1986		0.058	0.27	0.31	0.57	0.48	6.3	25	
Creaser et al. (1989)	50 km grid UK; All samples 77	< 89	ABSI	< 0.5 [< 0.5–6.4]	< 0.5 [< 0.5–7.8]	Only totals reported				277 [29–1365]	
	Reduced data-set 65	< 89		< 0.5 [0.5–2.11]	< 0.5 [0.5–2.4]	Only totals reported				191 [29–832]	
Creaser et al. (1990)	Urban soils (5 cities) 19	< 90	ABSI	0.7 [< 0.5–4.2]	2.4 [< 0.5–11]	Only totals reported				9980 [176–99 000]	
Stenhouse & Badsha (1990)	Different semi-urban sites 12	90	ABSO	3 [1–7]	< 1 [< 1–1]		4 [2–8]		33 [10–61]	58 [20–150]	8 [3–20]
Foxall & Lovett (1994)	South Wales; close to incinerator plant 42	91/93	N								66 [2.5–1745]
United States											
Kimbrough et al. (1977)	E. Missouri; Horse arena A	8/71	N	31.8–33×10^4	No further isomer-specific information						
	Arena A (excavated)	8/74		None	No further isomer-specific information						
	Arena C	8/74		0.22–0.85×10^4	No further isomer-specific information						
	Farmroad soil	9/74		0.61×10^4	No further isomer-specific information						

Table 3 (contd)

Reference	Origin; sample description (and no.)		Coll. period	Anal. meth.	PCDD concentration (ng/kg; ppt)							I-TEQ PCDD/PCDF
					TCDD 2378	PeCDD 12378	HxCDD 123478	123678	123789	HpCDD 1234678	OCDD	
United States (contd)												
Viswanathan et al. (1985)	E. Missouri; Denney's farm	27	NG	ACSO	46×10⁶– 9.6×10⁹		No further isomer-specific information					
	Other sites	22	NG		2 200– 1 500 000		No further isomer-specific information					
Nestrick et al. (1986)	Dow, Midland; Chlorophenol prod. area, top soil		83	ACSI	41–5 200		No further isomer-specific information					
	Waste incinerator area, top soil	10	83		18–4 300		No further isomer-specific information					
	Background, top soil	11	83		6.5–590		No further isomer-specific information					
	Various; Industrial areas of US cities, top soil	20	83		< 0.2–9.4		No further isomer-specific information					
Reed et al. (1990)	Elk River, MI			ABSI								
	Site 1 untilled*	1	9/88		ND	ND	ND	14	9.9	300	2300	
	Site 1 tilled*	1	9/88		ND	ND	ND	ND	ND	37	340	
	Site 2 untilled*	1	9/88		ND	ND	ND	ND	ND	78	680	
	Site 2 tilled*	1	9/88		ND	ND	ND	ND	8.7	360	3 300	
Rappe et al. (1995)	S. Mississippi; rural	36	94	ABSI	No further isomer-specific information						Range: 11–15 000	3.14 [0.08–22.6]
Lorber et al. (1996b)	Columbus, OH; MSWI, on site	4	95	ABSI	29	180	143	138	202	765	1495	
	MSWI, downwind off site	4	95		4	18	16	26	28	459	3893	
	City of Columbus; urban	14	95		2	3	3	6	6	112	892	
	Ohio; Rural	3	95		0.4	0.1	0.4	0.8	1.2	18	161	

Table 3 (contd)

Reference	Origin; sample description (and no.)		Coll. period	Anal. meth.	PCDD concentration (ng/kg; ppt)								
					TCDD 2378	PeCDD 12378	HxCDD 123478	123678	123789	HpCDD 1234678	OCDD	I-TEQ PCDD/PCDF	

Viet Nam

Matsuda et al. (1994)	Hanoi; background	5	89–91	ACSI	ND						66.3–578	
	Hue, Phu Loc; sprayed area	6	89–91		4.37–16.8	No further isomer-specific information					72.8–1 318	
	Ho Chi Minh; sprayed area	9	89–91		2.98–59.2	No further isomer-specific information					317–1 865	
	Tay Ninh; sprayed area	54	89–91		1.2–38.5	No further isomer-specific information					17–16 000	
	Song Be; sprayed area	11	89–91		6.0	No further isomer-specific information					11–880	
	Tam Nong; sprayed area	4	89–91		–	No further isomer-specific information					69	
	Dog Bin Kieu; sprayed area	6	89–91		–	No further isomer-specific information					180–380	
	Ca Mau; sprayed area	16	89–91		–	No further isomer-specific information					210–900	

Analytical methods: A, high-resolution gas chromatography; B, high-resolution mass spectrometry; C, low-resolution mass spectrometry; I, isomer-specific; O, others; N, no information; S, sophisticated clean-up; R, reduced clean-up; W, WHO-accepted laboratory

ND, not detected, detection limit in parentheses; [ ], range; +, contains 50% of detection limit

Data presented are means. Figures in parentheses are ranges. Levels of congeners not detected at known detection limits (for examples, 0.02 pg/m³) are presented as < 0.02

S, soluble; PB, particle bound; MWTP, municipal water treatment plant; CFP, chemical fertilizer plant; CWI, clinical waste incinerator; MSWI, municipal solid-waste incinerator; NG, not given

*German TEQ
*Sample depth, 0–20 cm
*Nordic TEQ
*Median values
*Cars per day
*Sample depth: 0–30 cm
*Sample depth, 0–2.5 cm

Table 4. PCDD/PCDFF content in various materials from different areas of Brazil

Area	Material	ng I-TEQ/kg
Amazon basin		
Eucalipto (eucalyptus trees)	Leaves ($n = 5$)	0.19
	< 2 mm ($n = 3$)[a]	0.04
	Soil ($n = 2$)	0.4
Capoeira (wood cut)	Leaves ($n = 5$)	0.07
	< 2 mm ($n = 3$)	0.08
	Soil ($n = 3$)	0.05
Mata natural 1 (natural forest)	Leaves ($n = 5$)	0.03
	< 2 mm ($n = 3$)	0.1
	Soil ($n = 2$)	0.05
Mata natural 2 (natural forest)	Leaves ($n = 5$)	0.02
	< 2 mm ($n = 3$)	0.02
	Soil ($n = 2$)	0.03
Mata degradada (new-grown forest)	Leaves ($n = 5$)	0.03
	< 2 mm ($n = 3$)	0.05
	Soil ($n = 2$)	0.1
Rio de Janeiro – industrial regions		
Niterói, hospital waste incineration	Soil (from plant)	23
	Soil (street nearby)	73
	Soil (reference)	3
São Gonçalo, metal industry	Soil (nearby)	35
	Soil (outer wall)	15
Santa Cruz, iron industry	Sludge	21
	Soil	27
	Leaves	77
	Soil beyond leaves	654
Rio de Janeiro – recreation areas		
Itaipuaçu	Leaves	2.6
	1. Soil layer	0.6
	2. Soil layer	1.8
Serra de Mauá	Leaves	0.6
	Soil	0.4
Saquarema	Leaves	0.4
	Soil (sand)	0.03
Cubatão, São Paulo – industrial region		
Ultrafertil (fertilizer production)	Leaves	10
	Soil	11
Eletropaulo (chlorochemistry plant)	Leaves	12
	Soil	54
Carbocloro (chlorochemistry plant)	Leaves	49
	Soil	341

From Krauss *et al.* (1995)
[a] Fraction < 2 mm (detritus plus soil particles)

Table 5. Concentrations of PCDDs/PCDFs in soil samples from former East and West Germany (ng I-TEQ/kg)

Soil type	East	West
For defined emitters — traffic, incinerators, landfills	2–14	1–160
Diffuse sources — green land, parks, playgrounds	1–9	0.8–1594
Background — forest soils, forest litter, green land	1–54	0.01–140

From Kujawa *et al.* (1995)

Table 6. 2,3,7,8-TCDD soil levels (in ng/kg) in the City of Midland, MI

	Range
Chlorophenol production site	
Locally elevated level area 1	52–52 000
Locally elevated level area 2	1000–34 000
Other sites	41–1 100
Chemical plant	
Waste incinerator site	18–4 300
Background area	ND–590
City of Midland	
Close to chemical plant	22–450
Further from chemical plant	0.6–9.2

From Nestrick *et al.* (1986)
ND, not detected

Table 7. 2,3,7,8-TCDD soil levels in industrialized areas of US cities (ng/kg)

Lansing, MI ($n = 2$)	ND (0.8)–3	Pittsburgh, PA	2.6
Gaylord, MI	ND (0.2)	Marcus Hook, PA	0.4
Detroit, MI ($n = 2$)	2.1–3.6	Philadelphia, PA	0.9
Chicago, IL ($n = 2$)	4.2–9.4	Clifton Heights, PA	ND (0.4)
Middletown, OH ($n = 2$)	ND (0.3)	Brooklyn, NY	2.6
Barberton, OH	5.6	South Charleston, WV	ND (0.4)
Akron, OH	6.3	Arlington, VA	ND (0.4)
Nashville, TN	0.8	Newport News, VA	0.4

From Nestrick *et al.* (1986)
ND, not detected; detection limits in parentheses

Table 8. PCDD/PCDF concentrations in Mississippi (USA) soil samples (ng/kg dry matter)

County	OCDD	I-TEQ	County	OCDD	I-TEQ	County	OCDD	I-TEQ
George	36	0.16	Jones	4 000	20.30	Perry	140	0.52
Jackson	98	0.42	Jones	590	1.31	Perry	18	0.17
Jackson	67	0.38	Jones	13 000	14.30	Wayne	39	0.17
Jackson	34	0.31	Jones	1 200	2.81	Wayne	210	7.15
Jackson	29	0.37	Lamar	110	0.64	Wayne	2 400	3.41
Jackson	20	0.27	Lamar	174	0.55	Wayne	11	0.08
Forrest	4 300	10.90	Lamar	500	1.42	Wayne	880	1.66
Forrest	260	1.12	Lamar	140	0.36	Greene	51	0.20
Forrest	200	1.05	Lamar	37	0.15	Greene	410	1.03
Forrest	450	0.93	Perry	7 100	8.09	Greene	3 500	5.26
Forrest	110	0.25	Perry	1 200	2.75	Greene	36	0.18
Jones	260	0.90	Perry	15 000	22.60	Greene	75	0.37

I-TEQ: Mean 3.14 Min 0.08
Median 0.77 Max 22.60

From Fiedler *et al.* (1995); Rappe *et al.* (1995)

Table 9. Concentrations of PCDDs in background cow's milk

Reference	Origin; sample description (and no.)	Coll. period	PCDD concentration (ng/kg fat)								I-TEQ PCDD/PCDF
			TCDD 2378	PeCDD 12378	HxCDD 123478	123678	123789	HpCDD 1234678	OCDD		
Canada											
Ryan et al. (1990)	6 cities (2% fat)	6	1985–88	1.9	NR	NR	NR	NR	NR	NR	10.0
France											
Fraisse et al. (1996)	57	1994	NR	NR	NR	NR	NR	NR	NR	1.74
Germany											
Beck et al. (1987)	Berlin	8	1987~	0.2	0.7	0.3	1.1	0.4	<2	<10	1.79
Fürst et al. (1990)	NR West.	10	1989~	0.4	1.2	0.8	4.0	0.8	6.2	11	3.83
Fürst et al. (1992a)	NR West.	120	1990	NR	NR	NR	NR	NR	NR	NR	1.38
Netherlands											
Liem et al. (1991b)	NR	1991	0.25	0.52	0.25	0.73	0.28	1.39	3.64	1.50
Russian Federation											
Khamitov et al. (1996)	Bashkortostan	15	1995	0.16	NR	NR	NR	NR	NR	NR	0.26
Spain											
Ramos et al. (1996)	Asturias	15	1995	ND	0.36	0.24	8.93	15.8[a]	7.21	136	3.94
Sweden											
Rappe et al. (1990b)	Malmö	1	1989	<0.4	0.49	0.3	1.5	<0.3	3.1	3.5	1.77
	Stockholm	1	1989	<0.1	<0.2	<0.2	0.3	<0.2	1.0	2	0.48
	Umeå	1	1989	<0.1	0.2	<0.2	0.3	<0.2	1.0	1.4	0.47
	Vaxjo	1	1989	<0.3	<0.2	<0.2	1.0	<0.2	3.0	4.9	1.08
	Gothenburg	1	1989	<0.2	<0.2	<0.2	1.0	0.2	1.8	1.6	0.82

Table 9 (contd)

Reference	Origin; sample description (and no.)		Coll. period	PCDD concentration (ng/kg fat)								I-TEQ
				TCDD 2378	PeCDD 12378	HxCDD 123478	123678	123789	HpCDD 1234678	OCDD		PCDD/PCDF
Switzerland												
Rappe et al. (1987b)	Bern (retail)	1	1986	<0.3	<1.0	<1.7	<1.7	<1.7	<1.6	<4.0		2.68
	Bowil (pool)	1	1986	<0.3	<1.4	<1.4	<1.4	<1.4	<1.5	<2.8		2.48
	Bowil	1	1986	<0.3	<1.83	<2.29	<2.29	<2.29	<1.51	<5.95		2.96
Schmid & Schlatter (1992)	Retail	9	1990–91	0.2	0.46	0.21	0.49	0.27	0.98	2.5		1.31
United Kingdom												
Harrison et al. (1996)	Derbyshire (4% fat assumed)	47	1991–93	1.25	2.25	5		1.75	3.25	11.75		3.64
Startin et al. (1990)	Rural farms (4% fat assumed)	7	1989	0.225	0.4		0.8	0.25	1.15	5.75		1.11
Wright & Startin (1995)	TDS	pool	1982	0.84	1.4	2.2	4.4	1.2	12	32		4.53
Wright & Startin (1995)	TDS	pool	1992	<0.40	0.80	0.50	0.95	0.56	6.6	51		2.02
USA												
Eitzer (1995)	Connecticut (4% fat assumed)	17	1991	0.425	0.16	0.775	0.8	0.375	2.35	19.25		0.99

NR, not reported; ND, not detected and detection limit not reported; TDS, total diet study; NR West., North Rhine Westphalia

[a] [Dubious concentration]

TEQ concentrations recalculated where possible assuming congeners that were not detected were present at the full value of the detection limit

Table 10. Summary of concentrations (ng/kg fat) of PCDDs in background cow's milk, reported in Table A1.10

| | TCDD | PeCDD | HxCDD | | | HpCDD | OCDD | I-TEQ |
	2378	12378	123478	123678	123789	1234678		PCDD/PCDF
Number of positives	10	13	10	16	11	15	15	23
Mean	0.58	0.72	0.57	2.0	0.58	3.4	19	2.3
Minimum	0.16	0.16	0.13	0.30	0.20	0.20	1.4	0.26
5th %tile	0.18	0.18	0.17	0.30	0.23	0.68	1.5	0.47
25th %tile	0.74	0.80	0.71	2.1	0.68	4.7	16	2.8
Median	0.33	0.49	0.30	0.97	0.38	2.4	4.9	1.7
75th %tile	0.21	0.40	0.24	0.71	0.28	1.1	2.9	1.1
95th %tile	1.6	1.7	1.6	6.0	1.5	8.6	76	4.5
Maximum	1.9	2.3	2.2	8.9	1.8	12	140	10.0

Table 11. Concentrations of PCDDs in milk products

Sample description	Origin	Reference	Coll. period	No.	PCDD concentration (ng/kg fat)							I-TEQ PCDD/PCDF
					TCDD 2378	PeCDD 12378	HxCDD 123478	123678	123789	HpCDD 1234678	OCDD	
Butter	Egypt	Malisch & Saad (1996)	1994–96	33	1.06	2.1	0.53	0.8	0.31	1.14	8.36	7.68
Butter	Germany, NR West.	Fürst et al. (1992a)	1990	22	NR	NR	NR	NR	NR	NR	NR	1.11
Butter	Germany, Berlin, retail	Beck et al. (1989a)	1987~	1	0.08	0.41	0.15	0.95	0.26	0.34	3.4	0.79
Butter	Germany, NR West.	Fürst et al. (1990)	1989~	5	<0.5	<0.5	<0.5	0.7	<0.5	1.7	11.6	1.76
Butter	Netherlands	Liem et al. (1991b)	1990~91		0.24	0.67	0.36	0.83	0.31	0.91	0.98	1.78
Butter	Norway	Biseth et al. (1990)	1989~	3	<0.5	0.35	0.26	1.0	0.41	1.0	4.6	1.38
Butter	Russian Federation, Baikalsk	Schecter et al. (1990a)	1988–89	1	<1.0	<0.49	<0.49	0.6	<0.49	1.0	17	3.37
Cheese	Germany	Fürst et al. (1992b)	1990	4	NR	NR	NR	NR	NR	NR	NR	1.83
Cheese	Germany, NR West.	Fürst et al. (1990)	1989~	10	0.5	0.6	0.3	0.8	0.5	2.3	10.5	2.17
Cheese	Netherlands	Liem et al. (1991b)	1990~91		0.22	0.5	0.24	0.72	0.22	1.16	3.77	1.41
Cheese	Russian Federation, Moscow	Schecter et al. (1990a)	1988–89	1	<1.0	<0.67	0.4	1.6	0.4	8.0	22	2.13
Cheese/butter	Russian Federation, Novosibirsk	Schecter et al. (1990a)	1988–89	1	<1.0	<0.5	<0.5	0.8	<0.5	2.0	15	1.78
Cream	Germany	Fürst et al. (1992a)	1990	22	NR	NR	NR	NR	NR	NR	NR	1.37
Cream	Russian Federation, Irkutsk	Schecter et al. (1990a)	1988–89	1	<1.0	<0.47	<0.47	0.9	<0.47	3.0	21	6.26
Mixed (TDS)	Spain, Basque	Startin (1996)	1994	8	0.51	0.5	0.59	0.94	0.55	3.14	14	2.30
Mixed (TDS)	United Kingdom	Wright & Startin (1995); MAFF (1995)	1982	pool	0.56	1.4	2.2	4.9	1.4	13	25	3.42
Mixed (TDS)	United Kingdom	Wright & Startin (1995); MAFF (1995)	1992	pool	0.17	0.28	0.22	0.34	0.29	0.95	3.6	0.75

NR, not reported; NR West., North Rhine Westphalia; MAFF, Ministry of Agriculture, Fisheries and Food
I-TEQ concentrations recalculated where possible assuming congeners that were not detected were present at the full value of the detection limit

Table 12. Concentrations of PCDDs in meat and meat products

Sample description	Origin	Reference	Coll. period	No.	PCDD concentration (ng/kg fat)							I-TEQ PCDD/PCDF
					TCDD 2378	PeCDD 12378	HxCDD 123478	123678	123789	HpCDD 1234678	OCDD	
Mixed (TDS)	Spain, Basque region	Startin (1996)	1994	8	<0.5	0.33	<0.5	0.85	0.5	8.7	50	1.64
Mixed (TDS)	United Kingdom	Wright & Startin (1995)	1982	pool	<0.44	0.88	1.5	2.3	0.8	13	51	2.81
Mixed (TDS)	United Kingdom	Wright & Startin (1995)	1992	pool	<0.12	0.44	0.30	0.70	<0.15	2.0	6.6	0.95
Beef	Germany, Berlin, retail	Beck et al. (1989a)	1987~	1	0.6	0.8	0.6	1.9	0.6	18	25	2.59
Beef	Germany, NR West.	Fürst et al. (1990)	1989~	3	<0.5	1.7	1.9	3.2	2.0	3.9	5.4	3.73
Beef	Russian Fed., Bashkortostan	Khamitov et al. (1996)	1995	8	0.12	NR	NR	NR	NR	NR	NR	0.20
Beef	Russian Fed., Irkutsk	Schecter et al. (1990a)	1988–89	1	<1.0	<0.67	<0.67	0.6	<0.67	5.2	21	5.84
Beef fat	Russian Fed., Novosibirsk	Schecter et al. (1990a)	1988–89	1	<1.0	<0.5	<0.5	1.0	<0.5	3	10.0	2.05
Beef	USA	Ferrario et al. (1996)	1993	63	0.05	0.35	0.46	1.4	0.53	4.50	4.80	0.89
Beef (hamburger)	Canada	Ryan et al. (1990)	1985–88	6	0	0	0	6.3	0	21.3	35.6	1.29
Beef fat	Netherlands	Liem et al. (1991b)	1990–91	pool	0.21	0.57	0.3	1.32	0.31	1.95	2.86	1.77
Beef fat	Viet Nam, Hanoi	Schecter et al. (1989a)	1985–87	1	1.6	1.3	2.1	4.1	2.1	0	0	3.61
Canned (unspecified)	Germany, NR West.	Fürst et al. (1990)	1989~	2	<0.5	<0.5	1.0	3.2	1.2	13.2	53	2.10
Liver (cow)	Netherlands	Liem et al. (1991b)	1990–91	pool	0.16	1.1	2.82	3.56	1.59	39.2	144	5.72
Goat	Netherlands	Liem et al. (1991b)	1990–91	pool	0.8	1.98	1.27	6.4	0.64	12.8	26.8	4.20

Table 12 (contd)

Sample description	Origin	Reference	Coll. period	No.	PCDD concentration (ng/kg fat)							I-TEQ PCDD/PCDF
					TCDD 2378	PeCDD 12378	HxCDD 123478	123678	123789	HpCDD 1234678	OCDD	
Horse fat	Netherlands	Liem et al. (1991b)	1990–91	pool	1.98	5.16	7.36	20.75	2.7	92.2	171	13.8
Horse liver	Netherlands	Liem et al. (1991b)	1990–91	pool	2.03	15.9	24.2	39.3	12	941	1751	61.2
Liver (pooled)	Netherlands	Liem et al. (1991b)	1990–91	pool	1.25	5.39	6.49	14.8	4.0	227	1017	30.7
Mutton fat	Netherlands	Liem et al. (1991b)	1990–91	pool	0.32	0.86	0.44	1.41	0.28	2.44	4.73	1.81
Offal (TDS)	UK	Wright & Startin (1995); MAFF (1995)	1982	pool	0.32	1.3	4.9	7.4	1.9	360	4400	19.0
Offal (TDS)	UK	Wright & Startin (1995); MAFF (1995)	1992	pool	0.81	1.7	2.9	2.6	1.3	30	200	9.86
Liver (pig)	Netherlands	Liem et al. (1991b)	1990–91	pool	0.24	0.73	3.41	4.4	1.29	120	3431	15.3
Pork	Germany, Berlin, retail	Beck et al. (1989a)	1987~	1	0.03	0.12	0.21	0.29	0.06	2.1	19	0.28
Pork	Germany, NR West.	Fürst et al. (1990)	1989~	3	< 0.5	< 0.5	< 0.5	< 0.5	< 0.5	0.7	8.2	1.20
Pork	Netherlands	Liem et al. (1991b)	1990–91	pool	0.07	0.07	0.18	0.54	0.1	3.82	44.8	0.42
Pork	Russian Fed., Baikalsk	Schecter et al. (1990a)	1988–89	1	< 1	< 0.5	< 0.5	< 0.5	< 0.5	2.0	16	1.97
Pork	Russian Fed., Bashkortostan	Khamitov et al. (1996)	1995	6	0.14	NR	NR	NR	NR	NR	NR	0.34
Pork fat	Viet Nam, Ho Chi Minh City	Schecter et al. (1990a)	1988–89	1	< 1.0	0.5	0.6	1.7	0.4	7.5	30	2.34
Pork sticks	Viet Nam, Ho Chi Minh City	Schecter et al. (1990a)	1988–89	1	< 1	0.5	0.7	1.4	0.3	8.4	28	2.31

Table 12 (contd)

Sample description	Origin	Reference	Coll. period	No.	PCDD concentration (ng/kg fat)							I-TEQ PCDD/PCDF
					TCDD 2378	PeCDD 12378	HxCDD 123478	123678	123789	HpCDD 1234678	OCDD	
Pork fat	Viet Nam, Song Be	Schecter et al. (1989a)	1986	1	0.6	0.9	0.4	1.2	0.8	13.2	64	2.65
Products	Netherlands	Liem et al. (1991b)	1990–91	pool	0.09	0.13	0.19	0.41	0.06	2.93	32.9	0.67
Products (TDS)	UK	Wright & Startin (1995); MAFF (1995)	1982	pool	0.15	0.34	1.5	2.1	0.33	19	111	1.44
Products (TDS)	UK	Wright & Startin (1995); MAFF (1995)	1992	pool	<0.04	0.11	0.23	0.34	0.13	2.9	18	0.40
Sausage	Moscow	Schecter et al. (1990a)	1988–89	1	<1	<0.51	<0.51	<0.51	<0.51	1.0	10	1.73
Sheep	Germany, Berlin, retail	Beck et al. (1989a)	1987~	1	0.01	0.5	0.3	1.5	0.4	15	68	1.65
Sheep	Germany, NR West.	Fürst et al. (1990)	1989~	2	<0.5	<0.5	0.8	3.0	0.7	11.4	19.3	2.43
Veal	Germany, NR West.	Fürst et al. (1990)	1989~	4	<0.5	3.1	1.9	5.3	1.8	14.4	22.3	7.68

NR, not reported; NR West., North Rhine Westphalia; TDS, total diet survey; MAFF, Ministry of Agriculture, Fisheries and Food
I-TEQ, concentrations recalculated where possible assuming congeners that were not detected were present at the full value of the detection limit

Table 13. Summary of concentrations (ng/kg fat) of PCDDs for meat and meat products reported in Table 12

	TCDD	PeCDD	HxCDD			HpCDD	OCDD	I-TEQ PCDD/PCDF
	2378	12378	123478	123678	123789	1234678		
Number of positives	24	29	31	34	30	36	36	39
Mean	0.54	1.9	2.4	5.0	1.6	62	350	6.5
Minimum	0.01	0.07	0.18	0.29	0.06	0.70	2.9	0.20
5th %tile	0.03	0.11	0.20	0.39	0.08	1.7	4.8	0.33
25th %tile	0.14	0.44	0.42	1.3	0.35	3.0	18	1.4
Median	0.30	0.86	1.0	2.5	0.75	12	29	2.3
75th %tile	0.70	1.7	2.5	5.8	1.9	22	79	5.8
95th %tile	1.9	5.4	6.9	17	4.2	260	2 200	22
Maximum	2.0	16	24	39	12	941	4 400	61

Table 14. Concentrations of PCDDs in poultry

Sample description	Origin	Reference	Sample year	No.	Concentration ng/kg fat							
					TCDD 2378	PeCDD 12378	HxCDD 123478	123678	123789	HpCDD 1234678	OCDD	I-TEQ PCDD/PCDF
Chicken fat, PCP contamination	Canada	Ryan et al. (1985a)	1980	26	ND	ND	[a]	27	ND	52	90	3.31
Chicken	Germany, Berlin, retail	Beck et al. (1989a)		1	0.3	0.7	0.5	2.8	0.6	6	52	2.25
Chicken	Germany, North Rhine Westphalia,	Fürst et al. (1990)	1989~	2	<0.5	1	0.6	1.8	0.6	4.5	16.5	2.53
Chicken fat	Netherlands	Liem et al. (1991b)	1990–91		0.29	0.53	0.4	1.84	0.64	6.73	25.6	1.62
Chicken	Russian Federation, Bashkortostan	Khamitov et al. (1996)	1995	10	1.02	NR	NR	NR	NR	NR	NR	4.54
Chicken (TDS)	United Kingdom	Wright & Startin (1995)	1982	pool	0.76	1.3	5.1	12	1.5	65	150	5.41
Chicken (TDS)	United Kingdom	Wright & Startin (1995)	1992	pool	<0.51	0.36	0.37	0.79	0.61	<4.5	10	1.68
Chicken fat	Viet Nam, Hanoi	Schecter et al. (1989a)	1986	1	1.0	0.6	[a]	1.0	1.2	<4.5	<15	2.94
Chicken liver	Viet Nam, Ho Chi Minh City	Schecter et al. (1990a)	1988–89	1	<1.0	2.4	2.6	9.7	3.7	34	42	10.2
Chicken	Vietnam, Ho Chi Minh City	Schecter et al. (1990a)	1988–89	1	<1.0	1.0	0.5	4.0	0.7	14	24	2.80
Chicken fat	Vietnam, Song Be	Schecter et al. (1989a)	1986	1	4.1	10	6.9	27	5.4	71	75	21.8

NR, not reported; ND, not detected and detection limit not reported; TDS, total diet survey; I-TEQ concentrations recalculated where possible assuming congeners that were not detected were present at the full value of the detection limit
[a] Included with 1,2,3,6,7,8-HxCDD

Table 15. Concentrations of PCDDs in poultry eggs

Sample description	Origin	Reference	Coll. period	No.	PCDD concentration (ng/kg fat)								I-TEQ PCDD/PCDF
					TCDD 2378	PeCDD 12378	HxCDD 123478	123678	123789	HpCDD 1234678	OCDD		
Chicken	Germany, Berlin, retail	Beck et al. (1989a)	1987~	1	0.2	0.4	1.3	1.4	0.5	0.4	12		1.52
Chicken	Netherlands	Liem et al. (1991b)	1990–91		0.27	0.76	0.44	1.49	0.68	7.1	70.9		2.02
Chicken	Spain, Basque region, TDS	Startin (1996)	1994	8	0.23	0.28	0.29	2.0	0.51	14	64		1.26
Chicken (TDS)	UK	Wright & Startin (1995)	1982	pool	0.65	2.7	8.6	18	6.3	120	720		8.26
Chicken (TDS)	UK	Wright & Startin (1995)	1992	pool	0.43	0.51	0.54	0.96	0.65	6.2	38		1.80
Duck	UK, rural	Lovett et al. (1996)	1993–94	7									0.7

TDS, total diet survey

Table 16. Concentrations of PCDDs in fish

Species	Origin	Reference	Coll. period	No.	Concentration ng/kg fat							I-TEQ PCDD/PCDF
					TCDD 2378	PeCDD 12378	HxCDD 123478	123678	123789	HpCDD 1234678	OCDD	
Barbel (river)	Germany	Frommberger (1991)	1988	1	5.1	8.3	1.0	4.7	1.1	4.1	9.0	39.2
Brown trout (river)	Germany	Frommberger (1991)	1988	1	1.4	1.3	< 1.3	0.6	< 0.2	0.7	< 5	10.6
Catfish (farmed)	USA	Cooper et al. (1996)	1995	1	2.2	3.6	1.9	4.2	2.3	11	48	5.0
Catfish (farmed)	USA	Cooper et al. (1996)	1995	1	32	16	1.4	5.7	14	8.8	49	42.9
Cod	Norway	Biseth et al. (1990)	1989~	2	< 29.4	< 17.6	< 14.7	< 14.7	< 29.4	< 29.4	353	59.6
Cod (retail)	Germany, Berlin	Beck et al. (1989a)		1	23	1.3	0.01	17	5.2	10	83	42.7
Eel	Germany	Frommberger (1991)	1988	1	3.1	3.5	2.4	14	2.6	15	60	15.2
Eel	Germany	Frommberger (1991)	1988	1	3.3	3.4	< 2.0	10	2.3	19	52	16.2
Herring	Norway	Biseth et al. (1990)	1989~	6	< 3.60	< 1.08	< 0.72	< 0.72	< 2.16	< 2.16	17.3	17.6
Herring, retail	Germany, Berlin	Beck et al. (1989a)		1	4.7	12	1.2	5.8	1.0	3.6	19	33.7
Lean sea fish	Netherlands	Liem et al. (1991b)	1990–91		16.3	6.61	2.38	7.11	4.10	22.9	213	48.6
Mackerel	Norway	Biseth et al. (1990)	1989~	3	< 1.57	< 0.47	< 0.31	< 0.31	< 0.94	< 0.94	16.6	3.49
Mixed	Russian Federation, Bashkortostan	Khamitov et al. (1996)	1995	13	0.11	NA	NA	NA	NA	NA	NA	0.18
Mixed (TDS)	Spain, Basque Region	Startin (1996)	1994	8	2.2	2.0	1.5	2.9	1.6	23	98	7.24
Mixed (TDS)	UK	Wright & Startin (1995); MAFF (1995)	1982	pool	0.79	1.2	0.61	3.6	1.5	14	57	5.29
Mixed (TDS)	UK	Wright & Startin (1995); MAFF (1995)	1992	pool	< 0.25	0.90	0.59	1.0	0.74	2.7	16	2.72

APPENDIX 1

Table 16 (contd)

Species	Origin	Reference	Coll. period	No.	Concentration ng/kg fat							
					TCDD 2378	PeCDD 12378	HxCDD 123478	123678	123789	HpCDD 1234678	OCDD	I-TEQ PCDD/PCDF
Mixed, freshwater	Germany, North Rhine Westphalia	Fürst (1990)	1989~	18	NA	9.7	2.4	14.9	1.8	9.9	19.3	30.5
Mixed, salt-water	Germany, North Rhine Westphalia	Fürst (1990)	1989~	15	6.5 (n = 6)	7.5	1.0	7.3	2.8	8.8	10.5	35.3
Redfish, retail	Germany, Berlin	Beck et al. (1989a)	1987~	1	2.8	6.5	0.5	8.4	1.3	3	11	30.6
Salmon (farmed)	Norway	Biseth et al. (1990)	1989~	4	<19.0	<4.76	<3.81	<3.81	<9.52	16.7	129	53.0

NA, not analyzed; TDS, total diet survey; MAFF, Ministry of Agriculture, Fisheries and Food

Table 17. Summary of concentrations (ng/kg fat) of PCDDs in fish reported in Table 16

	TCDD	PeCDD	HxCDD			HpCDD	OCDD	I-TEQ PCDD/PCDF
	2378	12378	123478	123678	123789	1234678		
Number of positives	14	15	13	15	14	16	18	19
Mean	7.4	5.6	1.3	7.1	3.0	11	70	25
Minimum	0.11	0.90	0.01	0.60	0.74	0.70	9.0	0.2
5th %tile	0.55	1.1	0.30	0.88	0.91	2.2	10	3.4
25th %tile	2.2	1.6	0.61	3.9	1.4	4.0	17	9.1
Median	3.2	3.6	1.2	5.8	2.0	9.9	49	31
75th %tile	6.2	7.9	1.9	9.2	2.8	15	77	41
95th %tile	26	13	2.4	16	8.3	23	230	54
Maximum	32	16	2.4	17	14	23	350	60

Table 18. Concentrations of PCDDs in miscellaneous foods

Sample description	Origin	Reference	Coll. period	No.	PCDD concentration (ng/kg fat)							I-TEQ PCDD/PCDF
					TCDD 2378	PeCDD 12378	HxCDD 123478	123678	123789	HpCDD 1234678	OCDD	
Bread (Mixed, TDS)	United Kingdom	Wright & Startin (1995)	1982	pool	< 0.23	< 0.31	< 0.26	0.87	0.70	9.9	55	1.27
Bread (Mixed, TDS)	United Kingdom	Wright & Startin (1995)	1992	pool	< 0.49	< 0.14	< 0.22	< 0.22	< 0.22	15	94	1.34
Cereal products (Mixed, TDS)	United Kingdom	Wright & Startin (1995)	1982	pool	< 0.14	< 0.16	0.55	4.45	2.7	10	50	1.76
Cereal products (Mixed, TDS)	United Kingdom	Wright & Startin (1995)	1992	pool	< 0.41	< 0.56	< 0.80	< 0.66	< 0.93	16	870	2.66
Cheesecake	United States, Mississippi	Fiedler et al. (1996)	1995	1	0.08	0.44	0.45	2.2	0.42	5	4	0.95
Cod liver oil	Germany, NRW	Fürst et al. (1990)	1989~	4	1.7	1.9	0.4	4.1	0.9	1.4	9.6	16.4
Fish oil	Germany, NRW	Fürst et al. (1990)	1989~	4	< 1.0	1.0	0.4	1.5	1.0	1.8	4.8	4.39
Fish oils	Netherlands	Liem et al. (1991b)	1990–91	5	0.53	1.17	0.65	1.2	1.46	6.19	14.9	2.24
Fish oil (dietary supplement)	Spain	Jiménez et al. (1996b)	1994	7	0.50	0.44	0.11	0.58	0.40	2.1	6.4	2.15
Hamburger	United States, Mississippi	Fiedler et al. (1996)	1995	1	< 0.05	0.22	0.18	0.97	0.25	3	3.9	0.47
Infant formula	Germany, NRW	Fürst et al. (1990)	1989~	10	< 0.5	0.4	0.3	0.3	0.3	2.2	25.8	1.11
Lard	Germany, NRW	Fürst et al. (1990)	1989~	4	< 0.5	< 0.5	< 0.5	0.3	< 0.5	2.8	16.0	1.23
Margarine	Germany, NRW	Fürst et al. (1990)	1989~	6	< 0.5	< 0.5	< 0.5	< 0.5	< 0.5	0.9	11.0	1.2

Table 18 (contd)

Sample description	Origin	Reference	Coll. period	No.	PCDD concentration (ng/kg fat)							
					TCDD	PeCDD	HxCDD			HpCDD	OCDD	I-TEQ PCDD/PCDF
					2378	12378	123478	123678	123789	1234678		
Margarine	Norway	Biseth et al. (1990)	1989~	4	<0.9	<0.2	<0.2	<0.2	<0.2	1.3	18	1.53
Mexican dish	United States, Mississippi	Fiedler et al. (1996)	1995	1	0.04	0.09	0.09	0.12	0.12	0.88	9.1	0.22
Mexican dish	United States, Mississippi	Fiedler et al. (1996)	1995	1	0.06	0.06	<0.08	<0.07	<0.08	0.37	2.8	0.19
Mexican dish	United States, Mississippi	Fiedler et al. (1996)	1995	1	<0.05	0.17	0.15	0.74	0.16	2.1	2.5	0.40
Nuts	Netherlands	Liem et al. (1991b)	1990–91	pool	0.17	ND	ND	ND	ND	0.88	7.25	0.20
Oils and fats (Mixed, TDS)	Spain, Basque region	Startin (1996)	1994	8	<0.22	<0.18	<0.25	<0.25	<0.25	1.48	17.7	0.24
Oils and fats (Mixed, TDS)	United Kingdom	Wright & Startin (1995)	1982	pool	0.15	0.17	0.57	1.3	1.5	11	50	1.26
Oils and fats (Mixed, TDS)	United Kingdom	Wright & Startin (1995)	1992	pool	<0.02	0.09	0.07	0.14	0.18	1.5	10	0.26
Vegetable oils	Netherlands	Liem et al. (1991b)	1990–91		<0.05	<0.05	<0.05	<0.05	<0.05	0.5	8.3	0.03

ND, not detected and detection limit not reported; TDS, total diet survey; NRW, North Rhine Westphalia

APPENDIX 2

TABLES ON OCCURRENCE (PCDFs)

Table 1. Concentrations of PCDFs in air

Reference	Origin; sample description (and no.)	Coll. period	Samp. meth. / Anal. meth.	TCDF 2378	PeCDF 12378	23478	HxCDF 123478	123678	123789	234678	HpCDF 1234678	1234789	OCDF 1234789
Austria													
Christmann et al. (1989b)	Brixlegg; ~280 m from Cu reclamation plant (1)	2/88	G/P / CSI	1.9	2.5	1.4	0.9	0.7	ND	0.7	3.0	ND	1.1
	(1)	5/88		2.0	2.1	0.9	0.8	0.8	ND	0.7	4.6	ND	ND
	(1)	6/88		1.9	1.3	0.6	0.4	0.3	ND	0.2	0.9	0.07	0.9
	(1)	7/88		2.0	2.3	1.0	0.7	0.7	ND	0.4	2.7	0.1	0.8
Belgium													
Wevers et al. (1992)	Antwerp; tunnel air (1)	91	G/P / BSN	0.0013	0.0072	0.0193	0.0073	0.0093	0.0143	0.0004	0.005	0.0007	0.0003
Canada													
Steer et al. (1990a)	SW Ontario; burning tyre dump	2/90	G/P / CSO										
	1 km downwind (5)							I-TEQ for PCDFs only, 0.012–2.2					
	3 km downwind (4)							I-TEQ for PCDFs only, 0.032–0.23					
Germany													
Bruckmann & Hackhe (1987)	Hamburg; Dump site (1)	2/85	G/P/S / BSI	<0.02	<0.02	<0.02	<0.02	<0.02	<0.02	<0.02	ND	ND	0.27
	Dump site, oil (1)	4/85		<0.1	–	–	–	–	–	–		<0.2*	<0.2
	Residential, west of dump (2)	4/85 3/86		<0.1–0.12	0.09	0.08	0.46	0.42	<0.03	0.09		<0.2–0.47*	<0.3–0.19
	Residential, highway, dump, industrial (5)	85–87		0.04–0.37	0.06–1.06	0.05–1.2	0.08–1.1	0.06–1.4	<0.01–0.33	0.02–0.80		1.0–5.1*	0.14–7.0
	Close to copper industry (2)	1 & 2/87		0.04–0.16	0.07–0.16	0.04–0.05	0.04	0.11–0.13	0.01	0.03–0.05		0.41–0.70*	0.1–0.25
	Industry, highway (2)	1 & 10/86		0.23–0.38	0.29–0.42	0.25–0.43	0.27–0.36	0.24–0.31	<0.02–0.05	0.10–0.12		2.0–3.6*	0.78–<2.6
	Industry, 2 MWI (2)	85–86		0.36–0.5	0.17–0.79	0.47	0.12–0.5	0.09–0.50	<0.03–0.08	0.05–0.36		0.20–4.2*	<0.06–<0.97
	Highway tunnel (2)	1/86		0.17–0.72	0.36–0.40	0.19	0.13–0.26	0.15–0.16	<0.05	<0.05–0.12		1.2–1.9*	<1.0–<1.3
	Suburb, highway (1)	9/86		0.04	0.06	<0.03	<0.03	0.12	<0.04	<0.04		0.59*	0.50
	Suburb (north) (1)	8/86		<0.02	<0.02	<0.02	0.03	<0.03	<0.03	<0.03		0.23*	0.10
	Suburb (13 km SE) (1)	4/86		0.04	0.04	0.03	0.03	0.03	<0.01	0.03		0.10*	<0.11
	Forest (20 km N) (1)	4/86		<0.05	<0.02	<0.02	<0.03	<0.03	<0.03	<0.03	ND	ND	<0.12

Table 1 (contd)

Reference	Origin; sample description (and no.)		Coll. period	Samp. meth. / Anal. meth.	PCDF concentration (pg/m³)									
					TCDF 2378	PeCDF 12378	23478	HxCDF 123478	123678	123789	234678	HpCDF 1234678	1234789	OCDF
Kirschner (1987)	Rhine-Ruhr; Mean of 11 sites/wide range of uses	(33)	85-86	G/P CSI	0.09	0.14	0.10	0.13	0.08	–	0.14	1.02² (total HpCDFs)		0.49
Christmann et al. (1989b)	Ambient air; Berlin-Dahlem	(10)	1/87	G/P CSI	ND	ND	ND	<0.1	<0.1	ND	ND	1.6	ND	0.2
	Bad-Kreuzberg	(1)	2/88		ND	ND	ND	ND	ND	ND	ND	0.3	ND	ND
	Gelsenkirchen	(5)	87-88		<0.1	<0.1	<0.1	<0.1	<0.1	ND	<0.1	0.7	ND	ND
	Recklinghausen	(3)	5-9/87		ND-0.2	ND	ND	ND-0.5	ND-0.5	ND	ND-0.6	ND-3.7	ND-0.6	ND-1.3
	Indoor air; PCP application	(1)			ND	ND	ND	0.5	1.0	0.2	0.4	19.5	ND	10.3
Päpke et al. (1989a)	Indoor air; PCP application	(1)	86	G/P BSI	<0.01	0.04	0.04	0.74	1.98	0.16	0.17	51.0	0.40	25.3
König et al. (1993)	Hessen; ambient air		90	G/P BSI										
	Rural	(21)			0.024	0.031	0.032	0.060	0.029	0.005	0.024	0.107	0.011	0.08
	Rural/industry	(21)			0.040	0.049	0.052	0.087	0.051	0.008	0.040	0.168	0.013	0.11
	Rural/industry	(21)			0.037	0.049	0.049	0.085	0.048	0.009	0.037	0.155	0.014	0.13
	Industry	(21)			0.065	0.104	0.098	0.157	0.108	0.021	0.083	0.553	0.029	0.48
	Industry	(21)			0.056	0.089	0.072	0.145	0.068	0.010	0.053	0.197	0.014	0.14
	Traffic	(21)			0.040	0.050	0.053	0.085	0.051	0.008	0.038	0.163	0.013	0.13
Hippelein et al. (1996)	Augsburg; ambient air (mean)			G/X BSI										
	March-April	(6)	92		0.027	0.023	0.023	0.023	0.016	–	0.023	0.062	0.010	<0.059
	April-May	(6)	92		0.015	0.013	0.013	0.011	<0.009	–	0.013	0.033	0.007	0.035
	June-July	(6)	92		<0.010	0.008	0.009	0.008	0.006	–	0.009	0.026	0.004	0.024
	July-September	(6)	92		0.009	0.007	0.009	<0.008	<0.006	–	0.010	0.033	0.004	<0.028
	Sept.-October	(6)	92		0.023	0.022	0.027	<0.029	<0.021	–	<0.023	0.064	0.012	0.064
	Oct.-November	(6)	92		0.037	0.035	0.038	0.038	0.025	–	0.030	0.086	0.017	0.079
	Nov.-January	(6)	92-93		0.063	0.091	0.080	0.080	0.057	–	0.048	0.180	0.029	0.120
	January-February	(6)	93		0.047	<0.051	0.059	0.050	0.039	–	0.044	0.120	0.018	0.098
	Mean of mean	(48)	92-93		0.029	0.031	0.032	0.031	0.022	–	0.025	0.076	0.012	0.063

Table 1 (contd)

Reference	Origin; sample description (and no.)		Coll. period	Samp. meth. / Anal. meth.	PCDF concentration (pg/m³)									
					TCDF	PeCDF		HxCDF				HpCDF		OCDF
					2378	12378	23478	123478	123678	123789	234678	1234678	1234789	
Menzel et al. (1966)	Workplace air;		95	G/P/Ps / N										
	Welding, MWI1 boiler pipes	(1)						Total 2,3,7,8-PCDF isomers, 833						
	Welding, MWI2 waste chute	(2)						Total 2,3,7,8-PCDF isomers, 238–1142						
	Milling, MWI1 boiler pipes	(1)						Total 2,3,7,8-PCDF isomers, 1451						
	Fitting, MWI1 waste chute	(2)						Total 2,3,7,8-PCDF isomers, 31 549–37 509						
	Fitting, MWI2 waste chute	(2)						Total 2,3,7,8-PCDF isomers, 897–2947						
	Air burning, MWI2 waste chute	(2)						Total 2,3,7,8-PCDF isomers, 415–8319						
	Cutting/welding, wood chip dryer	(1)						Total 2,3,7,8-PCDF isomers, 18						
	Open-air burning, power plant dem.	(2)						Total 2,3,7,8-PCDF isomers, 1651–2415						
	Open-air burning, metal reclamation 1	(2)						Total 2,3,7,8-PCDF isomers, 773–4804						
	Open-air burning, metal reclamation 2	(2)						Total 2,3,7,8-PCDF isomers, 2329–7825						
Japan														
Sugita et al. (1993)	Urban area; ambient air, mean summer	(2)	92	G/P / BSI	0.173	0.401	0.484	0.687	0.714	0.261	1.381	5.020	0.630	5.338
	Ambient air, mean winter	(2)			0.308	0.868	0.898	1.317	1.308	0.233	2.321	5.948	0.771	5.588

Table 1 (contd)

Reference	Origin; sample description (and no.)	Coll. period	Samp. meth. / Anal. meth.	PCDF concentration (pg/m³)									
				TCDF	PeCDF		HxCDF				HpCDF		OCDF
				2378	12378	23478	123478	123678	123789	234678	1234678	1234789	
Norway													
Oehme et al. (1991)	Tunnel air; *Northbound*	89	G/P CSI										
	Inlet, weekday (1)			0.053	0.075	0.063	0.061	0.048	0.004	0.042	0.12	0.012	0.28
	Outlet, weekday (1)			0.63	0.90	0.84	0.85	0.67	0.042	0.78	1.9	0.23	1.9
	Inlet, weekend (1)			0.12	0.067	0.045	0.10	0.074	<0.003	0.037	0.27	0.033	0.96
	Outlet, weekend (1)			0.191	0.82	0.62	0.44	0.38	0.037	0.17	1.2	0.17	3.5
	Southbound												
	Inlet, weekday (1)			0.14	0.079	0.075	0.11	0.087	0.011	0.057	0.33	0.046	1.1
	Outlet, weekday (1)			0.23	0.14	0.11	0.33	0.26	0.012	0.14	2.7	0.54	2.0
	Inlet, weekend (1)			0.060	0.054	0.035	0.16	0.12	0.013	0.039	0.63	0.11	2.2
	Outlet, weekend (1)			0.180	0.10	0.053	0.17	0.20	–	0.059	0.39	0.043	3.5
Schlabach et al. (1996)	Spitzbergen, arctic; ambient air (1) (1)	5/95 8/95	G/P BSI	0.0006 0.0005	0.0013 0.0016	0.0016 0.0007	0.0030 0.0014	0.0024 0.0014	0.0004 0.0007	0.0008 0.0004	– 0.0022	– 0.0013	– 0.0038
Poland													
Grochowalski et al. (1995)	Cracow centre;	3/95	G/P CSI										
	Market square (1)			0.38	0.26	0.51	0.79	0.6	0.25	0.58	5.55	1.35	7.5
	Mateczny crossroad (1)			3.75	4.25	7.4	8.8	7.5	2.65	9.9	110	42	220
Russian Federation													
Kruglov et al. (1996)	Oil fire; residential area	96	BSO										
	100 m downwind (1)			0.65	0.19	0.24	0.28	0.26	0.30	0.37	0.67	0.44	2.00
	100 m upwind (1)			0.42	0.13	0.16	0.12	0.10	0.05	0.08	0.21	0.05	0.22

Table 1 (contd)

Reference	Origin; sample description (and no.)		Coll. period	Samp. meth. / Anal. meth.	PCDF concentration (pg/m³)									
					TCDF	PeCDF		HxCDF				HpCDF		OCDF
					2378	12378	23478	123478	123678	123789	234678	1234678	1234789	
Spain														
Abad et al. (1996)	Catalonia (ambient air)		93–95	G/P / BSI										
	Urban, traffic	(8)			0.105	0.055	0.116	1.029	0.075	0.094	0.009	0.298	0.045	0.128
	Rural, near MWI	(12)			0.042	0.012	0.029	0.046	0.027	0.035	0.004	0.120	0.016	0.126
	Urban	(3)			0.313	0.030	0.063	0.180	0.073	0.097	< 0.001	0.387	0.043	1.213
	Urban	(3)			0.273	0.020	0.047	0.127	0.050	0.077	0.003	0.287	0.033	1.810
	MWI influence	(2)			0.535	0.115	0.230	0.595	0.210	0.315	0.015	3.425	0.335	126.8
	Industrial, MWI influence, traffic	(3)			0.377	0.027	0.127	0.413	0.217	0.387	0.020	1.380	0.200	4.090
	Heavy industry near MWI	(2)			0.205	0.015	0.035	0.080	0.030	0.040	< 0.001	0.220	0.020	1.550
	MWI	(2)			0.350	0.225	0.410	0.480	0.425	0.450	0.020	1.300	0.110	0.755
Sweden														
Rappe et al. (1989a)	Rörvik; ambient air			G / BSI										
	Wind WSW	(1)	9/85		< 0.003	0.002	0.002	0.002	0.002	< 0.001	0.002	0.024[f] (total HpCDFs)		0.026
		(1)	1/86		0.005	0.007	0.006	0.008	0.008	0.003	0.007	0.120[f] (total HpCDFs)		0.100
	Wind W, N & E	(1)	1/86		0.015	0.018	0.027	0.021	0.017	0.004	0.018	0.190[f] (total HpCDFs)		0.270
	Wind E & N	(1)	1/86		0.062	0.058	0.069	0.038	0.033	0.014	0.032	0.500[f] (total HpCDFs)		0.440
	Wind SE	(1)	2/86		0.008	0.011	0.009	0.011	0.011	0.004	0.015	0.200[f] (total HpCDFs)		–
	Wind NE	(1)	2/86		0.016	0.017	0.018	0.014	0.014	0.003	0.017	0.200[f] (total HpCDFs)		0.140
	Gothenburg; ambient air													
	Wind W, N & E	(1)	1/86		0.030	0.039	0.051	0.023	0.020	0.004	0.010	0.200[f] (total HpCDFs)		0.150
	Wind E & N	(1)	1/86		0.240	0.190	0.240	0.100	0.079	0.0017	0.084	1100[f] (total HpCDFs)		0.480
	Wind SE	(1)	2/86		0.011	0.019	0.021	0.019	0.018	0.006	0.022	0.260[f] (total HpCDFs)		0.360
United Kingdom														
Clayton et al. (1993)	Ambient; Cardiff	(42)	1/91–9/92	N / B	Mean (range) 2,3,7,8-isomers, 0.78 (ND–11)									
	Manchester	(43)	3/91–9/92		Mean (range) 2,3,7,8-isomers, 1.1 (ND–18)									
	London	(43)	1/91–11/92		Mean (range) 2,3,7,8-isomers, 0.48 (ND–7.1)									
	Stevenage	(43)	1/91–4/92		Mean (range) 2,3,7,8-isomers, 0.36 (ND–7.8)									

Table 1 (contd)

Reference	Origin; sample description (and no.)	Coll. period	Samp. meth. / Anal. meth.	PCDF concentration (pg/m³)									
				TCDF 2378	PeCDF 12378	23478	HxCDF 123478	123678	123789	234678	HpCDF 1234678	1234789	OCDF
United States													
Smith et al. (1989)	Niagara Falls; ambient air		G/P CSO										
	Downwind from industry (1)	11/86		0.33	0.1	0.13	0.22	0.14	ND	0.11	0.55		0.39
	(1)	11/86		3.81	0.61	1.92	ND	1.17	0.1	2.17	5.43		3.38
	(1)	1/86		0.28	0.03	ND	0.1	0.05	ND	ND	0.26		0.10
	Upwind from industry (1)	11/86		0.08	ND	ND	ND	0.02	ND	ND	ND	ND	0.12
	(1)	1/87		0.14	ND	ND	0.06	ND	ND	0.04	0.15	ND	0.12
	(1)	2/87		0.04	ND	ND	ND	ND	ND	ND	ND	ND	0.16
Edgerton et al. (1989)	Akron; 2 km from MWI	11–12/87	G/P BSN	0.20	0.026	0.032	0.100	0.055	0.039	<0.036	0.25	<0.035	0.19
				0.20	0.033	0.042	0.053	0.048	0.036	<0.021	0.24	<0.022	0.17
				0.19	0.029	0.034	0.095	0.092	0.020	<0.005	0.22	0.031	0.18
	Columbus;												
	3/4 km from RDF			0.32	0.032	<0.023	0.060	0.092	0.038	<0.028	0.20	<0.015	<0.31
	1/4 km from SSI			0.49	0.057	0.089	0.270	0.190	0.120	<0.012	0.47	<0.028	0.21
	Highway			<0.13	<0.036	<0.036	<0.034	<0.034	<0.034	<0.034	0.087	<0.013	<0.16
	Waldo; Background			0.13	0.021	<0.033	0.098	0.014	0.097	<0.008	0.22	0.019	0.077
Hahn et al. (1989)	Workplace air; Bottom ash conveyor	1/88	G/P/X N	0.069	0.012	ND	0.032	ND	ND	ND	0.107	ND	0.166
	Feed table floor			0.095	0.015	ND	0.052	ND	ND	ND	0.149	ND	0.254
Tiernan et al. (1989)	Dayton, OH; ambient air, near MWI	88	N	0.11	0.46	0.53	1.18	2.27	ND	ND	8.22	0.56	3.78
Kominsky & Kwoka (1989)	Boston;	9/86	G/Si CN										
	Office building (12)			<0.37–1.4		<0.012–1.9		<0.09–0.36				<0.39–1.5	<0.54–<1.8
	Ambient air (4)			<0.72–0.83		<0.23–1.2		<0.11–0.29				<0.51–1.5	<0.51–<2.8
Harless et al. (1990)	Green Bay, WI; ambient air (4)	89	G/P BSI	<0.01–0.04	0.02–0.09	<0.02–0.07	0.01–0.05	0.01–0.04	<0.01–0.02	<0.01–0.02	0.03–0.15	<0.01–0.01	0.02–0.2
Hunt & Maisel (1990)	Bridgeport, CT; ambient air (29)	87–88	G/P BSI	?0.078	0.031	0.047	0.106	0.039	0.007	0.087	0.212	0.033	0.211

Table 1 (contd)

Reference	Origin; sample description (and no.)		Coll. period	Samp. meth. / Anal. meth.	PCDF concentration (pg/m³)									
					TCDF	PeCDF		HxCDF				HpCDF		OCDF
					2378	13378	23478	123478	123678	123789	234678	1234678	1234789	
Maisel (1990)	Bridgeport MWI; Ambient, pre-operational	(22)	87–88	G/P BSI	ᵇ0.062	0.032	0.049	0.11	0.041	<0.010	0.10	0.22	0.031	–
Maisel & Hunt (1990)	Los Angeles, CA; Ambient	(1)	W/87	G/P BSI	0.021	0.077	0.077	0.150	0.250	<0.083	<0.069	<0.190	<0.018	0.056
Hunt & Maisel (1992)	S. California			G/P BSI										
	Session I	(6)	12/87		0.046	0.401	0.098	0.188	0.407	<0.070	<0.298	<1.162	<0.094	0.108
	Session II	(2)	12/87		<0.032	<0.016	<0.016	<0.044	<0.018	<0.012	<0.020	<0.140	<0.014	0.048
	Session III	(5)	7/88		<0.022	<0.068	<0.068	<0.060	<0.060	<0.060	<0.060	<0.160	<0.088	<0.073
	Session IV	(6)	7/88		<0.048	<0.050	<0.050	<0.068	<0.052	<0.046	<0.052	<0.272	<0.078	<0.148
	Session V	(7)	9/88		0.047	<0.034	<0.062	<0.080	<0.044	<0.020	<0.038	0.375	<0.054	0.546
	Session VI	(1)	11/88		0.011	<0.040	<0.044	<0.066	<0.066	<0.046	<0.066	0.251	<0.062	<0.436
	Session VII	(6)	3/89		0.107	<0.028	<0.012	<0.032	<0.034	<0.054	<0.042	<0.104	<0.026	0.187
	Mean, all sessions	(33)			0.048	<0.196	<0.074	<0.124	<0.204	<0.048	<0.090	<0.514	<0.066	<0.466

Analytical methods: All analyses use high-resolution gas chromatography; B, high-resolution mass spectrometry; C, low-resolution mass spectrometry; I, isomer-specific; O, others; N, no information; S, sophisticated clean-up (see Table 5 and Section 1.1.4 in monograph on PCDDs in this volume)

Sampling methods: G, glass fibre filter; P, polyurethane foam; X, XAD; C, carbon; Si, silica; Ps, personal sampling

ND, not detected; MWI, municipal waste incinerator; SSI, sewage sludge incinerator; RDF, refuse-derived fuel incinerator

Data presented are means. Figures in parentheses are ranges. Levels of congeners not detected at known detection limits (for examples, 0.02 pg/m³) are presented as <0.02

ᵃ Contains non-toxic isomers

ᵇ Including non-2,3,7,8-substituted isomers

Table 2. Concentrations of PCDFs in water

Reference	Origin; sample description (and no.)	Coll. period	Anal. meth.	TCDF 2378	PnCDF 12378	23478	HxCDF 123478	123678	123789	234678	HpCDF 1234678	1234789	OCDF
Canada													
Muir et al. (1995)	Downstream of pulp mill; river water, dissolved phase	NG	92–93 BN	0.09–0.10	–	–	–	–	–	–	–	–	–
Japan													
Matsumura et al. (1994)	Coastal seawater	(1)	NG BIS	0.050	0.020	0.035	0.028	0.020	<0.005	0.055	0.380	0.390	0.560
Russian Federation													
Fedorov (1993)	Chapaevsk; Artesian drinking water		6–9/92 N		70.0	70.0		23.5		1.8	16.3		39.4
Sweden													
Rappe et al. (1989b)	Bälinge, Uppsala; MWTP ingoing water	(1)	87 BIS	<3.7	<5.1	<6.1	<9	<6	<20	<10	23	<5	25
	Bälinge, Uppsala; MWTP outgoing water	(1)	87	<0.57	<0.33	<0.39	<1	<1	<1	<1	2	<1.2	<3.0
	Henriksdal, Stockholm; MWTP ingoing water	(1)	87	2.8	<1.6	<1.8	<8	<4	<8	<6	<7	<82	<65
	Henriksdal, Stockholm; MWTP outgoing water	(1)	87	<0.32	<0.22	<0.24	<1	<0.5	<1	<1	<2	<10	<20
	Järnsjön; Eman river	(1)	87	0.026	0.025	0.019	0.026	0.025	0.022	0.027	0.130	0.058	0.360
	Fliseryd; Eman river	(1)	87	0.022	0.013	0.014	0.021	0.019	<0.014	<0.012	0.083	0.030	0.150
	Filtered water; Eman river	(1)	87	<0.017	<0.011	<0.014	<0.024	<0.023	<0.029	<0.024	<0.011	<0.030	<0.059

Table 2 (contd)

Reference	Origin; sample description (and no.)	Coll. period	Anal. meth.	PCDF concentration (pg/L)									
				TCDF	PnCDF		HxCDF				HpCDF		OCDF
				2378	12378	23478	123478	123678	123789	234678	1234678	1234789	
Sweden (contd)													
Rappe et al. (1989b) (contd)	Blank; Laboratory (1)	87	BIS	< 0.016	< 0.011	< 0.014	< 0.033	< 0.032	< 0.039	< 0.032	< 0.015	< 0.040	< 0.099
Rappe et al. (1990a)	Ringhals, in; Sea cooling water (1)	89	BIS	0.016	0.0032	0.0034	0.0068	0.0021	< 0.005	< 0.004	0.025	< 0.007	0.026
	Ringhals, out; Sea cooling water (1)	89		0.013	0.0097	0.0068	0.0066	0.0020	< 0.006	< 0.004	0.019	< 0.007	< 0.015
	Ringhals, in; Sea cooling water (1)	89		0.0072	0.0020	0.0025	0.0021	0.0012	< 0.001	0.0019	0.010	< 0.002	0.020
	Ringhals, out; Sea cooling water (1)	89		0.0091	0.0021	0.0023	0.0025	0.0013	< 0.001	0.0012	0.012	< 0.002	0.018
	River Ljusnan (3)	89		0.011	0.0036–0.0073	0.0059–0.010	0.005–0.011	0.0038–0.0082	< 0.007	0.0047–0.0091	0.023–0.058	0.0003–0.004	0.018–0.044
	River Ljungan (1)	89		0.026	0.0079	0.0085	0.0095	0.0031	< 0.0006	0.002	0.099	< 0.0009	0.100
	Drinking water (1)	89		0.0096	< 0.0003	0.0023	0.0007	0.0006	< 0.0005	< 0.0004	0.0003	< 0.001	< 0.006
United States													
Meyer et al. (1989)	Lockport; Finished water, S (1)	8/86	C/BO S	1.2/1.2		< 1.1			< 0.7		< 0.8	< 0.8	0.8
	Finished water, PB (1)			< 0.8		< 2.0			< 1.1		< 1.2	< 1.2	< 0.5
	Blank; Distilled water, S (1)	9/86		< 1.4		< 1.0			< 0.8		< 3.7	< 3.7	< 1.5
	Distilled water, PB (1)			< 0.9		< 0.8			< 0.5		< 2.7	< 2.7	< 0.9
	Lockport; Finished water, S (1)	2/88		< 3.4		< 4.0			< 4.4		< 6.6	< 6.6	< 15
	Finished water, PB (1)			< 3.6		< 4.0			< 4.3		< 5.1	< 5.1	< 11
	Lockport; Finished water, S (1)	8/88		< 2.5		< 2.3			< 3.1		< 4.4	< 4.4	< 6.8
	Finished water, PB (1)			< 2.9		< 2.2			< 2.1		< 3.6	< 3.6	< 7.8

Table 2 (contd)

Reference	Origin; sample description (and no.)	Coll. period	Anal. meth.	PCDF concentration (pg/L)									
				TCDF	PnCDF		HxCDF				HpCDF		OCDF
				2378	12378	23478	123478	123678	123789	234678	1234678	1234789	
United States (contd)													
Meyer *et al.* (1989) (contd)	19 other locations; Finished water, S	(19)	86–87	ND (0.3–2.6)	ND (0.3–2.7)			ND (0.3–1.7)			ND (0.8–4.8)		ND (0.6–8.6)
	Finished water, PB	(19)		ND (0.3–2.7)	ND (0.4–2.6)			ND (0.3–1.7)			ND (0.7–12.4)		ND (0.5–48)

Analytical methods: All analyses use high-resolution gas chromatography; B, high-resolution mass spectrometry; N, no information; C, low-resolution mass spectrometry; I, isomer-specific; O, others; S, sophisticated clean-up (see Table 5 and Section 1.1.4 in monograph on PCDDs in this volume)

ND, not detected; detection limit in parentheses; MWTP, municipal water treatment plant; S, soluble; PB, particle-bound

Data presented are means. Figures in parentheses are ranges. Levels of congeners not detected at known detection limits (for examples, 0.02 pg/m³) are presented as < 0.02.

Table 3. Concentrations of PCDFs in soil

Reference	Origin; sample description (and no.)	Coll. period	Anal. meth.	PCDF concentration (ng/kg; ppt)									
				TCDF	PeCDF		HxCDF				HpCDF		OCDF
				2378	12378	23478	123478	123678	123789	234678	1234678	1234789	
Austria													
Boos et al. (1992)	Meadow; urban emission	90/91	CSI	ND	3.0	1.7	6.4	2.2	ND	1.9	11.3	ND	12.1
	Park; urban emission	90/91		ND	2.6	1.7	3.3	2.1	ND	ND	9.8	0.5	10.2
	Traffic island; heavy traffic	90/91		3.0	6.5	2.7	11.3	4.3	ND	ND	38.3	2.9	30.1
	Meadow; urban emission	90/91		6.1	4.2	2.2	2.7	3.6	ND	1.8	15.9	1.4	27.2
	Meadow; urban emission	90/91		ND	2.6	ND	1.3	2.1	ND	2.5	12.4	0.5	26.1
	Meadow; urban emission	90/91		ND	3.3	1.6	7.1	2.9	ND	2.8	16.6	1.8	20.9
	Meadow; urban emission	90/91		ND	1.7	ND	2.5	1.5	ND	3.9	26.2	4.2	45.6
	Park; urban emission	90/91		1.3	1.5	1.3	3.6	1.9	ND	5.4	12.0	ND	13.3
	Meadow; cable proc. plant	90/91		2.3	4.7	3.3	5.2	4.0	ND	5.5	19.0	1.8	30.1
	Meadow; cable proc. plant	90/91		3.8	13.4	5.3	14.0	5.2	1.2	3.2	18.5	4.1	12.8
	Meadow; cable proc. plant	90/91		2.2	2.3	2.8	3.2	2.9	ND	5.0	12.7	ND	3.5
	Meadow; diffuse emission	90/91		ND	2.7	1.7	5.1	3.2	2.8	4.1	13.5	ND	10.9
	Meadow; diffuse emission	90/91		ND	2.1	0.6	1.9	0.6	ND	ND	3.5	0.6	5.1
	Meadow; Diffuse emission, highway 100 m	90/91		ND	2.4	0.7	ND	ND	ND	ND	3.1	1.3	4.6
	Meadow; diffuse emission, highway 200 m	90/91		1.9	1.4	0.6	1.4	1.2	ND	ND	5.2	0.5	5.1
	Meadow; steel foundry	90/91		ND	1.7	0.8	1.8	0.8	ND	1.0	5.9	0.6	10.8
	Meadow; steel foundry	90/91		2.4	1.8	1.6	1.0	0.6	ND	1.2	5.7	0.5	6.8

Table 3 (contd)

Reference	Origin: sample description (and no.)	Coll. period	Anal. meth.	PCDF concentration (ng/kg; ppt) TCDF 2378	PeCDF 12378	PeCDF 23478	HxCDF 123478	HxCDF 123678	HxCDF 123789	HxCDF 234678	HpCDF 1234678	HpCDF 1234789	OCDF
Austria (contd)													
Boos et al. (1992) (contd)	Meadow; industry	90/91	CSI	ND	3.3	2.3	4.2	2.5	ND	ND	8.2	ND	7.2
	Meadow; Alpine background	90/91		ND	ND	ND	ND	ND	ND	ND	5.4	ND	6.0
	Urban outskirts; 2ndary Al smelter (1)	90/91		1.5	3.2	1.3	5.0	3.1	ND	2.6	20.3	1.3	52.7
	Urban outskirts; 2ndary Al smelter (1)	90/91		2.5	6.7	3.5	6.9	6.2	ND	6.0	26.5	1.8	56.0
	Urban outskirts; diffuse emission (1)	90/91		0.7	2.7	1.7	4.5	4.1	ND	9.6	20.8	0.8	11.3
	Meadow; highway 0.5 m (1)	90/91		ND	4.9	2.0	3.9	2.4	ND	2.8	12.2	1.7	13.0
	Industrial area; metal smelter (1)	90/91		12.0	7.3	11.1	9.3	6.9	ND	ND	85.0	ND	74.0
Canada													
Pearson et al. (1990)	Hamilton; vicinity incinerator (11)	83	CSO	No other isomers reported				No other isomers reported					4 (ND–33)
	Scarborough; vicinity incinerator (12)	87						No other isomers reported					43 (ND–230)
	Ontario; Rural soils (1)	83						No other isomers reported					ND
	Rural soils (26)	87						No other isomers reported					ND
	Rural soils (15)	88						No other isomers reported					ND
	Rural soils (1)	88						No other isomers reported					ND
	Ontario; Urban soils (2)	83						No other isomers reported					41 (ND–81)
	Urban soils (11)	87						No other isomers reported					19 (ND–160)
	Urban soils (15)	88						No other isomers reported					77 (ND–600)
	Urban soils (1)	88						No other isomers reported					ND

Table 3 (contd)

Reference	Origin; sample description (and no.)		Coll. period	Anal. meth.	PCDF concentration (ng/kg; ppt)									
					TCDF	PeCDF		HxCDF				HpCDF		OCDF
					2378	12378	23478	123478	123678	123789	234678	1234678	1234789	
China, People's Republic														
Wu et al. (1995)	Ya-Er Lake area; soil 1	(1)	91–94	CSI	0.17	ND	0.05	0.49	ND	ND	0.04	0.01	ND	0.15
	Ya-Er Lake area; soil 2	(1)	91–94		ND	0.19	ND	0.45	ND	ND	ND	0.03	ND	0.13
Finland														
Assmuth & Vartiainen (1995)	Sawmill; depth, 0–0.5 m; soil	(10)	NG	BSI	15–3000	ND–530	ND–1 000	7500–800 000	ND–180	ND	ND–2200	20 000–1 200 000	ND	23 000–1 200 000
Germany														
Schlesing (1989)	Herbic. plant; Boring d., 1 m	(?)	< 89	NSI	TCDF–HpCDF only totals reported									1 661 000
	Herbic. plant; Boring d., 2 m	(?)	< 89		TCDF–HpCDF only totals reported									19 600
	Herbic. plant; Boring d., 3 m	(?)	< 89		TCDF–HpCDF only totals reported									17 600
	Herbic. plant; Boring d., 4 m	(?)	< 89		TCDF–HpCDF only totals reported									11 200
	Herbic. plant; Boring d., 1 m	(1)	< 89		TCDF–HpCDF only totals reported									61 200
	Herbic. plant; Boring d., 2 m	(1)	< 89		TCDF–HpCDF only totals reported									42 000
	Herbic. plant; Boring d., 3 m	(1)	< 89		TCDF–HpCDF only totals reported									27 100
	Herbic. plant; Boring d., 4 m	(1)	< 89		TCDF–HpCDF only totals reported									–
	Herbic. plant; Boring d., 5 m	(1)	< 89		TCDF–HpCDF only totals reported									700
	Herbic. plant; Boring d., 6 m	(1)	< 89		TCDF–HpCDF only totals reported									1 600
	Herbic. plant; Boring d., 7 m	(1)	< 89		TCDF–HpCDF only totals reported									261 000
	Herbic. plant; Boring d., 8 m	(1)	< 89		TCDF–HpCDF only totals reported									500

Table 3 (contd)

Reference	Origin; sample description (and no.)	Coll. period	Anal. meth.	PCDF concentration (ng/kg; ppt)									
				TCDF	PeCDF		HxCDF				HpCDF		OCDF
				2378	12378	23478	123478	123678	123789	234678	1234678	1234789	
Germany (contd)													
Schlesing (1989) (contd)	Herbic. plant; Boring d. 9 m (1)	< 89		TCDF-HpCDF only totals reported									—
Hagenmaier et al. (1992)	Rastatt; site 1 (1)	87	BSI	24	25	20	36	21	4	18	110	12	80
	(1)	89		16	33	18	41	25	4	17	62	12	100
	Rastatt; site 2 (1)	87		5 000	8 240	5 240	7 010	3 880	740	3 280	20 900	2 860	14 200
	(1)	89		4 710	9 430	3 870	7 500	4 390	780	2 530	16 900	2 360	14 200
	Rastatt; site 3 (1)	87		440	780	480	880	470	70	370	2 200	280	1 700
	(1)	89		470	980	480	800	470	80	290	2 160	280	1 600
	Rastatt; site 4 (1)	87		250	420	300	610	330	70	260	1 770	220	1 400
	(1)	89		350	650	370	790	450	80	290	2 310	330	1 900
She & Hagenmaier (1996)	Rastatt; all samples[a] (77)	87	BSI	140 (10–13 300)	350 (10–25 000)	240 (3–13 100)	390 (15–21 200)	240 (9–11 500)	21 (1–1470)	180 (6–7940)	1 010 (51–63 600)	120 (3–9630)	880 (40–37 000)
Theisen et al. (1993)	Kieselrot Cu slag	92	BSI	6 800	28 000	14 200	94 100	83 300	14 200	64 200	1 674 600	150 300	314 000
	Close to Kieselrot sport ground; garden soil	92		15	72	36	231	204	33	160	2988	200	8 120
	Corresponding standard soil	92		2.5	2	1.8	2.9	2.4	0.3	2.5	15.8	< 0.2	< 9
McLachlan & Reissinger (1990)	Field 1; no sludge[a] (1)	89	CSI	0.64	0.72	0.88	0.57	0.45	0.06	0.39	3.0	0.20	2.8
	Field 2; sludge for 10 y[a] (1)	89		0.63	1.6	0.89	2.0	0.94	0.19	0.59	7.4	0.38	9
	Field 3; sludge for 30 y[a] (1)	89		2.1	4.2	2.7	5.4	3.2	0.70	1.3	19	1.1	29
	Meadow; sludge for 30 y[a] (1)	89		2.4	6.4	5.9	9.7	3.8	1.1	1.9	31	1.6	43
	Sewage sludge (1)	89		12	8.2	15	16	10	3.3	15	110	10	400

Table 3 (contd)

Reference	Origin; sample description (and no.)	Coll. period	Anal. meth.	TCDF 2378	PeCDF 12378	23478	HxCDF 123478	123678	123789	234678	HpCDF 1234678	1234789	OCDF
Germany (contd)													
Rotard et al. (1994)	Ploughland (14)	<94	CSI	1.8 (0.7–3.4)	1.8 (0.5–3.4)	1.7 (0.7–3.1)	1.7 (0.9–3.3)	1.4 (0.7–2.4)	0.7 (0.5–0.9)	1.3 (0.7–2.8)	9.5 (3.2–25)	1.0 (0.4–1.6)	18 (3.3–54)
	Grassland (7)	<94		2.2 (0.7–3.6)	2.7 (0.9–5.0)	2.6 (1.2–5.3)	2.6 (1.0–4.8)	1.9 (0.7–3.7)	1.1 (0.7–1.8)	2.2 (0.1–3.7)	13.1 (4.6–34)	1.7 (0.8–2.8)	23.8 (7.4–82)
	Deciduous forest (9)	<94		25.4 (7.2–68)	36 (5.9–93)	30 (5.6–86)	35 (3.7–129)	26 (3.3–83)	7.6 (1.0–27)	18.6 (2.1–54)	184 (25–697)	15.8 (2.3–63)	390 (47–2142)
	Coniferous forest (11)	<94		27.9 (10.0–61)	36 (10.5–108)	32 (8.1–97)	25 (5.4–89)	21 (5.4–77)	4.4 (ND–16)	17.2 (4.1–63)	140 (23–646)	10.3 (1.6–50)	167 (18–985)
Jordan													
Alawi et al. (1996a)	Landfill, Amman:												
	Sample 1 (1)	95	CSI	<10	644	494	377	372	<10	581	1280	<10	109
	Sample 2 (1)	95		<10	160	115	96	90	<10	145	327	<10	195
	Sample 3 (1)	95		<10	90	62	72	58	<10	80	387	<10	79
	Sample 4 (1)	95		<10	109	55	44	38	<10	53	156	<10	15
	Sample 5 (1)	95		19	42	111	27	51	<10	23	79	<10	16
	Sample 6 (1)	95		<10	<10	<10	<10	<10	<10	<10	36	<10	24
The Netherlands													
van Wijnen et al. (1992)	Scrap car dealer (4)	6/88	CSI	39–88	ND–53	37–80	44–100	52–120	ND	40–120	390–590	ND–28	150–860
	Cable burning (3)	6/88		210–8000	220–12 000	210–14 000	250–9 300	230–15 000	34–1 600	270–16 000	800–32 000	46–2 200	180–11 000
	Scrap metal dealer, cable burning (1)	6/88		370	340	560	980	2300	110	410	3700	360	12 000
	Scrap metal dealer, cable burning (2)	6/88		ND	ND	ND–310	400–6 000	ND	ND	ND	1200–5 400	ND	690–5 800
	Scrap car and open air cable burning (4)	6/88		100–5200	150–7 400	140–7 700	59–6 900	210–9 400	ND–680	150–11 000	470–15 000	ND–1300	330–5 100
	Scrap car and open air cable burning (3)	6/88		17 000–23 000	52 000–91 000	41 000–53 000	75 000–190 000	75 000–120 000	8 200–18 000	94 000–150 000	240 000–450 000	10 000–24 000	79 000–270 000

Table 3 (contd)

Reference	Origin: sample description (and no.)		Coll. period	Anal. meth.	PCDF concentration (ng/kg; ppt)									
					TCDF	PeCDF		HxCDF				HpCDF		OCDF
					2378	12378	23478	123478	123678	123789	234678	1234678	1234789	
The Netherlands (contd)														
van Wijnen et al. (1992) (contd)	Scrap car and open air cable burning	(3)	6/88		1 000–3 200	2 200–7 500	2 800–7 400	3 400–14 000	4 900–16 000	760–2 400	6 000–21 000	19 000–59 000	720–2 600	ND–36 000
Russian Federation														
Fedorov (1993)	Incinerator Ufa; near sect. N 15		10/90	N	36 500				No other isomers reported					
	Near sect. N 11		10/90		59 000				No other isomers reported					
Fedorov et al. (1993)	Chapaevsk; CFP on site	(3)	92–93	CN					Only total reported					2 200–67 000
	Chapaevsk; 1.5 km from CFP	(2)	92–93						Only total reported					2 200–6 350
	Chapaevsk; 2 km from CFP	(1)	92–93						Only total reported					910
	Chapaevsk; 3 km from CFP	(1)	92–93						Only total reported					600
	Chapaevsk; 6 km from CFP	(1)	92–93						Only total reported					225
	Chapaevsk; 7 km from CFP	(1)	92–93						Only total reported					50
	Chapaevsk; 8 km from CFP	(1)	92–93						Only total reported					< 5
	Chapaevsk; 12 km from CFP	(1)	92–93						Only total reported					< 5
Spain														
Jiménez et al. (1996a)	Madrid; SW, 400 m fr. CWI	(1)	93	BSO	4.64	0.88	0.74	0.97	0.40	0.73	0.42	1.01	0.12	2.02
	Madrid; SE, 1200 m fr. CWI	(1)	93		4.81	0.91	1.27	2.09	0.86	0.17	1.07	3.49	0.30	5.19
	Madrid; NE, 600 m fr. CWI	(1)	93		5.51	0.89	1.26	1.64	0.61	0.37	0.73	1.57	0.15	1.26
	Madrid; NW, 1200 m fr. CWI	(1)	93		5.46	0.44	0.70	0.84	0.42	0.72	0.36	0.92	–	–

Table 3 (contd)

Reference	Origin; sample description (and no.)	Coll. period	Anal. meth.	PCDF concentration (ng/kg; ppt)									
				TCDF	PeCDF		HxCDF				HpCDF		OCDF
				2378	12378	23478	123478	123678	123789	234678	1234678	1234789	
Spain (contd)													
Jiménez et al. (1996a) (contd)	Madrid; W, 2000 m fr. CWI	(1)	93 BSO	5.27	1.03	0.62	0.82	0.59	ND	0.41	ND	ND	1.56
	Madrid; SW, 2000 m fr. CWI	(1)	93	13.3	3.51	4.23	15.6	5.60	0.88	6.54	38.4	3.63	64.5
	Madrid; N, 2000 m fr. CWI	(1)	93	1.51	0.41	0.37	0.74	0.27	0.21	0.36	1.57	0.23	3.14
	Madrid; S, 1200 m fr. CWI	(1)	93	6.49	0.88	1.49	2.17	0.90	0.23	1.24	1.91	0.25	1.72
	Madrid; NE, 2600 m fr. CWI	(1)	93	2.92	0.66	0.55	1.03	0.40	0.27	0.52	1.46	0.10	1.52
	Madrid; NE, 2600 m fr. CWI	(1)	93	3.58	0.75	0.89	1.65	0.66	0.19	0.70	1.90	0.20	4.70
	Madrid; NE, 2600 m fr. CWI	(1)	93	5.45	1.20	0.96	1.36	0.59	0.54	0.62	1.63	0.17	1.98
	Madrid; NE, 3000 m fr. CWI	(1)	93	2.93	0.75	0.94	2.06	0.93	0.19	0.96	2.66	0.30	2.29
	Madrid; NE, 3000 m fr. CWI	(1)	93	1.27	0.40	0.40	0.56	0.25	0.17	0.29	0.94	0.08	3.04
	Madrid; NE, 3000 m fr. CWI	(1)	93	2.07	0.40	0.47	0.91	0.37	0.16	0.38	1.31	0.11	1.56
	Madrid, control; NW, 4500 m fr. CWI	(1)	93	2.36	0.37	0.44	0.53	0.19	0.22	0.25	0.66	0.11	0.66
	Madrid, control; NE, 4500 m fr. CWI	(1)	93	1.15	0.32	0.33	0.53	0.27	0.47	0.30	0.76	0.08	1.89
Schuhmacher et al. (1996)	Tarragona; 250 m fr. MSWI	(6)	<96 BSO	0.34	0.09	0.10	0.22	–	ND	0.17	0.51	–	0.84
	Tarragona; 500 m fr. MSWI	(6)	<96	0.69	0.20	0.12	0.23	0.09	0.06	0.15	0.64	0.09	0.85
	Tarragona; 750 m fr. MSWI	(6)	<96	1.28	0.21	0.33	1.18	0.43	0.15	0.61	3.60	0.31	3.88
	Tarragona; 1000 m fr. MSWI	(6)	<96	1.14	0.22	0.25	0.64	0.23	0.10	0.33	1.33	0.15	1.38

Table 3 (contd)

Reference	Origin; sample description (and no.)		Coll. period	Anal. meth.	PCDF concentration (ng/kg; ppt)									
					TCDF	PeCDF		HxCDF				HpCDF		OCDF
					2378	12378	23478	123478	123678	123789	234678	1234678	1234789	
Spain (contd)														
Schuhmacher et al. (1996) (contd)	Tarragona; NE fr. MSWI	(8)	<96	BSO	0.35	0.07	0.08	0.16	0.07	0.09	0.14	0.40	0.08	0.36
	Tarragona; SE fr. MSWI	(8)	<96		1.27	0.49	0.18	0.33	0.12	0.05	0.14	0.95	0.11	1.46
	Tarragona; SW fr. MSWI	(8)	<96		0.45	0.05	0.09	0.19	0.09	0.04	0.18	0.57	0.07	0.71
Sweden														
Rappe et al. (1991b)	Plant B; soil I	(1)	90	BSI	30 000	33 000	12 000	17 000	2 800	160	820	1 700	1 600	4 900
	Plant B; soil II	(1)	90		2 500	1 700	870	1 300	280	18	75	170	31	–
	Outside plant B; grassfield; soil III	(1)	90		17	7.6	3.9	11	2.1	<0.2	0.2	7.9	0.9	13
	Plant B; soil II	(1)	90		1300	910	420	680	140	24	42	240	110	1000
	Plant B; soil V	(1)	90		240	160	100	150	33	2	8.7	39	14	64
	Plant B; Cl; prod.; soil II	(1)	90		11 000	960	520	320	67	10	27	72	36	110
Taiwan														
Huang et al. (1992)	Electric wire incinerator site	(1)	89	BSI	2215	293	6630	1326	631	ND	837	541	41	86
	Electric wire incinerator site	(1)	89		68	58	786	157	89	ND	139	95	2	9
	Mainly magnetic card incinerator site	(1)	89		4	3	41	8	6	ND	17	8	–	1
	Mainly magnetic card incinerator site	(1)	89		6	5	116	23	7	ND	1	1	ND	ND
	Mainly magnetic card incinerator site	(1)	89		30	29	162	32	28	ND	37	16	–	–
	Mainly magnetic card incinerator site	(1)	89		8	1	12	2	3	ND	–	1	ND	–

Table 3 (contd)

Reference	Origin: sample description (and no.)		Coll. period	Anal. meth.	PCDF concentration (ng/kg; ppt)									
					TCDF	PeCDF		HxCDF				HpCDF		OCDF
					2378	12378	23478	123478	123678	123789	234678	1234678	1234789	
Taiwan (contd)														
Soong & Ling (1996)	PCP production plant site	(1)	<96	CSO	311	2 596	65	211	162	172	293	41 150	1 089	432 700
	PCP production plant site	(1)	<96		44 670	16 550	7 946	142 000	37 333	248 400	93 960	22 470 000	672 500	471 700 000
United Kingdom														
Kjeller et al. (1991)	Rothamsted (semi-rural); archived samples (0–23 cm depth)	(1)	1846	BSI	0.790	1.100	0.820	1.000	0.630	<0.01	0.680	3.300	0.250	2.900
		(1)	1856		0.450	0.590	0.460	0.640	0.380	<0.01	0.310	1.200	0.080	0.980
		(1)	1893		0.290	0.320	0.350	0.430	0.340	<0.01	0.540	1.500	0.087	1.100
		(1)	1914		0.420	0.680	0.500	0.650	0.460	<0.01	0.400	1.900	0.110	1.400
		(1)	1944		1.200	1.100	1.100	1.600	0.730	<0.01	0.500	3.200	0.660	7.600
		(1)	1956		0.740	1.000	0.830	1.100	0.750	<0.01	0.560	4.900	0.230	4.400
		(1)	1966		0.930	0.710	0.820	1.100	0.810	<0.02	0.650	3.600	0.280	3.900
		(1)	1980		0.870	0.930	0.790	1.100	0.710	<0.02	0.530	3.600	0.450	4.200
		(1)	1986		1.000	1.000	0.860	1.200	0.810	<0.01	0.530	4.200	0.310	5.200
Creaser et al. (1989)	50 km grid UK; all samples	(77)	<89	BSI	Only total reported									55 (<2–622)
	50 km grid UK; reduced data set	(65)	<89		Only total reported									27 (<2–144)
Creaser et al. (1990)	Urban soils (5 cities)	(19)	<90	BSI	Only total reported									196 (7.3–1100)
Stenhouse & Badsha (1990)	Different semi-urban sites	(12)	90	BSO	17 (3–50)	4 (1–10)	2 (1–5)		12 (3–30)				15 (3–39)	30 (10–90)
United States														
Reed et al. (1990)	Elk River, MI; site 1 untilled	(1)	9/88	BSI	ND	ND	ND	ND	ND	ND	7.1	72	ND	120
	Elk River, MI; site 1 tilled	(1)	9/88		ND	ND	ND	ND	ND	ND	ND	11	ND	ND
	Elk River, MI; site 2 untilled	(1)	9/88		ND	ND	ND	ND	ND	ND	ND	26	ND	60
	Elk River, MI; site 2 tilled	(1)	9/88		ND	ND	ND	ND	ND	ND	ND	80	ND	270

Table 3 (contd)

Reference	Origin; sample description (and no.)		Coll. period	Anal. meth.	PCDF concentration (ng/kg; ppt)									OCDF
					TCDF	PeCDF		HxCDF				HpCDF		
					2378	12378	23478	123478	123678	123789	234678	1234678	1234789	
United States (contd)														
Lorber et al. (1996b)	Columbus, OH; MSWI, on site[a]	(4)	95	BSI	86	140	200	197	209	12	157	641	58	184
	Columbus, OH; MSWI, downwind off site[a]	(4)	95		9	15	21	30	23	1	19	106	10	109
	Columbus, OH; Urban[a]	(14)	95		2	2	4	4	4	0.3	3	23	1	26
	Ohio; rural[a]	(3)	95		0.5	0.2	0.2	0.2	0.5	0.2	0.6	4.0	0.3	11
Viet Nam														
Matsuda et al. (1994)	Hue, Phu Loc; sprayed area	(6)	89–91	CSI	No other isomers reported									n.a
	Ho Chi Minh; sprayed area	(9)	89–91		No other isomers reported									n.a
	Tay Ninh; sprayed area	(54)	89–91		No other isomers reported									3.6–560
	Song Be; sprayed area	(11)	89–91		No other isomers reported									ND
	Tam Nong; sprayed area	(4)	89–91		No other isomers reported									ND
	Dog Bin Kieu; sprayed area	(6)	89–91		No other isomers reported									ND
	Hanoi; background	(5)	89–91		No other isomers reported									n.a.

Table 3 (contd)

Reference	Origin; sample description (and no.)	Coll. period	Anal. meth.	PCDF concentration (ng/kg; ppt)									
				TCDF	PeCDF		HxCDF				HpCDF		OCDF
				2378	12378	23478	123478	123678	123789	234678	1234678	1234789	
Viet Nam (contd)													
Matsuda *et al.* (1994) (contd)	Ca Mau; sprayed area (16)	89–91					No other isomers reported						ND

Analytical methods: All analyses use high-resolution gas chromatography; B, high-resolution mass spectrometry; C, low-resolution mass spectrometry; I, isomer-specific; O, others; N, no information; S, sophisticated clean-up; y, years;

ND, not detected; detection limit in parentheses

Data presented are means. Figures in parentheses are ranges. Levels of congeners not detected at known detection limits (for examples, 0.02 pg/m³) are presented as < 0.02.

CFP, Chemical fertilizer plant; CWI, clinical waste incinerator; MSWI, municipal solid-waste incinerator

*Sample depth: 0–30 m

*Sample depth: 0–20 m

*0–2.5 cm

*0–7.5 cm

Table 4. Concentrations of PCDFs in cow's milk

Reference	Origin; sample description (and no.)		Coll. period	PCDF concentration (ng/kg fat)									
				TCDF	PeCDF		HxCDF				HpCDF		OCDF
				2378	12378	23478	123478	123678	123789	234678	1234678	1234789	
Canada													
Ryan et al. (1990)	6 cities (2% fat)	(6)	85–88	73.3	ND	1.6	ND	ND	ND	ND	ND	NR	NR
Germany													
Beck et al. (1987)	Berlin	(8)	<87	0.7	0.2	1.4	0.9	0.8	NR	0.7	<0.5	NR	<1
Fürst et al. (1990)	North Rhine Westphalia	(10)	89–90	4.1	0.3	2.7	1.7	1.1	NR	1.3	1.5	NR	1.2
Netherlands													
Liem et al. (1991b)			91	0.43	0.06	1.2	0.68	0.58	<0.01	0.65	0.47	<0.01	0.08
Spain													
Ramos et al. (1996)	Asturias	(15)	95	0.34	0.18	0.97	2.04	1.16	ND	1.21	7.21	0.23	8.55
Sweden													
Rappe et al. (1990b)	Gothenburg	(1)	89	0.5	0.1	0.5	0.2	0.1	<0.1	<0.1	0.3	<0.2	<0.2
	Malmö	(1)	89	0.6	0.3	1.2	0.84	0.6	<0.2	0.3	0.5	<0.2	<1.5
	Stockholm	(1)	89	0.4	0.1	0.2	ND	0.4	<0.1	<0.1	0.2	<0.2	<0.3
	Umeå	(1)	89	0.4	0.1	0.2	<0.1	<0.1	<0.1	<0.1	0.2	<0.2	<0.3
	Vaxjo	(1)	89	0.43	0.3	0.7	0.3	0.2	<0.2	0.2	0.4	<0.3	<0.3
Switzerland													
Rappe et al. (1987b)	Bern (retail)	(1)	86?	<0.70	<0.50	2.10	<0.50	0.70	NR	<0.50	<3.00	NR	<5.0
	Bowil (pool)	(1)	86?	<0.49	<0.49	1.61	<0.40	<0.49	NR	<0.47	<1.87	NR	<2.10
	Bowil	(1)	86?	<0.80	<0.50	1.51	<0.60	<0.41	NR	<0.41	<2.98	NR	<2.98
Schmid & Schlatter (1992)	Retail	(9)	90–91	0.24	0.09	1.13	0.56	0.51	0.03	0.61	0.36	0.05	0.18

Table 4 (contd)

Reference	Origin; sample description (and no.)		Coll. period	PCDF concentration (ng/kg fat)									
				TCDF	PeCDF		HxCDF				HpCDF		OCDF
				2378	12378	23478	123478	123678	123789	234678	1234678	1234789	
United Kingdom													
Harrison et al. (1996)	Derbyshire (4% fat assumed)	(47)	91–93	0.25	0.25	0.75	0.5	0.25	0.25	0.25	0.25	0.25	0.25
Startin et al. (1990)	Rural farms (4% fat assumed)	(7)	89	0.2	0.125	0.8	0.425	0.3	0.2	0.3	0.5	0.65	1.025
Wright & Startin (1995)	TDS	Pool	82	6.6	0.21	2.2	1	0.83	<0.13	0.79	1.4	<0.11	1.2
	TDS	Pool	92	<0.37	<0.17	1.2	0.75	0.68	<0.14	0.65	0.69	0.13	23
United States													
Eitzer (1995)	Connecticut (4% fat assumed)	(17)	91	0.217	0.1	0.09	0.425	0.4	0.3	0.35	1.5	0.325	6.25

NR, not reported; ND, not detected and limit of detection not reported; TDS, Total Diet Dtudy

APPENDIX 3

GENETIC AND RELATED EFFECTS

Appendix 3A. Test system code words for genetic and related effects

End-point[a]	Code	Definition

NON-MAMMALIAN SYSTEMS

Prokaryotic systems

D	PRB	Prophage, induction, SOS repair test, DNA strand breaks, cross-links or related damage
D	ECB	*Escherichia coli* (or *E. coli* DNA), DNA strand breaks, cross-links or related damage; DNA repair
D	SAD	*Salmonella typhimurium*, DNA repair-deficient strains, differential toxicity
D	ECD	*Escherichia coli pol* A/W3110-P3478, differential toxicity (spot test)
D	ECL	*Escherichia coli pol* A/W3110-P3478, differential toxicity (liquid suspension test)
D	ERD	*Escherichia coli rec* strains, differential toxicity
D	BSD	*Bacillus subtilis rec* strains, differential toxicity
D	BRD	Other DNA repair-deficient bacteria, differential toxicity
G	BPF	Bacteriophage, forward mutation
G	BPR	Bacteriophage, reverse mutation
G	SAF	*Salmonella typhimurium*, forward mutation
G	SA0	*Salmonella typhimurium* TA100, reverse mutation
G	SA2	*Salmonella typhimurium* TA102, reverse mutation
G	SA3	*Salmonella typhimurium* TA1530, reverse mutation
G	SA4	*Salmonella typhimurium* TA104, reverse mutation
G	SA5	*Salmonella typhimurium* TA1535, reverse mutation
G	SA7	*Salmonella typhimurium* TA1537, reverse mutation
G	SA8	*Salmonella typhimurium* TA1538, reverse mutation
G	SA9	*Salmonella typhimurium* TA98, reverse mutation
G	SAS	*Salmonella typhimurium* (other miscellaneous strains), reverse mutation
G	ECF	*Escherichia coli* exclusive of strain K12, forward mutation
G	ECK	*Escherichia coli* K12, forward or reverse mutation
G	ECW	*Escherichia coli* WP2 *uvr*A, reverse mutation
G	EC2	*Escherichia coli* WP2, reverse mutation
G	ECR	*Escherichia coli* (other miscellaneous strains), reverse mutation
G	BSM	*Bacillus subtilis*, multigene test
G	KPF	*Klebsiella pneumoniae*, forward mutation
G	MAF	*Micrococcus aureus*, forward mutation

---

[a] Endpoints are grouped within each phylogenetic category as follows: A, aneuploidy; C, chromosomal aberrations; D, DNA damage, F, assays of body fluids; G, gene mutation; H, host-mediated assays; I, inhibition of intercellular communication; M, micronuclei; P, sperm morphology; R, mitotic recombination or gene conversion; S, sister chromatid exchange; T, cell transformation

Appendix 3A (contd)

End-point[a]	Code	Definition

NON-MAMMALIAN SYSTEMS (contd)

Lower eukaryotic systems

D	SSB	*Saccharomyces* species, DNA strand breaks, cross-links or related damage
D	SSD	*Saccharomyces* species, DNA repair-deficient strains, differential toxicity
D	SZD	*Schizosaccharomyces pombe*, DNA repair-deficient strains, differential toxicity
R	SCG	*Saccharomyces cerevisiae*, gene conversion
R	SCH	*Saccharomyces cerevisiae*, homozygosis by mitotic recombination or gene conversion
R	SZG	*Schizosaccharomyces pombe*, gene conversion
R	ANG	*Aspergillus nidulans*, genetic crossing-over
G	SCF	*Saccharomyces cerevisiae*, forward mutation
G	SCR	*Saccharomyces cerevisiae*, reverse mutation
G	SGR	*Streptomyces griseoflavus*, reverse mutation
G	STF	*Streptomyces coelicolor*, forward mutation
G	STR	*Streptomyces coelicolor*, reverse mutation
G	SZF	*Schizosaccharomyces pombe*, forward mutation
G	SZR	*Schizosaccharomyces pombe*, reverse mutation
G	ANF	*Aspergillus nidulans*, forward mutation
G	ANR	*Aspergillus nidulans*, reverse mutation
G	NCF	*Neurospora crassa*, forward mutation
G	NCR	*Neurospora crassa*, reverse mutation
G	PSM	*Paramecium* species, mutation
C	PSC	*Paramecium* species, chromosomal aberrations
A	SCN	*Saccharomyces cerevisiae*, aneuploidy
A	ANN	*Aspergillus nidulans*, aneuploidy
A	NCN	*Neurospora crassa*, aneuploidy

Plant systems

D	PLU	Plants, unscheduled DNA synthesis
G	ASM	*Arabidopsis* species, mutation
G	HSM	*Hordeum* species, mutation
G	TSM	*Tradescantia* species, mutation
G	PLM	Plants (other), mutation
S	VFS	*Vicia faba*, sister chromatid exchange
S	PLS	Plants (other), sister chromatid exchange
M	TSI	*Tradescantia* species, micronuclei
M	PLI	Plants (other), micronuclei
C	ACC	*Allium cepa*, chromosomal aberrations
C	HSC	*Hordeum* species, chromosomal aberrations
C	TSC	*Tradescantia* species, chromosomal aberrations
C	VFC	*Vicia faba*, chromosomal aberrations
C	PLC	Plants (other), chromosomal aberrations

Appendix 3A (contd)

End-point[a]	Code	Definition

NON-MAMMALIAN SYSTEMS (contd)

Insect systems

R	DMG	*Drosophila melanogaster*, genetic crossing-over or recombination
G	DMM	*Drosophila melanogaster*, somatic mutation (and recombination)
G	DMX	*Drosophila melanogaster*, sex-linked recessive lethal mutations
C	DMC	*Drosophila melanogaster*, chromosomal aberrations
C	DMH	*Drosophila melanogaster*, heritable translocation test
C	DML	*Drosophila melanogaster*, dominant lethal test
A	DMN	*Drosophila melanogaster*, aneuploidy

MAMMALIAN SYSTEMS

Animal cells in vitro

D	DIA	DNA strand breaks, cross-links or related damage, animal cells *in vitro*
D	RIA	DNA repair exclusive of unscheduled DNA synthesis, animal cells *in vitro*
D	URP	Unscheduled DNA synthesis, rat primary hepatocytes
D	UIA	Unscheduled DNA synthesis, other animal cells *in vitro*
G	GCL	Gene mutation, Chinese hamster lung cells exclusive of V79 *in vitro*
G	GCO	Gene mutation, Chinese hamster ovary cells *in vitro*
G	G9H	Gene mutation, Chinese hamster lung V79 cells, *hprt* locus
G	G9O	Gene mutation, Chinese hamster lung V79 cells, ouabain resistance
G	GML	Gene mutation, mouse lymphoma cells exclusive of L5178Y *in vitro*
G	G5T	Gene mutation, mouse lymphoma L5178Y cells, TK locus
G	G5I	Gene mutation, mouse lymphoma L5178Y cells, all other loci
G	GIA	Gene mutation, other animal cells *in vitro*
S	SIC	Sister chromatid exchange, Chinese hamster cells *in vitro*
S	SIM	Sister chromatid exchange, mouse cells *in vitro*
S	SIR	Sister chromatid exchange, rat cells *in vitro*
S	SIS	Sister chromatid exchange, Syrian hamster cells *in vitro*
S	SIT	Sister chromatid exchange, transformed animal cells *in vitro*
S	SIA	Sister chromatid exchange, other animal cells *in vitro*
M	MIA	Micronucleus test, animal cells *in vitro*
C	CIC	Chromosomal aberrations, Chinese hamster cells *in vitro*
C	CIM	Chromosomal aberrations, mouse cells *in vitro*
C	CIR	Chromosomal aberrations, rat cells *in vitro*
C	CIS	Chromosomal aberrations, Syrian hamster cells *in vitro*
C	CIT	Chromosomal aberrations, transformed animal cells *in vitro*
C	CIA	Chromosomal aberrations, other animal cells *in vitro*
A	AIA	Aneuploidy, animal cells *in vitro*
T	TBM	Cell transformation, BALB/c 3T3 mouse cells
T	TCM	Cell transformation, C3H 10T1/2 mouse cells
T	TCS	Cell transformation, Syrian hamster embryo cells, clonal assay
T	TFS	Cell transformation, Syrian hamster embryo cells, focus assay

Appendix 3A (contd)

End-point[a]	Code	Definition

MAMMALIAN SYSTEMS (contd)

Animal cells in vitro *(contd)*

T	TPM	Cell transformation, mouse prostate cells
T	TCL	Cell transformation, other established cell lines
T	TRR	Cell transformation, RLV/Fischer rat embryo cells
T	T7R	Cell transformation, SA7/rat cells
T	T7S	Cell transformation, SA7/Syrian hamster embryo cells
T	TEV	Cell transformation, other viral enhancement systems
T	TVI	Cell transformation, treated *in vivo*, scored *in vitro*

Human cells in vitro

D	DIH	DNA strand breaks, cross-links or related damage, human cells *in vitro*
D	RIH	DNA repair exclusive of unscheduled DNA synthesis, human cells *in vitro*
D	UHF	Unscheduled DNA synthesis, human fibroblasts *in vitro*
D	UHL	Unscheduled DNA synthesis, human lymphocytes *in vitro*
D	UHT	Unscheduled DNA synthesis, transformed human cells *in vitro*
D	UIH	Unscheduled DNA synthesis, other human cells *in vitro*
G	GIH	Gene mutation, human cells *in vitro*
S	SHF	Sister chromatid exchange, human fibroblasts *in vitro*
S	SHL	Sister chromatid exchange, human lymphocytes *in vitro*
S	SHT	Sister chromatid exchange, transformed human cells *in vitro*
S	SIH	Sister chromatid exchange, other human cells *in vitro*
M	MIH	Micronucleus test, human cells *in vitro*
C	CHF	Chromosomal aberrations, human fibroblasts *in vitro*
C	CHL	Chromosomal aberrations, human lymphocytes *in vitro*
C	CHT	Chromosomal aberrations, transformed human cells *in vitro*
C	CIH	Chromosomal aberrations, other human cells *in vitro*
A	AIH	Aneuploidy, human cells *in vitro*
T	TIH	Cell transformation, human cells *in vitro*

Body fluid and host-mediated assays

F	BFA	Body fluids from animals, microbial mutagenicity
F	BFH	Body fluids from humans, microbial mutagenicity
H	HMA	Host-mediated assay, animal cells in animal hosts
H	HMH	Host-mediated assay, human cells in animal hosts
H	HMM	Host-mediated assay, microbial cells in ahimal hosts

Animals in vivo

D	DVA	DNA strand breaks, cross-links or related damage, animal cells *in vivo*
D	RVA	DNA repair exclusive of unscheduled DNA synthesis, animal cells *in vivo*
D	UPR	Unscheduled DNA synthesis, rat hepatocytes *in vivo*
D	UVC	Unscheduled DNA synthesis, hamster cells *in vivo*
D	UVM	Unscheduled DNA synthesis, mouse cells *in vivo*

Appendix 3A (contd)

End-point[a]	Code	Definition

MAMMALIAN SYSTEMS (contd)

Animals in vivo *(contd)*

D	UVR	Unscheduled DNA synthesis, other rat cells *in vivo*
D	UVA	Unscheduled DNA synthesis, other animal cells *in vivo*
G	GVA	Gene mutation, animal cells *in vivo*
G	MST	Mouse spot test
G	SLP	Mouse specific locus test, postspermatogonia
G	SLO	Mouse specific locus test, other stages
S	SVA	Sister chromatid exchange, animal cells *in vivo*
M	MVM	Micronucleus test, mice *in vivo*
M	MVR	Micronucleus test, rats *in vivo*
M	MVC	Micronucleus test, hamsters *in vivo*
M	MVA	Micronucleus test, other animals *in vivo*
C	CBA	Chromosomal aberrations, animal bone-marrow cells *in vivo*
C	CLA	Chromosomal aberrations, animal leucocytes *in vivo*
C	CCC	Chromosomal aberrations, spermatocytes treated *in vivo*, spermatocytes observed
C	CGC	Chromosomal aberrations, spermatogonia treated *in vivo*, spermatocytes observed
C	CGG	Chromosomal aberrations, spermatogonia treated *in vivo*, spermatogonia observed
C	COE	Chromosomal aberrations, oocytes or embryos treated *in vivo*
C	CVA	Chromosomal aberrations, other animal cells *in vivo*
C	DLM	Dominant lethal test, mice
C	DLR	Dominant lethal test, rats
C	MHT	Mouse heritable translocation test
A	AVA	Aneuploidy, animal cells *in vivo*
T	TVI	Cell transformation, treated *in vivo*, scored *in vitro*

Humans in vivo

D	DVH	DNA strand breaks, cross-links or related damage, human cells *in vivo*
D	UBH	Unscheduled DNA synthesis, human bone-marrow cells *in vivo*
D	UVH	Unscheduled DNA synthesis, other human cells *in vivo*
S	SLH	Sister chromatid exchange, human lymphocytes *in vivo*
S	SVH	Sister chromatid exchange, other human cells *in vivo*
M	MVH	Micronucleus test, human cells *in vivo*
C	CBH	Chromosomal aberrations, human bone-marrow cells *in vivo*
C	CLH	Chromosomal aberrations, human lymphocytes *in vivo*
C	CVH	Chromosomal aberrations, other human cells *in vivo*
A	AVH	Aneuploidy, human cells *in vivo*

Test systems not shown on activity profiles

D	BID	Binding (covalent) to DNA *in vitro*
D	BIP	Binding (covalent) to RNA or protein *in vitro*

Appendix 3A (contd)

End-point[a]	Code	Definition
		Test systems not shown on activity profiles (contd)
D	BVD	Binding (covalent) to DNA, animal cells *in vivo*
D	BVP	Binding (covalent) to RNA or protein, animal cells *in vivo*
D	BHD	Binding (covalent) to DNA, human cells *in vivo*
D	BHP	Binding (covalent) to RNA or protein, human cells *in vivo*
I	ICR	Inhibition of intercellular communication, animal cells *in vitro*
I	ICH	Inhibition of intercellular communication, human cells *in vitro*
P	SPF	Sperm morphology, F1 mice *in vivo*
P	SPM	Sperm morphology, mice *in vivo*
P	SPR	Sperm morphology, rats *in vivo*
P	SPH	Sperm morphology, humans *in vivo*

Appendix 3B: 1. Summary table of genetic and related effects of 2,7-dichlorodibenzo-*para*-dioxin

Non-mammalian systems				Mammalian systems			
				In vitro		*In vivo*	
Proka-ryotes	Lower eukaryotes	Plants	Insects	Animal cells	Human cells	Animals	Humans
D G	D R G A	D G C	R G C A	D G S M C A T I	D G S M C A T I	D G S M C DL A	D S M C A
−¹				−¹			

A, aneuploidy; C, chromosomal aberrations; D, DNA damage; DL, dominant lethal mutation; G, gene mutation; I, inhibition of intercellular communication; M, micronuclei; R, mitotic recombination and gene conversion; S, sister chromatid exchange; T, cell transformation

In completing the table, the following symbols indicate the consensus of the Working Group with regard to the results for each end-point:

+   considered to be positive for the specific end-point and level of biological complexity
+¹   considered to be positive, but only one valid study was available to the Working Group
−   considered to be negative
−¹   considered to be negative, but only one valid study was available to the Working Group
?   considered to be equivocal or inconclusive (e.g. there were contradictory results from different laboratories; there were confounding exposures; the results were equivocal)

Appendix 3B: 2. Summary table of genetic and related effects of 2,3,7,8-TCDD

Non-mammalian systems				Mammalian systems			
Proka-ryotes	Lower eukaryotes	Plants	Insects	In vitro		In vivo	
				Animal cells	Human cells	Animals	Humans
D G	D R G A	D G C	R G C A	D G S M C A T I	D G S M C A T I	D G S M C DL A	D S M C A
–				?　　　　　–¹ ?	–¹ 　+¹ +¹　　?	+　–　–¹ –¹	–¹　　　–

A, aneuploidy; C, chromosomal aberrations; D, DNA damage; DL, dominant lethal mutation; G, gene mutation; I, inhibition of intercellular communication; M, micronuclei; R, mitotic recombination and gene conversion; S, sister chromatid exchange; T, cell transformation

In completing the table, the following symbols indicate the consensus of the Working Group with regard to the results for each end-point:

+　considered to be positive for the specific end-point and level of biological complexity

+¹　considered to be positive, but only one valid study was available to the Working Group

–　considered to be negative

–¹　considered to be negative, but only one valid study was available to the Working Group

?　considered to be equivocal or inconclusive (e.g. there were contradictory results from different laboratories; there were confounding exposures; the results were equivocal)

Appendix 3B: 3. Summary table of genetic and related effects of octachlorodibenzo-*para*-dioxin

Non-mammalian systems				Mammalian systems			
				In vitro		*In vivo*	
Prokaryotes	Lower eukaryotes	Plants	Insects	Animal cells	Human cells	Animals	Humans
D G	D R G A	D G C	R G C A	D G S M C A T I	D G S M C A T I	D G S M C DL A	D S M C A
$-^1$							

A, aneuploidy; C, chromosomal aberrations; D, DNA damage; DL, dominant lethal mutation; G, gene mutation; I, inhibition of intercellular communication; M, micronuclei; R, mitotic recombination and gene conversion; S, sister chromatid exchange; T, cell transformation

In completing the table, the following symbols indicate the consensus of the Working Group with regard to the results for each end-point:

+   considered to be positive for the specific end-point and level of biological complexity

$+^1$ considered to be positive, but only one valid study was available to the Working Group

–   considered to be negative

$-^1$ considered to be negative, but only one valid study was available to the Working Group

?   considered to be equivocal or inconclusive (e.g. there were contradictory results from different laboratories; there were confounding exposures; the results were equivocal)

Appendix 3B: 4. Summary table of genetic and related effects of 2,3,4,7,8-PeCDF

Non-mammalian systems				Mammalian systems			
				In vitro		*In vivo*	
Proka-ryotes	Lower eukaryotes	Plants	Insects	Animal cells	Human cells	Animals	Humans
D G	D R G A	D G C	R G C A	D G S M C A T I	D G S M C A T I	D G S M C DL A	D S M C A
					$+^I$ $+^I$		

A, aneuploidy; C, chromosomal aberrations; D, DNA damage; DL, dominant lethal mutation; G, gene mutation; I, inhibition of intercellular communication; M, micronuclei; R, mitotic recombination and gene conversion; S, sister chromatid exchange; T, cell transformation

In completing the table, the following symbols indicate the consensus of the Working Group with regard to the results for each end-point:

+   considered to be positive for the specific end-point and level of biological complexity

$+^I$ considered to be positive, but only one valid study was available to the Working Group

–   considered to be negative

$–^I$ considered to be negative, but only one valid study was available to the Working Group

?   considered to be equivocal or inconclusive (e.g. there were contradictory results from different laboratories; there wer   e confounding exposures; the results were equivocal)

APPENDIX 3C

ACTIVITY PROFILES FOR
GENETIC AND RELATED EFFECTS

Methods

The x-axis of the activity profile (Waters *et al.*, 1987, 1988) represents the bioassays in phylogenetic sequence by end-point, and the values on the y-axis represent the logarithmically transformed lowest effective doses (LED) and highest ineffective doses (HID) tested. The term 'dose', as used in this report, does not take into consideration length of treatment or exposure and may therefore be considered synonymous with concentration. In practice, the concentrations used in all the in-vitro tests were converted to μg/ml, and those for in-vivo tests were expressed as mg/kg bw. Because dose units are plotted on a log scale, differences in the relative molecular masses of compounds do not, in most cases, greatly influence comparisons of their activity profiles. Conventions for dose conversions are given below.

Profile-line height (the magnitude of each bar) is a function of the LED or HID, which is associated with the characteristics of each individual test system — such as population size, cell-cycle kinetics and metabolic competence. Thus, the detection limit of each test system is different, and, across a given activity profile, responses will vary substantially. No attempt is made to adjust or relate responses in one test system to those of another.

Line heights are derived as follows: for negative test results, the highest dose tested without appreciable toxicity is defined as the HID. A single dose tested with a negative result is considered to be equivalent to the HID. Similarly, for positive results, the LED is recorded. If the original data were analysed statistically by the author, the dose recorded is that at which the response was significant ($p < 0.05$). If the available data were not analysed statistically, the dose required to produce an effect is estimated as follows: when a dose-related positive response is observed with two or more doses, the lower of the doses is taken as the LED; a single dose resulting in a positive response is considered to be equivalent to the LED.

In order to accommodate both the wide range of doses encountered and positive and negative responses on a continuous scale, doses are transformed logarithmically, so that effective (LED) and ineffective (HID) doses are represented by positive and negative numbers, respectively. The response, or logarithmic dose unit (LDUij), for a given test system i and chemical j is represented by the expressions

$LDU_{ij} = -\log_{10}$ (dose), for HID values; LDU ≤ 0

and   (1)

$LDU_{ij} = -\log_{10}$ (dose $\times 10^{-5}$), for LED values; LDU ≥ 0.

These simple relationships define a dose range of 0 to –5 logarithmic units for ineffective doses (1–100 000 μg/mL or mg/kg bw) and 0 to +8 logarithmic units for effective doses (100 000–0.001 μg/mL or mg/kg bw). A scale illustrating the LDU values is shown in **Figure 1**. Negative responses at doses less than 1 μg/mL (mg/kg bw) are set equal to 1. Effectively, an LED value $\geq$ 100 000 or an HID value ≤ 1 produces an LDU = 0; no quantitative information is gained from such extreme values. The dotted lines at the levels of log dose units 1 and –1 define a 'zone of uncertainty' in which positive results are reported at such high doses (between 10 000 and 100 000 μg/mL or mg/kg bw) or negative results are reported at such low doses (1 to 10 μg/ml or mg/kg bw) as to call into question the adequacy of the test.

Fig. 1. Scale of log dose units used on the y-axis of activity profiles

Positive (μg/mL or mg/kg bw)		Log dose units	
0.001	....	8	----
0.01	....	7	--
0.1	....	6	--
1.0	....	5	--
10	....	4	--
100	....	3	--
1000	....	2	--
10 000	....	1	--
100 000	.... 1	0	----
	.... 10	-1	--
	.... 100	-2	--
	.... 1000	-3	--
	.... 10 000	-4	--
	.... 100 000	-5	----

Negative
(μg/mL or mg/kg bw)

In practice, an activity profile is computer generated. A data entry programme is used to store abstracted data from published reports. A sequential file (in ASCII) is created for each compound, and a record within that file consists of the name and Chemical Abstracts Service number of the compound, a three-letter code for the test system (see below), the qualitative test result (with and without an exogenous metabolic system), dose (LED or HID), citation number and additional source information. An abbreviated citation for each publication is stored in a segment of a record accessing both the test data file and the citation file. During processing of the data file, an average of the logarithmic values of the data subset is calculated, and the length of the profile line represents this average value. All dose values are plotted for each profile line, regardless of whether results are positive or negative. Results obtained in the absence of an exogenous metabolic system are indicated by a bar (–), and results obtained in the presence of an exogenous metabolic system are indicated by a caret (∧). When all results for a given assay are either positive or negative, the mean of the LDU values is plotted as a solid line; when conflicting data are reported for the same assay (i.e. both positive and negative results), the majority data are shown by a solid line and the minority data by a dashed line (drawn to the extreme conflicting response). In the few cases in which the numbers of positive and negative results are equal, the solid line is drawn in the positive direction and the maximal negative response is indicated with a dashed line. Profile lines are identified by three-letter code words representing the commonly used tests. Code words for most of the test systems in current use in genetic toxicology were defined for the US Environmental Protection Agency's GENE-TOX Program (Waters, 1979; Waters & Auletta, 1981). For *IARC Monographs* Supplement 6, Volume 44 and subsequent volumes, including this publication, codes were redefined in a manner that should facilitate inclusion of additional tests. Naming conventions are described below.

Data listings are presented in the text and include end-point and test codes, a short test code definition, results, either with or without an exogenous metabolic system, the associated LED or HID value and a short citation. Test codes are organized phylogenetically and by end-point from left to right across each activity profile and from top to bottom of the corresponding data listing. End-points are defined as follows: A, aneuploidy; C, chromosomal aberrations; D, DNA damage; F, assays of body fluids; G, gene mutation; H, host-mediated assays; I, inhibition of intercellular communication; M, micronuclei; P, sperm morphology; R, mitotic recombination or gene conversion; S, sister chromatid exchange; and T, cell transformation.

Dose conversions for activity profiles

Doses are converted to μg/mL for in-vitro tests and to mg/kg bw per day for in-vivo experiments.

1. In-vitro test systems
    (a) Weight/volume converts directly to μg/ml.
    (b) Molar (M) concentration × molecular weight = mg/mL = 10^3 μg/mL; mM concentration × molecular weight = μg/mL.
    (c) Soluble solids expressed as % concentration are assumed to be in units of mass per volume (i.e. 1% = 0.01 g/mL = 10 000 μg/mL; also, 1 ppm = 1 μg/mL).
    (d) Liquids and gases expressed as % concentration are assumed to be given in units of volume per volume. Liquids are converted to weight per volume using the density (D) of the solution (D = g/mL). Gases are converted from volume to mass using the ideal gas law, PV = nRT. For exposure at 20–37 °C at standard atmospheric pressure, 1% (v/v) = 0.4 μg/ml × molecular weight of the gas. Also, 1 ppm (v/v) = 4×10^{-5} μg/mL × molecular weight.

(e)   In microbial plate tests, it is usual for the doses to be reported as weight/plate, whereas concentrations are required to enter data on the activity profile chart. While remaining cognisant of the errors involved in the process, it is assumed that a 2.7-ml volume of top agar is delivered to each plate and that the test substance remains in solution within it; concentrations are derived from the reported weight/plate values by dividing by this arbitrary volume if the actual top agar volume is not reported. For spot tests, a 1-ml volume is used in the calculation.

(f)   Conversion of particulate concentrations given in $\mu g/cm^2$ is based on the area (A) of the dish and the volume of medium per dish; i.e. for a 100-mm dish: $A = \pi R^2 = \pi \times (5 \text{ cm})^2 = 78.5 \text{ cm}^2$. If the volume of medium is 10 mL, then 78.5 cm^2 = 10 mL and 1 cm^2 = 0.13 mL.

2.   In-vitro systems using in-vivo activation

For the body fluid-urine (BF-) test, the concentration used is the dose (in mg/kg bw) of the compound administered to test animals or patients.

3.   In-vivo test systems

(a)   Doses are converted to mg/kg bw per day of exposure, assuming 100% absorption. Standard values are used for each sex and species of rodent, including body weight and average intake per day, as reported by Gold et al. (1984). For example, in a test using male mice fed 50 ppm of the agent in the diet, the standard food intake per day is 12% of body weight, and the conversion is dose = 50 ppm × 12% = 6 mg/kg bw per day.

Standard values used for humans are: weight—males, 70 kg; females, 55 kg; surface area, 1.7 m^2; inhalation rate, 20 L/min for light work, 30 L/min for mild exercise.

(b)   When reported, the dose at the target site is used. For example, doses given in studies of lymphocytes of humans exposed in vivo are the measured blood concentrations in μg/mL.

Codes for test systems

For specific nonmammalian test systems, the first two letters of the three-letter code word define the test organism (e.g. SA- for *Salmonella typhimurium*, EC- for *Escherichia coli*). If the species is not known, the convention used is -S-. The third letter may be used to define the tester strain (e.g. SA8 for *S. typhimurium* TA1538, ECW for *E. coli* WP2*uvr*A). When strain designation is not indicated, the third letter is used to define the specific genetic end-point under investigation (e.g. --D for differential toxicity, --F for forward mutation, --G for gene conversion or genetic crossing-over, --N for aneuploidy, --R for reverse mutation, --U for unscheduled DNA synthesis). The third letter may also be used to define the general end-point under investigation when a more complete definition is not possible or relevant (e.g. --M for mutation, --C for chromosomal aberration). For mammalian test systems, the first letter of the three-letter code word defines the genetic end-point under investigation: A-- for aneuploidy, B-- for binding,

C-- for chromosomal aberration, D-- for DNA strand breaks, G-- for gene mutation, I-- for inhibition of intercellular communication, M-- for micronucleus formation, R-- for DNA repair, S-- for sister chromatid exchange, T-- for cell transformation and U-- for unscheduled DNA synthesis.

For animal (i.e. non-human) test systems *in vitro*, when the cell type is not specified, the code letters -IA are used. For such assays *in vivo*, when the animal species is not specified, the code letters -VA are used. Commonly used animal species are identified by the third letter (e.g. --C for Chinese hamster, --M for mouse, --R for rat, --S for Syrian hamster).

For test systems using human cells *in vitro*, when the cell type is not specified, the code letters -IH are used. For assays on humans *in vivo*, when the cell type is not specified, the code letters -VH are used. Otherwise, the second letter specifies the cell type under investigation (e.g. -BH for bone marrow, -LH for lymphocytes).

Some other specific coding conventions used for mammalian systems are as follows: BF- for body fluids, HM- for host-mediated, --L for leukocytes or lymphocytes *in vitro* (-AL, animals; -HL, humans), -L- for leukocytes *in vivo* (-LA, animals; -LH, humans), --T for transformed cells.

Note that these are examples of major conventions used to define the assay code words. The alphabetized listing of codes must be examined to confirm a specific code word. As might be expected from the limitation to three symbols, some codes do not fit the naming conventions precisely. In a few cases, test systems are defined by first-letter code words, for example: MST, mouse spot test; SLP, mouse specific locus mutation, postspermatogonia; SLO, mouse specific locus mutation, other stages; DLM, dominant lethal mutation in mice; DLR, dominant lethal mutation in rats; MHT, mouse heritable translocation.

The genetic activity profiles and listings were prepared in collaboration with Integrated Laboratory System (ILS) under contract to the United States Environmental Protection Agency; ILS also determined the doses used. The references cited in each genetic activity profile listing can be found in the list of references in the appropriate monograph.

References

Garrett, N.E., Stack, H.F., Gross, M.R. & Waters, M.D. (1984) An analysis of the spectra of genetic activity produced by known or suspected human carcinogens. *Mutat. Res.*, **134**, 89–111

Gold, L.S., Sawyer, C.B., Magaw, R., Backman, G.M., de Veciana, M., Levinson, R., Hooper, N.K., Havender, W.R., Bernstein, L., Peto, R., Pike, M.C. & Ames, B.N. (1984) A carcinogenic potency database of the standardized results of animal bioassays. *Environ. Health Perspect.*, **58**, 9–319

Waters, M.D. (1979) *The GENE-TOX program*. In: Hsie, A.W., O'Neill, J.P. & McElheny, V.K., eds, *Mammalian Cell Mutagenesis: The Maturation of Test Systems* (Banbury Report 2), Cold Spring Harbor, NY, CSH Press, pp. 449–467

Waters, M.D. & Auletta, A. (1981) The GENE-TOX program: genetic activity evaluation. *J. chem. Inf. comput. Sci.*, **21**, 35–38

Waters, M.D., Stack, H.F., Brady, A.L., Lohman, P.H.M., Haroun, L. & Vainio, H. (1987) Appendix 1: Activity profiles for genetic and related tests. In: *IARC Monographs on the Evaluation of the Carcinogenic Risk of Chemicals to Humans*, Suppl. 6, *Genetic and Related Effects: An Updating of Selected* IARC Monographs *from Volumes 1 to 42*, Lyon, IARC, pp. 687–696

Waters, M.D., Stack, H.F., Brady, A.L., Lohman, P.H.M., Haroun, L. & Vainio, H. (1988) Use of computerized data listings and activity profiles of genetic and related effects in the review of 195 compounds. *Mutat. Res.*, **205**, 295–312

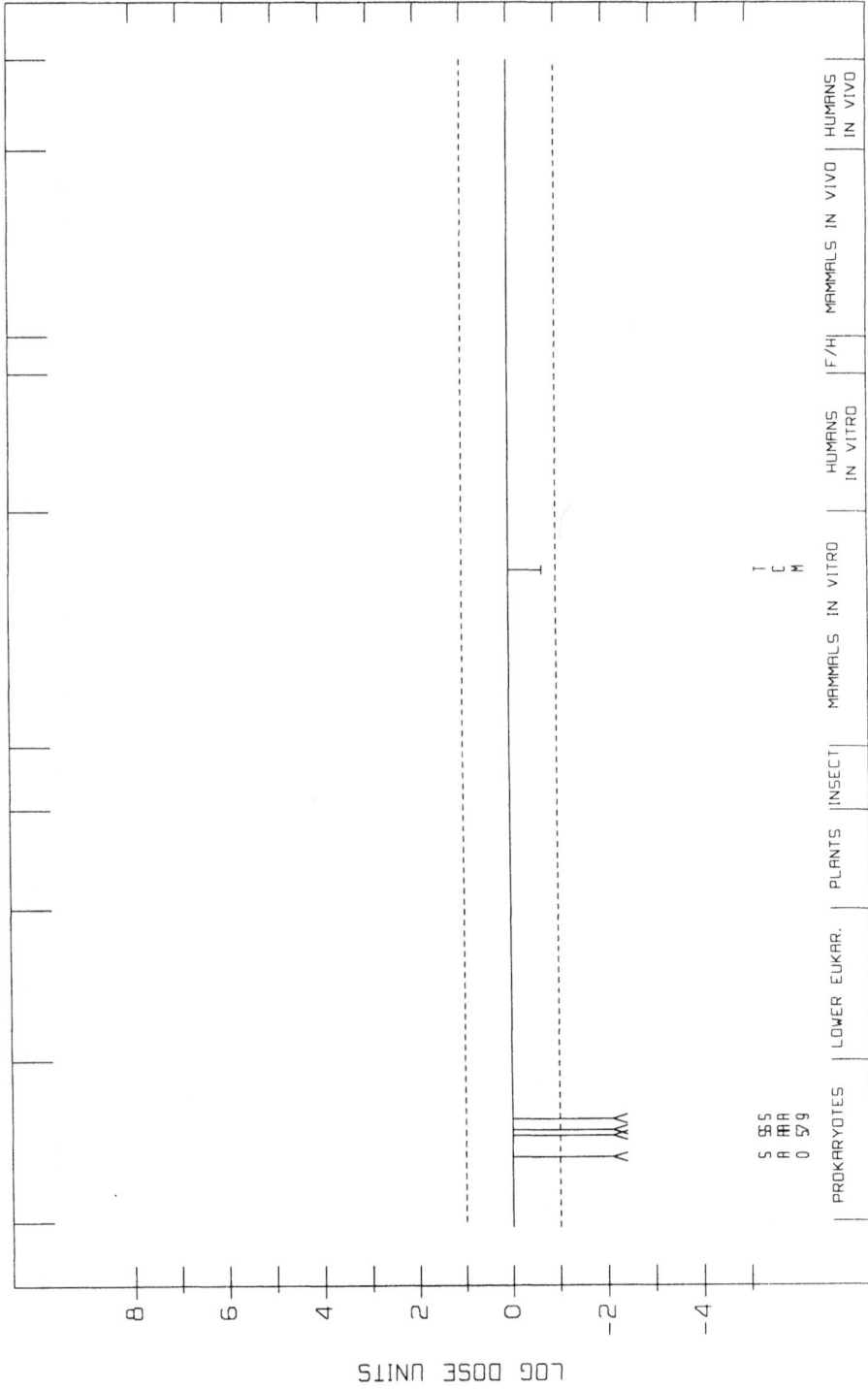

DICHLORODIBENZO-p-DIOXIN, 2,7-   33857-26-0

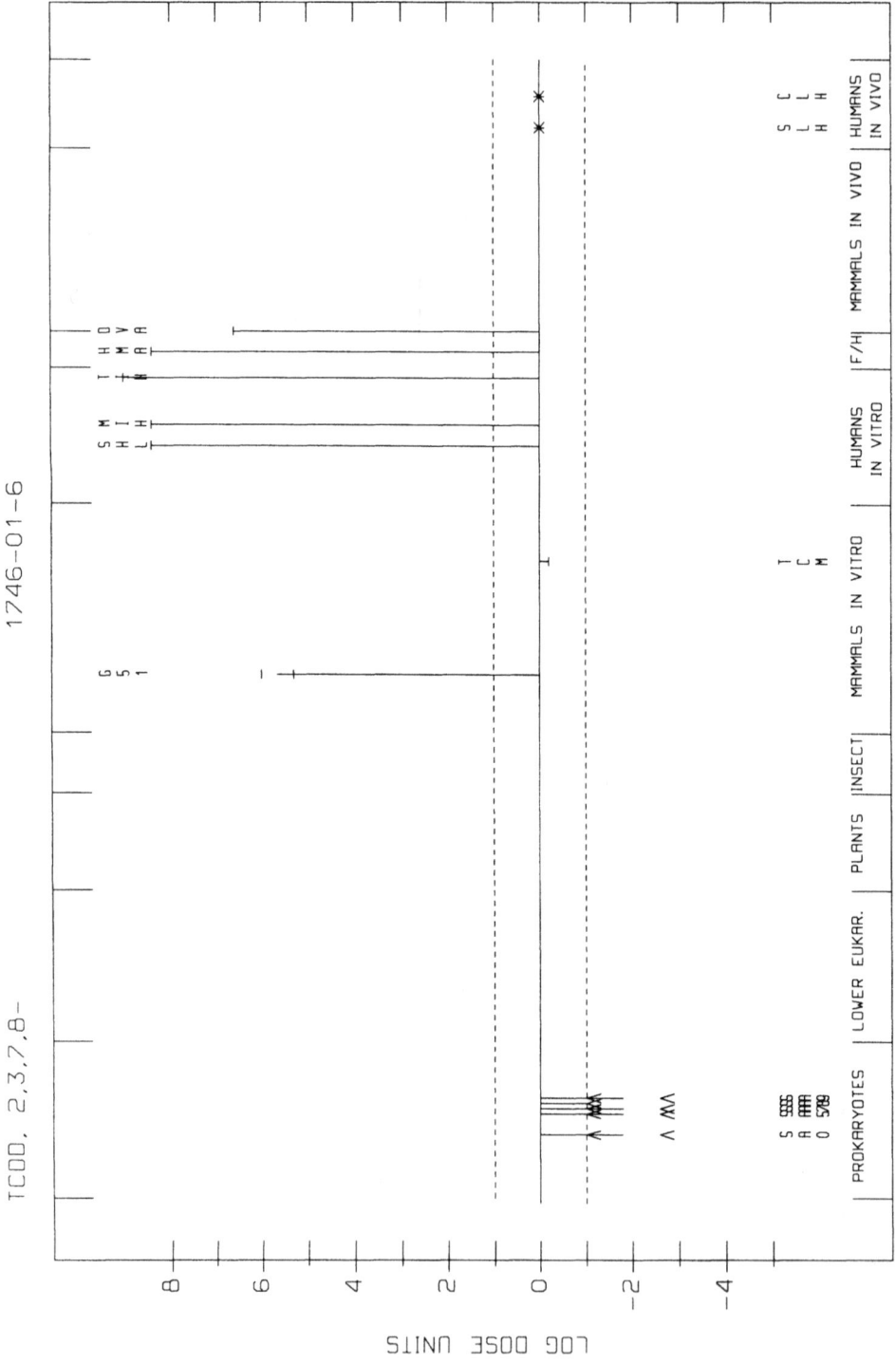

1746-01-6

TCDD, 2,3,7,8-

LOG DOSE UNITS

PROKARYOTES | LOWER EUKAR. | PLANTS | INSECT | MAMMALS IN VITRO | HUMANS IN VITRO | F/H | MAMMALS IN VIVO | HUMANS IN VIVO

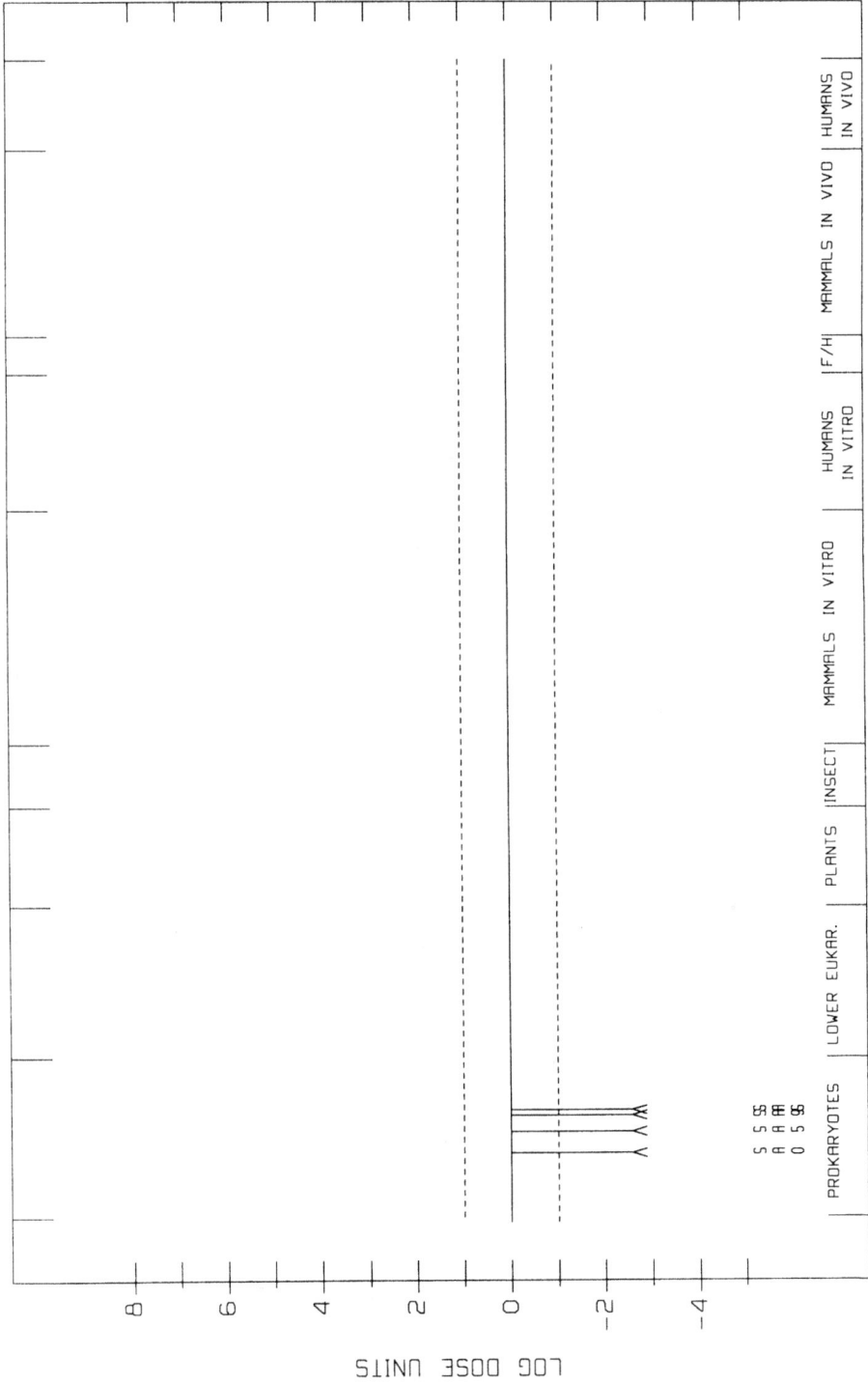

OCTACHLORODIBENZO-p-DIOXIN

3268-87-9

LOG DOSE UNITS

PROKARYOTES | LOWER EUKAR. | PLANTS | INSECT | MAMMALS IN VITRO | HUMANS IN VITRO | F/H | MAMMALS IN VIVO | HUMANS IN VIVO

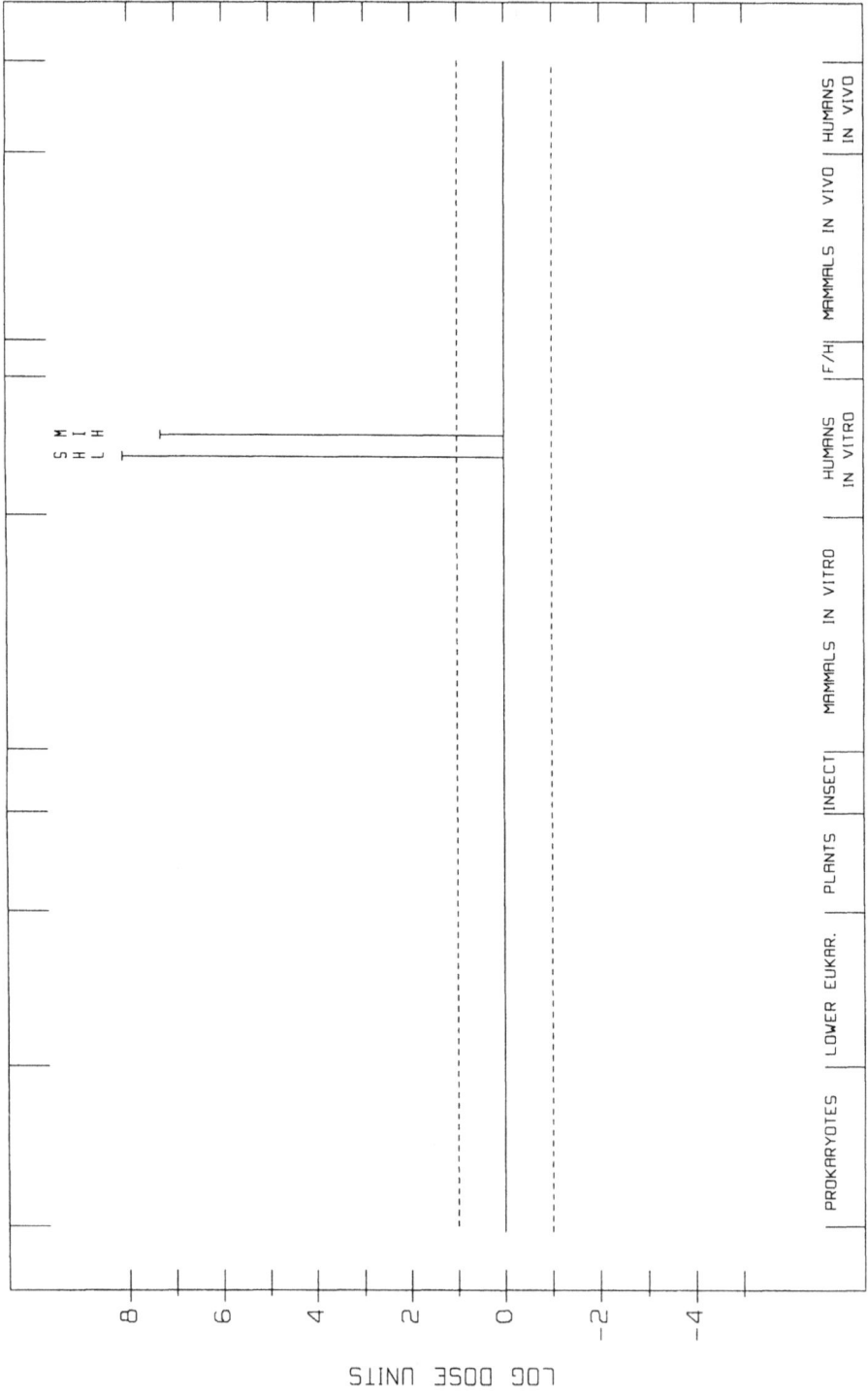

PeCDF, 2,3,4,7,8—

57117-31-4

LOG DOSE UNITS

REFERENCES

Abad, E., Caixach, J. & Rivera, J. (1996) Analysis of PCDD/PCDF from emissions sources and ambient air in Northeast of Spain. *Organohalogen Compounds*, **28**, 175–180

Abbott, B.D. (1995) Review of the interaction between TCDD and glucocorticoids in embryonic palate. *Toxicology*, **105**, 365–373

Abbott, B.D. (1996) Developmental toxicity of dioxin: searching for the cellular and molecular basis of morphological responses. In: Kavlock, R.J., ed., *Drug Toxicity in Embryonic Development*, Section III, *Pathogenesis and Mechanisms of Drug Toxicity in Development*, Berlin, Springer Verlag

Abbott, B.D. & Birnbaum, L.S. (1989a) TCDD alters medial epithelial cell differentiation during palatogenesis. *Toxicol. appl. Pharmacol.*, **99**, 276–286

Abbott, B.D. & Birnbaum, L.S. (1989b) Cellular alterations and enhanced induction of cleft palate after coadministration of retinoic acid and TCDD. *Toxicol. appl. Pharmacol.*, **99**, 287–301

Abbott, B.D. & Birnbaum, L.S. (1990a) TCDD-induced altered expression of growth factors may have a role in producing cleft palate and enhancing the incidence of clefts after coadministration of retinoic acid and TCDD. *Toxicol. appl. Pharmacol.*, **106**, 418–432

Abbott, B.D. & Birnbaum, L.S. (1990b) Effects of TCDD on embryonic ureteric epithelial EGF receptor expression and cell proliferation. *Teratology*, **41**, 71–84

Abbott, B.D. & Birnbaum, L.S. (1991) TCDD exposure of human embryonic palatal shelves in organ culture alters the differentiation of medial epithelial cells. *Teratology*, **43**, 119–131

Abbott, B.D., Birnbaum, L.S. & Pratt, R.M. (1987) TCDD-induced hyperplasia of the ureteral epithelium produces hydronephrosis in murine fetuses. *Teratology*, *35*, 329–334

Abbott, B.D., Diliberto, J.J. & Birnbaum, L.S. (1989) 2,3,7,8-Tetrachlorodibenzo-*p*-dioxin alters embryonic palatal medial epithelial cell differentiation *in vitro*. *Toxicol. appl. Pharmacol.*, **100**, 119–131

Abbott, B.D., Perdew, G.H. & Birnbaum, L.S. (1994a) Ah receptor in embryonic mouse palate and effects of TCDD on receptor expression. *Toxicol. appl. Pharmacol.*, **126**, 16–25

Abbott, B.D., Perdew, G.H., Fantel, A.G. & Birnbaum, L.S. (1994b) Gene expression in human palatal shelves exposed to TCDD in organ culture. *Teratology*, **49**, 378

Abbott, B.D., Perdew, G.H., Buckalew, A.R. & Birnbaum, L.S. (1994c) Interactive regulation of Ah and glucocorticoid receptors in the synergistic induction of cleft palate by 2,3,7,8-tetrachlorodibenzo-*p*-dioxin and hydrocortisone. *Toxicol. appl. Pharmacol.*, **128**, 138–150

Abbott, B.D., Probst, M.R. & Perdew, G.H. (1994d) Immunohistochemical double-staining for Ah receptor and Arnt in human embryonic palatal shelves. *Teratology*, **50**, 361–366

Abernethy, D.J. & Boreiko, C.J. (1987) Promotion of C3H/10T1/2 morphological transformation by polychlorinated dibenzo-*p*-dioxin isomers. *Carcinogenesis*, **8**, 1485–1490

Abernethy, D.J., Greenlee, W.F., Huband, J.C. & Boreiko, C.J. (1985) 2,3,7,8-Tetrachloro-dibenzo-*p*-dioxin (TCDD) promotes the transformation of C3H/10T1/2 cells. *Carcinogenesis*, **6**, 651–653

Abid, A., Bouchon, I., Siest, G. & Sabolovic, N. (1995) Glucuronidation in the Caco-2 human intestinal cell line: induction of UDP-glucuronosyltransferase 1*6. *Biochem. Pharmacol.*, **50**, 557–561

Abraham, K., Krowke, R. & Neubert, D. (1988) Pharmacokinetics and biological activity of 2,3,7,8-tetrachlorodibenzopdioxin. 1. Dose-dependent tissue distribution and induction of hepatic ethoxyresorufin O-deethylase in rats following a single injection. *Arch. Toxicol.*, **62**, 359–368

Abraham, K., Wiesmuller, T., Brunner, H., Krowke, R., Hagenmaier, H. & Neubert, D. (1989) Absorption and tissue distribution of various polychlorinated dibenzopdioxins and dibenzo-furans (PCDDs and PCDFs) in the rat. *Arch. Toxicol.*, **63**, 193–202

Abraham, K., Hille, A., Ende, M. & Helge, H. (1994) Intake and fecall excretion of PCDDs, PCDFs, HCB and PCBs (138, 153, 180) in a breast-fed and formula-fed infant. *Chemosphere*, **29**, 2279–2286

Abraham, K., Steuerwald, U., Päpke, O., Ball, M., Lis, A., Weihe, P. & Helge, H. (1995a) Concentrations of PCDDs, PCDFs and PCBs in human perinatal samples from Faroe Islands and Berlin. *Organohalogen Compounds*, **26**, 213–218

Abraham, K., Alder, L., Beck, H., Mathar, W., Palavinskas, R., Steuerwald, U. & Weihe, P. (1995b) Organochlorine compounds in human milk and pilot whale from Faroe Islands. *Organohalogen Compounds*, **26**, 63–7

Ackermann, M.F., Gasiewicz, T.A., Lamm, K.R., Germolec, D.R., & Luster, M.I. (1989) Selective inhibition of polymorphonuclear neutrophil activity by 2,3,7,8- tetrachlorodibenzo-*p*-dioxin. *Toxicol. appl. Pharmacol.*, **101**, 470–480

Adriaens, P., Fu, Q. & Grbic-Galic, D. (1995) Bioavailability and transformation of highly chlorinated dibenzo-*p*-dioxins and dibenzofurans in anaerobic soils and sediments. *Environ. Sci. Technol.*, **29**, 2252–2260

Ahlborg, U.G., Håkansson, H., Waern, F. & Hanberg, A. (1988) *Nordisk Dioxinrisk Bedömning* (Nordic dioxin risk evaluation) (Nord 49), Copenhagen, Nordic Council of Ministers

Ahlborg, U.G., Hakansson, H., Lindstrom, G. & Rappe, C. (1990) Studies on the retention of individual polychlorinated dibenzofurans (PCDFs) in the liver of different species. *Chemosphere*, **20**, 1235

Ahlborg, U.G., Brouwer, A., Fingerhut, M.A., Jacobson, J.L., Jacobson, S.W., Kennedy, S.W., Kettrup, A.A.F., Koeman, J.H., Poiger, H., Rappe, C., Safe, S.H., Seegal, R.F., Tuomisto, J. & van den Berg, M. (1992a) Impact of polychlorinated dibenzo-*p*-dioxins, dibenzofurans and biphenyls on human and environmental health, with special emphasis on application of the toxic equivalency factor concept. *Europ. J. Pharmacol.-environ. Toxicol. Pharmacol. Sect.*, **228**, 179–199

Ahlborg, U.G., Kimbrough, R.D. & Yrjänheikki, E.J. (1992b) Tolerable daily intake of PCDDs and PCDFs. *Tox. Subst. J.*, **12**, 101–131

Alaluusua, S., Lukinmaa, P.L., Pohjanvirta, R., Unkila, M. & Tuomisto, J.(1993) Exposure to 2,3,7,8-tetrachlorodibenzo-*para*-dioxin leads to defective dentin formation and pulpal perfo-ration in rat incisor tooth. *Toxicology*, **81**, 1–13

Alawi, M.A., Wichmann, H., Lorenz, W. & Bahadir, M. (1996a) Dioxins and furans in the Jordanian environment. Part 1: Preliminary study on a municipal landfill site with open combustion nearby Amman - Jordan. *Chemosphere*, **32**, 907–912

Alawi, M.A., Wichmann, H., Lorenz, W. & Bahadir, M. (1996b) Dioxins and furans in the Jordanian environment. Part 2: Levels of PCDD and PCDF in human milk samples from Jordan. *Chemosphere*, **33**, 2469–2474

Albrecht, E., Böllmann, U., Ecker P., Mair, K., Reifenhäuser, W., Schreiner, M., Wegenke, M. & Kalbfus, W. (1993) Examination of agricultural areas which have been treated with PCDD/F containing sewage sludge, and emission measurements from the firing installations of a waste water treatment plant. *Organohalogen Compounds*, **12**, 295–300

Albro, P.W. (1979) Problems in analytic methodology: sample handling, extraction, and cleanup. *Ann. N.Y. Acad. Sci.*, **320**, 19–27

Alder, L., Beck, H., Mathar, W. & Palavinskas, R. (1994) PCDDs,PCDFs, PCBs and other organochlorine compounds in human milk. Levels and their dynamics in Germany. *Organohalogen Compounds*, **21**, 39–44

Alexandrou, N., Miao, Z., Colquhoun, M. & Pawliszyn, J. & Jennison, C. (1992) Supercritical fluid extraction and cleanup with capillary GC-ion trap mass spectrometry for determination of polychlorinated dibenzo-*p*-dioxins and dibenzofurans in environmental samples. *J. chromatogr. Sci.*, **30**, 351–357

Allen, J.R. & Lalich, J.J. (1962) Response of chickens to prolonged feeding of crude 'toxic fat'. *Proc. Soc. exp. Biol. Med.*, **109**, 48–51

Allen, J.R., VanMiller, J.P. & Norback, D.H. (1975) Tissue distribution, excretion and biological effects of [^{14}C]tetrachlordibenzo-*p*-dioxin in rats. *Food Cosmet. Toxicol.*, **13**, 501–505

Allen, J.R., Barsotti, D.A., Van Miller, J.P., Abrahamson, L.J. & Lalich, J.J. (1977) Morphological changes in monkeys consuming a diet containing low levels of 2,3,7,8-tetrachloro-dibenzo-*p*-dioxin. *Food Cosmet. Toxicol.*, **15**, 401–410

Allen, J.R., Barsotti, D.A., Lambrecht, L.K. & Van Miller, J.P. (1979) Reproductive effects of halogenated aromatic hydrocarbons on nonhuman primates. *Ann. N. Y. Acad. Sci.*, **320**, 419–425

Alsharif, N.Z., Hassoun, E., Bagchi, M., Lawson, T. & Stohs, S.J. (1994a) The effects of anti-TNF-α antibody and dexamethasone on TCDD-induced oxidative stress in mice. *Pharmacology*, **48**, 127–136

Alsharif, N.Z., Schlueter, W.J. & Stohs, S.J. (1994b) Stimulation of NADPH-dependent reactive oxygen species formation and DNA damage by 2,3,7,8-tetrachlorodibenzo-*p*-dioxin in rat peritoneal lavage cells. *Arch. environ. Contam. Toxicol.*, **26**, 392–397

Alvarez, R. (1991) Standard reference materials for dioxins and other environmental pollutants. *Sci. total Environ.*, **104**, 1–7

Ambidge, P.F., Cox, E.A., Creaser, C.S., Greenberg, M., de M. Gem, M.G., Gilbert, J., Jones, P.W., Kibblewhite, M.G., Levey, J., Lisseter, S.G., Meredith, T.J., Smith, L., Smith, P., Startin, J.R., Stenhouse, I. & Whitworth, M. (1990) Acceptance criteria for analytical data on polychlorinated dibenzo-*p*-dioxins and polychlorinated dibenzofurans. *Chemosphere*, **21**, 999–1006

American Conference of Governmental Industrial Hygienists (1995) *Threshold Limit Values and Biological Exposure Indices for 1995–1996*, Cincinnati, OH

Andrews, J.S., Jr, Garrett, W.A., Jr, Patterson, D.G., Jr, Needham, L.L., Roberts, D.W., Bagby, J.R., Anderson, J.E., Hoffman, R.E. & Schramm, W. (1989) 2,3,7,8-Tetrachlorodibenzo-*p*-dioxin levels in adipose tissue of persons with no known exposure and in exposed persons. *Chemosphere*, **18**, 499–506

Antonsson, A.-B., Runmark, S. & Mowrer, J. (1989) Dioxins in the work environment in steel mills. *Chemosphere*, **19**, 699–704

Aoki, Y., Satoh, K., Sato, K. & Suzuki, K.T. (1992) Induction of glutathione *S*-transferase P-form in primary cultured rat liver parenchymal cells by coplanar polychlorinated biphenyl congeners. *Biochem. J.*, **281**, 539–543

Aoki, Y., Matsumoto, M. & Suzuki, K.T. (1993) Expression of glutathione *S*-transferase P-form in primary cultured rat liver parenchymal cells by coplanar polychlorinated biphenyl congeners is suppressed by protein kinase inhibitors and dexamethasone. *FEBS Lett.*, **333**, 114–118

Aschengrau, A. & Monson, R.R. (1989) Paternal military service in Vietnam and risk of spontaneous abortion. *J. occup. Med.*, **31**, 618–623

Aschengrau, A. & Monson, R.R. (1990) Paternal military service in Vietnam and risk of late adverse pregnancy outcomes. *Am. J. public Health*, **10**, 1218–1224

Ashe, W.F. & Suskind, R.R. (1950) *Reports on Chloracne Cases, Monsanto Chemical Co., Nitro, West Virginia, October 1949 and April 1950*, Cincinnati, OH, Department of Environmental Health, College of Medicine, University of Cincinnati

Asman, D.C., Takimoto, K., Pitot, H.C., Dunn, T.J. & Lindahl, R. (1993) Organization and characterization of the rat class 3 aldehyde dehydrogenase gene. *J. biol. Chem.*, **268**, 12530–12536

Asp S., Riihimäki V., Hernberg S. & Pukkala E. (1994) Mortality and cancer morbidity of Finnish chlorophenoxy herbicide applicators: an 18-year prospective follow-up. *Am. J. ind. Med.*, **26**, 243–253

Assennato, G., Cervino, D., Emmet, E.A., Longo, G. & Merlo, F. (1989) Follow-up of subjects who developed chloracne following TCDD exposure at Seveso. *Am. J. ind. Med.*, **16**, 119–125

Assmuth, T.M. & Vartiainen, T. (1995) Analysis of toxicological risks from local contamination by PCDDs and PCDFs: importance of isomer distribution and toxic equivalents. *Chemosphere*, **31**, 2853–2861

Astroff, B. & Safe, S. (1988) Comparative antiestrogenic activities of 2,3,7,8-tetrachlorodibenzo-*p*-dioxin and 6-methyl-1,3,8-trichlorodibenzofuran in the female rat. *Toxicol. appl. Pharmacol.*, **95**, 435–443

Astroff, B. & Safe, S. (1990) 2,3,7,8-Tetrachlorodibenzo-*p*-dioxin as an antiestrogen: effect on rat uterine peroxidase activity. *Biochem. Pharmacol.*, **39**, 485–488

Astroff, B. & Safe, S. (1991) 6-Alkyl-1,3,8-trichlorodibenzofurans as antiestrogens in female Sprague-Dawley rats. *Toxicology*, **69**, 187–197

Astroff, B., Rowlands, C., Dickerson, R. & Safe, S. (1990) 2,3,7,8-Tetrachlorodibenzo-*p*-dioxin inhibition of 17 beta-estradiol-induced increases in rat uterine epidermal growth factor receptor binding activity and gene expression. *Mol. cell. Endocrinol.*, **72**, 247–252

Astroff, B., Eldridge, B. & Safe, S. (1991) Inhibition of 17β-estradiol-induced and constitutive expression of the cellular protooncogene c-*fos* by 2,3,7,8-tetrachlorodibenzo-*p*-dioxin (TCDD) in the female uterus. *Toxicol. Lett.*, **56**, 305–315

Axelson, A. & Sundell, L. (1974) Herbicide exposure, mortality and tumor incidence. An epidemiological investigation on Swedish railroad workers. *Work environ. Health*, **11**, 21–28

Axelson, A., Sundell, L., Andersson, K., Edling, C., Hogstedt, C. & Kling, H. (1980) Herbicide exposure and tumor mortality. An updated epidemiologic investigation on Swedish railroad workers. *Scand J. Work Environ. Health*, **6**, 73–79

Baader, E.W. & Bauer, H.J. (1951) Industrial intoxication due to pentachlorophenol. *Ind. Med. Surg.*, **20**, 286–290

Badesha, J.S., Maliji, G. & Flaks, B. (1995) Immunotoxic effects of exposure of rats to xenobiotics via maternal lactation. Part I. 2,3,7,8-Tetrachlorodibenzo-*p*-dioxin. *Int. J. exp. Pathol.*, **76**, 425–439

Bagchi, D., Shara, M.A., Bagchi, M., Hassoun, E.A. & Stohs, S.J. (1993) Time-dependent effects of 2,3,7,8-tetrachlorodibenzo-*p*-dioxin on serum and urine levels of malondialdehyde, formaldehyde, acetaldehyde, and acetone in rats. *Toxicol. appl. Pharmacol.*, **123**, 83–88

Baker, T.K., Kwiatkowski, A.P., Madhukar, B.V. & Klaunig, J.E. (1995) Inhibition of gap junctional intercellular communication by 2,3,7,8-tetrachlorodibenzo-*p*-dioxin (TCDD) in rat hepatocytes. *Carcinogenesis*, **16**, 2321–2326

Ball, Dr & Düwel, U. (1996) Sampling and analysis of dioxins. *VDI Berichte*, **1298**, 97–115 (in German)

Banks, Y.B. & Birnbaum, L.S. (1991) Absorption of 2,3,7,8-tetrachlorodibenzo-*p*-dioxin (TCDD) after low dose dermal exposure. *Toxicol. appl. Pharmacol.*, **107**, 302–310

Banks, Y.B., Brewster, D.W. & Birnbaum, L.S. (1990) Age-related changes in dermal absorption of 2,3,7,8-tetrachlorodibenzopdioxin and 2,3,4,7,8-pentachlorodibenzofuran. *Fundam. appl. Toxicol.*, **15**, 163–173

Barker, C.W., Fagan, J.B. & Pasco, D.S. (1992) Interleukin-1beta suppresses the induction of P4501A1 and P4501A2 messenger RNAs in isolated hepatocytes. *J. biol. Chem.* **267**, 8050–8055

Barrett, J.C. (1993) Mechanisms of multistep carcinogenesis and carcinogen risk assessment. *Environ. Health Perspect.*, **100**, 9–20

Barsotti, D.A., Abrahamson, L.J. & Allen, J.R. (1979) Hormonal alterations in female rhesus monkeys fed a diet containing 2,3,7,8-tetrachlorodibenzo-*p*-dioxin. *Bull. environ. Contam. Toxicol.*, **21**, 461–469

Barthel, E. (1981) Increased risk of lung cancer in pesticide-exposed male agricultural workers. *J. Toxicol. environ. Health*, **8**, 1027–1040

Bastomsky, G.H. (1977) Enhanced thyroxine metabolism and high uptake goiter in rats after single dose of 2,3,7,8-tetrachlorodibenzo-*p*-dioxin. *Endocrinology*, **101**, 292–296

Battershill, J.M. (1994) Review of the safety assessment of polychlorinated biphenyls (PCBs) with particular reference to reproductive toxicity. *Hum. exp. Toxicol.*, **13**, 581–597

Bauer, H., Schulz, K. & Spiegelburg, W. (1961) Industrial poisoning in the manufacture of chlorophenol compounds. *Arch. Gewerbepath. Gewerbehyg.*, **18**, 538–555

Baughman, R. & Meselson, M. (1973a) An improved analysis for tetrachlorodibenzo-*p*-dioxins. In: Blair, E.H., ed., *Chlorodioxins — Origin and Fate (Advances in Chemistry, Ser. 120)*, Washington DC, American Chemical Society, pp. 92–104

Baughman, R. & Meselson, M. (1973b) An analytical method for detecting TCDD (dioxin): levels of TCDD in samples from Vietnam. *Environ. Health Perspectives*, **5**, 27–35

Baughman, R.W. & Newton, L. (1972) *Analysis of Two Hexachlorophene and Two 2,4,5-Trichlorophenol Samples for Tetrachlorodibenzo-p-dioxins*, Cambridge, MA, Harvard University

Bauman, J.W., Goldsworthy, T.L., Dunn, C.S. & Fox, T.R. (1995) Inhibitory effects of 2,3,7,8-tetrachlorodibenzo-*p*-dioxin on rat hepatocyte proliferation induced by 2/3 partial hepatectomay. *Cell Prolif.*, **28**, 437–451

van Bavel, B., Järemo, M., Karlsson, L. & Lindström, G. (1996) Development of a solid phase carbon trap for simultaneous determination of PCDDs, PCDFs, PCBs, and pesticides in environmental samples using SFE-LC. *Analyt. Chem.*, **68**, 1279-1283

Beatty, P.W., Vaughn, W.K. & Neal, R.A. (1978) Effect of alteration of rat hepatic mixed-function oxidase (MFO) activity on the toxicity of 2,3,7,8-tetrachlorodibenzo-*p*-dioxin (TCDD). *Toxicol. appl. Pharmacol.*, **45**, 513–519

Becher, C., Skaare, J.U., Polder, A., Sletten, B., Rossland, O.J., Hansen, H.K. & Ptashekas, J. (1995) PCDDs, PCDFs, and PCBs in human milk from different parts of Norway and Lithuania. *J. Toxicol. environ. Health*, **46**, 133–148

Becher, H., Flesch-Janys, D., Kauppinen, T., Kogevinas, M., Steindorf, K., Manz, A. & Wahrendorf, J. (1996) Cancer mortality in German male workers exposed to phenoxy herbicides and dioxins. *Cancer Causes Control*, **7**, 312–321

Beck, H., Eckart, K., Kellert, M., Mathar, W., Rühl, C.-S. & Wittkowski, R. (1987) Levels of PCDFs and PCDDs in samples of human origin and food in the Federal Republic of Germany. *Chemosphere*, **16**, 1977–1982

Beck, H., Eckart, K., Mathar, W. & Wittkowski, R. (1989a) PCDD and PCDF body burden from food intake in the Federal Republic of Germany. *Chemosphere*, **18**, 417–424

Beck, H., Eckart, K., Mathar, W. & Wittkowski, R. (1989b) Levels of PCDDs and PCDFs in adipose tissue of occupationally exposed workers. *Chemosphere*, **18**, 507–516

Beck, H., Eckart, K., Mathar, W. & Wittkowski, R. (1989c) Dependence of PCDD and PCDF levels in human milk on various parameters in the Federal Republic of Germany. *Chemosphere*, **18**, 1063–1066

Beck, H., Dross, A., Mathar, W. & Wittkowski, R. (1990a) Influence of different regional emissions and cardboard containers on levels of PCDD, PCDF and related compounds in cow milk. *Chemosphere*, **21**, 789–798

Beck, H., Dross, A., Kleemann, W.J. & Mathar, W. (1990b) PCDD and PCDF concentrations in different organs from infants. *Chemosphere*, **20**, 903–910

Beck, H., Dross, A. & Mathar, W. (1992) Dependence of PCDD and PCDF levels in human milk on various parameters in Germany. II. *Chemosphere*, **25**, 1015–1020

Beck, H., Kleemann, W.J., Mathar, W. & Palavinskas, R. (1994) PCDD and PCDF levels in different organs from infants. II. *Organohalogen Compounds*, **21**, 259–264

Beebe, L.E., Anver, M.R., Riggs, C.W., Fornwald, L.W. & Anderson, L.M. (1995a) Promotion of *N*-nitrosodimethylamine-initiated mouse lung tumors following single or multiple low dose exposure to 2,3,7,8-tetrachlorodibenzo-*p*-dioxin. *Carcinogenesis*, **16**, 1345–1349

Beebe, L.E., Fornwald, L.W., Diwan, B.A., Anver, M.R. & Anderson, L.M. (1995b) Promotion of *N*-nitrosodiethylamine-initiated hepatocellular tumors and hepatoblastomas by 2,3,7,8-tetrachlorodibenzo-*p*-dioxin or Aroclor 1254 in C57BL/6, DBA/2, and B6D2F1 mice. *Cancer Res.*, **55**, 4875–4880

Berghard, A., Gradin, K., Pongratz, I., Whitelaw, M. & Poellinger, L. (1993) Cross-coupling of signal transduction pathways: the dioxin receptor mediates induction of cytochrome P-450IA1 expression via a protein kinase C-dependent mechanism. *Mol. cell. Biol.*, **13**, 677–689

Bergqvist, P.-A., Bergex, S., Hallbäck, H., Rappe, C. & Slorach, S.A. (1989) Dioxins in cod and herring from the seas around Sweden. *Chemosphere*, **19**, 513–516

Bergqvist, P.-A., Strandberg, B., Bergek, S. & Rappe, C. (1993) Lipid reduction during the analyses of PCDDs, PCDFs and PCBs in environmental samples using semipermeable membrane technique. *Organohalogen Compounds*, **11**, 41–44

Bergschicker, R., Bräunlich, A., Heuchert, G., Kersten, N. & Päpke, O. (1994) *Dioxin and Heavy Metals Occurrence in Old Plants of Primary and Secondary Copper Smelters, Presentation at the 34th Anniversary of the German Society of Occupational Medicine and Environmental Medicine, Wiesbaden, 16–19 May 1994*, Lübeck, Germany, Institute of Occupational Medicine at Medical University of Lübeck (in German)

Berkers, J.A., Hassing, I., Spenkelink, B., Brouwer, A. & Blaauboer, B.J. (1995) Interactive effects of 2,3,7,8-tetrachlorodibenzo-*p*-dioxin and retinoids on proliferation and differentiation in cultured human keratinocytes: quantification of crosslinked envelope formation. *Arch. Toxicol.*, **69**, 368–378

Berry, D.L., DiGiovanni, J., Juchau, M.R., Bracken, W.M., Gleason, G.L. & Slaga, T.J. (1978) Lack of tumor-promoting ability of certain environmental chemicals in a two-stage mouse skin tumorigenesis assay. *Res. Commun. chem. Pathol. Pharmacol.*, **20**, 101–108

Bertazzi, P.A. & di Domenico, A. (1994) Chemical, environmental, and health aspects of the Seveso, Italy, accident. In: Schecter, A., ed., *Dioxin and Health*, New York, Plenum Press, pp. 587–632

Bertazzi, P.A., Zocchetti, C., Pesatori, A.C., Guercilena, S., Sanarico, M. & Radice, L. (1989) Ten-year mortality study of the population involved in the Seveso incident in 1976. *Am. J. Epidemiol.*, **129**, 1187–1199

Bertazzi, P.A., Zocchetti, C., Pesatori, A.C., Guercilena, S., Consonni, D., Tironi, A. & Landi, M.T. (1992) Mortality of a young population after accidental exposure to 2,3,7,8-tetrachlorodibenzo-*p*-dioxin. *Int. J. Epidemiol.*, **21**, 118–123

Bertazzi, P.A., Pesatori, A.C., Consonni, D., Tironi, A., Landi, M.T. & Zocchetti, C. (1993) Cancer incidence in a population accidentally exposed to 2,3,7,8-tetrachlorodibenzo-*para*-dioxin. *Epidemiology*, **4**, 398–406

Bertazzi, P.A., Pesatori, A.C. & Landi, M.T. (1996) Cancer mortality, 1976–1991, in the population exposed to 2,3,7,8-tetrachlorodibenzo-*p*-dioxin. *Organohalogen compounds*, **30**, 294–296

Bestervelt, L.L., Nolan, C.J., Cai, Y., Maimansomsuk, P., Mousigian, C.A. & Piper, W.N. (1991) Tetrachlorodibenzo-*para*-dioxin alters rat hypothalamic endorphin and mu-opioid receptors. *Neurotoxicol. Teratol.*, **13**, 495–497

Bestervelt, L.L., Cai, Y., Piper, D.W., Nolan, C.J., Pitt, J.A. & Piper, W.N. (1993a) TCDD alters pituitary–adrenal function. I. Adrenal responsiveness to exogenous ACTH. *Neurotoxicol. Teratol.*, **15**, 365–370

Bestervelt, L.L., Pitt, J.A., Nolan, C.J. & Piper, W.N. (1993b) TCDD alters pituitary-adrenal function II: evidence for decreased bioactivity of ACTH. *Neurotoxicol. Teratol.*, **15**, 371–376

Bhattacharyya, K.K., Brake, P.B., Eltom, S.E., Otto, S.A. & Jefcoate, C.R. (1995) Identification of a rat adrenal cytochrome P450 active in polycyclic hydrocarbon metabolism as rat CYP1B1. Demonstration of a unique tissue-specific pattern of hormonal and aryl hydrocarbon receptor-linked regulation. *J. biol. Chem.*, **270**, 11595–11602

Biegel, L. & Safe, S. (1990) Effects of 2,3,7,8-tetrachlorodibenzo-*p*-dioxin (TCDD) on cell growth and the secretion of the estrogen-induced 34-, 52- and 160-kDa proteins in human breast cancer cells. *J. steroid Biochem. mol. Biol.*, **37**, 725–732

Bignert, A., Olsson, M., de Wit, C., Litzén, K., Rappe, C. & Reutergårdh, L. (1994) Biological variation — an important factor to consider in ecotoxicological studies based on environmental samples. *Fresenius J. anal. Chem.*, **348**, 76–85

van Birgelen, A.P.J.M., Van der Kolk, J., Fase, K.M., Bol, I,. Poiger, H., Brouwer, A. & Van den Berg, M. (1994) Toxic potency of 3,3′,4,4′,5-pentachlorobiphenyl relative to and in combination with 2,3,7,8-tetrachlorodibenzo-*p*-dioxin in a subchronic feeding study in the rat. *Toxicol. appl. Pharmacol.*, **127**, 209–221

van Birgelen, A.P.J.M., Van der Kolk, J., Fase, K.M., Bol, I., Poiger, H., Brouwer, A. & Van den Berg, M. (1995a) Subchronic dose–response study of 2,3,7,8-tetrachlorodibenzo-*p*-dioxin in female Sprague-Dawley rats. *Toxicol. appl. Pharmacol.*, **132**, 1–13

van Birgelen, A.P., Smit, E.A., Kampen, I.M., Groeneveld, C.N., Fase, K.M., Van der Kolk, J., Poiger, H., Van den Berg, M., Koeman, J.H. & Brouwer, A. (1995b) Subchronic effects of 2,3,7,8-TCDD or PCBs on thyroid hormone metabolism: use in risk assessment. *Eur. J. Pharmacol.*, **293**, 77–85

van Birgelen, A.P.J.M., Fase, K.M., van der Kolk, J., Poger, H., Brouwer, A., Seinen, W. & Van den Berg, M. (1996a) Synergistic effect of 2,2′,4,4′,5,5′-hexachlorobiphenyl and 2,3,7,8-tetrachlorodibenzo-*p*-dioxin on hepatic porphyrin levels in the rat. *Environ. Health Perspectives*, **104**, 550–557

van Birgelen, A.P.J.M., DeVito, M.J., Akins, J.M., Ross, D.G., Diliberto, J.J. & Birnbaum, L.S. (1996b) Relative potencies of polychlorinated dibenzo-*p*-dioxins, dibenzofurans, and byphenyls derived from hepatic porphyrin accumulation in mice. *Toxicol. appl. Pharmacol.*, **138**, 98–109

Birmingham, B. (1990) Analysis of PCDD and PCDF patterns in soil samples: use in the estimation of the risk of exposure. *Chemosphere*, **20**, 807–814

Birmingham, B., Thorpe, B., Frank, R., Clement, R., Tosine, H., Fleming, G., Ashman, J., Wheeler, J., Ripley, B.D. & Ryan, J.J. (1989) Dietary intake of PCDD and PCDF from food in Ontario, Canada. *Chemosphere*, **19**, 507–512

Birnbaum, L.S. (1986) Distribution and excretion of 2,3,7,8-tetrachlorodibenzopdioxin in congenic strains of mice which differ at the Ah locus. *Drug Metab. Dispos.*, **14**, 34–40

Birnbaum, L.S. (1991) Developmental toxicity of TCDD and related compounds: Species sensitivities and differences. In: *Biological Basis for Risk Assessment of Dioxins and Related Compounds* (Banbury Report 35), CSH Press, Cold Spring Harbor, NY, pp. 51–67

Birnbaum, L.S. (1995a) Workshop on perinatal exposure to dioxin-like compounds. V. Immunologic effects. *Environ. Health Perspectives*, **103** (Suppl. 2), 157–160

Birnbaum, L.S. (1995b) Developmental effects of dioxins. *Environ. Health Perspectives*, **103** (Suppl. 7), 89–94

Birnbaum, L.S. (1996) Developmental effects of dioxins and related endocrine disrupting chemicals. *Toxicol. Lett.*, **82/83**, 743–750

Birnbaum, L.S. & Abbott, B.D. (1997) Effect of dioxin on growth factor and receptor expression in developing palate. In: *Methods in Developmental Toxicology and Biology*, Berlin, Blackwell Wissenchafts-Verlag, pp. 51–63

Birnbaum, L.S. & Couture, L.A. (1988) Disposition of octachlorodibenzo-*p*-dioxin (OCDD) in male rats. *Toxicol. appl. Pharmacol.*, 93, 22–30

Birnbaum, L.S., Decad, G.M. & Matthews, H.B. (1980) Disposition and excretion of 2,3,7,8-tetrachlorodibenzofuran in the rat. *Toxicol. appl. Pharmacol.*, 55, 342–352

Birnbaum, L.S., Decad, G.M., Matthews, H.B. & McConnell, E.E. (1981) Fate of 2,3,7,8-tetrachlorodibenzofuran in the monkey. *Toxicol. appl. Pharmacol.*, 57, 189–196

Birnbaum, L.S., Harris, M.W., Miller, C.P., Pratt, R.M. & Lamb, J.C. (1986) Synergistic interaction of 2,3,7,8-tetrachlorodibenzo-*p*-dioxin and hydrocortisone in the induction of cleft palate in mice. *Teratology*, 33, 29–35

Birnbaum, L.S., Harris, M.W., Barnhart, E.R. & Morrissey, R.E. (1987a) Teratogenicity of three polychlorinated dibenzofurans in C57BL/6N mice. *Toxicol. appl. Pharmacol.*, 90, 206–216

Birnbaum, L.S., Harris, M.W., Crawford, D.D. & Morrissey, R.E. (1987b) Teratogenic effects of polychlorinated dibenzofurans in combination in C57BL/6N mice. *Toxicol. appl. Pharmacol.*, 91, 246–255

Birnbaum, L.S., Harris, M.W., Stocking, L., Clark, A.M. & Morrissey, R.E. (1989) Retinoic acid and 2,3,7,8-tetrachlorodibenzo-*p*-dioxin (TCDD) selectively enhance teratogenesis in C57BL/6N mice. *Toxicol. appl. Pharmacol.*, 98, 487–500

Birnbaum, L.S., McDonald, M.M., Blair, P.C., Clark, A.M. & Harris, M.W. (1990) Differential toxicity of 2,3,7,8-tetrachlorodibenzo-*p*-dioxin (TCDD) in C57BL/6J mice congenic at the Ah locus. *Fundam. appl. Toxicol.*, 15, 186–200

Bisanti, L., Bonetti, F., Caramaschi, F., Del Corno, G., Favaretti, C., Giambelluca, S.E., Marni, E., Montesarchio, E., Puccinelli, V., Remotti, G., Volpato, C., Zambrelli, E. & Fara, G.M. (1980) Experiences from the accident of Seveso. *Acta Morphol. Acad. Sci. Hung.*, 28, 139–157

Biseth, A., Oehme, M. & Færden, K. (1990) Levels of polychlorinated dibenzo-*p*-dioxins and polychlorinated dibenzofurans in selected Norwegian foods. In: *Proceedings of the 10th International Conference on Organohalogen Compounds (Dioxin 90)*

Bjerke, D.L. & Peterson, R.E. (1994) Reproductive toxicity of 2,3,7,8,-tetrachlorodibenzo-*p*-dioxin in male rats: different effects of *in utero* versus lactational exposure. *Toxicol. appl. Pharmacol.*, 127, 241–249

Bjerke, D.L., Brown, T.J., MacLusky, N.J., Hochberg, R.B. & Peterson, R.E. (1994) Partial demasculinization and feminization of sex behavior in male rats by in utero and lactational exposure to 2,3,7,8-tetrachlorodibenzo-*p*-dioxin is not associated with alterations in estrogen receptor binding or volumes of sexually differentiated brain nuclei. *Toxicol. appl. Pharmacol.*, 127, 258–267

Blair, A., Grauman, D.J., Lubin, J.H. & Fraumeni, J.F., Jr (1983) Lung cancer and other causes of death among licensed pesticide applicators. *J. natl Cancer Inst.*, 71, 31–37

Blankenship, A.L., Suffia, M.C., Matsumura, F., Walsh, K.J. & Wiley, L.M. (1993) 2,3,7,8-tetrachlorodibenzo-*p*-dioxin (TCDD) accelerates differentiation of murine preimplantation embryos in vitro. *Reprod. Toxicol.*, 7, 255–261

Blaylock, B.L., Holladay, S.D., Comment, C.E., Heindel, J.J.& Luster, M.I. (1992) Exposure to tetrachlorodibenzo-*p*-dioxin (TCDD) alters fetal thymocyte maturation. *Toxicol. appl. Pharmacol.*, **112**, 207–213

Bleiberg, J., Wallen, M., Brodkin, R. & Applebaum, I.L. (1964) Industrially acquired porphyria. *Arch. Dermatol.*, **89**, 793–797

Bobet, E., Berard, M.F. & Dann, T. (1990) The measurement of PCDD and PCDF in ambient air in southwestern Ontario. *Chemosphere*, **20**, 1439–1445

Bolm-Audorff, U., Menzel, H.M., Murzen, R., Päpke, O., Turcer, E. & Vater, U. (1994) Dioxin and furan occurrence due to employment in solid-waste incinerator. *Verhandl. Arbeitsmed.*, **34**, 105–108 (in German)

Bolt, A., & de Jong, A.P.J.M. (1993) Ambient air dioxin measurement in the Netherlands. *Chemosphere*, **27**, 73–81

Bombick, D.W., Madhukar, B.V., Brewster, D.W. & Matsumura, F. (1985) TCDD (2,3,7,8-tetrachlorodibenzo-*p*-dioxin) causes increases in protein kinases particularly protein kinase C in the hepatic plasma membrane of the rat and the guinea pig. *Biochem. biophys. Res. Commun.*, **127**, 296–302

Bond, G.G., Ott, M.G., Brenner, F.E. & Cook, R.R. (1983) Medical and morbidity surveillance findings among employees potentially exposed to TCDD. *Br. J. ind. Med.*, **40**, 318–324

Bond, G.G., Cook, R.R., Brenner, F.E. & McLaren, E.A. (1987) Evaluation of mortality patterns among chemical workers with chloracne. *Chemosphere*, **16**, 2117–2121

Bond, G.G., McLaren, E.A., Lipps, T.E. & Cook, R.R. (1989a) Update of mortality among chemical workers with potential exposure to the higher chlorinated dioxins. *J. occup. Med.*, **31**, 121–123

Bond, G., McLaren, E., Brenner, F. & Cook, R. (1989b) Incidence of chloracne among chemical workers potentially exposed to chlorinated dioxins. *J. occup. Med.*, **31**, 771–774

Bookstaff, R.C., Moore, R.W. & Peterson, R.E. (1990a) 2,3,7,8-Tetrachlorodibenzo-*p*-dioxin increases the potency of androgens and estrogens as feedback inhibitors of luteinizing hormone secretion in male rats. *Toxicol. appl. Pharmacol.*, **104**, 212–224

Bookstaff, R.C., Kamel, F., Moore, R.W., Bjerke, D.L. & Peterson, R.E. (1990b) Altered regulation of pituitary gonadotropin-releasing hormone (GnRH) receptor number and pituitary responsiveness to GnRH in 2,3,7,8-tetrachlorodibenzo-*p*-dioxin-treated male rats. *Toxicol. appl. Pharmacol.*, **105**, 78–92

Boos, R., Himsl, A., Wurst, F., Prey, T., Scheidl, K., Sperka, G. & Gläser, O. (1992) Determination of PCDDs and PCDFs in soil samples from Salzburg, Austria. *Chemosphere*, **25**, 283–291

Boreiko, C.J,. Abernethy, D.J., Rickert, D.E. & Stedman, D.B. (1989) Effect of growth state, tumor promoters, and transformation upon intercellular communication between C3H/-10T1/2 murine fibroblasts. *Carcinogenesis*, **10**, 113–121

Böske, J., Dreier, M. & Päpke, O. (1995) Polychlorinated dibenzodioxins and dibenzofurans in the blood of employees in a municipal solid-waste incinerator. *Arbeitsmed. Sozialmed. Umweltm.*, **30**, 352–354 (in German)

Bouwman, C.A., Seinen, W., Koppe, J.G. & van der Berg, M. (1992) Effects of 2,3,7,8-tetrachlorodibenzo-*p*-dioxin or 2,2′, 4,4′, 5,5′-hexachlorobiphenyl on vitamin K-dependent blood coagulation in female germfree WAG/Rij rats. *Toxicology*, **75**, 109–120

Bowes, G.W., Mulvihill, M.J., Simoneit, B.R.T., Burlingame, A.L. & Risebrough, R.W. (1975) Identification of chlorinated dibenzofurans in American polychlorinated biphenyls. *Nature*, **256**, 305–307

Bowman, R.E., Schantz, S.L., Weerasinghe, N.C.A., Gross, M. & Barsotti, D. (1989a) Chronic dietary intake of 2,3,7,8-tetrachlorodibenzo-*p*-dioxin (TCDD) at 5 or 25 parts per trillion in the monkey: TCDD kinetics and dose-effect estimate of reproductive toxicity. *Chemosphere*, **18**, 243–252

Bowman, R.E., Schantz, S.L. & Gross, M.L. (1989b) Behavioral effects in monkeys exposed to 2,3,7,8-TCDD transmitted maternally during gestation and for four months of nursing. *Chemosphere*, **18**, 235–242

Bradfield, C.A., Kende, A.S. & Poland, A. (1988) Kinetic and equilibrium studies of Ah receptor-ligand binding: use of [^{125}I]-2-iodo-7,8-dibromodibenzo-*p*-dioxin. *Mol. Pharmacol.*, **34**, 229

Brewster, D.W. & Birnbaum, L.S. (1987) Disposition and excretion of 2,3,4,7,8-pentachlorodibenzofuran in the rat. *Toxicol. appl. Pharmacol.*, **90**, 243–252

Brewster, D.W. & Birnbaum, L.S. (1988) Disposition of 1,2,3,7,8-pentachlorodibenzofuran in the rat. *Toxicol. appl. Pharmacol.*, **95**, 490–498

Brewster, D.W., Elwell, M.R. & Birnbaum, L.S. (1988) Toxicity and disposition of 2,3,4,7,8-pentachlorodibenzofuran (4PeCDF) in the rhesus monkey (*Macaca mulatta*). *Toxicol. appl. Pharmacol.*, **93**, 231–246

Brewster, D.W., Banks, Y.B., Clark, A.M. & Birnbaum, L.S. (1989) Comparative dermal absorption of 2,3,7,8-tetrachlorodibenzo-*p*-dioxin and three polychlorinated dibenzofurans. *Toxicol. appl. Pharmacol.*, **197**, 156–166

Bröker, G. (1996) Standardization of dioxin-range of measurements. *VDI Berichte*, **1298**, 117–132 (in German)

Broman, D., Näf, C., Rolff, C. & Zebühr, Y. (1990) Analysis of polychlorinated dibenzo-p-dioxins (PCDD) and polychlorinated dibenzofurans (PCDF) in soil and digested sewage sludge from Stockholm, Sweden. *Chemosphere*, **21**, 1213–1220

Broman, D., Näf, C., Rolff, C. & Zebühr, Y. (1991) Occurrence and dynamics of polychlorinated dibenzo-*p*-dioxins and dibenzofurans and polycyclic aromatic hydrocarbons in the mixed surface layer of remote coastal and offshore waters in the Baltic. *Environ. Sci. Technol.*, **25**, 1850–1864

Broman, D., Näf, C. & Zebühr, Y. (1992) Occurrence and dynamics of polychlorinated dibenzo-*p*-dioxins ans dibenzofurans and other combustion related organic pollutants in the aquatic environment of the Baltic. *Chemosphere*, **25**, 125–128

Brouwer, A., Håkansson, H., Kukler, A., Van den Berg, K.J. & Ahlborg, U.G. (1989) Marked alterations in retinoid homeostasis of Sprague-Dawley rats induced by a single i.p. dose of 10 mg/kg of 2,3,7,8-tetrachlorodibenzo-*p*-dioxin. *Toxicology*, **58**, 267–283

Brouwer, A., Ahlborg, U.G., Van den Berg, M., Birnbaum, L.S., Boersma, E.R., Bosveld, B., Denison, M.S., Gray, L.E., Hagmar, L., Holene, E., Huisman, M., Jacobson, S.W., Jacobson, J.L., Koopman-Esseboom, C., Koppe, J.G., Kulig, B.M., Morse, D.C., Muckle, G., Peterson, R.E., Sauer, P.J.J., Seegal, R.F., Smits-Van Prooije, A.E., Touwen, B.C.L., Weisglas-Kuperus, N. & Winneke, G. (1995) Functional aspects of developmental toxicity of polyhalogenated aromatic hydrocarbons in experimental animals and human infants. *Environ. Toxicol. Pharmacol.*, **293**, 1–40

Brown, D.P. (1987) Mortality of workers exposed to polychlorinated biphenyls — an update. *Arch. environ. Health*, **42**, 333–339

Bruckmann, P. & Hackhe, K.-H. (1987) Emission measurements of PCDDs and PCDFs in places with different air quality in Hamburg. *VDI-Berichte*, **634**, 165–191 (in German)

Bryant, P.L., Clark, G., Probst, M.R. & Abbott, B.D. (1995) Expression of Ah receptor and ARNT in mouse embryonic urinary tract. *Toxicologist*, **15**, 349

Bryant, P.L., Clark, G. & Abbott, B.D. (1996) Effects of TCDD on EGF, TGFa, and EGF receptor in embryonic mouse urinary tract epithelia. *Teratology*, **53**, 106–107

Buchmann, A., Stinchcombe, S., Körner, W., Hagenmaier, H. & Bock, K.W. (1994) Effects of 2,3,7,8-tetrachloro- and 1,2,3,4,6,7,8-heptachlorodibenzo-*p*-dioxin on the proliferation of preneoplastic liver cells in the rat. *Carcinogenesis*, **15**, 1143–1150

Buckland, S.J., Hannah, D.J. & Taucher, J.A. (1990a) Levels of polychlorinated dibenzo-*p*-dioxins and dibenzofurans in the breast milk of New Zealand mothers. In: *Organohalogen Compounds*, **1**, 225–226

Buckland, S.J., Hannah, D.J., Taucher, J.A. & Weston, R.J. (1990b) The migration of poly-chlorinated dibenzo-*p*-dioxins and dibenzofurans into milks and cream from bleached paper-board packaging. *Organohalogen Compounds*, **3**, 223–226

Buckland, S.J., Dye, E.A., Leathem, S.V. & Taucher, J.A. (1994) The levels of PCDDs and PCDFs in soil samples collected from conservation areas following bush fires. *Organo-halogen Compounds*, **20**, 85–89

Buckland, S.J., Ellis, H.K. & Salter, R.T. (1996) Assessment of the New Zealand environment for levels of PCDDs, PCDFs, PCBs and other organochlorine contaminants. *Organohalogen Compounds*, **28**, 140–144

Buckley-Kedderis, L., Diliberto, J.J., Linko, P., Goldstein, J.A. & Birnbaum, L.S. (1992) Dispo-sition of 2,3,7,8-tetrabromodibenzo-*p*-dioxin in the rat: biliary excretion and induction of cytochromes CYP1A1 and CYP1A2. *Toxicol. appl. Pharmacol.*, **111**, 163

Bueno de Mesquita, H.B., Doornbos, G., van der Kuip, D.A.M., Kogevinas, M. & Winkelmann, R. (1993) Occupational exposure to phenoxy herbicides and chlorophenols and cancer mortality in The Netherlands. *Am. J. ind. Med.*, **23**, 289–300

Burbach K.M., Poland A. & Bradfield C.A. (1992) Cloning of the Ah receptor cDNA reveals a distinctive ligand-activated transcription factor. *Proc. natl Acad. Sci. USA*, **89**, 8185–8189

Burka, L.T., McGown, S.R. & Tomer, K.B. (1990) Identification of the biliary metabolites of 2,3,7,8-tetrachlorodibenzofuran in the rat. *Chemosphere*, **21**, 1231–1242

Burkhard, L.P. & Kuehl, D.W. (1986) *n*-Octanol/water partition coefficients by reverse phase liquid chromatography/mass spectrometry for eight tetrachlorinated planar molecules. *Chemosphere*, **15**, 163–167

Burleson, G.R., Lebrec, H., Yang, Y.G., Ibanes, J.D., Pennington, K.N. & Birnbaum, L.S. (1996) Effect of 2,3,7,8-tetrachlorodibenzo-*p*-dioxin (TCDD) on influenza virus host resis-tance in mice. *Fundam. appl. Toxicol.*, **29**, 40–47

Buser, H.-R. (1991) Review of methods of analysis for polychlorinated dibenzodioxins and dibenzofurans. In: Rappe, C., Buser, H.-R., Dodet, B. & O'Neill, I.K., eds, *Environmental Carcinogens: Methods of Analysis and Exposure Measurement. Vol. 11: Polychlorinated Dioxins and Dibenzofurans* (IARC Scientific Publications No. 108), Lyon, IARC, pp. 105–146

Buser, H.-R. & Bosshardt, H.P. (1976) Determination of polychlorinated dibenzo-*p*-dioxins and dibenzofurans in commercial pentachlorophenols by combined gas chromatography-mass spectrometry. *J. Assoc. off. anal. Chem.*, **59**, 562–569

Buser, H.R. & Rappe, C. (1978) Identification of substitution patterns in polychlorinated di-benzo-*p*-dioxins (PCDDs) by mass spectrometry. *Chemosphere*, **7**, 199–211

Buser, H.R., Bosshardt, H.P. & Rappe, C. (1978a) Identification of polychlorinated dibenzo-*p*-dioxin isomers found in fly ash. *Chemosphere*, **7**, 165–172

Buser, H.R., Bosshardt, H.P. & Rappe, C. (1978b) Formation of polychlorinated dibenzofurans (PCDFs) from the pyrolysis of PCBs. *Chemosphere*, **7**, 109–119

Büsser, M.-T. & Lutz, W.K. (1987) Stimulation of DNA synthesis in rat and mouse liver by various tumor promoters. *Carcinogenesis*, **8**, 1433–1437

Buu-Hoi, N.P., Chanh, P.-H., Sesque, G., Azum-Gelade, M.C. & Saint-Ruf, G. (1972) Organs as targets of 'dioxin' (2,3,7,8-tetrachlorodibenzo-*p*-dioxin) intoxication. *Naturwissenschaften*, **59**, 174–175

Calvert, G.M., Sweeney, M.H., Morris, J.A., Fingerhut, M.A., Hornung, R.W. & Halperin, W.E. (1991) Evaluation of chronic bronchitis, chronic obstructive pulmonary disease, and venti-latory function among workers exposed to 2,3,7,8-tetrachlorodibenzo-*p*-dioxin. *Am. Rev. respir. Dis.*, **144**, 1302–1306

Calvert, G.M., Hornung, R.W., Sweeney, M.H., Fingerhut, M.A. & Halperin, W.E. (1992) Hepatic and gastrointestinal effects in an occupational cohort exposed to 2,3,7,8-tetrachloro-dibenzo-*para*-dioxin. *J. Am. med. Assoc.*, **267**, 2209–2214

Calvert, G.M., Sweeney, M.H., Fingerhut, M.A., Hornung, R.W. & Halperin, W.E. (1994) Eva-luation of porphyria cutanea tarda in U.S. workers exposed to 2,3,7,8-tetrachlorodibenzo-*p*-dioxin. *Am. J. ind. Med.*, **25**, 559–571

Calvert G.M., Wille, K.K., Sweeney, M.H., Fingerhut, M.A. & Halperin, W.E. (1996) Eva-luation of serum lipid concentrations among U.S. workers exposed to 2,3,7,8-tetrachloro-dibenzo-*p*-dioxin. *Arch. environ. Health*, **51**, 100–107

Cantoni, L., Dal Fiume, D., Ferraroli, A., Salmona, M. & Ruggieri, R. (1984) Different suscep-tibility of mouse tissues to porphyrogenic effect of 2,3,7,8-tetrachlorodibenzo-*p*-dioxin. *Toxicol. Lett.*, **20**, 201–210

Cantor, K.P., Blair, A., Everett, G., Gibson, R., Burmeister, L.F., Brown, L.M., Schuman, L. & Dick, F.R. (1992) Pesticides and other agricultural risk factors for non-Hodgkin's lymphoma among men in Iowa and Minnesota. *Cancer Res.*, **52**, 2447–2455

Caramaschi, F., Del Caino, G., Favaretti, C., Giambelluca, S.E., Montesarchio, E. & Fara, G.M. (1981) Chloracne following environmental contamination by TCDD in Seveso, Italy. *Int. J. Epidemiol.*, **10**, 135–143

Carban, M.J., III, Flood, L.P., Cambpell, B.D. & Busbee, D.L. (1995) Effects of benzo(*a*)pyrene and tetrachlorodibenzo(p)dioxin on fetal dolphin kidney cells: inhibition of proliferation and initiation of DNA damage. *Chemosphere*, **30**, 187–198

Carlé, J., Nygren, M., Younes, M., Ersboell, A., Startin, J. & Yrjánheikki, E., eds, (1995) *Quality Assessment of PCB, PCDD and PCDF Analysis: Third Round of WHO-Coordinated Study* (Environmental Health in Europe No. 2), Bilthoven, WHO European Centre for Envi-ronmental and Health

Carpenter, G. (1987) Receptors for epidermal growth factor and other polypeptide mitogens. *Ann. Rev. Biochem.*, **56**, 881–914

Carrier, F., Owens, R.A., Nebert, DW. & Puga, A. (1992) Dioxin-dependent activation of murine Cyp1a-1 gene transcription requires protein kinase-C-dependent phosphorylation. *Mol. cell. Biol.*, **12**, 1856–1863

Carrier, G., Brunet, R.C. & Brodeur, J. (1995a) Modeling of the toxicokinetics of polychlorinated dibenzo-p-dioxins and dibenzofurans in mammalians, including humans. I. Nonlinear distribution of PCDD/PCDF body burden between liver and adipose tissues. *Toxicol. appl. Pharmacol.*, **131**, 253-266

Carrier, G., Brunet, R.C. & Brodeur, J. (1995b) Modeling of the toxicokinetics of polychlorinated dibenzo-p-dioxins and dibenzofurans in mammalians, including humans. II. Kinetics of absorption and disposition of PCDDs/PCDFs. *Toxicol. appl. Pharmacol.*, **131**, 267-276

Carver, L.A., Jackiw, V. & Bradfield, C.A. (1994) The 90-kDa heat shock protein is essential for Ah receptor signaling in a yeast expression system. *J. biol. Chem.i*, **269**, 30109–30112.

Centers for Disease Control Veterans Health Studies (1988) Serum 2,3,7,8-tetrachlorodibenzo-*p*-dioxin levels in U.S. Army Vietnam-era veterans. *J. Am. med. Assoc.*, **260**, 1249–1254

Centers for Disease Control Vietnam Experience Study (1988a) Health status of Vietnam veterans. II. Physical health. *J. Am. med. Assoc.*, **259**, 2708–2714

Centers for Disease Control Vietnam Experience Study (1988b) Health status of Vietnam veterans. I. Psychosocial characteristics. *J. Am. med. Assoc.*, **259**, 2701–2707

Centers for Disease Control Vietnam Experience Study (1988c) Postservice mortality among Vietnam veterans. *J. Am. med. Assoc.*, **257**, 790–795

Centers for Disease Control Vietnam Experience Study (1988d) Health status of Vietnam veterans. III. Reproductive outcomes and child health. *J. Am. med. Assoc.*, **259**, 2715–2719

Chang, K.J., Lu, F.J., Tung, T.C. & Lee, T.P. (1980) Studies on patients with polychlorinated biphenyl poisoning. 2. Determination of urinary coproporphyrin, uroporphyrin, L aminolevulinic acid and porphobilinogen. *Res. Commun. chem. Pathol. Pharmacol.*, **30**, 547–554

Chao, W.-Y. & Hsu, C.-C. (1994) Middle ear abnormalities in Yu-Cheng children. *Organohalogen Comp.*, **21**, 501–502

Chapman, D.E. & Schiller, C.M. (1985) Dose-related effects of 2,3,7,8-tetrachlorodibenzo-*p*-dioxin (TCDD) in C57BL/6J and DBA/2J mice. *Toxicol. appl. Pharmacol.*, **78**, 147–157

Chen, P.H. & Hites, R.A. (1983) Polychlorinated biphenyls and dibenzofurans retained in the tissues of a deceased patient with yucheng in Taiwan. *Chemosphere*, **12**, 1507–1516

Chen, Y.C. & Hsu, C.C. (1994) Effects of prenatal exposure to PCBs on the neurological function of children: A neuropsychological and neurophysiological study. *Dev. Med. Child Neurol.*, **36**, 312–320

Chen, H.S. & Perdew, G.H. (1994) Subunit composition of the heterodimeric cytosolic aryl hydrocarbon receptor complex. *J. biol. Chem.*, **269**, 27554–27558

Chen, R.-C., Chang, Y.-C., Chang, K.-J., Lu, F.-J. & Tung, T.-C. (1981) Peripheral neuropathy caused by chronic polychlorinated biphenyls poisoning. *J. formosan Med. Assoc.*, **80**, 47–54

Chen, R.-C., Chang, Y.-C., Tung, T.-C. & Chang, K.-J. (1983) Neurological manifestations of chronic polychlorinated biphenyls poisoning. *Proc. natl Sci. Counc. ROC (A)*, **7**, 87–91

Chen, R.-C., Tang, S.-Y., Miyata, H., Kashimoto, T., Chang, Y.-C., Chang, K.-J. & Tung, T.-C. (1985a) Polychlorinated biphenyl poisoning: correlation of sensory and motor nerve conduction, neurologic symptoms, and blood levels of polychlorinated biphenyls, quaterphenyls and dibenzofurans. *Environ. Res.*, **37**, 340–348

Chen, P.H., Wong, C.-K., Rappe, C. & Nygren, M. (1985b) Polychlorinated biphenyls, dibenzofurans and quaterphenyls in toxic rice-bran oil and in the blood and tissues of patients with PCB poisoning (Yu-Cheng) in Taiwan. *Environ. Health Perspectives*, **59**, 59–65

Chen, Y.C.J., Guo, Y.L.L. & Hsu, C.C. (1992) Cognitive development of children prenatally exposed to polychlorinated biphenyls (Yu-Cheng children) and their siblings. *J. formosan Med. Assoc.*, **91**, 704–707

Chen Y.-C.J., Yu, M.L., Rogan, W.J., Gladen, B.C. & Hsu, C.C. (1994) A 6-year follow-up of behavior and activity disorders in the Taiwan Yu-Cheng children. *Am. J. public Health*, **84**, 415–421

Chia, L.G. & Chu, F.L. (1984) Neurological studies on polychlorinated biphenyl (PCB)-poisoned patients. *Am. J. ind. Med.*, **5**, 117–126

Chia, L.G. & Chu, F.L. (1985) A clinical and electrophysiological study of patients with polychlorinated biphenyl poisoning. *J. Neurol. Neurosurg. Psychiat.*, **48**, 894–901

Choi, E.J., Toscano, D.G., Ryan, J.A., Riedel, N. & Toscano, W.A., Jr (1991) Dioxin induces transforming growth factor-alpha in human keratinocytes. *J. biol. Chem.*, **266**, 9591–9597

Christian, B.J. & Peterson, R.E. (1983) Effects of 2,3,7,8-tetrachlorodibenzo-*p*-dioxin on [^{3}H]-thymidine incorporation into rat liver deoxyribonucleic acid. *Toxicology*, **8**, 133–146

Christmann, W., Kasiske, D., Klöppel, K.D., Bartscht, H. & Rotard, W. (1989a) Combustion of polyvinylchloride. An important source for the formation of PCDD/PCDF. *Chemosphere*, **19**, 387–392

Christmann, W., Klöppel, K.D., Partscht, H. & Rotard, W. (1989b) Determination of PCDD/-PCDF in ambient air. *Chemosphere*, **19**, 521–526

Clar, G.C. & Taylor, M.J. (1994) Tumor necrosis factor involvement in the toxicity of TCDD: the role of endotoxin in the response. *Exp. clin. Immunogenet.*, **11**, 136–141

Clark, D.A., Gauldie, J., Szewczuk, M.R. & Sweeney, G. (1981) Enhanced suppressor cell activity as a mechanism of immunosuppression by 2,3,7,8-tetrachlorodibenzo-*p*-dioxin (41275) *Proc. Soc. exp. Biol. Med.*, **168**, 290–299

Clark, D.A., Sweeney, G., Safe, S., Hancock, E., Kilburn, D.G.& Gauldie, J. (1983) Cellular and genetic basis for suppression of cytotoxic T-cell generation by haloaromatic hydrocarbons. *Immunopharmacology*, **6**, 143–153

Clark, G.A., Tritscher, A., Maronpot, R., Foley, J. & Lucier, G. (1991a) Tumor promotion by TCDD in female rats. In: Gallo, M.A., Scheuplein, R.J. & van der Heijden, K.A., eds, *Biological Basis for Risk Assessment of Dioxins and Related Compounds* (Banbury Report 35), Cold Spring Harbor, NY, CSH Press, pp. 389–404

Clark, G.C., Taylor, M.J., Tritscher, A.M. & Lucier, G.W. (1991b) Tumor necrosis factor involvement in 2,3,7,8-tetrachlorodibenzo-*p*-dioxin-mediated endotoxin hypersensitivity in C57BL/6J mice congenic at the Ah locus. *Toxicol. appl. Pharmacol.*, **111**, 422–431

Clark, G.C., Blank, J.A., Germolec, D.R. & Luster M.I. (1991c) 2,3,7,8-Tetrachlorodibenzo-*p*-dioxin stimulation of tyrosine phosphorylation in B lymphocytes: potential role in immunosuppression. *Mol. Pharmacol.*, **39**, 495–501

Clayton, P., Davis, B., Duarte-Davidson, R., Halsall, C., Jones, K.C. & Jones, P. (1993) PCDDs and PCDFs in ambient UK urban air. *Organohalogen Compounds*, **12**, 89–93

Clement, R.E. (1991) Ultratrace dioxin and dibenzofuran analysis: 30 years of advances. *Analyt. Chem.*, **63**, 1130–1137

Clement, R.E. & Tosine, H.M. (1988) The gas chromatography/mass spectrometry determination of chlorodibenzo-*p*-dioxins and dibenzofurans. *Mass Spec. Rev.*, **7**, 593–636

Clench-Aas, J., Bartonova, A., Oehme, M. & Lindstrøm, G. (1992) PCDD and PCDF in human milk from Scandinavia, with special emphasis on Norway. *J. Toxicol. environ. Health*, **37**, 73–83

van Cleuvenbergen, R., Schoeters, J., Wevers, M., De Fré, R. & Rymen, T. (1993) Soil contamination with PCDDs and PCDFs at some typical locations in Flanders. *Organohalogen Compounds*, **12**, 243–246

Cochrane, W.P., Singh, J., Miles, W., Wakeford, B. & Scott, J. (1982) Analysis of technical and formulated products of 2,4-dichlorophenoxy acetic acid for the presence of chlorinated dibenzo-*p*-dioxins. In: Hutzinger, O., Frei, R.W., Merian, E. & Pocchiari, F., eds, *Chlorinated Dioxins and Related Products. Impact on the Environment*, Oxford, Pergamon Press, pp. 209–213

Coggon, D., Pannett, B., Winter, P.D., Acheson, E.D. & Bonsall, J. (1986) Mortality of workers exposed to 2 methyl-4-chlorophenoxyacetic acid. *Scand. J. Work Environ. Health*, **12**, 448–454

Coggon, D., Pannett, B. & Winter, P. (1991) Mortality and incidence of cancer at four factories making phenoxy herbicides. *Br. J. ind. Med.*, **48**, 173–178

Cohen, G.M., Bracken, W.M., Iyer, R.P., Berry, D.L., Selkirk, J.K. & Slaga, T.J. (1979) Anti-carcinogenic effects of 2,3,7,8-tetrachlorodibenzo-*p*-dioxin on benzo(*a*)pyrene and 7,12-dimethylbenz(*a*)anthracene tumor initiation and its relationship to DNA binding. *Cancer Res.*, **39**, 4027–4033

Collins, J.J., Strauss, M.E., Levinskas, G.J. & Conner, P.R. (1993) The mortality experience of workers exposed to 2,3,7,8-tetrachlorodibenzo-*p*-dioxin in a trichlorophenol process accident. *Epidemiology*, **4**, 7–13

Connor, M.J., Phvel, S.M., Sakamoto, M. & Nanthur, J. (1994) The *hr* locus and the toxicity of 2,3,7,8-tetrachlorodibenzo-*p*-dioxin (TCDD) in newborn mice. *Arch. Toxicol.*, **69**, 87–90

Constable, J.D. & Hatch, M.C. (1985) Reproductive effects of herbicide exposure in Vietnam: recent studies by the Vietnamese and others. *Teratog. Carcinog. Mutag.*, **5**, 231–250

Cook, R.R., Townsend, J.C., Ott, M.G. & Silverstein, L.G. (1980) Mortality experience of employees exposed to 2,3,7,8-tetrachlorodibenzo-*p*-dioxin (TCDD). *J. occup. Med.*, **22**, 530–532

Cook, R.R., Bond, G.G., Olson, R.A., Ott, M.G. & Gondek, M.R. (1986) Evaluation of the mortality experience of workers exposed to the chlorinated dioxins. *Chemosphere*, **15**, 1769–1776

Cook, J.C., Dold, K.M. & Greenlee, W.F. (1987) An in vitro model for studying the toxicity of 2,3,7,8-tetrachlorodibenzo-*p*-dioxin to human thymus. *Toxicol. appl. Pharmacol.*, **89**, 256–268

Cooper, K.R., Bergek, S., Fiedler, H., Hjelt, M., Bonner, M.S., Howell, F.G. & Rappe, C. (1996) PCDDs, PCDFs and PCBs in farm raised catfish from southeast United States. *Organohalogen Compounds*, **28**, 197–202

Cordier, S., Le, T.B.T., Verger, P., Bard, D., Le, C.D., Larouze, B., Dazza, M.C., Hoang, T.Q. & Abenhaim, L. (1993) Viral infections and chemical exposures as risk factors for hepato-cellular carcinoma in Vietnam. *Int. J. Cancer*, **55**, 196–201

Corrao, G., Calleri, M., Carle, F., Russo, R., Bosia, S. & Piccioni, P. (1989) Cancer risk in a cohort of licensed pesticide users. *Scand. J. Work Environ. Health*, **15**, 203–209

Couture, L.A., Abbott, B.D. & Birnbaum, L.S. (1990a) A critical review of the developmental toxicity and teratogenicity of 2,3,7,8-tetrachlorodibenzo-*p*-dioxin: recent advances toward understanding the mechanism. *Teratology*, **42**, 619–627

Couture, L.A., Harris, M.W. & Birnbaum, L.S. (1990b) Characterization of the peak period of sensitivity for the induction of hydronephrosis in C57BL/6N mice following exposure to 2,3,7,8-tetrachlorodibenzo-*p*-dioxin. *Fundam. appl. Toxicol.*, **15**, 142–150

Couture-Haws, L., Harris, M.W., Clark, A.M. & Birnbaum, L.S. (1991) Evaluation of the persis-tence of hydronephrosis induced in mice following in utero and/or lactational exposure to 2,3,7,8-tetrachlorodibenzo-*p*-dioxin (TCDD). *Toxicol. appl. Pharmacol.*, **107**, 402–412

Creaser, C.S., Fernandes, A.R., Al-Haddad, A., Harrad, S.J., Homer, R.B., Skett, P.W. & Cox, E.A. (1989) Survey of background levels of PCDDs and PCDFs in UK soil. *Chemosphere*, **18**, 767–776

Creaser, C.S., Fernandes, A.R., Harrad, S.J. & Cox, E.A. (1990) Levels and sources of PCDDs and PCDFs in urban British soils. *Chemosphere*, **21**, 931–938

Crow, K. *et al.* (1978) Chloracne: the chemical disease. *New Scientist*, **78**, 78–80

Crummett, W.B., Lamparski, L.L. & Nestrick, T.J. (1986) Review and trends in the analysis for PCDD/PCDF. *Toxicol. environ. Chem.*, **12**, 111–135

Cummings, A.M. & Metcaff, J.L. (1995) Induction of endometriosis in mice: a new model sensitive to estrogen. *Reprod. Toxicol.*, **9**, 233–238

Cummings, A.M., Metcalf, J.L. & Birnbaum, L. (1996) Promotion of endometriosis by 2,3,7,8-tetrachlorodibenzo-*p*-dioxin in rats and mice: time–dose dependence and species compa-rison. *Toxicol. appl. Pharmacol.*, **138**, 131–139

Curtis, L.R., Kerkvliet, N.I., BaecherSteppan, L. & Carpenter, H.M. (1990) 2,3,7,8-Tetrachloro-dibenzo-*p*-dioxin pretreatment of female mice altered tissue distribution but not hepatic metabolism of a subsequent dose. *Fundam. appl. Toxicol.*, **14**, 523–531

Dahl, P., Lindström, G., Wiberg, K. & Rappe, C. (1995) Absorption of polychlorinated bi-phenyls, dibenzo-*p*-dioxins and dibenzofurans by breast-fed infants. *Chemosphere*, **30**, 2297–2306

Dahmane, N., Charron, G., Lopes, C., Yaspo, M.-L., Manoury, C., Decorte, L., Sinet, P.-M., Bloch, M. & Delabar, J.-M. (1995) Down syndrome-critical region contains a gene homo-logous to *Drosophila sim* expressed during rat and human central nervous system deve-lopment. *Proc. natl Acad. Sci. USA*, **92**, 9191–9195

D'Argy, R., Bergman, J. & Dencker, L. (1989) Effects of immunosuppressive chemicals on lymphoid development in foetal thymus organ culture. *Pharmacol. Toxicol.*, **64**, 33–38

Davis, D. & Safe, S. (1988) Immunosuppressive activities of polychlorinated dibenzofuran con-geners: quantitative structure–activity relationships and interactive effects. *Toxicol. appl. Pharmacol.*, **94**, 141–149

Davis, D. & Safe, S. (1989) Dose-response immunotoxicities of commercial polychlorinated biphenyls (PCBs) and their interaction with 2,3,7,8-tetrachlorodibenzo-*p*-dioxin. *Toxicol. Lett.*, **48**, 35–43

Davis, D. & Safe, S. (1991) Halogenated aryl hydrocarbon-induced suppression of the in vitro plaque-forming cell response to sheep red blood cells is not independent on the Ah receptor. *Immunopharmacology*, **21**, 183–190

Decad, G.M., Birnbaum, L.S. & Matthews, H.B. (1981a) 2,3,7,8-Tetrachlorodibenzofuran tissue distribution and excretion in guinea pigs. *Toxicol. appl. Pharmacol.*, **57**, 231–240

Decad, G.M., Birnbaum, L.S. & Matthews, H.B. (1981b) Distribution and excretion of 2,3,7,8-tetrachlorodibenzofuran in C57BL/6J and DBA/2J mice. *Toxicol. appl. Pharmacol.*, **59**, 564–573

DeCaprio, A.P., McMartin, D.N., O'Keefe, P.W., Rej, R., Silkworth, J.B. & Kaminsky, L.S. (1986) Subchronic oral toxicity of 2,3,7,8-tetrachlorodibenzo-*p*-dioxin in the guinea pig: comparisons with a PCB-containing transformer fluid pyrolysate. *Fundam. appl. Toxicol.*, **6**, 454–463

De Haan, L.H.J., Simons, J.-W.F.A., Bos, A.T., Aarts, J.M.M.J.G., Denison, M.S. & Brouwer, A. (1994) Inhibition of intercellular communication by 2,3,7,8-tetrachlorodibenzo-*p*-dioxin and dioxin-like PCBs in mouse hepatoma cells (Hepa1c1c7): involvement of the Ah receptor. *Toxicol. appl. Pharmacol.*, **129**, 283–293

De Haan, L.H.J., Halfwerk, S., Hovens, S.E.L., De Roos, B., Koeman, J.H. & Brouwer, A. (1996) Inhibition of intercellular communication and induction of ethoxyresorufin-*O*-deethylase activity by polychlorobiphenyls, -dibenzo-*p*-dioxins and -dibenzofurans in mouse hepa1c1c7 cells. *Environ. Toxicol. Pharmacol.*, **1**, 27–37

Deister, U. & Pommer, R. (1991) Distribution of PCDD/F in the vicinity of the hazardous waste incinerator at Schwabach. *Chemosphere*, **23**, 1643–1651

De Jongh, J., DeVito, M., Nieboer, R., Birnbaum, L. & Van den Berg, M. (1995) Induction of cytochrome P450 isoenzymes after toxicokinetic interactions between 2,3,7,8-tetrachlorodibenzo-*p*-dioxin and 2,2',4,4',5,5'-hexachlorobiphenyl in the liver of the mouse. *Fundam. appl. Toxicol.*, **25**, 264–270

Della Porta, G., Dragani, T.A. & Sozzi, G. (1987) Carcinogenic effects of infantile and long-term 2,3,7,8-tetrachlorodibenzo-*p*-dioxin treatment in the mouse. *Tumori*, **73**, 99–107

Dencker L., Hassoun, R., d'Argy, R. & Alm G. (1985) Fetal thymus organ culture as an in vitro model for the toxicity of 2,3,7,8-tetrachloro-dibenzo-*p*-dioxin and its congeners. *Mol. Pharmacol.*, **27**, 133–140

Denis, M., Cuthill, S., Wikström, A.-C., Poellinger, L. & Gustafsson, J.-Å. (1988) Association of the dioxin receptor with the mr 90,000 heat shock protein: a structural kinship with the glucocorticoid receptor. *Biochem. Biophys. Res. Commun.*, **155**, 801–807

Denison, M.S. & Whitlock, J.P., Jr (1995) Xenobiotic-inducible transcription of cytochrome P450 genes. *J. biol. Chem.*, **270**, 18175–18178

Denison, M.S., Fisher, J.M. & Whittlock, J.P., Jr (1988) The DNA recognition site for the dioxin-Ah receptor complex. *J. Biol. Chem.*, **263**, 17221–17224

DePetrillo, P.B. & Kurl, R.N. (1993) Stimulation of protein kinase C by 2,3,7,8-tetrachlorodibenzo-*p*-dioxin (TCDD) in rat thymocytes. *Toxicol. Lett.*, **69**, 31–36

Deutsche Forschungsgemeinschaft (1996) *List of MAK and BAT Values 1996* (Report No. 32), Weinheim, VCH Verlagsgesellschaft, pp. 86, 120

DeVito, M.J. & Birnbaum, L.S. (1995) The importance of pharmacokinetics in determining the relative potency of 2,3,7,8-tetrachlorodibenzo-*p*-dioxin and 2,3,7,8-tetrachlorodibenzofuran. *Fund. appl. Toxicol.*, **24**, 145–148

DeVito, M.J., Thomas, T., Martin, E., Umbreit, T.H. & Gallo, M.A. (1992) Antiestrogenic action of 2,3,7,8-tetrachlorodibenzo-p-dioxin: tissue-specific regulation of estrogen receptor in CD1 mice. *Toxicol. appl. Pharmacol.*, **113**, 284–292

DeVito, M.J., Ma, S., Babish, J.G., Menache, M. & Birnbaum, L.S. (1994) Dose–response relationships in mice following subchronic exposure to 2,3,7,8-tetrachlorodibenzo-*p*-dioxin: CYP1A1, CYP1A2, estrogen receptor, and protein tyrosine phosphorylation. *Toxicol. appl. Pharmacol.*, **124**, 82–90

Dewailly, E., Tremblay-Rousseau, H., Carrier, G., Groulx, S., Gingras, S., Boggess, K., Stanley, J. & Weber, J.P. (1991) PCDDs, PCDFs and PCBs in human milk of women exposed to a PCB fire and of women of the general population of the Province of Québec — Canada. *Chemosphere*, **23**, 1831–1835

Dickins, M., Seefeld, M.D. & Peterson, R.E. (1981) Enhanced liver DNA synthesis in partially hepatectomized rats pretreated with 2,3,7,8-tetrachlorodibenzo-*p*-dioxin. *Toxicol. appl. Pharmacol.*, **58**, 389–398

di Domenico, A. & Zapponi, G.A. (1986) 2,3,7,8-Tetrachlorodibenzo-p-dioxin (TCDD) in the environment: human health risk estimation and its application to the Seveso case as an example. *Reg. Toxicol. Pharmacol.*, **6**, 248–260

di Domenico, A., Ferri, F., Fulgenzi, A.R., Iacovella, N., La Rocca, C., Miniero, R., Rodriguez, F., Scotto di Tella, E., Silvestri, S., Tafani, P., Turrio Baldassarri, L. & Volpi, F. (1993a) Polychlorinated biphenyl, dibenzodioxin, and dibenzofuran occurence in the general environment in Italy. *Chemosphere*, **27**, 83–90

di Domenico, A., De Felip, E., Ferri, F., Iacovella, N., La Rocca, C., Lupi, C., Miniero, R., Rodriguez, F., Scotto di Tella, E., Silvestri, S., Turrio Baldassarri, L. & Volpi, F. (1993b) Polychlorinated dibenzodioxins, dibenzofurans, and biphenyls in the soil of an area neighboring a contaminated industrial site. *Organohalogen Compounds*, **12**, 247–250

DiGiovanni, J., Viaje, A., Berry, D.L., Slaga, T.J. & Juchau, M.R. (1977) Tumor-initiating ability of 2,3,7,8-tetrachlorodibenzo-*p*-dioxin (TCDD) and Arochlor 1254 in the two-stage system of mouse skin carcinogenesis. *Bull. environ. Contam. Toxicol.*, **18**, 552–557

DiGiovanni, J., Decina, P.C. & Diamond, L. (1983) Tumor initiating activity of 9- and 10-fluoro-7,12-dimethylbenz[*a*]anthracene (DMBA) and the effect of 2,3,7,8-tetrachlorodibenzo-*p*-dioxin on tumor initiation by monofluoro derivatives of DMBA in SENCAR mice. *Carcinogenesis*, **4**, 1045–1049

Diliberto, J.J., Akubue, P.I., Luebke, R.W. & Birnbaum, L.S. (1995) Dose-response relationships of tissue distribution and induction of CYP1A1 and CYP1A2 enzymatic activities following acute exposure to 2,3,7,8-tetrachlorodibenzo-*p*-dioxin (TCDD) in mice. *Toxicol. appl. Pharmacol.*, **130**, 197–208

Diliberto, J.J., Jackson, J.A. & Birnbaum, L.S., (1996) Comparison of 2,3,7,8-tetrachlorodibenzo-*p*-dioxin (TCDD) disposition following pulmonary, oral, dermal, and parenteral exposures to rats. *Toxicol. appl. Pharmacol.*, **138**, 158-168

Döhr, O., Vogel, C. & Abel, J. (1994) Modulation of growth factor expression by 2,3,7,8-tetrachlorodibenzo-*p*-dioxin. *Exp. clin. Immunogenet.*, **11**, 142–148

Dolwick, K.M., Swanson, H.I. & Bradfield, C.A. (1993) In vitro analysis of Ah receptor domains involved in ligand-activated DNA recognition. *Proc. natl Acad. Sci. USA*, **90**, 8566–8570

Donovan, J.W., MacLennan, R. & Adena, M. (1984) Vietnam service and the risk of congenital anomalies. A case control study. *Med. J. Aust.*, **140**, 394–397

Dooley, R.K. & Holsapple, M.P. (1988) Elucidation of cellular targets responsible for 2,3,7,8-tetrachloro-dibenzo-*p*-dioxin (TCDD)-induced suppression of antibody responses. I. The role of the B lymphocyte. *Immunopharmacology*, **16**, 167–180

Dooley, R.K., Morris, D.L. & Holsapple, M.P. (1990) Elucidation of cellular targets responsible for tetrachlorodibenzo-p-dioxin (TCDD)-induced suppression of antibody responses. II. The role of the T-lymphocyte. *Immunopharmacology*, **19**, 47–58

Döring, J., Damberg, M., Gamradt, A. & Oehme, M. (1992) Screening method based on the determination of perchlorinated aromatics for surface soil contaminated by copper slag containing high levels of polychlorinated dibenzofurans and dibenzo-*p*-dioxins. *Chemosphere*, **25**, 755–762

Dorschkind, K. (1994) Transcriptional control points during lymphopoiesis. *Cell*, **79**, 751–753

Doss, M., Sauer, H., Von Tiepermann, R. & Colombi, A.M. (1984) Development of chronic hepatic porphyria (porphyria cutanea tarda) with inherited uroporphyrinogen decarboxylase deficiency under exposure to dioxin. *Int. J. Biochem.*, **16**, 369–373

Doyle, B.W., Drum, D.A. & Lauber, J.D. (1985) The smoldering question of hospital wastes. *Pollut. Eng.*, **17**, 35–39

Dragan, Y.P., Rizvi, T., Xu, Y.-H., Hully, J.R., Bawa, N., Campbell, H.A., Maronpot, R.R. & Pitot, H.C. (1991) An initiation-promotion assay in rat liver as a potential complement to the 2-year carcinogenesis bioassay. *Fundam. appl. Toxicol.*, **16**, 525–547

Dragan, Y.P., Xu, X.-H., Goldsworthy, T.L., Campbell, H.A., Maronpot, R.R. & Pitot, H.C. (1992) Characterization of the promotion of altered hepatic foci by 2,3,7,8-tetrachlorodibenzo-*p*-dioxin in the female rat. *Carcinogenesis*, **13**, 1389–1395

Dragani, T. A., Canzian, F., Manenti, G. & Pierotti, M.A. (1996) Hepatocarcinogenesis: a polygenic model of inherited predisposition to cancer. *Tumori*, **82**, 1–5

Drenth, H.J., Seinen, W. & Van Den Berg, M. (1996) Effects of TCDD and PCB#126 on aromatase (CYP19) activity in the human choriocarcinoma cell line JEG-3. *Organohalogen Compounds*, **29**, 204–208

Drutel, G., Kathmann, M., Heron, A., Schwartz, J.-C. & Arrang, J.-M. (1996) Cloning and selective expression in brain and kidney of ARNTZ homologous to the Ah receptor nuclear translocator (ARNT). *Biochem. Biophys. Res. Comm.*, **225**, 333–339

Duarte-Davidson, R., Harrad, S.J., Allen, S., Sewart, A.S. & Jones, K.C. (1993) The relative contribution of individual polychlorinated biphenyls (PCBs), polychlorinated dibenzo-*p*-dioxins (PCDDs) and polychlorinated dibenzo-*p*-furans (PCDFs) to toxic equivalent values derived for bulked human adipose tissue samples from Wales, United Kingdom. *Arch. environ. Contam. Toxicol.*, **24**, 100–107

Durrin, L.K. & Whitlock, J.P., Jr (1987) *In situ* protein-DNA interactions at a dioxin-responsive enhancer associated with the cytochrome P_1-450 gene. *Mol. cell. Biol.*, **7**, 3008–3011

Dyke, P. & Colman, P. (1995) Dioxins in ambient air, bonfire night 1994. *Organohalogen Compounds*, **24**, 213–216

Ebner, K., Brewster, D.W. & Matsumura, F. (1988) Effects of 2,3,7,8-tetrachlorodibenzo-*p*-dioxin on serum insulin and glucose levels in the rabbit. *J. environ. Sci. Health*, **B23**, 427–438

Ebner, K., Matsumura, F., Enan, E. & Olsen, H. (1993) 2,3,7,8-Tetrachlorodibenzo-*p*-dioxin (TCDD) alters pancreatic membrane tyrosine phosphorylation following acute treatment. *J. biochem. Toxicol.*, **8**, 71–81

ECETOC (1992) *Exposure of Man to Dioxins: A Perspective on Industrial Waste Incineration* (Technical Report No. 49), Brussels, European Centre for Ecotoxicology and Toxicology of Chemicals

Edgerton, S.A., Czuczwa, J.M., Rench, J.D., Hodanbosi, R.F. & Koval, P.J. (1989) Ambient air concentrations of polychlorinated dibenzo-p-dioxins and dibenzofurans in Ohio: sources and health risk assessment.*Chemosphere*, **18**, 1713–1730

Egeland, G.M., Sweeney, M.H., Fingerhut, M.A., Wille, K.K., Schnorr, T.M. & Halperin, W.E. (1994) Total serum testosterone and gonadotropins in workers exposed to dioxin. *Am. J. Epidemiol.*, **139**, 272–281

Eitzer, B.D. (1995) Polychlorinated dibenzo-*p*-dioxins and dibenzofurans in raw milk samples from farms located near a new resource recovery incinerator. *Chemosphere*, **30**, 1237–1248

Eitzer, B.D. & Hites, R.A. (1989) Dioxins and furans in the ambient atmosphere: a baseline study. *Chemosphere*, **18**, 593-598

Eldridge, S.R., Gould, M.N. & Butterworth, B.E. (1992) Genotoxicity of environmental agents in human mammary epithelial cells. *Cancer Res.*, **52**, 5617–5621

Ema, M., Sogawa, K., Watanabe, Y., Chujoh, Y., Matsushita, N., Gotoh, O., Funae, Y. & Fujii-Kuriyama, Y. (1992) cDNA cloning and structure of mouse putative Ah receptor. *Biochem. Biophys. Res. Commun.*, **184**, 246–253

Ema, M., Ohe, N., Suzuki, M., Mimura, J., Sogawa, K., Ikawa, S. & Fujii-Kuriyama, Y. (1994) Dioxin binding activities of polymorphic forms of mouse and human arylhydrocarbon receptors. *J. biol. Chem.*, **269**, 27337–27343

Emi, Y., Ikushiro, S. & Iyanagi, T. (1995) Drug-responsive and tissue-specific alternative expression of multiple first exons in rat UDP-glucuronosyl transferase family 1 (UGT1) gene complex. *J. Biochem. (Tokyo)*, **117**, 392–399

Emi, Y., Ikushiro, S. & Iyanagi, T. (1996) Xenobiotic responsive element-mediated transcriptional activation in the UDP-glucuronosyltransferase family 1 gene complex. *J. biol. Chem.*, **271**, 3952–3958

Enan, E. & Matsumura, F. (1994a) 2,3,7,8-Tetrachlorodibenzo-*p*-dioxin (TCDD)-induced changes in glucose transporting activity in guinea pigs, mice, and rats *in vivo* and *in vitro*. *J. biochem. Toxicol.*, **9**, 97–106

Enan, E. & Matsumura, F. (1994b) Significance of TCDD-induced changes in protein phosphorylation in the adipocyte of male guinea pigs. *J. biochem. Toxicol.*, **9**, 159–170

Enan, E. & Matsumura, F. (1995a) Regulation by 2,3,7,8-tetrachlorodibenzo-*p*-dioxin (TCDD) of the DNA binding activity of transcriptional factors via nuclear protein phosphorylation in guinea pig adipose tissue. *Biochem. Pharmacol.*, **50**, 1199–1206

Enan, E. & Matsumura, F. (1995b) Evidence for a second pathway in the action mechanism of 2,3,7,8-tetrachlorodibenzo-*p*-dioxin (TCDD). *Biochem. Pharmacol.*, **49**, 249–261

Enan, E., Liu, P.C. & Matsumura, F. (1992) 2,3,7,8-Tetrachlorodibenzo-*p*-dioxin causes reduction of glucose transporting activities in the plasma membranes of adipose tissue and pancreas from the guinea pig. *J. biol. Chem.*, **267**, 19785–19791

Erickson, J.D., Mulinare, J., McClain, P.W., Fitch, T.G., James, L.M., McClearn, A.B. & Adams, M.J., Jr (1984) Vietnam veterans'risks for fathering babies with birth defects. *J. Am. med. Assoc.*, **252**, 903–912

Eriksson, P. (1988) Effects of 3,3′,4,4′-tetrachlorobiphenyl in the brain of the neonatal mouse. *Toxicology*, **69**, 43–48

Eriksson, M., Hardell, L., Berg, N.O., Moller, T. & Axelson, O. (1981) Soft-tissue sarcomas and exposure to chemical substances: a case-referent study. *Br. J. ind. Med.*, **38**, 27–33

Eriksson, M., Hardell, L. & Adami, H.-O. (1990) Exposure to dioxins as a risk factor for soft tissue sarcoma: a population-based case-control study. *J. natl Cancer Inst.*, **82**, 486–490

Eriksson, M., Hardell, L., Malker, H. & Weiner J. (1992) Malignant lymphoproliferative diseases in occupations with potential exposure to phenoxyacetic acids or dioxins: a register-based study. *Am. J. ind. Med.*, **22**, 305–312

European Commission (1992) Fifteenth Commission Directive 92/86/EEC of 21 October 1992 adapting to technical progress Annexes II, III, IV, V and VII of Council Directive 76/768/EEC on the approximation of the laws of the Member States relating to cosmetic products. *Off. J. Eur. Communities*, **L 325**

European Commission (1994) Council directive 94/67/EC of 16 December 1994 on the incineration of hazardous waste. *Off. J. Eur. Comm.*, **L365**, 34

Evans, G.R., Webb, K.B., Knutsen, A.P., Roodman, S.T., Roberts, D.W., Bägby, J.R., Garrett, W.A. & Andrews, J.S. (1988) A medical follow-up of the health effects of long-term exposure to 2,3,7,8-tetrachlorodibenzo-*p*-dioxin. *Arch. environ. Health*, **43**, 273–278

Ewers, U., Wittsiepe, J., Schrey, P., Engelhart, S., Bernsdorf, U. & Selenka, F. (1994) Blood levels of PCDDs/PCDFs in allotment gardeners in Duisburg. *Gesundh.-Wes.*, **56**, 467–471 (in German)

Fabarius, G., Wilken, M., Borgas, M. & Zeschmar-Lahl, B. (1990) Release of organic pollutants during accidental fires. *Organohalogen Compounds*, **3**, 373–377

Facchetti, S., Balasso, A., Fichtner, C., Frare, G., Leoni, A., Mauri, C. & Vasconi, M. (1986) Studies on the absorption of TCDD by plant species. In: Rappe, C., Choudhary, G. & Keith, L.H., eds, *Chlorinated Dioxins and Dibenzofurans in Perspective*, Chelsea, MI, Lewis Publishers, pp. 225–239

Faerden, K. (1991) *Dioxins in Food* (SNT-report 4), Olso, Norwegian Food Control Authority (in Norwegian)

Fagan, J.B., Pastewka, J.V., Chalberg, S.C., Gozukara, E., Guengerich, F.P. & Gelboin, H.V. (1986) Noncoordinate regulation of the mRNAs encoding cytochromes P-450$_{BNF/MC-B}$ and P-450$_{ISF/BNF-G}$. *Arch. Biochem. Biophys.*, **244**, 261–272

Fahrig, R. (1993) Genetic effects of dioxins on the spot test with mice. *Environ. Health Perspectives*, **101** (Suppl. 3), 257–261

Faith, R.E. & Moore, J.A. (1977) Impairment of thymus-independent immune functions by exposure of developing immune system to 2,3,7,8-tetrachlorodibenzo-*p*-dioxin (TCDD). *J. Toxicol. environ. Health*, **3**, 451–464

Fan, F. & Rozman, K.K. (1994) Relationship between acute toxicity of 2,3,7,8-tetrachlorodibenzo-*p*-dioxin (TCDD) and disturbance of intermediary metabolism in the Long-Evans rat. *Arch. Toxicol.*, **69**, 73–78

Fan, F. & Rozman, K.K. (1995) Short- and long-term biochemical effects of 2,3,7,8-tetrachlorodibenzo-*p*-dioxin in female Long-Evans rats. *Toxicol. Lett.*, **75**, 209–216

Fan, F., Pinson, D.M. & Rozman, K.K. (1995) Immunomodulatory effect of 2,3,7,8-tetrachloro-dibenzo-*p*-dioxin tested by the popliteal lymph node assay. *Toxicol. Pathol.*, **23**, 513–517

Fauvarque, J. (1996) The chlorine industry. *Pure appl. Chem.*, **68**, 1713–1720

Fedorov, L. (1993) Ecological problems in Russia caused by dioxin emissions from chemical industry. *Chemosphere*, **27**, 91–95

Fedorov, L.A., Tyler, A.O., Jones, P.H. & Vasjuchin, P.M. (1993) Levels and profiles of PCDDs and PCDFs in soils and sediments from Chapaevsk, Samara Province, Russia. *Organohalogen Compounds*, **12**, 195–198

Fehringer, N.V., Walthers, S.M., Kozara, R.J. & Schneider, L.F. (1985) Survey of 2,3,7,8-tetra-chlorodibenzo-*p*-dioxin in fish from the Great Lakes and selected Michigan rivers. *J. agric. Food Chem.*, **33**, 626–630

Fernandez, P. & Safe, S. (1992) Growth inhibitory and antimitogenic activity of 2,3,7,8-tetra-chlorodibenzo-*p*-dioxin (TCDD) in T47D human breast cancer cells. *Toxicol. Lett.*, **61**, 185–197

Fernandez-Salguero, P., Pineau, T., Hilbert, D.M., McPhail, T., Lee, S.S.T., Kimura, S., Nebert, D.W., Rudikoff, S., Ward, J.M. & Gonzalez, F.J. (1995) Immune system impairment and hepatic fibrosis in mice lacking the dioxin-binding Ah receptor. *Science*, **268**, 722–726

Ferrario, J., Byrne, C., McDaniel, D., Dupuy, A. & Harless, R. (1996) Determination of 2,3,7,8-chlorine-substituted dibenzo-p-dioxins and -furans at the part per trillion level in United States beef fat using high resolution gas chromatography/high-resolution mass spectrometry. *Anal. Chem.*, **68**, 647–652

Fett, M.J., Adena, M.A., Cobbin, D.M. & Dunn, M. (1987a) Mortality among Australian conscripts of the Vietnam conflict era. I. Death from all causes. *Am. J. Epidemiol.*, **125**, 869–877

Fett, M.J., Nairn, J.R., Cobbin, D.M. & Adena, M.A. (1987b) Mortality among Australian conscripts of the Vietnam conflict era. II. Causes of death. *Am. J. Epidemiol.*, **125**, 878–884

Fiedler, H., Lau, C., Cooper, K., Andersson, R., Kulp, S.-E., Rappe, C., Howell, F. & Bonner, M. (1995) PCDD/PCDF in soil and pine needle samples in a rural area in the United States of America. *Organohalogen Compounds*, **24**, 285–292

Fiedler, H., Lau, C., Bonner, M.S., Cooper, K.R., Anderson, R., Bergek, S., Hjelt, M. & Rappe, C. (1996) PCDD/PCDF in Mexican food. *Organohalogen Compounds*, **28**, 105–110

Field, B. & Kerr, C. (1979) Herbicide use and incidence of neural-tube defects. *Lancet*, **i**, 1341–1342

Filippini, G., Bordo, B., Crenna, P., Massetto, N., Musicco, M. & Boeri, R. (1981) Relationship between clinical and electrophysiological findings and indicators of heavy exposure to 2,3,7,8-tetrachlorodibenzo-*p*-dioxin. *Scand. J. Work Environ. Health*, **7**, 257–262

Fine, J.S., Gasiewicz, T.A. & Silverstone, A.E. (1988) Lymphocyte stem cell alterations following perinatal exposure to 2,3,7,8-tetrachlorodibenzo-*p*-dioxin. *Mol. Pharmacol.*, **35**, 15–25

Fine, J.S., Gasiewicz, T.A. & Silverstone, A.E. (1989) Lymphocyte stem cell alterations following perinatal exposure to 2,3,7,8-tetrachlorodibenzo-*p*-dioxin. *Mol. Pharmacol.*, **35**, 18–25.

Fine, J.S., Gasiewicz, T.A., Fiore, N.C. & Silverstone, A.E. (1990a) Prothymocyte activity is reduced by perinatal 2,3,7,8-tetrachlorodibenzo-*p*-dioxin exposure. *J. exp. Pharmacol. Ther.*, **255**, 1–5

Fine, J.S., Silverstone, A.E. & Gasiewicz, T.A. (1990b) Impairment of prothymocyte activity by 2,3,7,8-tetrachloro-dibenzo-*p*-dioxin. *J. Immunol.*, **144**, 1169–1176

Fingerhut, M.A., Sweeney, M.H., Patterson, D.G., Piacitelli, L.A., Morris, J.A., Marlow, D.A., Hornung, R.W., Cameron, L.W., Connally, L.B., Needham, L.L. & Halperin, W.E. (1989) Levels of 2,3,7,8-tetrachlorodibenzo-*p*-dioxin in the serum of U.S. chemical workers exposed to dioxin contaminated products: interim results. *Chemosphere*, **19**, 835–840

Fingerhut, M.A., Halperin, W.E., Marlow, D.A., Piacitelli, L.A., Honchar, P.A., Sweeney, M.H., Greife, A.L., Dill, P.A., Steenland, K. & Suruda, A.J. (1991a) Cancer mortality in workers exposed to 2,3,7,8-tetrachlorodibenzo-*p*-dioxin. *New Engl. J. Med.*, **324**, 212–218

Fingerhut, M.A., Halperin, W.E., Marlow, D.A., Piacitelli, L.A., Honchar, P.A., Sweeney, M.H., Greife, A.L., Dill, P.A., Steenland, K. & Suruda, A.J. (1991b) *Mortality Among U.S. Workers Employed in the Production of Chemicals Contaminated with 2,3,7,8-Tetrachloro-dibenzo-p-dioxin (TCDD)* (NTIS PB 91-125971), Cincinnati, OH, United States Department of Health and Human Services, National Institute for Occupational Safety and Health

Fiorella, P.D., Olson, J.R. & Napoli, J.L. (1995) 2,3,7,8-Tetrachlorodibenzo-*p*-dioxin induces diverse retinoic acid metabolites in multiple tissues of the Sprague Dawley rat. *Toxicol. appl. Pharmacol.*, **134**, 222–228

Firestone, D. (1973) Etiology of chick edema disease. *Environ. Health Perspectives*, **5**, 59–66

Firestone, D., Niemann, R.A., Schneider, L.F., Gridley, J.R. & Brown, D.E. (1986) Dioxin residues in fish and other foods. In: Rappe, C., Chaudhary, G. & Keith, L.H., eds, *Chlorinated Dioxins and Dibenzofurans in Perspective*, Chelsea, MI, Lewis Publishers, pp. 355–365

Firestone, D., Fehringer, N.V., Walters, S.M., Kozara, R.J., Ayres, R.J., Ogger, J.D., Schneider, L.F., Glidden, R.M., Ahlrep, J.R., Brown, P.J., Ford, S.E., Davy, R.A., Gulick, D.J., McCullough, B.H., Sittig, R.A., Smith, P.V., Syvertson, C.N. & Barber, M.R. (1996) TCDD residues in fish and shellfish from US waterways. *J Am. off. anal. Chem. int*, **79**, 1174–1183

Fitchett, J.E. & Hay, E.D. (1989) Medial edge epithelium transforms to mesenchyme after embryonic palatal shelves fuse. *Dev. Biol.*, **131**, 455–474

Flesch-Janys, D., Berger, J., Gurn, P., Manz, A., Nagel, S., Waltsgott, H. & Dwyer, J.H. (1995) Exposure to polychlorinated dioxins and furans (PCDD/F) and mortality in a cohort of workers from a herbicide-producing plant in Hamburg, Federal Republic of Germany. *Am. J. Epidemiol.*, **142**, 1165–1176

Flesch-Janys, D., Becher, H., Gurn, P., Jung, D., Konietzko, J., Manz, A. & Päpke, O. (1996a) Elimination of polychlorinated dibenzo-*p*-dioxins and dibenzofurans in occupationally exposed persons. *J. Toxicol. environ. Health*, **47**, 363–378

Flesch-Janys, D., Berger, J., Gurn, P., Manz, A., Nagel, S., Waltsgott, H. & Dwyer, J.H. (1996b) Erratum. *Am. J. Epidemiol.*, **144**, 716

Flodström, S. & Ahlborg, U.G. (1989) Tumour promoting effects of 2,3,7,8-tetrachlorodibenzo-*p*-dioxin (TCDD) — Effects of exposure duration, administration schedule and type of diet. *Chemosphere*, **19**, 779–783

Flodström, S. & Ahlborg, U. (1991) Promotion of hepatocarcinogenesis in rats by PCDDs and PCDFs. In: Gallo, M.A., Schleuplein, R. & van der Heijden, K., eds, *Biological Basis for Risk Assessment of Dioxins and Related Compounds* (Banbury Report 35), Cold Spring Harbor, NY, CSH Press, pp. 405–414

Flodström, S., Busk, L., Kronevi, T. & Ahlborg, U.G. (1991) Modulation of 2,3,7,8-tetrachloro-dibenzo-*p*-dioxin and phenobarbital-induced promotion of hepatocarcinogenesis in rats by the type of diet and vitamin A deficiency. *Fundam. appl. Toxicol.*, **16**, 375–391

Fortunati, G.U., Banfi, C. & Pasturenzi, M. (1994) Soil sampling. *Fresenius J. analyt. Chem.*, **348**, 86-100

Fox, A.J. & Collier, P.F. (1976) Low mortality rates in industrial cohort studies due to selection for work and survival in the industry. *Br. J. prev. soc. Med.*, **30**, 225–230

Fox, T.R., Best, L.L., Goldsworthy, S. M., Mills, J. J. & Goldsworthy, T.L. (1993) Gene expression and cell proliferation in rat liver after 2,3,7,8-tetrachlorodibenzo-*p*-dioxin exposure. *Cancer Res.*, **53**, 2265–2271

Foxall, C.D. & Lovett, A.A. (1994) The relationship between soil PCB and PCDD/DF concentrations in the vicinity of a chemical waste incinerator in South Wales, UK. *Organohalogen Compounds*, **20**, 35–40

Fraisse, D., Schnepp, B., Mort-Bontemps, C. & Le Querrec, F. (1996) Levels of polychloro-dibenzo-dioxins (PCDDs) and polychlorodibenzo-furans (PCDFs) in milk in France. *Organohalogen Compounds*, **28**, 209–212

Frankenhaeuser, M., Manninen, H., Kojo, I., Ruuskanen, J., Vartiainen, T., Vesterinen, R. & Virkki, J. (1993) Organic emissions from co-combustion of mixed plastics with coal in a burning fluidized bed boiler. *Chemosphere*, **27**, 309–316

Frazier, D.E., Silverstone, A.E., Soults J.A. & Gasiewicz, T.A. (1994a) The thymus does not mediate 2,3,7,8-tetrachlorodibenzi-p-dioxin elicited alterations in bone marrow lymphocyte stem cells. *Toxicol. appl. Pharmacol.*, **124**, 242–247

Frazier, D.E., Silverstone, A.E. & Gasiewicz, T.A. (1994b) 2,3,7,8-Tetrachlorodibenzo-*p*-dioxin induced thymic atrophy and lymphocyte stem cell alterations by mechanisms independent of the estrogen receptor. *Biochem. Pharmacol.*, **47**, 2039–2048

Fries, G.F. & Marrow, G.S. (1975) Retention and excretion of 2,3,7,8-tetra-chlorodibenzo-*p*-dioxin by rats. *J. agric. Food Chem.*, **23**, 265–269

Friesel, P., Sievers, S., Fiedler, H., Gras, B., Lau, C., Reich, T., Rippen, G., Schacht, U. & Vahrenholt, F. (1996) Dioxin mass balance for the City of Hamburg, Germany. Part 4: Follow up study — trends of PCDD/PCDF fluxes. *Organohalogen Compounds*, **28**, 89–94

Friesen, K.J., Vilk, J. & Muir, D.C.G. (1990) Aqueous solubilities of selected 2,3,7,8-substituted polychlorinated dibenzofurans (PCDFs). *Chemosphere*, **20**, 27–32

Friesen, K.J., Foga, M.M. & Loewen, M.D. (1996) Aquatic photodegradation of polychlorinated dibenzofurans: rates and photoproduct analysis. *Environ. Sci. Technol.*, **30**, 2504–2510

Frommberger, R. (1990) Polychlorinated dibenzo-*p*-dioxins and polychlorinated dibenzofurans in cumulative samples of human milk from Baden-Württemberg, FRG. *Chemosphere*, **20**, 333–342

Frommberger, R. (1991) Polychlorinated dibenzo-*p*-dioxins and polychlorinated dibenzofurans in fish from South-west Germany: River Rhine and Neckar. *Chemosphere*, **22**, 29–38

Fujii-Kuriyama, Y., Imataka, H., Sogawa, K., Yasumoto, K.-I. & Kiguchi, Y. (1992) Regulation of Cyp1A1 expression. *Fed. Am. Soc. exp. Biol. J.*, **6**, 706–710

Fujisawa-Sehara, A., Sogawa, K., Nishi, C. & Fujii-Kuriyama, Y. (1986) Regulatory DNA elements localized remotely upstream from the drug-metabolizing cytochrome P-450c gene. *Nucleic Acids Res.*, **14**,1465–1477

Fujisawa-Sehara, A., Yamane, M. & Fujii-Kuriyama, Y. (1988) A DNA-binding factor specific for xenobiotic responsive elements of P-450c gene exists as a cryptic form in cytoplasm: its possible translocation to nucleus. *Proc. natl Acad. Sci. USA*, **85**, 5859–5863

Funseth, E. & Ilbäck, N.-G. (1992) Effects of 2,3,7,8-tetrachlorodibenzo-*p*-dioxin on blood and spleen natural killer (NK) cell activity in the mouse. *Toxicol. Lett.*, **60**, 247–256

Funseth, E. & Ilbäck, N.-G. (1994) Coxsackievirus B3 infection alters the uptake of 2,3,7,8-tetrachlorodibenzo-*p*-dioxin into various tissues of the mouse. *Toxicology*, **90**, 29–38

Fürst, P. & Wilmers, K. (1995) PCDD/F levels in dairy products 1994 versus 1990. *Organohalogen Compounds*, **26**, 101–104

Fürst, P., Meemken, H.-A., Krüger, C. & Groebel, W. (1987) Polychlorinated dibenzodioxins and dibenzofurans in human milk samples from western Germany. *Chemosphere*, **16**, 1983–1988

Fürst, P., Krüger, C., Meemken, H.-A. & Groebel, W. (1989) PCDD and PCDF levels in human milk — dependence on the period of lactation. *Chemosphere*, **18**, 439–444

Fürst, P., Fürst, C. & Groebel, W. (1990) Levels of PCDDs and PCDFs in food-stuffs from the Federal Republic of Germany. *Chemosphere*, **20**, 787–792

Fürst, P., Fürst, C. & Wilmers, K. (1992a) Survey of dairy products for PCDDs, PCDFs, PCBs and HCB. *Chemosphere*, **25**, 1039–1048

Fürst, P., Fürst, C. & Wilmers, K. (1992b) PCDDs and PCDFs in human milk — statistical evaluation of a 6-years survey. *Chemosphere*, **25**, 1029–1038

Fürst, P., Krause, G.H.M., Hein, D., Delschen, T. & Wilmers, K (1993) PCDD/PCDF in cow's milk in relation to their levels in grass and soil. *Chemosphere*, **27**, 1349–1357

Gaido, K.W. & Maness, S.C. (1994) Regulation of gene expression and acceleration of differentiation in human keratinocytes by 2,3,7,8-tetrachlorodibenzo-*p*-dioxin. *Toxicol. appl. Pharmacol.*, **127**, 199–208

Gaido, K.W., Maness, S.C., Leonard, L.S. & Greenlee, W.F. (1992) 2,3,7,8-Tetrachlorodibenzo-*p*-dioxin-dependent regulation of transforming growth factors-a and b$_2$ expression in a human keratinocyte cell line involves both transcriptional and post-transcriptional control. *J. biol. Chem.*, **267**, 24591–24595

Gallagher, J.E., Everson, R.B., Lewtas, J., George, M. & Lucier, G.W. (1994) Comparison of DNA adduct levels in human placenta from polychlorinated biphenyl exposed women and smokers in which CYP 1A1 levels are similarly elevated. *Teratog. Carcinog. Mutag.*, **14**, 183–192

Gälli, R., Krebs, J., Kaft, M. & Good, M. (1992) PCDDs and PCDFs in soil samples from Switzerland. *Chemosphere*, **24**, 1095–1102

Gasiewicz, T.A. & Neal, R.A. (1979) 2,3,7,8-Tetrachlorodibenzo-*p*-dioxin tissue distribution, excretion, and effects on clinical chemical parameters in guinea pigs. *Toxicol. appl. Pharmacol.*, **51**, 329–339

Gasiewicz, T.A., Holscher, M.A. & Neal, R.A. (1980) The effect of total parenteral nutrition on the toxicity of 2,3,7,8-tetrachlorodibenzo-*p*-dioxin in the rat. *Toxicol. appl. Pharmacol.*, **54**, 469–488

Gasiewicz, T.A., Geiger, L.E., Rucci, G. & Neal, R.A. (1983) Distribution, excretion, and metabolism of 2,3,7,8-tetrachlorodibenzo-*p*-dioxin in C57BL/6J, DBA/2J, and B6D2F1/J mice. *Drug Metab. Dispos.*, **11**, 397–403

Gehrs, B. & Smialowicz R. (1994) Effects of in utero TCDD exposure to phenotypic subpopulations of rat fetal thymocytes (Abstract). *Toxicologist*, **14**, 382

Gehrs, B.D., Riddle, M.M., Williams, W.C. & Smialowicz, R.J. (1995) Effects of perinatal 2,3,7,8-TCDD exposure on the developing immune system of the F344 rat (Abstract). *Toxicologist*, **15**, 104

Geiger, L.E. & Neal, R.A. (1981) Mutagenicity testing of 2,3,7,8-tetrachlorodibenzo-*p*-dioxin in Histidine Auxotrophs of *Salmonella typhimurium*. *Toxicol. appl. Pharmacol.*, **59**, 125–129

George, L., Sund, C., Sund, K.G. & Baller, J. (1993) Assessment of dioxin-related health risks for the Melbourne metropolitan area. *Aust. J. public Health*, **17**, 162–168

Germolec, D.R., Henry, E.C., Maronpot, R., Foley, J.F., Adams, N.H., Gasiewicz, T.A., & Luster, M.I. (1996) Induction of CYP1A1 and ALDH-3 in lymphoid tissues from Fisher 344 rats exposed to 2,3,7,8-tetrachlorodibenzo-*p*-dioxin (TCDD). *Toxicol. appl. Pharmacol.*, **137**, 57–66

Geyer, H.J., Scheuntert, I., Rapp, K., Kettrup, A., Korte, F., Greim, H. & Rozman, K. (1990) Correlation between acute toxicity of 2,3,7,8-tetrachlorodibenzo-*p*-dioxin (TCDD) and total body fat content in mammals. *Toxicology*, **65**, 97–107

Giavini, E.M., Prati, M. & Vismara, C. (1982) Effects of 2,3,7,8-tetrachlorodibenzo-*p*-dioxin administered to pregnant rats during the preimplantation period. *Environ. Res.*, **29**, 185–189

Giavinni, E., Prati, M. & Vismara, C. (1983) Embryotoxic effects of 2,3,7,8-tetrachlordibenzo-*p*-dioxin administered to female rats before mating. *Environ. Res.*, **31**, 105–110

Gierthy, J.F. & Crane, D. (1985) *In vitro* bioassay for dioxin-like activity based on alterations in epithelial cell proliferation and morphology. *Fundam. appl. Toxicol.*, **5**, 754–759

Gierthy, J.F. & Lincoln, D.W. (1988) Inhibition of postconfluent focus production in cultures of MCF-7 breast cancer cells by 2,3,7,8-tetrachlorodibenzo-*p*-dioxin. *Breast Cancer Res.*, **12**, 227–233

Gierthy, J.F., Lincoln, D.W., Gillespie, M.B., Seeger, J.I., Martinez, H.L., Dickerman, H.W. & Kumar, S.A. (1987) Suppression of estrogen-regulated extracellular plasminogen activator activity of MCF-7 cells by 2,3,7,8-tetrachlorodibenzo-*p*-dioxin. *Cancer Res.*, **47**, 6198–6203

Gierthy, J.F., Bennett, J.A., Bradley, L.M. & Cutler, D.S. (1993) Correlation of *in vitro* and *in vivo* growth suppression of MCF-7 human breast cancer by 2,3,7,8-tetrachlorodibenzo-*p*-dioxin. *Cancer Res.*, **53**, 3149–3153

Gillespie, W.J. & Gellman, L. (1989) Dioxin in pulp and paper products: incidence and risk. In: *Bleaching: a TAPPI Press Anthology, TAPPI Proceedings. Bleach Plant Operation*, pp. 658–663

Gillner, M., Brittebo, E.B., Brandt, I., Soderkvist, P., Appelgren, L.E. & Gustafsson, J.A. (1987) Uptake and specific binding of 2,3,7,8-tetrachlorodibenzo-*p*-dioxin in the olfactory mucosa of mice and rats. *Cancer Res.*, **47**, 4150–4159

Gillner, M., Bergman, J., Cambilleau, C., Alexandersson, M., Fernström, B. & Gustafsson, J.-Å. (1993) Interactions of indolo(3,2-*b*)carbazoles and related polycyclic aromatic hydrocarbons with specific binding sites for 2,3,7,8-tetrachlorodibenzo-*p*-dioxin in rat liver. *Mol. Pharmacol.*, **44**, 336–345

Gilman, A., Newhook, R. & Birmingham, B. (1991) An updated assessment of the exposure of Canadians to dioxins and furans. *Chemosphere*, **23**, 1661–1667

Gladen, B.C., Rogan, W.J., Ragan, N.B. & Spierto, F.W. (1988) Urinary porphyrins in children exposed transplacentally to polyhalogenated aromatics in Taiwan. *Arch. environ. Health*, **43**, 54–58

Gladen, B.C., Taylor, J.S., Wu, Y.-C., Ragan, N.B., Rogan, W.J. & Hsu, C.-C. (1990) Dermatological findings in children exposed transplacentally to heat-degraded polychlorinated biphenyls in Taiwan. *Br. J. Dermatol.*, **122**, 799–808

Glidden, R.M., Brown, P.J., Sittig, R.A., Syvertson, C.N. & Smith, P.V. (1990) Determination of 2,3,7,8-tetrachlorodibenzo-*p*-dioxin and 2,3,7,8-tetrachlorodibenzofuran in cow's milk. *Chemosphere*, **20**, 1619–1624

Gochfeld, M., Nygren, M., Hansson, M., Rappe, C., Velez, H., Ghent-Guenther, T., Wilson, W.P. & Kahn, P.C. (1989) Correlation of adipose and blood levels of several dioxin and dibenzofuran congeners in agent orange exposed Viet Nam veterans. *Chemosphere*, **18**, 517–524

Gohl, G., Lehmköster, T., Münzel, P.A., Schrenk, D., Viebahn, R. & Bock, K.W. (1996) TCDD-inducible plasminogen activatory inhibitor type 2 (PAI-2) in human hepatocytes, HepG2 and monocytic U937 cells. *Carcinogenesis*, **17**, 443–449

Goldey, E.S., Kehn, L.S., Lau, C., Rehnberg, G.L. & Crofton, K.M. (1995) Developmental exposure to polychlorinated biphenyls (Aroclor 1254) reduces circulating thyroid hormone concentrations and causes hearing deficits in rats. *Toxicol. appl. Pharmacol.*, **135**, 77–88

Goldey, E.S., Lau, C., Kehn, L.S. & Crofton, K.M. (1996) Developmental dioxin exposure: Disruption of thyroid hormones and ototoxicity. *Fundam. appl. Toxicol.*, **30**, 225

Goldman, P.J. (1972) Critically acute chloracne caused by trichlorophenol decomposition products. *Arbeitsmed. Sozialmed. Arbeitshyg.*, **7**, 12–18

Goldstein, J.A. & Linko, P. (1984) Differential induction of two 2,3,7,8-tetrachlorodibenzo-*p*-dioxin-inducible forms of cytochrome P-450 in extrahepatic versus hepatic tissues. *Mol. Pharmacol.*, **25**, 185–191

Goldstein, J.A. & Safe, S. (1989) Mechanism of action and structure-activity relationships for the chlorinated dibenzo-*p*-dioxins and related compounds. In: Kimbrough, R.D. & Jensen, A.A., eds, *Halogenated Biphenyls, Terphenyls, Napthalenes, Dibenzodioxins and Related Products*, New York, Elsevier , pp. 239–293

Goldstein, J.A., Hickman, P., Bergman, H. & Vos, J.G. (1973) Hepatic porphyria induced by 2,3,7,8-tetrachlorodibenzo-*p*-dioxin (TCDD). *Res. Commun. chem. Path. Pharmacol.*, **6**, 919–928

Goldstein, J.A., Linko, P. & Bergman, H. (1982) Induction of porphyria in the rat by chronic versus acute exposure to 2,3,7,8-tetrachlorodibenzo-*p*-dioxin. *Biochem. Pharmacol.*, **31**, 1607–1613

González, F.J. & Nebert, D.W. (1985) Autoregulation plus upstream positive and negative control regions associated with transcriptional activation of the mouse cytochrome P_1-450 gene. *Nucleic Acids Res.*, **13**, 7269–7288

González, M.J., Jiménez, B., Hernández, L.M., Rivera, J. & Eljarrat, E. (1994) PCDDs and PCDFs in soils near a clinical waste incinerator in Madrid, Spain. Chemometric comparison with other pollution sources. *Organohalogen Compounds*, **20**, 107–110

González, M.J., Jiménez, B., Hernández, L.M. & Gonnord, M.F. (1996) Levels of PCDDs and PCDFs in human milk from populations in Madrid and Paris. *Bull. environ. Contam. Toxicol.*, **56**, 197–204

González, C.A., Kogevinas, M., Huici, A., Gadea, E., Ladona, M., Bosch, A. & Bleda, M.J. (1997) Blood levels of polychlorinated dibenzodioxins, polychlorinated dibenzofurans and polychlorinated biphenyls in the general population of a Spanish Mediterranean city. *Chemosphere* (in press)

Goodman, D.G. & Sauer, R.M. (1992) Hepatotoxicity and carcinogenicity in female Sprague-Dawley rats treated with 2,3,7,8-tetrachlorordibenzo-*p*-dioxin (TCDD): a pathology Working Group Reevaluation. *Regul. Toxicol. Pharmacol.*, **15**, 245–252

Gordon, C.J., Gray, L.E., Jr, Monteiro-Riviere, N.A. & Miller, D. B. (1995) Temperature regulation and metabolism in rats exposed perinatally to dioxin: permanent change in regulated body temperature. *Toxicol. appl. Pharmacol.*, **133**, 172–176

Gordon, C.J., Ying, Y. & Gray, L.E. (1996) Autonomic and behavioral thermoregulation in golden hamsters exposed perinatally to dioxin. *Toxicol. appl. Pharmacol.*, **137**, 120–125

Górski, J.R. & Rozman, K. (1987) Dose-response and time course of hypothyroxinemia and hypoinsulinemia and characterization of insulin hypersensitivity in 2,3,7,8-tetrachlorodibenzo-*p*-dioxin (TCDD)-treated rats. *Toxicology*, **44**, 297–307

Górski, T., Konopka, L. & Brodzki, M. (1984) Persistence of some polychlorinated dibenzo-*p*-dioxins and polychlorinated dibenzofurans of pentachlorophenol in human adipose tissue. *Roczn. Pnstw. Zakl. Hig.*, **35**, 297–301

Górski, J.R., Weber, L.W.D. & Rozman, K. (1990) Reduced gluconeogenesis in 2,3,7,8-tetrachlorodibenzo-*p*-dioxin (TCDD)-treated rats. *Arch. Toxicol.*, **64**, 66–71

Göttlicher, M. & Wiebel, F.J. (1991) 2,3,7,8-Tetrachlorodibenzo-*p*-dioxin causes unbalanced growth in 5L rat hepatoma cells. *Toxicol. appl. Pharmacol.*, **111**, 496–503

Göttlicher, M., Cikryt, P. & Wiebel, F.J. (1990) Inhibition of growth by 2,3,7,8-tetrachlorodibenzo-*p*-dioxin in 5L rat hepatoma cells is associated with the presence of Ah receptor. *Carcinogenesis*, **11**, 2205–2210

Götz, R., Enge, P., Friesel, P., Roch, K., Kjeller, L.-O., Kulp, S.E. & Rappe, C. (1994) Sampling and analysis of water and suspended particulate matter of the River Elbe for polychlorinated dibenzo-*p*-dioxins (PCDDs) and dibenzofurans (PCDFs). *Chemosphere*, **28**, 63–74

Government of Canada (1993) *Polychlorinated Dibenzodioxins and Polychlorinated Dibenzofurans.* Canadian Environmental Protection Act. Priority Substances List. (Assessment Report No. 1), Canada, Health and Welfare

Gradin, K., Wilhelmsson, A., Poellinger, L. & Berghard, A. (1996) Nonresponsiveness of normal human fibroblasts to dioxin correlates with the presence of a constitutive xenobiotic response element-binding factor. *J. biol. Chem.*, **268**, 4061–4068

Gradin, K., McGuire, J., Wenger, R.H., Kvietikova, I., Whitelaw, M.L., Toftgård, R., Tora, L., Gassmann, M. & Poellinger, L. (1996) Functional interference between hypoxia and dioxin signal transduction pathways: competition for recruitement of the Arnt transcription factor. *Mol. Cell. Biol.*, **16**, 5221–5231

Graham, M., Hileman, F., Kirk, D., Wendling, J. & Wilson, J. (1985) Background human exposure to 2,3,7,8-TCDD. *Chemosphere*, **14**, 925–928

Graham, M.J., Lucier, G.W., Linko, P., Maronpot, R. R. & Goldstein, J.A. (1988) Increases in cytochrome P-450 mediated 17 β-estradiol 2-hydroxylase activity in rat liver microsomes after both acute administration and subchronic administration of 2,3,7,8-tetrachlorodibenzo-*p*-dioxin in a two-stage hepatocarcinogenesis model. *Carcinogenesis*, **9**, 1935–1941

Gray, L.E. & Kelce, W.R. (1996) Latent effects of pesticides and toxic substances on sexual differentiation of rodents. *Toxicol. ind. Health*, **12**, 515–531

Gray, L.E., Jr & Ostby, J.S. (1995) In utero 2,3,7,8-tetrachlorodibenzo-*p*-dioxin (TCDD) alters reproductive morphology and function in female rat offspring. *Toxicol. appl. Pharmacol.*, **133**, 285–294

Gray, L.E., Kelce, W.R., Monosson, E., Ostby, J.S. & Birnbaum, L.S. (1995a) Exposure to TCDD during development permanently alters reproductive function in male LE rats and hamsters: reduced ejaculated and epididymal sperm numbers and sex accessory gland weights in offspring with normal androgenic status. *Toxicol. appl. Pharmacol.*, **131**, 108–118

Gray, L.E., Ostby, J., Wolf, C., Miller, D.B., Kelce, W.R., Gordon, C.J & Birnbaum, L. (1995b) Functional developmental toxicity of low doses of 2,3,7,8-tetrachlorodibenzo-*p*-dioxin and a dioxin-like PCB (169) in Long Evans rats and Syrian hamsters: Reproductive, behavioral and thermoregulatory alterations. *Organohalogen Compounds*, **25**, 33–38

Greenlee, W.F., Dold, K.M., Irons, R.D. & Osborne, R. (1985) Evidence for direct action of 2,3,7,8-tetrachlorodibenzo-*p*-dioxin (TCDD) on thymic epithelium. *Toxicol. appl. Pharmacol.*, **79**, 112–120

Grehl, H., Grahmann, F., Claus, D. & Neundörfer, B. (1993) Histologic evidence for a toxic polyneuropathy due to exposure to 2,3,7,8-tetrachlorodibenzo-*p*-dioxin (TCDD) in rats. *Acta neurol. scand.*, **88**, 354–357

Greig, J.B., Jones, G., Butler, W.H. & Barnes, J.M. (1973) Toxic effects of 2,3,7,8-tetrachlorodibenzo-*p*-dioxin. *Food Cosmet. Toxicol.*, **11**, 585–595

Grochowalski, A., Wybraniec, S. & Ryszard, C. (1995) Determination of PCDFs/PCDDs in ambient air from Cracow City, Poland. *Organohalogen Compounds*, **24**, 153–156

Gronemeyer, H. & Laudet, V. (1995) Transcription factors. 3: Nuclear receptors. *Prot. Profile*, **2**, 1173–1308

Gross, M.L., Lay, J.O., Jr, Lyon, P.A., Lippstreu, D., Kangas, N., Harless, R.L., Taylor, S.E. & Dupuy, A.E., Jr (1984) 2,3,7,8-Tetrachlorodibenzo-*p*-dioxin levels in adipose tissue of Vietnam veterans. *Environ. Res.*, **33**, 261–268

Grubbs, W.D., Wolfe, W.H., Michalek, J.E., Williams, D.E., Lustik, M.B., Brockman, A.S., Henderson, S.C., Burnett, F.R., Land, R.J., Osborne, D.J., Rocconi, V.K., Schreiber, M.E., Miner, J.C., Henriksen, G. L. & Swaby, J.A. (1995) *Air Force Health Study: An Epidemiologic Investigation of Health Effects in Air Force Personnel Following Exposure to Herbicides* (Report number AL-TR-920107)

Guo, Y.L., Lai, T.J., Ju, S.H., Chen, Y.C. & Hsu, C.C. (1993) Sexual developments and biological findings in Yu-Cheng children. In: *Proceedings of the 13th International Symposium on Chlorinated Dioxins and Related Compounds (Dioxin '93), September 20-24, 1993, Vienna, Austria*

Guo, Y.L., Lin, C.J., Yao, W.J., Ryan, J.J. & Hsu, C.C. (1994) Musculoskeletal changes in children prenatally exposed to polychlorinated biphenyls and related compounds (Yu-Cheng children). *J. Toxicol. environ. Health*, **41**, 83–93

Gupta, B.N., Vos, J.G., Moore, J.A., Zinkl, J.G. & Bullock, B.C. (1973) Pathologic effects of 2,3,7,8-tetrachlorodibenzo-*p*-dioxin in laboratory animals. *Environ. Health Perspectives*, **5**, 125–140

Gupta, C., Hattori, A., Betschart, J.M., Virji, M.A. & Shinozuka, H. (1988) Modulation of epi-dermal growth factor receptors in rat hepatocytes by two liver tumor-promoting regimens, a choline-deficient and a phenobarbital diet. *Cancer Res.*, **48**, 1162–1165

Guzelian, P.S. (1985) Clinical evaluation of liver structure and function in humans exposed to halogenated hydrocarbons. *Environ. Health Perspectives*, **60**, 159–164

Ha, M.C., Cordier, S., Bard, D., Thuy, L.T.B., Hao, H.A., Quinh, H.T., Dai, L.C., Abenhaim, L. & Phuong, N.T.N. 1996) Agent Orange and the risk of gestational trophoblastic disease in Vietnam. *Arch. environ. Health*, **51**, 368–374

Hagenmaier, H. (1986) Determination of 2,3,7,8-tetrachlorodibenzo-*p*-dioxin in commercial chlorophenols and related compounds. *Fresenius Z. anal. Chem.*, **325**, 603–606

Hagenmaier, H. & Brunner, H. (1987) Isomer specific analysis of pentachlorophenol and sodium pentachlorophenate for 2,3,7,8-substituted PCDD and PCDF at sub-ppb level. *Chemosphere*, **16**, 1759–1864

Hagenmaier, H., Brunner, H., Knapp, W. & Weberuß, U. (1985) Study of the content of poly-chlorinated dibenzodioxins, polychlorinated dibenzofurans and derived chlorinated hydro-carbons in waste-water plants. *UBA-Bericht*, **103**, 03 305 (in German)

Hagenmaier, H.P., Brunner, H., Haag, R. & Kraft, M. (1986) Selective determination of 2,3,7,8-tetrachlorodibenzo-*p*-dioxin in the presence of a large excess of other polychlorinated di-benzodioxins and polychlorinated dibenzofurans. *Fresenius J. analyt. Chem.*, **323**, 24–28

Hagenmaier, H., Dawidowsky, N., Weberruss, U., Hertzinger, O., Schwind, K.H., Thoma, H., Essers, U., Bühler, U. & Greiner, R. (1990a) Emissions of polyhalogenated dibenzodioxins and dibenzofurans from combustion-engines. *Organohalogen Compounds*, **2**, 329–334

Hagenmaier, H., Wiesmuller, T., Golor, G., Krowke, R., Helge, H. & Neubert, D. (1990b) Transfer of various polychlorinated dibenzopdioxins and dibenzofurans (PCDDs and PCDFs) via placenta and through milk in a marmoset monkey. *Arch. Toxicol.*, **64**, 601–615

Hagenmaier, H., She, J. & Lindig, C. (1992) Persistence of polychlorinated dibenzo-*p*-dioxins and polychlorinated dibenzofurans in contaminated soil at Maulach and Rastatt in Southwest Germany. *Chemosphere*, **25**, 1449–1456

Hagmar, L., Lindén, K., Nilsson, A., Norrving, B., Åkesson, B., Schütz, A. & Möller, T. (1992) Cancer incidence and mortality among Swedish Baltic Sea fishermen. *Scand. J. Work Environ. Health*, **18**, 217–224

Hahn, J.L., von dem Fange, H.P. & Westerman, G. (1989) A comparison of ambient and work-place dioxin levels from testing in and around modern resource recovery facilities with predicted ground level concentrations of dioxins from stack emission testing with corres-ponding workplace health risk. *Chemosphere*, **19**, 629–636

Håkansson, H. & Hanberg, A. (1989) The distribution of [^{14}C]-2,3,7,8-tetrachlorodibenzo-*p*-dioxin (TCDD) and its effect on the vitamin A content in parenchymal and stellate cells of rat liver. *J. Nutr.*, **119**, 573–580

Håkansson, H., Manzoor, E. & Ahlborg, U.G. (1990) Interaction between dietary vitamin A and single oral doses of 2,3,7,8-tetrachlorodibenzo-*p*-dioxin (TCDD) on the TCDD-induced toxi-city and on the vitamin A status in the rat. *J. Nutr. Sci. Vitaminol.*, **37**, 239–255

Håkansson, H., Johansson, L., Manzoor, E. & Ahlborg, U.G. (1991a) Effects of 2,3,7,8-tetra-chlorodibenzo-*p*-dioxin (TCDD) on the vitamin A status of Hartley guinea pigs, Sprague-Dawley rats, C57BL/6 mice, DBA/2 mice, and golden Syrian hamsters. *J. nutr. Sci. Vita-minol.*, **37**, 117–138

Håkansson, H., Manzoor, E. & Ahlborg, U.G. (1991b) Interaction between dietary vitamin A and single oral doses of 2,3,7,8-tetrachlorodibenzo-*p*-dioxin (TCDD) on the TCDD-induced toxicity and on the vitamin A status in the rat. *J. nutr. Sci. Vitaminol.*, **37**, 239–255

Hallett, D.J. & Kornelsen, P.J. (1992) Persistence of 2,3-dichlorophenol, 2,3,4-trichlorophenol, 2,3,7,8-tetrachlorodibenzo-p-dioxin, and 2,3,7,8-tetrachlorodibenzofuran in soils of a forest ecosystem treated with 2,4-d/2,4,5-t-herbicide in eastern Canada. *Organohalogen Compounds*, **9**, 87–88

Hanberg, A., Kling, L. & Håkansson, H. (1996) Effect of 2,3,7,8-tetrachlorodibenzo-*p*-dioxin (TCDD) on the hepatic stellate cell population in the rat. *Chemosphere*, **32**, 1225–1233

Hanify, J.A., Metcalf, P., Nobbs, C.L. & Worsley, K.J. (1981) Aerial spraying of 2,4,5-T and human birth malformations: an epidemiological investigation. *Science*, **212**, 349–351

Hankinson, O. (1994) The role of the aryl hydrocarbon receptor nuclear translocator protein in aryl hydrocarbon receptor action. *Trends Endocrinol. Metab.*, **5**, 240–244

Hanneman, W.H., Legare, M.E., Barhoumi, R., Burghardt, R.C., Safe, S. & Tiffany-Castiglioni, E. (1996) Stimulation of calcium uptake in cultured rat hippocampal neurons by 2,3,7,8-tetrachlorodibenzo-*p*-dioxin. *Toxicology*, **112**, 19–28

Hansen, E.S., Hasle, H. & Lander, F. (1992) A cohort study on cancer incidence among Danish gardeners. *Am. J. ind. Med.*, **21**, 651–660

Hansen-Stottrup, E., Hasle, H. & Lander, F. (1992) A cohort study on cancer incidence among Danish gardeners. *Am. J. ind. Med.*, **21**, 651–660

Hanson, C.D. & Smialowicz, R.J. (1994) Evaluation of the effect of low-level 2,3,7,8-tetrachlorodibenzo-*p*-dioxin exposure on cell mediated immunity. *Toxicology*, **88**, 213–224

Hansson, M., Rappe, C., Gochfeld, M., Velez, H., Wilson, W.P., Ghent-Guenther, T. & Kahn, P.C. (1989) Effects of fasting on blood levels of 2,3,7,8-TCDD and related compounds. *Chemosphere*, **18**, 525–530

Hansson, M., Grimstad, T. & Rappe, C. (1995) Occupational exposure to polychlorinated dibenzo-*p*-dioxins and dibenzofurans in a magnesium production plant. *Occup. environ. Med.*, **52**, 823–826

Hansson, M., Barregård, L., Sällsten, G., Svensson, B.-G. & Rappe, C. (1997) Polychlorinated dibenzo-*p*-dioxin and dibenzofuran levels and patterns in PVC and chloralkali industry workers. *Occup. environ. Med.* (in press)

Hapgood, J., Cuthill, S., Söderkvist, P., Wilhelmsson, A., Pongratz, I., Tukey, R.H., Johnson, E.F., Gustafsson, J. & Poellinger, L. (1991) Liver cells contain constitutive DNase I-hypersensitive sites at the xenobiotic response elements 1 and 2 (XRE1 and -2) of the rat cytochrome P-450IA1 gene and a constitutive, nuclear XRE-binding factor that is distinct from the dioxin receptor. *Mol. cell. Biol.*, **11**, 4314–4323

Hardell, L. (1977) Soft tissue sarcomas and exposure to phenoxyacetic acids — a clinical observation. *Läkartidningen*, **74**, 2853–2854 (in Swedish)

Hardell, L. (1979) Malignant lymphoma of histiocytic type and exposure to phenoxyacetic acids or chlorophenols (Letter to the Editor). *Lancet*, **i**, 55–56

Hardell, L. (1981) The relation of soft-tissue sarcoma, malignant lymphoma and colon cancer to phenoxy acids, chlorophenols and other agents. *Scand. J. Work Environ. Health*, **7**, 119–130

Hardell, L. & Eriksson, M. (1988) The association between soft-tissue sarcoma and exposure to phenoxyacetic acids. A new case-referent study. *Cancer*, **62**, 652–656

Hardell, L. & Sandström, A. (1979) Case–control study: soft-tissue sarcomas and exposure to phenoxyacetic acids or chlorophenols. *Br. J. Cancer*, **39**, 711–717

Hardell, L., Eriksson, M., Lenner, P. & Lundgren, E. (1981) Malignant lymphoma and exposure to chemicals, especially organic solvents, chlorophenols and phenoxy acids: a case-control study. *Br. J. Cancer*, **43**, 169–176

Hardell, L., Johansson, B. & Axelson, O. (1982) Epidemiological study of nasal and naso-pharyngeal cancer and their relation to phenoxy acid or chlorophenol exposure. *Am. J. ind. Med.*, **3**, 247–257

Hardell, L., Bengtsson, N.O., Jonsson, U., Eriksson, S. & Larsson, L.G. (1984) Aetiological aspects on primary liver cancer with special regard to alcohol, organic solvents and acute intermittent porphyria — an epidemiological investigation. *Br. J. Cancer*, **50**, 389–397

Hardell, L., Eriksson, M., Axelson, O. & Fredriksson, M. (1991) Dioxin and mortality from cancer (Letter to the Editor). *New Engl. J. Med.*, **324**, 1810–1811

Hardell, L., Fredrikson, M., Eriksson, M., Hansson, M. & Rappe, C. (1995) Adipose tissue concentrations of dioxins and dibenzofurans in patients with malignant lymphoproliferative diseases and in patients without a malignant disease. *Eur. J. Cancer Prev.*, **4**, 225–229

Hardell, L., van Bavel, B., Lindström, G., Fredrikson, M. & Liljegren, G. (1996) Higher concen-trations of specific polychlorinated biphenyl congeners and chlordanes in adipose tissue from non-Hodgkin's lymphoma patients compared with controls without a malignant disease. *International Symposium. Dioxins and Furans: Epidemiologic Assessment of Cancer Risks and Other Human Health Effects, 1-8 November 1996* (Abstracts), Heidelberg, Deutsches Krebsforschungszentrum, pp. 10–11

Harless, R.L., Oswald, E.O., Lewis, R.G., Dupuy, A.E., McDaniel, D.D. & Tai, H. (1982) Deter-mination of 2,3,7,8-tetrachlorodibenzo-*p*-dioxin in fresh water fish. *Chemosphere*, **11**, 193–198

Harless, R.L., Lewis, R.G., McDaniel, D.D. & Dupuy, A.E., Jr (1990) Sampling and analysis for polychlorinated dibenzo-*p*-dioxins and dibenzofurans in ambient air. *Organohalogen Com-pounds*, **4**, 179–182

Harper, N., Conner, K. & Safe, S. (1993) Immunotoxic potencies of polychlorinated biphenyl (PCB), dibenzofuran (PCDF) and dibenzo-*p*-dioxin (PCDD) congeners in C57BL/6 and DBA/2 mice. *Toxicology*, **80**, 217–227

Harper, N., Wang, X., Liu, H. & Safe, S. (1994) Inhibition of estrogen-induced progesterone receptor in MCF-7 human breast cancer cells by aryl hydrocarbon (Ah) receptor agonists. *Mol. cell. Endocrinol.*, **104**, 47–55

Harper, N., Steinberg, M., Thomsen, J. & Safe, S. (1995) Halogenated aromatic hydrocarbon-induced suppression of the plaque-forming cell response in B6C3F1 splenocytes cultured with allogenic mouse serum: Ah receptor structure activity relationships. *Toxicology*, **99**, 199–206

Harris, L., Preat, V. & Farber, E. (1987) Patterns of ligand binding to normal, regenerating, pre-neoplastic, and neoplastic rat hepatocytes. *Cancer Res.*, **47**, 3954–3958

Harris, M.W., Moore, J.A., Vos, J.G. & Gupta, B.N. (1973) General biological effects of TCDD in laboratory animals. *Environ. Health Perspectives*, **5**, 101–109

Harris, M., Zacharewski, T. & Safe, S. (1990) Effects of 2,3,7,8-tetrachlorodibenzo-*p*-dioxin and related compounds on the occupied nuclear estrogen receptor in MCF-7 human breast cancer cells. *Cancer Res.*, **50**, 3579–3584

Harrison, N., Gem, M.G. de M., Startin, J.R., Wright, C., Kelly, M. & Rose, M. (1996) PCDDs and PCDFs in milk from farms in Derbyshire, UK. *Chemosphere*, **32**, 453–460

Hashiguchi, I., Toriya, Y., Anan, H., Maeda, K., Akamine, A., Aono, M., Fukuyama, H. & Okumura, H. (1995) An epidemiologic examination on the prevalence of the periodontal diseases and oral pigmentation in Yusho patients. *Fukuoka Igaku Zasahi*, **86**, 256–260 (in Japanese)

Hashimoto, S., Matsuda, M., Wakimoto & T., Tatsukawa, R. (1995a) Simple sampling and analysis of PCDDs and PCDFs in Japanese coastal sea water. *Chemosphere*, **30**, 1979–1986

Hashimoto, S., Yamamoto, T., Yasuhara, A. & Morita, M. (1995b) PCDD, PCDF, planar and other PCB levels in human milk in Japan. *Chemosphere*, **31**, 4067–4075

Hass, R.J. & Friesen, M.D. (1979) Qualitative and quantitative methods for dioxin analysis. *Ann. N.Y. Acad. Sci.*, **320**, 28–42

Hassoun, E.A. & Stohs, S.J. (1996) TCDD, endrin and lindane induced oxidative stress in fetal and placental tissues of C57BL/6J and DBA/2J mice. *Comp. Biochem. Physiol.*, **115**, 11–18

Hassoun, E.A., Bagchi, D. & Stohs, S.J. (1995) Evidence of 2,3,7,8-tetrachlorodibenzo-*p*-dioxin (TCDD)-induced tissue damage in fetal and placental tissues and changes in amniotic fluid lipid metabolites of pregnant CF1 mice. *Toxicol. Lett.*, **76**, 245–250

Hayes, C.L., Spink, D.C., Spink, B.C., Cao, J.Q., Walker, N.J. & Sutter, T.R. (1996) 17 beta-estradiol hydroxylation catalyzed by human cytochrome P450 1B1. *Proc. natl Acad. Sci. USA.*, **93**, 9776–9781

Health Council of the Netherlands (1996) *Dioxins. Polychlorinated Dibenzo-p-dioxins, Dibenzo-furans and Dioxin-like Polychlorinated Biphenyls* (No. 1996/10E), Rijswijk

Hébert, C.D. & Birnbaum, L.S. (1987) The influence of aging on intestinal absorption of TCDD in rats. *Toxicol. Lett.*, **37**, 47–55

Hébert, C.D., Harris, M.W., Elwell, M.R. & Birnbaum, L.S. (1990a) Relative toxicity and tumor-promoting ability of 2,3,7,8-tetrachlorodibenzo-*p*-dioxin (TCDD), 2,3,4,7,8-penta-chlorodibenzofuran (PCDF), and 1,2,3,4,7,8-hexachlorodibenzofuran (HCDF) in hairless mice. *Toxicol. appl. Pharmacol.*, **102**, 362–377

Hébert, C.D., Cao, Q.-L. & Birnbaum, L.S. (1990b) Role of transforming growth factor β in the proliferative effect of 2,3,7,8-tetrachlorodibenzo-*p*-dioxin on human squamous carcinoma cells. *Cancer Res.*, **50**, 7190–7197

Hébert, C.D., Cao, Q.-L. & Birnbaum, L.S. (1990c) Inhibition of high-density growth arrest in human squamous carcinoma cells by 2,3,7,8-tetrachlorodibenzo-*p*-dioxin (TCDD). *Carcino-genesis*, **11**, 1335–1342

de Heer, C., Schuurman, H.-J., Vos, J.G. & Van Loveren, H. (1994a) Lymphodepletion of the thymus cortex in rats after single oral dosis intubation of 2,3,7,8-tetrachlorodibenzo-*p*-dioxin. *Chemosphere*, **29**, 2295–2299

de Heer, C., Verlaan, A.P.J., Penninks, A. H., Vos, J.G., Schuurman, H.-J. & Van Loveren, H. (1994b) Time course of 2,3,7,8-tetrachlorodibenzo-*p*-dioxin (TCDD)-induced thymic athropy in the Wistar rat. *Toxicol. appl. Pharmacol.*, **128**, 97–104

de Heer, C., Schuurman, H.-J., Djien Liem, A.K., Penninks, A. H., Vos, J. G. & Van Loveren, H. (1995) Toxicity of 2,3,7,8-tetrachlorodibenzo-*p*-dioxin (TCDD) to the human thymus after implantation in SCID mice. *Toxicol. appl. Pharmacol.*, **134**, 296–304

Heida, H., van der Oost, R. & van den Berg, M. (1995) The Volgermeerpolder revisited. Dioxins in sediments, topsoil, and eel. *Organohalogen compounds*, **24**, 281–284

Hembrock-Heger, A. (1990) PCDD/PCDF-levels in soils and plants of Northrhine-Westfalia. *Organohalogen Compounds*, **1**, 475–478

Hemming, H., Bager, Y., Flodström, S., Nordgren, I., Kronevi, T., Ahlborg, U.G. & Wärngård, L. (1995) Liver tumour promoting activity of 3,4,5,3',4'-pentachlorobiphenyl and its interaction with 2,3,7,8-tetrachlorodibenzo-*p*-dioxin. *Eur. J. Pharmacol.*, **292**, 241–249

Hempel, J., Harper, K. & Lindahl, R. (1989) Inducible (class 3) aldehyde dehydrogenase from rat hepatocellular carcinoma and 2,3,7,8-tetrachlorodibenzo-*p*-dioxin-treated liver: distant relationship to the class 1 and 2 enzymes from mammalian liver cytosol/mitochondria. *Biochemistry*, **28**, 1160–1167

Henck, J.W., New, M.A., Kociba, R.J. & Rao, K.S. (1981) 2,3,7,8-Tetrachlorodibenzo-*p*-dioxin: acute oral toxicity in hamsters. *Toxicol. appl. Pharmacol.*, **59**, 405–407

Henriksen, G.L. & Michalek, J.E. (1996) Serum dioxin, testosterone, and gonodotrophins in veterans of Operation Ranch Hand (Letter). *Epidemiology*, **7**, 454–455

Henriksen, G.L., Michalek, J.E., Swaby, J.A. & Rahe, A.J. (1996) Serum dioxin, testosterone, and gonodotrophins in veterans of Operation Ranch Hand. *Epidemiology*, **7**, 352–357

Henry, E.C. & Gasiewicz, T.A. (1987) Changes in thyroid hormones and thyroxine glucuronidation in hamsters compared with rats following treatment with 2,3,7,8-tetrachlorodibenzo-*p*-dioxin. *Toxicol. appl. Pharmacol.*, **89**, 165–174

Henry, E.C. & Gasiewicz, T.A. (1993) Transformation of the aryl hydrocarbon receptor to a DNA-binding form is accompanied by release of the 90 kDa heat-shock protein and increased affinity for 2,3,7,8-tetrachlorodibenzo-*p*-dioxin. *Biochem. J.*, **294**, 95–101

Her Majesty's Stationery Office (1989) *Dioxins in the Environment* (Pollution Paper No. 27), London

Hertzman, C., Teschke, K., Dimich-Ward, H. & Ostry, A. (1988) Validity and reliability of a method for restrospective evaluation of chlorophenate exposure in the lumber industry. *Am. J. ind. Med.*, **14**, 703–713

Hertzmann, C., Teschke, K., Ostry, A., Herschler, R., Dimich-Ward, H., Kelly, S., Spinelli, J.J., Gallagher, R.P., McBride, M. & Marion, S.A. (1997) Mortality and cancer incidence among sawmill workers exposed to chlorophenate wood preservatives. *Am. J. public Health*, **87**, 71–79

Hiester, E., Bruckmann, P., Böhm, R., Eynck, P., Gerlach, A., Mülder, W. & Ristow, H. (1995) Pronounced decrease of PCDD/PCDF burden in ambient air. *Organohalogen Compounds*, **24**, 147–152

Hiles, R.A. & Bruce, R.D. (1976) 2,3,7,8-Tetrachlorodibenzo-*p*-dioxin elimination in the rat: first order or zero order? *Food Cosmet. Toxicol.*, **14**, 599–600

Hinsdill, R.D., Couch, D.L. & Speirs, R.S. (1980) Immunosuppression in mice induced by dioxin (TCDD) in feed. *J. environ. Pathol. Toxicol.*, **4**, 401–425

Hippelein, M., Kaupp, H., Dörr, G., McLachlan, M. & Hutzinger, O. (1996) Baseline contamination assessment for a new resource recovery facility in Germany. Part II: Atmospheric concentrations of PCDD/F. *Chemosphere*, **38**, 1605–1616

Hirakawa, H., Matsueda, T., Iida, T., Fukamachi, K., Takahashi, K., Nagayama, J. & Nagata, T. (1991) Coplanar PCBs, PCDFs and PCDDs in the subcutaneous adipose tissue of the yusho patients and normal controls. *Fukuoka Igaku Zasshi*, **82**, 274–279

Hirakawa, H., Iida, T, Matsueda, T., Nakagawa, R., Hori, T. & Nagayama, J. (1995) Comparison of concentrations of PCDDs, PCDFs, PCBs and other organohalogen compounds in human milk of primiparas and multiparas. *Organohalogen Compounds*, **26**, 197–200

Hirose, K., Morita, M., Ema, M., Mimura, J., Hamada, H., Fujii, H., Saijo, Y., Gotoh, O., Sogawa, K. & Fujii-Kuriyama, Y. (1996) cDNA Cloning and tissue-specific expression of a novel basic helix-loop-helix/PAS factor (Arnt2) with close sequence similarity to the aryl hydrocarbon receptor nuclear translocator (Arnt). *Mol. Cell. Biol.*, **16**, 1706–1713

Hoang, T.Q., Le, C.D. & Le, T.H.T. (1989) Effects of geographical conditions, soil movement and other variables on the distribution of 2,3,7,8-TCDD levels in adipose tissues from Vietnam: preliminary observations. *Chemosphere*, **18**, 967–974

Hoar, S.K., Blair, A., Holmes, F.F., Boysen, C.D., Robel, R.J., Hoover, R. & Fraumeni, J.F., Jr (1986) Agricultural herbicide use and risk of lymphoma and soft-tissue sarcoma. *J. Am. med. Assoc.*, **256**, 1141–1147

Hochstein, J.R., Aulerich, R.J. & Bursian, S.J. (1988) Acute toxicity of 2,3,7,8-tetrachlorodibenzo-*p*-dioxin to mink. *Arch. environ. Contam. Toxicol.*, **17**, 33–37

Hoffman, R.E., Stehr-Green, P.A., Webb, K.B., Evans, R.G., Knutsen, A.P., Schram, W.F., Staake, J.L., Gibson, B.B. & Steinberg, K.K. (1986) Health effects of long-term exposure to 2,3,7,8-tetrachlorodibenzo-*p*-dioxin. *J. Am. med. Assoc.*, **255**, 2031–2038

Hoffman, E.C., Reyes, H., Chu, F.-F., Sander, F., Conley, L.H., Brooks, B.A. & Hankinson, O. (1991) Cloning of a factor required for the activity of the Ah (dioxin) receptor. *Science*, **252**, 954–958

Hogstedt, C. & Westerlund, S. (1980) Cohort studies of cause of death of forestry workers with and without exposure to phenoxyacid preparations. *Läkaridningen*, **77**, 1828–1830 (in Swedish)

Holladay, S.D., Lindstrom, P., Blaylock, C.D., Comment, C.E., Germolec, D.R., Heindell, J.J. & Luster, M.I. (1991) Perinatal thymocyte antigen expression and postnatal immune development altered by gestational exposure to tetrachlorodibenzo-*p*-dioxin (TCDD.) *Teratology*, **44**, 385–393

Holmes, S.J., Jones, K.C. & Miller, C.E. (1995) PCDD/F contamination of the environment at Bolsover, UK. *Organohalogen Compounds*, **24**, 373–377

Holoubek, I., Kocan, A., Petrik, J., Holoubková, I., Korinek, X. & Bezacinsky, M. (1991) The fate of selected organic compounds in the environment. Part VII. PCBs, PCDDs and PCDFs in ambient air in Czechoslovakia — 1990. *Chemosphere*, **23**, 1345–1348

Holsapple, M.P. (1995) Immunotoxicity of halogenated aromatic hydrocarbons. In: Smialowicz, R.J. & Holsapple, M,P., eds, *Experimental Immunotoxicology*, Boca Raton, FL, CRC Press, pp. 265–305

Holsapple, M.P., Dooley, R.K., McNerney, P.J. & McCay, J.A. (1986a) Direct suppression of antibody responses by chlorinated dibenzodioxins in cultured spleen cells from (C57BL/6 × C3H) F1 and DBA/2 mice. *Immunopharmacology*, **12**, 175–186

Holsapple, M.P., McCay, J.A. & Barnest, D.W. (1986b) Immunosuppression without liver induction by subchronic exposure to 2,7-dichlorodibenzo-*p*-dioxin in adult female B6C3F1 mice. *Toxicol. appl. Pharmacol.*, **83**, 445–455

Holsapple, M.P., Morris, D.L., Wood, St.C. & Snyder, N.K. (1991a) 2,3,7,8-tetrachlorodibenzo-*p*-dioxin-induced changes in immunocompetence: Possible mechanisms. *Ann. Rev. Pharmacol. Toxicol.*, **31**, 73–100

Holsapple, M.P., Snyder, N.K., Wood, S.C. & Morris, D.L. (1991b) A review of 2,3,7,8-tetra-chlordibenzo-*p*-dioxin-induced changes in immuncompetence: 1991 update. *Toxicology*, **69**, 219–255

Homberger, E., Reggiani, G., Sambeth, J. & Wipf, H. (1979) *The Seveso Accident: Its Nature, Extent and Consequences*, Givaudan Research Company/Hoffmann-La Roche & Co.

Hong, R., Taylor, K. & Abonour, R. (1989) Immune abnormalities associated with chronic TCDD exposure in Rhesus. *Chemosphere*, **18**, 313–320

Hooiveld, M., Heederik, D. & Bueno de Mesquita, H.B. (1996a) Preliminary results of the second follow-up of a Dutch cohort of workers occupationally exposed to phenoxy herbicides, chlorophenols and contaminants. *Organohalogen Compounds*, **30**, 185–189

Hooiveld, M., Heederik, D. & Bueno de Mesquita, H.B. (1996b) Second follow-up of a Dutch cohort of workers occupationally exposed to phenoxy herbicides, chlorophenols and contaminants (Abstract). In: *International Symposium, 7–8 November 1996. Dioxins and Furans: Epidemiologic Assessment of Cancer Risks and Other Human Health Effects*, Heidelberg, Deutsches Krebsforschungszentrum, p. 11

Hori, S., Obana, H., Kashimoto, T., Otake, T., Nishimura, H., Ikegami, N., Kunita, N. & Uda, H. (1982) Effect of polychlorinated biphenyls and polychlorinated quaterphenyls in cynomolgus monkey (*Macaca fascicularis*). *Toxicology*, **24**, 123–139

Hosoya, K., Kimata, K., Fukunishi, K., Tanaka, N., Patterson, D.G., Jr, Alexander, L.R., Barnhart, E.R. & Barr, J. (1995) Photodecomposition of 1,2,3,4- and 2,3,7,8-tetrachlorodi-benzo-*p*-dioxin (TCDD) in water-alcohol media on a solid support. *Chemosphere*, **31**, 3687–3698

House R.V., Lauer, L.D. & Murray, M.J. (1990) Examination of immune parameters and host resistance mechanisms in B6C3F1 mice following adult exposure to 2,3,7,8-tetrachloro-dibenzo-*p*-dioxin. *J. Toxicol. environ. Health*, **31**, 203–215

Hryhorczuk, D.O., Orris, P., Kominsky, J.R., Melius, J., Burton, W. & Hinkamp, D.L. (1986) PCB, PCDF, and PCDD exposure following a transformer fire: Chicago. *Chemosphere*, **15**, 1297–1303

Hsieh, S.-F., Yen, Y.-Y., Lan, S.-J., Hsieh, C.-C., Lee, C.-H. & Ko, Y.-C. (1996) A cohort study on mortality and exposure to polychlorinated biphenyls. *Arch. environ. Health*, **51**, 417–424

Hsu, S.-T., Ma, C.-I., Hsu, S.K.-H., Wu, S.-S., Hsu, N.H.-M., Yeh, C.-C. & Wu, S.-B. (1985) Discovery and epidemiology of PCB poisoning in Taiwan: a four-year follow-up. *Environ. Health Perspectives*, **59**, 5–10

Hsu, C.-C., Yu, M.-L.M., Chen, Y.-C.J., Guo, Y.-L.L. & Rogan, W.J. (1994) The Yu-cheng rice oil poisoning incident. In: Schecter, A., ed., *Dioxins and Health*, New York, Plenum Press, pp. 661–684

Huang, C.-W., Miyata, H., Lu, J.-R., Ohta, S., Chang, T. & Kashimoto, T. (1992) Levels of PCBs, PCDDs and PCDFs in soil samples from incineration sites for metal reclamation in Taiwan. *Chemosphere*, **24**, 1669–1676

Hudson, L.G., Toscano, W.A., Jr & Greenlee, W.F. (1985) Regulation of epidermal growth factor binding in a human keratinocyte cell line by 2,3,7,8-tetrachlorodibenzo-p-dioxin. *Toxicol. appl. Pharmacol.*, **77**, 251–259

Hudson, L.G., Toscano, W.A., Jr & Greenlee, W.F. (1986) 2,3,7,8-Tetrachlorodibenzo-*p*-dioxin (TCDD) modulated epidermal growth factor (EGF) binding to basal cells from a human keratinocyte cell line. *Toxicol. appl. Pharmacol.*, **82**, 481–492

Huisman, M., Koopman-Esseboom, C., Fidler, V., Hadders-Algra, M., van der Paauw, C.G., Tuinstra, L.G., Weisglas-Kuperus, N., Sauer, P.J., Touwen, B.C. & Boersma, E.R. (1995a) Perinatal exposure to polychlorinated biphenyls and dioxins and its effect on neonatal neurological development. *Early hum. Dev.*, **41**, 111–127.

Huisman, M., Koopman-Esseboom, C., Lanting, C.I., van der Paauw, C.G., Tuinstra, L.G.M., Fidler, V., Weisglas-Kuperus, N., Sauer, P.J., Boersma, E.R., Boersma, E.R. & Touwen B.C. (1995b) Neurological condition in 18-month-old children preinatially exposed to polychlorinated biphenyls and dioxins. *Early hum. Dev.*, **43**, 165–176

Hülster, A. & Marschner, H. (1993) Transfer of PCDD/PCDF from contaminated soils to food and fodder crop plants. *Chemosphere*, **27**, 439–446

Hülster, A., Müller, J.F. & Marschner, H. (1994) Soil-plant transfer of polychlorinated dibenzo-*p*-dioxins and dibenzofurans to vegetables of the cucumber family (*Cucurbitaceae*). *Environ. Sci. Technol.*, **28**, 1110–1115

Hunt, G.T. & Maisel, B.E. (1990) Atmospheric PCDDs/PCDFs in wintertime in a northeastern US urban coastal environment. *Chemosphere*, **20**, 1455–1462

Hunt, G.T. & Maisel, B.E. (1992) Atmospheric concentrations of PCDDs/PCDFs in southern California. *J. Air Waste Manag. Assoc.*, **42**, 672–680

Hushka, D.R. & Greenlee, W.F. (1995) 2,3,7,8-Tetrachlorodibenzo-*p*-dioxin inhibits DNA synthesis in rat primary hepatocytes. *Mutat. Res.*, **33**, 89–99

Huteau, B., Gonnord, M.F., Gille, P., Fraisse, D. & Bard, D. (1990a) PCDD and PCDF levels in human adipose tissue in France. *Organohalogen Compounds*, **1**, 243–245

Huteau, B., Gonnord, M.F., Gille, P. & Fraisse, D. (1990b) New data on PCDDs and PCDFs levels in South Vietnamese adipose tissues. *Organohalogen Compounds*, **1**, 239–241

Huuskonen, H., Unkila, M., Pohjanvirta, R. & Tuomisto, J. (1994) Developmental toxicity of 2,3,7,8-tetrachlorodibenzo-*p*-dioxin (TCDD) in the most TCDD-resistant and -susceptible rat strains. *Toxicol. appl. Pharmacol.*, **124**, 174–180

Huwe, J.K., Feil, V.J. & Larsen, G.L. (1996) Identification of the major metabolites of 1,4,7,8-tetrachlorodibenzo-*p*-dioxin in rats. *Organohalogen Compounds*, **29**, 462–467

IARC (1977a) *IARC Monographs on the Evaluation of the Carcinogenic Risk of Chemicals to Man*, Vol. 15, *Some Fumigants, the Herbicides 2,4-D and 2,4,5-T, Chlorinated Dibenzodioxins and Miscellaneous Industrial Chemicals*, Lyon, pp. 41–102

IARC (1977b) *IARC Monographs on the Evaluation of the Carcinogenic Risk of Chemicals to Man*, Vol. 15, *Some Fumigants, the Herbicides 2,4-D and 2,4,5-T, Chlorinated Dibenzodioxins and Miscellaneous Industrial Chemicals*, Lyon, pp. 273–299

IARC (1977c) *IARC Monographs on the Evaluation of the Carcinogenic Risk of Chemicals to Man*, Vol. 15, *Some Fumigants, the Herbicides 2,4-D and 2,4,5-T, Chlorinated Dibenzodioxins and Miscellaneous Industrial Chemicals*, Lyon, pp. 115–138

IARC (1979a) *IARC Monographs on the Evaluation of the Carcinogenic Risk of Chemicals to Humans*, Vol. 20, *Some Halogenated Hydrocarbons*, Lyon, pp. 349–367

IARC (1979b) *IARC Monographs on the Evaluation of the Carcinogenic Risk of Chemicals to Humans*, Vol. 20, *Some Halogenated Hydrocarbons*, Lyon, pp. 241–257

IARC (1979c) *IARC Monographs on the Evaluation of the Carcinogenic Risk of Chemicals to Humans*, Vol. 20, *Some Halogenated Hydrocarbons*, Lyon, pp. 155–178

IARC (1979d) *IARC Monographs on the Evaluation of the Carcinogenic Risk of Chemicals to Humans*, Vol. 19, *Some Monomers, Plastics and Synthetic Elastomers, and Acrolein.*, Lyon, pp. 402–438

IARC (1983) *IARC Monographs on the Evaluation of the Carcinogenic Risk of Chemicals to Humans*, Vol. 30, *Miscellaneous Pesticides*, Lyon, pp. 271–282

IARC (1986a) *IARC Monographs on the Evaluation of the Carcinogenic Risk of Chemicals to Humans*, Vol. 41, *Some Halogenated Hydrocarbons and Pesticide Exposures*, Lyon, pp. 357–406

IARC (1986b) *IARC Monographs on the Evaluation of the Carcinogenic Risk of Chemicals to Humans*, Vol. 41, *Some Halogenated Hydrocarbons and Pesticide Exposures*, Lyon, pp. 319–356

IARC (1987a) *IARC Monographs on the Evaluation of Carcinogenic Risks to Humans*, Suppl. 7, *Overall Evaluations of Carcinogenicity: An Updating of* IARC Monographs *Volumes 1–42*, Lyon, pp. 350–354

IARC (1987b) *IARC Monographs on the Evaluation of Carcinogenic Risks to Humans*, Suppl. 7, *Overall Evaluations of Carcinogenicity: An Updating of* IARC Monographs *Volumes 1–42*, Lyon, pp. 156–160

IARC (1987c) *IARC Monographs on the Evaluation of Carcinogenic Risks to Humans*, Suppl. 7, *Overall Evaluations of Carcinogenicity: An Updating of* IARC Monographs *Volumes 1–42*, Lyon, pp. 154–156

IARC (1987d) *IARC Monographs on the Evaluation of Carcinogenic Risks to Humans*, Suppl. 7, *Overall Evaluations of Carcinogenicity: An Updating of* IARC Monographs *Volumes 1–42*, Lyon, pp. 321–326

IARC (1987e) *IARC Monographs on the Evaluation of Carcinogenic Risks to Humans*, Suppl. 7, *Overall Evaluations of Carcinogenicity: An Updating of* IARC Monographs *Volumes 1–42*, Lyon, pp. 373–376

IARC (1987f) *IARC Monographs on the Evaluation of Carcinogenic Risks to Humans*, Suppl. 7, *Overall Evaluations of Carcinogenicity: An Updating of* IARC Monographs *Volumes 1–42*, Lyon, pp. 91–92

IARC (1987g) *IARC Monographs on the Evaluation of Carcinogenic Risks to Humans*, Suppl. 7, *Overall Evaluations of Carcinogenicity: An Updating of* IARC Monographs *Volumes 1–42*, Lyon, pp. 200–201

IARC (1987h) *IARC Monographs on the Evaluation of Carcinogenic Risks to Humans*, Suppl. 7, *Overall Evaluations of Carcinogenicity: An Updating of* IARC Monographs *Volumes 1–42*, Lyon, pp. 120–122

IARC (1987i) *IARC Monographs on the Evaluation of Carcinogenic Risks to Humans*, Suppl. 7, *Overall Evaluations of Carcinogenicity: An Updating of* IARC Monographs *Volumes 1–42*, Lyon, pp. 92–93

IARC (1991) *IARC Monographs on the Evaluation of Carcinogenic Risks to Humans*, Vol. 53, *Occupational Exposures in Insecticide Application and Some Pesticides*, Lyon, pp. 441–466

IARC (1994a) *IARC Monographs on the Evaluation of Carcinogenic Risks to Human*, Vol. 59, *Hepatitis Viruses*, Lyon, pp. 45–164

IARC (1994b) *IARC Monographs on the Evaluation of Carcinogenic Risks to Human*, Vol. 59, *Hepatitis Viruses*, Lyon, pp. 165–221

Ideo, G., Ballati, G., Bellobuno, A. & Bissanti, L. (1985) Urinary D-glucaric excretion in the Seveso area, polluted by tetrachlorodibenzo-*p*-dioxin (TCDD): five years of experience. *Environ. Health Perspectives*, **60**, 151–157

Ignatieva, L.P., Komornikova, N.V., Tarasova, E.N. & Somov, L.P. (1993) Quantitative estimation of the levels of polychlorinated compounds in natural environments of the Pribaikal. *Organohalogen Compounds*, **12**, 367–368

Ikeda, M. & Yoshimura, T. (1996) Survival of patients. In: Kuratsune, M., Yoshimura, H., Hori, Y., Okumura, M. & Masuda, Y., eds, *Yusho — A Human Disaster Caused by PCBs and Related Compounds*, Fukuoka, Kyushu University Press, pp. 316–323

Ikeda, M., Kuratsune, M., Nakamura, Y. & Hirohata, T. (1986) A cohort study on mortality of Yusho patients — a preliminary report. *Fukuoka Acta med.*, **78**, 297–300

Ikeya, K., Jaiswal, A.K., Owens, R.A., Jones, J.E., Nebert, D.W. & Kimura, S. (1989) Human *CYP1A2*. Sequence, gene structure comparison with the mouse and rat orthologous gene, and differences in liver 1A2 mRNA expression. *Mol. Endocrinol.*, **3**, 1399–1408

Ilic, P., Knöfel, S. & Sachs-Paulus, N. (1994) Pollution of municipal sewage sludges by polychlorinted dioxins/furans and polychlorinated biphenyls in the area of the Frankfurt Regional Co-operative Association. *Abwasser*, **41**, 448–454

Ioannou, Y.M., Birnbaum, L.S. & Matthews, H.B. (1983) Toxicity and distribution of 2,3,7,8-tetrachlorodibenzofuran in male guinea pigs. *J. Toxicol. environ. Health*, **12**, 541–553

Isaac, D.D. & Andrew, D.J. (1996) Tubologenesis in Drosophila: a requirement for the tracheless gene product. *Genes Dev.*, **10**, 103–117

Ito, S.I., Ito, M., Cho, J.-J., Shimotohno, K. & Tajima, K. (1991) Massive sero-epidemiological survey of hepatitis C virus: clusterung of carriers on the southwest coast of Tsushima, Japan. *Jpn. J. Cancer Res.*, **82**, 1–3

Jackson, J.A., Diliberto, J.J. & Birnbaum, L.S. (1993) Estimation of octanol-water partition coefficients and correlation with dermal absorption for several polyhalogenated aromatic hydrocarbons. *Fundam. appl. Toxicol.*, **21**, 334–344

Jager, J. (1993) PCDD/F and PCB emission from steel producing, processing and reclamation plants with varying input. *Toxicol. environ. Chem.*, **40**, 201–211

Jain, S., Dolwick, K.M., Schmidt, J.V. & Bradfield, C.A. (1994) Potent transactivation domains of the Ah receptor and the Ah receptor nuclear translocator map to their carboxyl termini. *J. biol. Chem.*, **269**, 31518–31524

Jaiswal, A.K. (1994) Human NAD(P)H:quinone oxidoreductase: gene structure, activity and tissue-specific expression. *J. biol. Chem.*, **269**, 14502–14508

Jan, Y.N. & Jan, L.Y. (1993) HLH proteins, fly neurogenesis, and vertebrate myogenesis. *Cell*, **75**, 827–830

Jansing, P.J. & Korff, R. (1992) Dioxinintoxication and resulting health impairment. A study of workers exposed to 2,3,7,8-TCDD. *Zbl. Arbeitsmed.*, 42, 494–497 (in German)

van Jaarsveld, J.A. & Schutter, M.A.A. (1992) Modelling the long-range transport and deposition of dioxins; first results for the North Sea and surrounding countries. *Organohalogen Compounds*, **9**, 299–303

van Jaarsveld, J.A. & Schutter, M.A.A. (1993) Modelling the long-range transport and deposition of dioxins; first results for NW Europe. *Chemosphere*, **27**, 131–139

Jennings, A.M., Wild, G., Ward, J.D. & Milford Ward, A. (1988) Immunological abnormalities 17 years after accidental exposure to 2,3,7,8-tetrachlorodibenzo-*p*-dioxin. *Br. J. ind. Med.*, **45**, 701–704

Jensen, A.A. (1987) Polychlorobiphenyls (PCBs), polychlorodibenoz-p-dioxins (PCDDs), and polychlorodibenzofurans (PCDFs) in human milk, blood and adipose tissue. *Sci. total Environ.*, **64**, 259–293

Jensen, A.A., Grove, A. & Hoffmann, L. (1995) Sources of dioxin-contamination and presence of dioxins in the environment (Report from Environmental Board No. 81), Dansk Teknologisk Institut, Miljøteknik, Miljø- og Energiministeriet Miljøstyrelsen (in Danish)

Jiménez, B., Hernández, L.M., González, M.J., Eljarrat, E., Caixach, J. & Rivera, J. (1995) Levels of PCDDs and PCDFs in serum samples of non exposed individuals living in Madrid (Spain). *Organohalogen Compounds*, **26**, 249–253

Jiménez, B., Eljarrat, E., Hernández, L.M., Rivera, J. & Gonzáles, M.J. (1996a) Polychlorinated dibenzo-*p*-dioxins and dibenzofurans in soils near a clinical waste incinerator in Madrid, Spain. Chemometric comparison with other pollution sources and soils. *Chemosphere*, **32**, 1327–1348

Jiménez, B., Wright. C., Kelly, M. & Startin, J. R. (1996b) Levels of PCDDs, PCDFs and non-ortho PCBs in dietary supplement fish oils obtained in Spain. *Chemosphere*, **32**, 461–467

Jirasek, L., Kalensky, K., Kubec, K., Pazderova, J. & Lukas, E. (1974) Chronic poisoning by 2,3,7,8-tetrachlorodibenzo-*p*-dioxin. *Cesk. Dermatol.*, **49**, 145–157

Jobb, B., Uza, M., Hunsinger, R., Roberts, K., Tosine, H., Clement, R., Bobbie, B., LeBel, G., Williams, D. & Lau, B. (1990) A survey of drinking water supplies in the Province of Ontario for dioxins and furans. *Chemosphere*, **20**, 1553–1558

Jödicke, B., Ende, M., Helge, H. & Neubert, D. (1992) Fecal excretion of PCDDs/PCDFs in a 3-month-old breast-fed infant. *Chemosphere*, **25**, 1061–1065

Johansen, H.R., Alexander, J., Rossland, O.J., Plantin, S., Løvik, M., Gaarder, P.I., Gdynia, W., Bjerve, K.S. & Becher, G. (1996) PCDDs, PCDFs, and PCBs in human blood in relation to consumption of crabs from a contaminated fjord area in Norway. *Environ. Health Perspectives*, **104**, 756–764

Johnson, E.S., Parsons, W., Weinberg, C.R., Shore, D.L., Mathews, J., Patterson, D.G., Jr & Needham, L.L. (1992a) Current serum levels of 2,3,7,8-tetrachlorodibenzo-*p*-dioxin in phenoxy acid herbicide applicators and characterization of historical levels. *J. natl Cancer Inst.*, 84, 1648–1653

Johnson, R., Tietge, J. & Botts, S. (1992b) Carcinogenicity of 2,3,7,8-TCDD to Medaca (Abstract No. 476). *Toxicologist*, **12**, 138

Johnson, L., Dickerson, R., Safe, S.H., Nyberg, C.L., Lewis, R.P. & Welsh, T.H., Jr (1992c) Reduce Leydig cell volume and function in adult rats exposed to 2,3,7,8-tetrachlorodibenzo-*p*-dioxin without a significant effect on spermatogenesis. *Toxicology*, **76**, 103–118

Johnson, L., Wilker, C.E., Safe, S.H., Scott, B., Dean, D.D. & White, P.H. (1994) 2,3,7,8-tetrachlorodibenzo-p-dioxin reduces the number, size, and organelle content of Leydig cells in adult rat testes. *Toxicology*, **89**, 49–65

Johnson, K., Cummings, A.M. & Birnbaum, L.S. (1996) Assessing the structure activity relationship of polyhalogenated aromatic hydrocarbons using endometriosis as an endpoint. *Organohalogen Compounds*, **29**, 268–671

Jones, G. & Greig, J.B. (1975) Pathological changes in the liver of mice given 2,3,7,8-TCDD. *Experientia*, **31**, 1315–1317

Jones, K.G. & Sweeney, G.D. (1980) Dependence of the porphyrinogenic effect of 2,3,7,8-tetra-chlorodibenzo(p)dioxin upon inheritance of aryl hydrocarbon hydroxylase responsiveness. *Toxicol. appl. Pharmacol.*, **53**, 42–49

Jones, R.E. & Chelsky, M. (1986) Further discussion concerning porphyria cutanea tarda and TCDD exposure. *Arch. environ. Health*, **41**, 100–103

Jones, K.G., Cole, F.M. & Sweeney, G.D. (1981) The role of iron in the toxicity of 2,3,7,8-tetra-chlorodibenzo-*p*-dioxin (TCDD). *Toxicol. appl. Pharmacol.*, **61**, 74–88

Jones, P.B., Galeazzi, D.R., Fisher, J.M. & Whitlock, J.P., Jr (1985) Control of cytochrome P$_1$-450 gene expression by dioxin. *Science*, **227**, 1499–1502

Jones, P.B., Durrin, L.K., Fisher, J.M. & Whitlock, J.P., Jr (1986a) Control of gene expression by 2,3,7,8-tetrachlorodibenzo-*p*-dioxin: multiple dioxin-responsive domains 5'-ward of the cytochrome P$_1$-450 gene. *J. biol. Chem.*, **261**, 6647–6650

Jones, P.B., Durrin, L.K., Galeazzi, D.R. & Whitlock, J.P., Jr (1986b) Control of cytochrome P$_1$-450 gene expression: analysis of a dioxin-responsive enhancer system. *Proc. natl Acad. Sci. USA*, **83**, 2802–2806

Jones, M.K., Weisenburger, W.P., Sipes, G. & Russell, D.H. (1987) Circadian alterations in prolactin, corticosterone, and thyroid hormone levels and down-regulation of prolactin receptor activity by 2,3,7,8-tetrachlorodibenzo-*p*-dioxin. *Toxicol. appl. Pharmacol.*, **87**, 337–350

de Jong, A.P.J.M. & Liem, A.K.D. (1993) Gas chromatography-mass spectrometry in ultra trace analysis of polychlorinated dioxins and related compounds. *Trends analyt. Chem.*, **12**, 115–124

de Jong, A.P.J.M., Liem, A.K.D. & Hoogerbrugge, R. (1993) Review: study of polychlorinated dibenzodioxins and furans from municipal waste incinerator emissions in the Netherlands: analytical methods and levels in the environment and human food chain. *J. Chromatogr.*, **643**, 91–106

Jurek, M.A., Powers, R.H., Gilbert, L.G. & Aust, S.D. (1990) The effect of TCDD on acyl CoA: retinol acyl transferase activity and vitamin A accumulation in the kidney of male Sprague Dawley rats. *J. biochem. Toxicol.*, **5**, 155–160

Jürgens, H.-J. & Roth, R., (1989) Case study and proposed decontamination steps of the soil and groundwater beneath a closed herbicide plant in Germany. *Chemosphere*, **18**, 1163–1169

Kahn, P.C., Gochfeld, M., Nygren, M., Hansson, M., Rappe, C., Velez, H., Ghent-Guenther, T. & Wilson, W.P. (1988) Dioxins and dibenzofurans in blood and adipose tissue of Agent Orange-exposed Vietnam veterans and matched controls. *J. Am. med. Assoc.*, **259**, 1661–1667

Kamimura, H., Koga, N., Oguri, K., Yoshimura, H., Honda, Y. & Nakano, M. (1988) Enhanced faecal excretion of 2,3,4,7,8-pentachlorodibenzofuran in rats by a long-term treatment with activated charcoal beads. *Xenobiotica*, **18**, 585–592

Kang, H.K., Watanabe, K.K., Breen, J., Remmers, J., Conomos, M.G., Stanley, J. & Flicker, M. (1991) Dioxins and dibenzofurans in adipose tissue of U.S. Vietnam veterans and controls. *Am. J. public Health*, **81**, 344–349

Kärenlampi, S.O., Eisen, H.J., Hankinson, O. & Nebert, D.W. (1983) Effects of cytochrome P_1-450 inducers on the cell-surface receptors for epidermal growth factor, phorbol 12,13-dibutyrate, or insulin of cultured mouse hepatoma cells. *J. biol. Chem.*, **258**, 10378–10383

Karras, J.G. & Holsapple, M.P. (1994a) Inhibition of calcium-dependent B cell activation by 2,3,7,8-tetrachlorodibenzo-*p*-dioxin. *Toxicol. appl. Pharmacol.*, **125**, 264–270

Karras, J.G. & Holsapple, M.P. (1994b) Mechanisms of 2,3,7,8-tetrachlorodibenzo-*p*-dioxin (TCDD)-induced disruption of B-lymphocyte signaling in the mouse: a current perspective. *Exp. clin. Immunogenet.*, **11**, 110–118

Karras, J.G., Conrad, D.H. & Holsapple, M.P. (1995) Effects of 2,3,7,8-tetrachlorodibenzo-*p*-dioxin (TCDD) on interleukin-4-mediated mechanisms of immunity. *Toxicol. Lett.*, **75**, 225–233

Karras, J.G., Morris, D.L., Matulka, R.A., Kramer, C.M. & Holsapple, M.P. (1996) 2,3,7,8-tetra-chloro-dibenzo-*p*-dioxin (TCDD) elevates basal B-cell intracellular calcium concentration and suppresses surface Ig- but not CD40-induced antibody secretion. *Toxicol. appl. Pharmacol.*, **137**, 275–284

Kashimoto, T., Miyata, H., Fukushima, S., Kunita, N., Ohi, G. & Tung, T.-C. (1985) PCBs, PCQs and PCDFs in blood of Yusho and Yu-Cheng patients. *Environ. Health Perspectives*, **59**, 73–78

Katz, L.B., Theobald, H.M., Bookstaff, R.C. & Peterson, R.E. (1984) Characterization on the enhanced paw edema response to carrageenan and dextran in 2,3,7,8-tetrachlorodibenzo-*p*-dioxin -treated rats. *J. Pharmacol. exp. Ther.*, **230**, 670–677

Kaune, A., Lenoir, D., Nikolai, U. & Kettrup, A. (1993) Indicator parameters for PCDD/F as a possible means to monitor emissons of toxicity equivalents from waste incinerators. *Central Eur. J. public Health*, **1**, 123–124

Kauppinen, T., Kogevinas, M., Johnson, E., Becher, H., Bertazzi, P.-A., Bueno de Mesquita, H.B., Coggon, D., Green, L., Littorin, M., Lynge, E., Mathews, J., Neuberger, M., Osman, J., Pannett, B., Pearce, N., Winkelmann, R. & Saracci, R. (1993) Chemical exposure in manufacture of phenoxy herbicides and chlorophenols and in spraying of phenoxy herbicides. *Am. J. ind. Med.*, **23**, 903–920

Keenan, R.E., Paustenbach, D.J., Wenning, R.J. & Parsons, A.H. (1991) Pathology reevaluation of the Kociba *et al.* (1978) bioassay of 2,3,7,8-TCDD: implications for risk assessment. *J. Toxicol. environ. Health*, **34**, 279–296

Kelling, C.K., Christian, B.J., Inhorn, S.L. & Peterson, R.E. (1985) Hypophagia-induced weight loss in mice, rats, and guinea pigs treated with 2,3,7,8-tetrachlorodibenzo-*p*-dioxin. *Fundam. appl. Toxicol.*, **5**, 700–712

Kelling, C.K., Menahan, L.A. & Peterson, R.E. (1987) Effects of 2,3,7,8-tetrachlorodibenzo-*p*-dioxin treatment on mechanical function of the rat heart. *Toxicol. appl. Pharmacol.*, **91**, 497–501

Kerkvliet, N.I. (1994) Immunotoxicology of dioxins and related chemicals. In: Schechter, A., ed., *Dioxins and Health*, New York, Plenum Press, pp. 199–225

Kerkvliet, N.I. & Brauner, J.A. (1987) Mechanisms of 1,2,3,4,6,7,8-heptachlorodibenzo-*p*-dioxin (HpCDD)-induced humoral immune suppression: evidence of primary defect in T-cell regulation. *Toxicol. appl. Pharmacol.*, **87**, 18–31

Kerkvliet, N.J. & Brauner, J.A. (1990) Flow cytometric analysis of lymphocyte subpopulations in the spleen and thymus of mice exposed to a acute immunosuppressive dose of 2,3,7,8-tetrachlorodibenzo-*p*-dioxin (TCDD). *Environ. Res.*, **52**, 146–154

Kerkvliet, N.I. & Burleson, G.R. (1994) Immunotoxicity of TCDD and related halogenated aromatic hydrocarbons. In: Dean, J.H., Luster, M.I., Munson, A.E., & Kimber, I., eds, *Immunotoxicology and Immunopharmacology*, 2nd Ed., New York, Raven Press, pp. 97–121

Kerkvliet, N.I. & Oughton, J.A. (1993) Acute inflammatory response to sheep red blood cell challenge in mice treated with 2,3,7,8-tetrachlorodibenzo-*p*-dioxin (TCDD): phenotypic and functional analysis of peritoneal excudate cells. *Toxicol. appl. Pharmacol.*, **119**, 248–257

Kerkvliet, N.I., Brauner, J.A. & Matlock J.P. (1985) Humoral immunotoxicity of polychlorinated diphenyl ethers, phenoxyphenols, dioxins and furans present as contaminations of technical grade pentachlorophenol. *Toxicology*, **36**, 307–324

Kerkvliet, N.J. Steppan, L.B., Brauner J.A., Deyo, J.A, Henderson, M.C., Tomar, R.S. & Buhlert, D.R. (1990a) Influence of the Ah locus on the humoral immunotoxicity of 2,3,7,8-tetrachlorodibenzo-*p*-dioxin: evidence for Ah-receptor-dependent and Ah-receptor-independent mechanisms of immunosuppression. *Toxicol. appl. Pharmacol.*, **105**, 26–36

Kerkvliet, N.I., Beacher-Steppan, L., Smith, B.B., Youngberg, J.A., Henderson, M.C. & Buhlert, D.R. (1990b) Role of the Ah locus in suppression of cytotoxic T lymphocyte activity by halogenated aromatic hydrocarbons (PCDs and TCDD): structure-activity, relationships and effects in C57Bl/6 mice congenic at the Ah locus. *Fundam. appl. Toxicol.*, **14**, 532–541

Ketchum, N.S. & Akhtar, F.Z. (1996) *The Air Force Health Study: an Epidemiologic Investigation of Health Effects in Air Force Personnel Following Exposure to Herbicides, Mortality Update 1996* (Interim Technical Report AL/AO-TR-1996-0068), Brooks Air Force Base, Texas. Armstrong Laboratory

Kew, G.A., Schaum, J.L., White, P. & Evans, T.T. (1989) Review of plant uptake of 2,3,7,8-TCDD from soil and potential influences of bioavailability. *Chemosphere*, **18**, 1313–1318

Khamitov, R.Z. & Maystrenko, V.N. (1994) Chlorinated dioxins and dibenzofurans — first results of systematic monitoring of Bashkortostan Republic. *Organohalogen Compounds*, **20**, 145–146

Khamitov, R.Z. & Maystrenko, V.N. (1995) PCDD/PCDF and related compounds; the Bashkortostan Republic situation. *Organohalogen Compounds*, **24**, 309–312

Khamitov, R.Z., Simonova, N.I., Maksimov, G.G. & Maystrenko, V.N. (1996) Chlorinated dioxin and dibenzofuran levels in food from Bashkortosan Republic, Russia. *Organohalogen Compounds*, **28**, 171–174

Kharatt, I. & Saatcioglu, F. (1996) Antiestrogenic effects of 2,3,7,8-tetrachlorodibenzo-*p*-dioxin are mediated by direct transcriptional interference with the liganded estrogen receptor. *J. Biol. Chem.*, **271**, 10533–10537

Khera, K.S. (1992) Extraembryonic tissue changes induced by 2,3,7,8-tetrachlorodibenzo-*p*-dioxin and 2,3,4,7,8-pentachlorodibenzofuran with a note on direction of maternal blood flow in the labyrinth of C57BL/6N mice. *Teratology*, **45**, 611–627

Khera, K.S. & Ruddick, J.A. (1973) Polychlorinated dibenzo-*p*-dioxins: perinatal effects and the dominant lethal test in Wistar rats. *Adv. Chem.*, **120**, 70–84

Kieselrot-Studie (1991) Minister für Arbeit, Gesundheit und Soziales des Landes Nordrhein-Westfalen

Kieaitwong, S., Nguyen, L.V., Herbert, V.R., Hackett, M., Miller, G.C., Mülle, M.J. & Mitzel, R. (1990) Photolysis of chlorinated dioxins in organic solvents and on soils. *Environ. Sci. technol.*, **24**, 1575–1580

Kim, H.M., Choi, I.P. & Holsapple, M.P. (1994) Direct exposure to 2,3,7,8-tetrachlorodibenzo-*p*-dioxin (TCDD) increases infectivity of human erythrocytes to a malarial parasite. *Life Sci.*, **54**, 215–220

Kimbrough, R.D., Coleman, D., Carter, C. D., Liddle, J.A., Cline, R.E. & Philipps, P.E. (1977) Epidemiology and pathology of a tetrachlorodibenzodioxin poisoning episode. *Arch. environ. Health*, **32**, 77–86

Kimbrough, R.D., Falk, H., Stehr, P. & Fries, G. (1984) Health implication of 2,3,7,8-tetrachlorodibenzodioxin (TCDD) contamination of residential soil. *J. Toxicol. environ. Health*, **14**, 47–93

Kimmig, J. & Schulz, K.H. (1957a) Chlorinated aromatic cyclic ethers as the cause of so-called chloracne. *Naturwissenschaften*, **44**, 337–338

Kimmig, J. & Schulz, K.H. (1957b) Occupational chloracne caused by aromatic cyclic ethers. *Dermatologica*, **115**, 540–546

Kimura, S., Gonzalez, F.J. & Nebert, D.W. (1986) Tissue-specific expression of the mouse dioxin-inducible P_1450 and P_3450 genes: differential transcriptional activation and mRNA stability in liver and extrahepatic tissues. *Mol. cell. Biol.*, **6**, 1471–1477

Kirschmer, P. (1987) Measurement of PCDD/PCDF emissions in North-Rhine Westphalia. *VDI-Berichte*, **634**, 145–163 (in German)

Kitchin, K.T. & Woods, J.S. (1979) 2,3,7,8-Tetrachlorodibenzo-*p*-dioxin (TCDD) effects on hepatic microsomal cytochrome P-448-mediated enzyme activities. *Toxicol. appl. Pharmacol.*, **47**, 537–546

Kjeller, L.-O., Rappe, C., Jones, K.C. & Johnston, A.E. (1990) Evidence for increases in the environmental burden of polychlorinated dibenzo-p-dioxins and furans (PCDD/PCDFs) over the last century. *Organohalogen Compounds*, **1**, 433–436

Kjeller, L.-O., Jones, K.C., Johnston, A.E. & Rappe, C. (1991) Increases in the polychlorinated dibenzo-*p*-dioxin and furan content of soils and vegetation since the 1840s. *Environ. Sci. Technol.*, **25**, 1619–1627

Kleeman, J.M., Moore, R.W. & Peterson, R.E. (1990) Inhibition of testicular sterodiogenesis in 2,3,7,8-tetrachlorodibenzo-*p*-dioxin-treated rats: evidence that the key lesion occurs prior to or during pregneneolone formation. *Toxicol. appl. Pharmacol.*, **106**, 112–125

Kleopfer, R.D., Yue, K.T. & Bunn, W.W. (1985) Determination of 2,3,7,8-tetrachlorodibenzo-*p*-dioxin in soil. In: Keith, L.H., Rappe, C. & Choudhary, G., eds., *Chlorinated Dioxins and Dibenzofurans in the Total Environment II,* Boston, Butterworth, pp. 367–375

Kline, J., Stein, Z. & Susser, M. (1989) *Conception to Birth: Epidemiology of Prenatal Development*, New York, Oxford University Press

Knutson, J.C. & Poland, A. (1980) 2,3,7,8-Tetrachlorodibenzo-*p*-dioxin: failure to demonstrate toxicity in twenty-three cultured cell tpes. *Toxicol. appl. Pharmacol.*, **54**, 377–383

Kociba, R. (1984) Evaluation of the carcinogenic and mutagenic potential of 2,3,7,8-TCDD and other chlorinated dioxins. In: Poland, A. & Kimbrough, R.D., *Biological Mechanisms of Dioxin Action* (Banbury Report No. 18), Cold Spring Harbor Laboratory, NY

Kociba, R.J., Keeler, P.A., Park, C.N. & Gehring, P.J. (1976) 2,3,7,8-Tetrachlorodibenzo-*p*-dioxin: results of a 13-week oral toxicity study in rats. *Toxicol. appl. Pharmacol.*, **35**, 553–574

Kociba, R.J, Keyes, D.G., Beyer, J.E., Carreon, R.M., Wade, C.E., Dittenber, D.A., Kalnins, R.P., Frauson, L.E., Park, C.N., Barnard, S.D., Hummel, R.A. & Humiston, C.G. (1978) Results of a two-year chronic toxicity and oncogenicity study of 2,3,7,8-tetrachlorodibenzo-*p*-dioxin in rats. *Toxicol. appl. Pharmacol.*, **46**, 279–303

Kociba, R.J., Keyes, D.G., Beyer, J.E., Carreon, R.M. & Gehring, P.J. (1979) Long-term toxicologic studies of 2,3,7,8-tetrachlorodibenzo-*p*-dioxin (TCDD) in laboratory animals. *Ann. N.Y. Acad. Sci.*, **320**, 397–404

Koga, N., Ariyoshi, N., Nakashima, H. & Yoshimura, H. (1990) Purification and characterization of two forms of 2,3,4,7,8-pentachlorodibenzofuran-inducible cytochrome P-450 in hamster liver. *J. Biochem.*, **107**, 826–833

Kogevinas, M., Saracci, R., Winkelman, R., Johnson, E.S., Bertazzi, P.A., Bueno de Mesquita, H.B., Kauppinen, T., Littorin, M., Lynge, E., Neuberger, M. & Pearce, N. (1993) Cancer incidence and mortality in women occupationally exposed to chlorophenoxy herbicides, chlorophenols and dioxins. *Cancer Causes Control.*, **4**, 547–553

Kogevinas, M., Kauppinen, T., Winkelman, R., Becher, H., Bertazzi, P.A., Bueno de Mesquita, H.B., Coggon, D., Green, L., Johnson, E., Littorin, M., Lynge, E., Marlow, D.A., Mathews, J.D., Neuberger, M., Benn, T., Pannett, B., Pearce, N. & Saracci, R. (1995) Soft tissue sarcoma and non-Hodgkin's lymphoma in workers exposed to phenoxy herbicides, chlorophenols, and dioxins: two nested case–control studies. *Epidemiology*, **6**, 396–402

Kogevinas, M., Becher, H., Benn, T., Bertazzi, P.A., Boffetta, P., Bueno de Mesquita, H.B., Coggon, D., Colin, D., Flesch-Janys, D., Fingerhut, M., Green, L., Kauppinen, T., Littorin, M., Lynge, E., Mathews, J.D., Neuberger, M., Pearce, N. & Saracci, R. (1997) Cancer mortality in workers exposed to phenoxy herbicides, chlorophenols and dioxins: An expanded and updated international cohort study. *Am. J. Epidemiol.* (in press)

Kohn, M.C., Lucier, G.W., Clark, G.C., Sewall, C., Tritscher, A.M. & Portier, C.J. (1993) A mechanistic model of effects of dioxin on gene expression in the rat liver. *Toxicol. appl. Pharmacol.*, **120**, 138–154

Kohn, M.C., Sewall, C.H., Lucier, G.W. & Portier, C.J. (1996) A mechanistic model of effects of dioxin on thyroid hormones in the rat. *Toxicol. appl. Pharmacol.*, **136**, 29–48

Koistinen J., Paasivirta J. & Vuorinen P.J. (1989) Dioxins and other planar polychloroaromatic compounds in Baltic, Finnish and Arctic fish samples. *Chemosphere*, **19**, 527–530

Kominsky, J.R. & Kwoka, C.D. (1989) Background concentrations of polychlorinated dibenzofurans (PCDFs) and polychlorinated dibenzo-p-dioxins (PCDDs) in office buildings in Boston, Massachusetts. *Chemosphere*, **18**, 599–608

König, J., Theisen, J., Günther, W.J., Liebl, K.H. & Büchen, M. (1993) Ambient air levels of polychlorinated dibenzofurans and dibenzo(*p*)dioxins at different sites in Hessen. *Chemosphere*, **26**, 851–861

Koopman-Esseboom, C., Huisman, M., Weisglas-Kuperus, N., Boersma, E.R., de Ridder, M.A., Van der Paauw, C.G., Tuinstra, L.G. & Sauer, P.J. (1994a) Dioxin and PCB levels in blood and human milk in relation to living areas in The Netherlands. *Chemosphere*, **29**, 2327–2338

Koopman-Esseboom, C., Morse, D.C., Weisglas-Kuperus, N., Lutkeschipholt, I.J., Van der Paauw, C.G., Tuinstra, L.G., Brouwer, A. & Sauer, P.J. (1994b) Effects of dioxins and poly-chlorinated biphenyls on thyroid hormone status of pregnant women and their infants. *Pediatr. Res.*, **36**, 468–473

Koopman-Esseboom, C., Huisman, M., Touwen, B.C.L., Boersma, E.R., Brouwer, A., Sauer, P.J. & Weisglas-Kuperus, N. (1995a) Effects of PCB/Dioxin exposure and feeding type on the infant's visual recognition memory. In: *Effects of Perinatal Exposure to PCBs and Dioxins on Early Human Development*, Rotterdam, Erasmus Universiteit Rotterdam, pp. 75–86

Koopman-Esseboom, C., Weisglas-Kuperus, N., de Ridder, M.A.J., van der Paauw, C.G., Tuinstra, L.G. & Sauer, P.J.(1995b) Effects of PCB/Dioxin exposure and feeding type on the infant's visual recognition memory. In: *Effects of Perinatal Exposure to PCBs and Dioxins on Early Human Development*, Rotterdam, Erasmus Universiteit Rotterdam, pp. 107–121

Koopman-Esseboom, C., Weisglas-Kuperus, N., de Ridder, M.A.J., Paauw, C.G.van der, Tuinstra, L.G. & Sauer, P.J. (1996) Effects of polychlorinated biphenyl/dioxin exposure and feeding type on the infant's mental and psychomotor development. *Pediatrics*, **97**, 700–706

Körner, W., Dawidowsky, N. & Hagenmaier, H. (1993) Fecal excretion rates of PCDDs and PCDFs in two breast-fed infants. *Chemosphere*, **27**, 157–162

Körner, W., Hanf, V., Faust, A., Temmen, R., Tinneberg, H.-R. & Hagenmaier, H. (1994) Concentrations and profiles of PCDDs and PCDFs in human mammary carcinoma tissue. *Chemosphere*, **29**, 2339–2347

Korte, M., Stahlman, R. & Neubert, D. (1990) Induction of hepatic monooxygenases in female rats and offspring in correlation with TCDD tissue concentrations after single treatment during pregnancy. *Chemosphere*, **20**, 1193

Korte, M., Stahlmann, R., Kubicki-Muranyi, M., Gleichmann, E. & Neubert, D. (1991a) Poly-halogenated dibenzo-*p*-dioxins and dibenzofurans and the immune system. 3. No effect of 2,3,7,8-TCDD in the popliteal lymph node assay (PLNA) in rats. *Arch. Toxicol.*, **65**, 656–660

Korte, M., Stahlmann, R., Thiel, R., Nagao, T., Chahoud, I., van Loveren, H., Vos, J.G. & Neubert, D. (1991b) Resistance to *Trichinella spiralis* infection, induction of hepatic mono-oxygenases, and concentrations in thymus and liver in rats after perinatal exposure to 2,3,7,8-tetrachlorodibenzo-*p*-dioxin. *Chemosphere*, **23**, 1845–1854

Koshakji, R.P., Harbison, R.D. & Bush, M.T. (1984) Studies on the metabolic fate of [^{14}C]-2,3,7,8-tetrachlorodibenzo-*p*-dioxin (TCDD) in the mouse. *Toxicol. appl. Pharmacol.*, **73**, 69–77

Kraemer, S.A., Arthur, K.A., Denison, M.S., Smith, W.L. & DeWitt, D.L. (1996) Regulation of prostaglandin endoperoxide H synthase-2 expression by 2,3,7,8,-tetrachlorodibenzo-*p*-dioxin. *Arch. Biochem. Biophys.*, **330**, 319–328

Kramer, C.M., Johnson, K.W., Dooley, R.K. & Holsapple, M.P. (1987) 2,3,7,8-Tetrachloro-dibenzo-*p*-dioxin (TCDD) enhances antibody production and protein kinase activity in murine B cells. *Biochem. biophys. Res. Comm.*, **145**, 25–33

Krauss, P., Mahnke, K. & Freire, L. (1995) Determination of PCDD/F and PCB in forest soils from Brazil. *Organohalogen Compounds*, **24**, 357–361

Krauthacker B., Reiner E., Lindstrom G. & Rappe C. (1989) Residues of polychlorinated-di-benzodioxins, -dibenzofurans and -biphenyls in human milk samples collected in a continental town in Croatia, Yugoslavia. *Arh. hig. rada. toksikol.*, **40**, 9–14

de Krey, G.K. & Kerkvliet, N.I. (1995) Suppression of cytotoxic T lymphocyte activity by 2,3,7,8-tetrachlorodibenzo-*p*-dioxin occurs in vivo, but not in vitro, and is independent of corticosterone elevation. *Toxicology*, **97**, 105–112

Krishnan, V. & Safe, S. (1993) Polychlorinated biphenyls (PCBs), dibenzo-*p*-dioxins (PCDDs) and dibenzofurans (PCDFs) as antiestrogens in MCF-7 human breast cancer cells: quantitative structure-activity relationships. *Toxicol. appl. Pharmacol.*, **120**, 55–61

Krishnan, V., Narasimhan, T.R. & Safe, S. (1992) Development of gel staining techniques for detecting the secretion of procathepsin D (52-kDa protein) in MCF-7 human breast cancer cells. *Anal. Biochem.*, **204**, 137–142

Krishnan, V., Wang, X. & Safe, S. (1994) ER/Sp1 complexes mediate estrogen-induced cathepsin D gene expression in MCF-7 human breast cancer cells. *J. biol. Chem.*, **269**, 15912–15917

Krishnan, V., Porter, W., Santostefano, M., Wang, X. & Safe, S. (1995) Molecular mechanism of inhibition of estrogen-induced cathepsin D gene expression by 2,3,7,8-tetrachlorodibenzo-*p*-dioxin (TCDD) in MCF-7 cells. *Mol. cell. Biol.*, **15**, 6710–6719

Krowke, R. & Neubert, D. (1990) Comparison of cleft palate frequency and TCDD concentration in mice at different stages of development. *Chemosphere*, **20**, 1177

Krowke, R., Abraham, K., Wiesmuller, T., Hagenmaier, H. & Neubert, D. (1990) Transfer of various PCDDs and PCDFs via the placenta and mothers milk to marmoset offspring. *Chemosphere*, **20**, 1065

Krueger, N., Neubert, B., Helge, H. *et al.* (1990) Induction of caffeine-demethylations by 2,3,7,8-TCDD in Marmoset monkeys measured with a $^{14}CO_2$ breath-test. *Chemosphere*, **20**, 1173–1176

Kruglov, E.A., Amirova, Z.K. & Loshkina, E.A. (1996) PCDDs and PCDFs in snow coat of an industrial city as a result of oil incineration at accident place. *Organohalogen Compounds*, **28**, 228–231

Kuehl, D.W., Butterworth, B.C., McBride, A., Kroner, S. & Bahnick, D. (1989) Contamination of fish by 2,3,7,7-tetrachlorodibenzo-*p*-dioxin: a survey of fish from major watersheds in the United States. *Chemosphere*, **18**, 1997–2014

Kujawa, M., Raab, M. & Haberland, W. (1995) Environmental levels of PCDD/PCDF in soils of Brandenburg, Germany. *Organohalogen Compounds*, **24**, 319–321

Kupfer, D., Mani, C., Lee, C.A. & Rifkind, A.B. (1994) Induction of tamoxifen-4-hydroxylation by 2,3,7,8-tetrachlorodibenzo-*p*-dioxin (TCDD), β-naphthoflavone (bNF), and phenobarbital (PB) in avian liver: identification of P450 TCDD$_{AA}$ as catalyst of 4-hydroxylation induced by TCDD and βNF. *Cancer Res.*, **54**, 3140–3144

Kuratsune, M. (1972) An abstract of results of laboratory examinations of patients with Yusho and of animal experiments. *Environ. Health Perspectives*, **5**, 129–136

Kuratsune, M. (1989) Yusho, with reference to Yu-Cheng. In: Kimbrough, R.D. & Jensen, A.A., eds, *Halogenated Biophenyls, Terphenyls, Naphthalenes, Dibenzodioxins and Related Products*, 2nd Ed. New York, Elsevier Science Publishers, pp. 381–400

Kuratsune, M., Yoshimura, T., Matsuzaka, J. & Yamaguchi, A. (1972) Epidemiologic study on Yusho, a poisoning caused by ingestion of rice oil contaminated with a commercial brand of polychlorinated biphenyls. *Environ. Health Perspectives*, **1**, 119–128

Kuriowa, Y., Murai, Y. & Santa, T. (1969) Neurological and nerve conduction velocity studies of 23 patients with chlorobiphenyls poisoning. *Fukuoka Acta med.*, **60**, 462–463

Kurl, R.N., Abraham, M. & Olnes M.J. (1993) Early effects of 2,3,7,8-tetrachlorodibenzo-p-dioxin (TCDD) on rat thymocytes *in vitro*. *Toxicology*, **77**, 103–114

Kurokawa, Y. (1997) Research group on risk assessment of dioxins. Interim report on risk assessment of dioxins (in Japanese). In: *Joint Expert Committee on Evaluation of Risks of Dioxins, Air Quality Guideline of WHO/EURO*, Bilthoven, Ministry of Health and Welfare (in press)

Kurokawa, Y., Matsueda, T., Nakamura, M., Takada, S. & Fukamachi, K. (1994) Distributions of atmospheric coplanar PCBs, polychlorinated dibenzo-p-dioxins and dibenzofurans between vapor phase and particle phase. *Organohalogen Compounds*, **20**, 91–94

Kuroki, H., Masuda, Y., Yoshihara, S. & Yoshimura, H. (1980) Accumulation of polychlorinated dibenzofurans in the livers of monkeys and rats. *Food Cosmet. Toxicol.*, **18**, 387–392

Kuroki, J., Koga, N. & Yoshimura, H. (1986) High affinity of 2,3,4,7,8-pentachlorodibenzofuran to cytochrome P-450 in the hepatic microsomes of rats. *Chemosphere*, **15**, 731

Kuroki, H., Hattori, R., Haraguchi, K. & Masuda, Y. (1989) Metabolism of 2,8-dichlorodibenzofuran in rats. *Chemosphere*, **19**, 803

Kuroki, H., Haraguchi, K. & Masuda, Y. (1990) Metabolism of polychlorinated dibenzofurans (PCDFs) in rats. *Chemosphere*, **20**, 1065

LaFleur, L., Bousquet, T., Ramage, K., Brunck, B., Davis, T., Luksemburg, W. & Peterson, B. (1990) Analysis of TCDD and TCDF on the ppq-level in milk and food sources. *Chemosphere*, **20**, 1657–1662

Lai, T.J., Chen, Y.C., Chou, W.J., Guo, Y.L., Ko, H.C. & Hsu, C.C. (1993) Cognitive development in Yu-Cheng children. In: *Proceedings of the 13th International Symposium on Chlorinated Dioxins and Related Compounds (Dioxin '93), September 20-24, 1993, Vienna, Austria*

Lai, T.J., Guo, Y.L., Yu, M.L., Ko, H.C. & Hsu, C.C. (1994) Cognitive development in Yu-Cheng children. *Chemosphere*, **29**, 2405–2411

Lamb, J.C., IV, Harris, M.W., McKinney, J.D. & Birnbaum, L.S. (1986) Effects of thyroid hormones on the induction of cleft palate by 2,3,7,8-tetrachlorodibenzo-p-dioxin (TCDD) in C57BL/6N mice. *Toxicol. appl. Pharmacol.*, **84**, 115–124

Lamparski, L.L., Nestrick, T.J. & Crummett, W.B. (1991) Method 4: determination of specific halogenated dibenzo-p-dioxin and dibenzofuran isomers in environmental and biological matrices by gas chromatography-mass spectrometry. In: Rappe, C., Buser, H.-R., Dodet, B. & O'Neill, I.K., eds, *Environmental Carcinogens: Methods of Analysis and Exposure Measurement. Vol. 11: Polychlorinated Dioxins and Dibenzofurans* (IARC Scientific Publications No. 108), Lyon, IARC, pp. 251–279

Lampi, P., Vartiainen, T. & Tuomisto, J. (1990) Population exposure to chlorophenols, dibenzo-p-dioxins and dibenzofurans after a prolonged ground water pollution by chlorophenols. *Chemosphere*, **20**, 625–634

Lan, S.-J., Yen, Y.-Y., Ko, Y.-C. & Chen, E.-R. (1989) Growth and development of permanent teeth germ of transplacental Yu-Cheng babies in Taiwan. *Bull. environ. Contam. Toxicol.*, **42**, 931–934

Lan, S.-J., Yen, Y.-Y., Lan, J.-L., Chen, E.-R. & Ko, Y.-C. (1990) Immunity of PCB trans-placental Yu-Cheng children in Taiwan. *Bull. environ. Contam. Toxicol.*, **44**, 224–229

Landers, J.P., Birse, L.M., Nakai, J.S., Winhall, M.J. & Bunce, N.J. (1990) Chemically induced hepatic cytosol from the Sprague-Dawley rat: evidence for specific binding of 2,3,7,8-tetra-chlorodibenzo-*p*-dioxin to components kinetically distinct from the Ah receptor. *Toxicol. Lett.*, **51**, 295–302

Landi, M.T., Bertazzi, P.A., Consonni, D., Needham, L., Patterson, D., Mocarelli, P., Brambilla, P., Lucier, G. & Caporaso, N.E. (1996) TCDD blood levels, population characteristics, and individual accident experience. *Organohalogen Compounds*, **30**, 290–293

Lang, D.S., Becker, S., Clark, G.C., Devlin, R.B. & Koren, H.S. (1994) Lack of direct immuno-suppressive effects of 2,3,7,8-tetrachlorodibenzo-p-dioxin (TCDD) on human peripheral blood lymphocytes subsets *in vitro*. *Arch. Toxicol.*, **68**, 296–302

Lans, M.C., Klasson-Wehler, E., Willemsen, M., Meussen, E., Safe, S. & Brouwer, A. (1993) Structure-dependent competitive interaction of hydroxy-polychlorobiphenyls, -dibenzo-*p*-dioxins and -dibenzofurans with human transthyretin. *Chem.-biol. Interactions*, **88**, 7–21

Lans, M.C., Spiertz, C., Brouwer, A. & Koeman, J. H. (1994) Different competition of thyroxine binding to transthyretin and thyroxine-binding globulin by hydroxy-PCBs, PCDDs and PCDFs. *Eur. J. Pharmacol.*, **270**, 129–136

Larsen, G.L., Feil, V.J., Hakk, H., Huwe, J.K. & Petroske, E. (1996) Polychlorodibenzo-p-dioxin metabolism. *Organohalogen Compounds*, **28**, 491–494

Lawrence, B.P., Leid, M. & Kerkvliet, N.I. (1996) Distribution and behavior of the Ah receptor in murine lymphocytes. *Toxicol. appl. Pharmacol.*, **138**, 275–284

Le, C.D., Le, B.T., , Dinh, Q.M., Hoang, T.Q. & Le, H.T. (1995) Remarks on the dioxin levels in human pooled blood from various localities of Vietnam. *Organohalogen Compounds*, **26**, 161–167

LeBel, G.L., Williams, D.T., Benoit, F.M. & Goddard, M. (1990) Polychlorinated dibenzo-dioxins and dibenzofurans in human adipose tissue samples from five Ontario municipalities. *Chemosphere*, **21**, 1465–1475

Lebrec, H. & Burleson, G.R. (1994) Influenza virus host resistance models in mice and rats: uti-lization for immune function assessment and immunotoxicology. *Toxicology*, **91**, 179–188

Lee, I.P. & Dixon, R.L. (1978) Factors influencing reproduction and genetic toxic effects on male gonads. *Environ. Health Perspectives*, **24**, 117–127

Lee, D.C., Barlow, K.D. & Gaido, K.W. (1996) The actions of 2,3,7,8-tetrachlorodibenzo-*p*-dioxin on transforming growth factor-b2 promoter activity are localized to the TATA box binding region and controlled through a tyrosine kinase-dependent pathway. *Toxicol. appl. Pharmacol.*, **137**, 90–99

Leung, H.-W., Wendling, J.M., Orth, R., Hileman, F. & Paustenbach, D.J. (1990) Relative distribution of 2,3,7,8-tetrachlorodibenzo-*p*-dioxin in human hepatic and adipose tissues. *Toxicol. Lett.*, **50**, 275–282

Levine, J. (1992) Global biomass burning. *Organohalogen Compounds*, **20**, 287

Li, X. & Rozman, K.K. (1995) Subchronic effects of 2,3,7,8-tetrachlorodibenzo-*p*-dioxin (TCDD) and their reversibility in male Sprague Dawley rats. *Toxicology*, **97**, 133–140

Li, H., Dong, L. & Whitlock, J.P., Jr (1994) Transcriptional activation function of the mouse Ah receptor nuclear translocator. *J. biol. Chem.*, **269**, 28098–28105.

Li, X., Weber L.W.D. & Rozman, K.K. (1995a) Toxicokinetics of 2,3,7,8-tetrachlorodibenzo-*p*-dioxin in female Sprague-Dawley rats including placental and lactational transfer to fetuses and neonates. *Fundam. appl. Toxicol.*, **27**, 70–76

Li, X., Johnson, D.C. & Rozman, K.K. (1995b) Effects of 2,3,7,8-tetrachlorodibenzo-p-dioxin (TCDD) on estrous cyclicity and ovulation in female Sprague-Dawley rats. *Toxicol. Lett.*, **78**, 219–222

Li, X., Johnson, D.C. & Rozman, K.K. (1995c) Reproductive effects of 2,3,7,8-tetrachloro-dibenzo-*p*-dioxin (TCDD) in female rats: ovulation, hormonal regulation and possible mechanism(s). *Toxicol. appl. Pharmacol.*, **133**, 321–327

Liehr, J.G. (1990) Genotoxic effects of estrogens. *Mutat. Res.*, **238**, 269–276

Liehr, J.G. & Roy, D. (1990) Free radical generation by redox cycling of estrogens. *Free Rad. Biol. Med.*, **8**, 415–423

Liem, A.K.D. & van Zorge, J.A. (1995) Dioxins and related compounds: status and regulatory aspects. *Environ. Sci. Poll. Res.*, **2**, 46–56

Liem, A.K.D., de Jong, A.P.J.M., Theelen, R.M.C., van Wijnen, J.H., Beijen, P.C., van der Schee, H.A., Vaessen, H.A.M.G., Kleter, G. & van Zorge, J.A. (1991a) Occurrence of dioxins and related compounds in Dutch foodstuffs - Part 1: Sampling strategy and analytical results. In: *Proceedings of the 11th International Symposium on Chlorinated Dioxins and Related Compounds, September 23-27*

Liem, A.K.D., Theelen, R.M.C., Slob, W. and van Wijnen, J.H. (1991b) *Dioxins and Planar PCBs in Food. Levels in Food Products and Intake by the Dutch Population* (RIVM Report 730501.034), Bilthoven, RIVM

Liem, A.K.D., Hoogerbrugge, R., Kootstra, P.R., van der Velde, E.G. & de Jong, A.P.J.M. (1991c) Occurrence of dioxins in cow's milk in the vicinity of municipal waste incinerators and a metal reclamation plant in the Netherlands. *Chemosphere*, **23**, 1675–1684

Liem, A.K.D., Albers, J.M.C., Baumann, R.A., van Beuzekom, A.C., den Hartog, R.S., Hoogerbrugge, R., de Jong, A.P.J.M. & Marsman, J.A. (1995) PCBs, PCDDs, PCDFs and organochlorine pesticides in human milk in the Netherlands. Levels and trends. *Organo-halogen Compounds*, **26**, 69–74

Ligon, W.V. & May, R.J. (1986) Determination of selected chlorodibenzofurans and chlorodibenzodioxins using two-dimensional gas chromatography/mass spectrometry. *Anal. Chem.*, **56**, 558–561

Lin, F.H., Clark, G., Birnbaum, L.S., Lucier, G.W. & Goldstein, J.A. (1991a) Influence of the Ah locus on the effects of 2,3,7,8-tetrachlorodibenzo-*p*-dioxin on the hepatic epidermal growth factor receptor. *Mol. Pharmacol.*, **39**, 307–313

Lin, F.H., Stohs, S.J., Birnbaum, L.S., Clark, G., Lucier, G.W. & Goldstein, J.A. (1991b) The effects of 2,3,7,8-tetrachlorodibenzo-*p*-dioxin (TCDD) on the hepatic estrogen and glucocorticoid receptors in congenic strains of Ah responsive and Ah nonresponsive C57BL/6 mice. *Toxicol. Pharmacol. appl.*, **108**, 129–139

Lin, H.-H., Hsu, H.-Y., Chang, M.-H., Hong, K.-F., Young, Y.-C., Lee, T.-Y., Chen, P.-J. & Chen, D.-S. (1991c) Low prevalence of hepatitis C virus and infrequent perinatal or spouse infection in pregnant women in Taiwan. *J. med. Virol.*, **35**, 237–240

Lin, W.-Q. & White, K.L., Jr (1993a) Mouse Hepa 1c1c[7] hepatoma cells produce complement component C3; 2,3,7,8-tetrachlorodibenzo-*p*-dioxin fails to modulate this capacity. *J. Toxicol. environ. Health*, **39**, 27–41

Lin, W.-Q. & White, K.L., Jr (1993b) Production of complement component C3 in vivo following 2,3,7,8-tetrachlorodibenzo-*p*-dioxin exposure. *J. Toxicol. environ. Health*, **39**, 273–285

Lin, W.-Q. & White, K.L., Jr (1993c) Modulation of liver intracellular C3 in mice by 2,3,7,8-tetrachlorodibenzo-*p*-dioxin. *J. Toxicol. environ. Health*, **39**, 107–119

Lincoln, D.W., II, Kampcik, S.J. & Gierthy, J.F. (1987) 2,3,7,8-Tetrachlorodibenzo-*p*-dioxin (TCDD) does not inhibit intercellular communication in Chinese hamster V79 cells. *Carcinogenesis*, **8**, 1817–1820

Linden, J., Pohjanvirta, R., Rahko, T. & Tuomisto, J. (1991) TCDD decreases rapidly and persistently serum melatonin concentration without morphologically affecting the pineal gland in TCDD-resistant Han/Wistar rats. *Pharmacol. Toxicol.*, **69**, 427–432

Lindstrom, G., Hooper, K., Petreas, M., Stephens, R. & Gilman, A. (1995) Workshop on perinatal exposure to dioxin-like compounds. I. Summary. *Environ. Health Perspectives*, **103**, 135–142

Littlewood, T.D. & Evan, G.I. (1995) Transcription factors. 2: Helix-loop-helix proteins. *Prot. Profile*, **2**, 621–702

Littorin, M., Hansson, M., Rappe, C. & Kogevinas, M. (1994) Dioxins in blood from Swedish phenoxy herbicide workers. *Lancet*, **344**, 611–612

Liu, P.C.C. & Matsumura, F. (1995) Differential effects of 2,3,7,8-tetrachlorodibenzo-*p*-dioxin on the 'adipose-type' and 'brain-type' glucose transporters in mice. *Mol. Pharmacol.*, **47**, 65–73

Lorber, M., Braverman, C., Gehring, P., Winters, D., Sovocool, W. (1996a) Soil and air monitoring in the vicinity of a municipal solid waste incinerator. Part II: Air monitoring. *Organohalogen Compounds*, **28**, 146-151

Lorber, M., Braverman, C., Gehring, P., Winters, D. & Sovocool, W. (1996b) Soil and air monitoring in the vicinity of a municipal solid waste incinerator, Part I: Soil monitoring. *Organohalogen Compounds*, **28**, 255–261

van Loveren, H., Schuurman, H.-J., Kampinga, J. & Vos, J.G. (1991) Reversibility of thymic atrophy induced by 2,3,7,8-tetrachlorodibenzo-*p*-dioxin (TCDD) and bis(tri-*n*-butylin)oxide (TBTO). *Int. J. Immunopharmacol.*, **13**, 369–377

Lovett, A.A., Foxall, C.D., Creaser, C.S. & Chewe, D. (1996) PCB and PCDD/F concentrations in egg and poultry meat samples from urban and rural areas in Wales and England. *Organohalogen Compounds*, **28**, 160–165

Lü, Y.C. & Wong, P.N. (1984) Dermatological, medical, and laboratory findings of patients in Taiwan and their treatments. *Am. J. ind. Med.*, **5**, 81–115

Lü, Y.C. & Wu, Y.C. (1985) Clinical findings and immunological abnormalities in Yu-Cheng patients. *Environ. Health Perspectives*, **59**, 17–29

Lu, Y.-F., Sun, G., Wang, X. & Safe, S. (1996) Inhibition of prolactin receptor gene expression by 2,3,7,8-tetrachlorodibenzo-*p*-dioxin in MCF-7 human breast cancer cells. *Arch. Biochem. Biophys.*, **332**, 35–40

Lucier, G.W. (1991) Humans are a sensitive species to some of the biochemical effects of structural analogs of dioxin. *Environ. Toxicol. Chem.*, **10**, 727–735

Lucier, G.W., Tritscher, A., Goldsworthy, T., Foley, J., Clark, G., Goldstein, J. & Maronpot, R. (1991) Ovarian hormones enhance 2,3,7,8-tetrachlorodibenzo-*p*-dioxin-mediated increases in cell proliferation and preneoplastic foci in a two-stage model for rat hepatocarcinogenesis. *Cancer Res.*, **51**, 1391–1397

Luebke, R.W., Copeland, C.B., Diliberto, J.J., Akubue, P.I., Andrews, D.L., Riddle, M.M., Williams, W.C. & Birnbaum, L.S. (1994) Assessment of host resistance to *Trichinella spiralis* in mice following preinfection exposure to 2,3,7,8-TCDD. *Toxicol. appl. Pharmacol.*, **125**, 7–16

Luksemburg, W. (1991) Method 10: Determination of polychlorinated dibenzo-*p*-dioxins and polychlorinated dibenzofurans in pulp and paper industry wastewaters, solid wastes, ashes and bleached pulps. In: Rappe, C., Buser, H.-R., Dodet, B. & O'Neill, I.K., eds, *Environmental Carcinogens: Methods of Analysis and Exposure Measurement. Vol. 11: Polychlorinated Dioxins and Dibenzofurans* (IARC Scientific Publications No. 108), Lyon, IARC, pp. 399–426

Lundberg, K. (1991) Dexamethasone and 2,3,7,8-tetrachlorodibenzo-*p*-dioxin can induce atrophy by different mechanisms in mice. *Biochem. biophys. Res. Communications*, **178**, 16–23

Lundberg, K., Grönvik, K.-O., Goldschmidt,.T.J., Klareskog, L. & Dencker, L. (1990a) 2,3,7,8-Tetrachlorodibenzo-*p*-dioxin (TCDD) alters intrathymic T-cell development in mice. *Chem.-biol. Interact.*, **74**, 179–193

Lundberg, K., Dencker, L. & Grönvik, K.-O. (1990b) Effects of 2,3,7,8-tetrachlorodibenzo-*p*-dioxin (TCDD) treatment in vivo on thymocyte functions in mice after activation in vitro. *Int. J. Immunopharmacol.*, **12**, 459–466

Lundberg, K., Grönvik, K.-O. & Dencker, L. (1991) 2,3,7,8-tetrachlorodibenzo-*p*-dioxin (TCDD) induced suppression of the local response. *Int. J. Immunopharmacol.*, **13**, 357–368

Lundberg, K., Dencker, L. & Grönvik, K.-O. (1992) 2,3,7,8-Tetrachlorodibenzo-p-dioxin (TCDD) inhibits the activation of antigen-specific T-cells in mice. *Int. J. Immunopharmacol.*, **14**, 699–705

Lundgren, K., Andries, M., Thompson, C. & Lucier, G.W. (1986) Dioxin treatment of rats results in increased in vitro induction of sister chromatid exchanges by alpha-naphthoflavone: an animal model for human exposure to halogenated aromatics. *Toxicol. appl. Pharmacol.*, **85**, 189–195

Lundgren, K., Collman, G.W., Wang-Wuu, S., Tiernan, T., Taylor, M., Lucier, G.W. & Thompson, C.L. (1988) Cytogenic and chemical detection of human exposure to polyhalogenated aromatic hydrocarbons. *Environ. mol. Mutag.*, **11**, 1–11

Luster, M.I., Boorman, G.A., Dean, J.H., Harris, M.W., Luebke, R.W., Padarathsingh, M.L. & Moore, J.A. (1980) Examination of bone marrow, immunologic parameters and host susceptibility following pre- and postnatal exposure to 2,3,7,8-tetrachlorodibenzo-*p*-dioxin (TCDD). *Int. J. Immunopharmacol.*, **2**, 301–310

Lynge, E. (1993) Cancer in phenoxy herbicide manufactoring workers in Denmark, 1947–87. An update. *Cancer Causes Control*, **4**, 261–272

Ma, X. & Babish, J.G. (1993) Acute 2,3,7,8-tetrachlorodibenzo-*p*-dioxin exposure results in enhanced tyrosylphosphorylation and expression of murine hepatic cyclin dependent kinases. *Biochem. biophys. Res. Commun.*, **197**, 1070–1077

Ma, Q. & Whitlock, J.P., Jr (1996) The aromatic hydrocarbon receptor modulates the Hepa 1c1c7 cell cycle and differentiated state independewntly of dioxin. *Mol. Cell. Biol.*, **16**, 2144–2150

Mably, T.A., Theobald, H.M., Ingall, G.B. & Peterson, R.E. (1990) Hypergastrinemia is associated with decreased gastric acid secretion in 2,3,7,8-tetrachlorodibenzo-*p*-dioxin treated rats. *Toxicol. appl. Pharmacol.*, **106**, 518–528

Mably, T.A., Moore, R.W., Goy, R.W. & Peterson, R.E. (1992a) In utero and lactational exposure of male rats to 2,3,7,8-tetrachlorodibenzo-*p*-dioxin. 2. Effects on sexual behavior and the regulation of luteinizing hormone secretion in adulthood. *Toxicol. appl. Pharmacol.*, **114**, 108–117

Mably, T.A., Bjerke, D.L., Moore, R.W., Gendron-Fitzpatrick, A. & Peterson, R.E. (1992b) In utero and lactational exposure of male rats to 2,3,7,8-tetrachlorodibenzo-*p*-dioxin. 3. Effects on spermatogenesis and reproductive capability. *Toxicol. appl. Pharmacol.*, **114**, 118–126

Mably, T.A., Moore, R.W. & Peterson, R.E. (1992c) In utero and lactational exposure of male rats to 2,3,7,8-tetrachlorodibenzo-*p*-dioxin. 1. Effects on androgenic status. *Toxicol. appl. Pharmacol.*, **114**, 97–107

Mackay, D., Shiu, W.Y. & Ma, K.C. (1991) *Illustrated Handbook of Physical-Chemical Properties and Environmental Fate for Organic Chemicals*, Vol. II, *Polynuclear Aromatic Hydrocarbons, Polychlorinated Dioxins, and Dibenzofurans*, Boca Raton, Lewis Publishers

MacKenzie, S.A., Thomas, T., Umbreit, T.H. & Gallo, M.A. (1992) The potentiation of 2,3,7,8-tetrachlorodibenzo-*p*-dioxin toxicity by tamoxifen in female CD1 mice. *Toxicol. appl. Pharmacol.*, **116**, 101–109

Madhukar, B.V., Brewster, D.W. & Matsumura, F. (1984) Effects of in vivo-administered 2,3,7,8-tetrachlorodibenzo-*p*-dioxin on receptor binding of epidermal growth factor in the hepatic plasma membrane of rat, guinea pig, mouse, and hamster. *Proc. natl Acad. Sci. USA*, **84**, 7407–7411

Madhukar, B.V., Ebner, K., Matsumura, F., Bombick, D.W., Brewster, D.W. & Kawamoto, T. (1988) 2,3,7,8-Tetrachlorodibenzo-*p*-dioxin causes an increase in protein kinases associated with epidermal growth factor receptor in the hepatic plasma membrane. *J. biochem. Toxicol.*, **3**, 261–277

Maier, E.A., Griepink, B. & Fortunati, U. (1994) Round table discussions: outcome and recommendations. *Fresenius J. analyt. Chem.*, **348**, 171–179

Maier, E.A., Van Cleuvenbergen, R., Kramer, G.N., Tuinstra, L.G.M.T. & Pauwels, J. (1995) BCR (non-certified) reference materials for dioxins and furans in milk powder. *Fresenius J. analyt. Chem.*, **352**, 179–183

Maisel, B.E. (1990) Comparison of pre- and post-operational ambient PCDDs/PCDFs levels in the vicinity of municipal solid waste (MSW) incinerators. *Organohalogen Compounds*, **4**, 413–418

Maisel, B.E. & Hunt, G.T. (1990) Background concentrations of PCDDs/PCDFs in ambient air. A comparison of toxic equivalency factor (TEF) models. *Chemosphere*, **20**, 771–778

Malisch, R. & Saad, M.M. (1996) PCDD/PCDF in butter samples from Egypt. *Organohalogen Compounds*, **28**, 281–285

Mantovani, A., Vecchi, A., Luini, W., Sironi, M., Candiani, G.P., Spreafico, F. & Garattini, S. (1980) Effect of 2,3,7,8-tetrachlorodibenzo-*p*-dioxin on macrophage and natural killer cell-mediated cytotoxicity in mice. *Biomedicine*, **32**, 200–204

Manz, A., Berger, J., Dwyer, J.H., Flesch-Janys, D., Nagel, S. & Waltsgott, H. (1991) Cancer mortality among workers in chemical plant contaminated with dioxin. *Lancet*, **338**, 959–964

Marinovich, M., Sirtori, C.R., Galli, C.L. & Paoletti, R. (1983) The binding of 2,3,7,8-tetra-chlorodibenzodioxin to plasma lipoproteins may delay toxicity in experimental hyper-lipidemia. *Chem.-biol. Interact.*, **45**, 393–399

Maronpot, R.R., Foley, J.F., Takahashi, K., Goldsworthy, T., Clark, G., Tritscher, A., Portier, C. & Lucier, G. (1993) Dose response for TCDD promotion of hepatocarcinogenesis in rats ini-tiated with DEN: histologic, biochemical, and cell proliferation endpoints. *Environ. Health. Perspectives*, **101**, 634–642

Martin, J.V. (1984) Lipid abnormalities in workers exposed to dioxin. *Br. J. ind. Med.*, **41**, 254–256

Mason, G., Farrell, K., Keys, B., Piskorska-Pliszczynska, J., Safe, L. & Safe, S. (1986) Poly-chlorinated dibenzo-*p*-dioxins: Quantitative in vitro and in vivo structure-activity relation-ships. *Toxicology*, **41**, 21–31

Massa, T., Esmaeili, A, Fortmeyer, H., Schlatterer, B., Hagenmaier, H. & Chandra, P. (1992) Cell transforming and oncogenic activity of 2,3,7,8-tetrachloro- and 2,3,7,8-tetrabromo-dibenzo-*p*-dioxin. *Anticancer Res.*, **12**, 2053–2060

Masten, S.A. & Shiverick, K.T. (1995) The Ah receptor recognizes DNA binding sites for the B cell transcription factor, BSAP: A possible mechanism for dioxin mediated alteration of CD19 gene expression in human B lymphocytes. *Biochem. biophys. Res. Communications*, **212**, 27–34

Mastroiacovo, P., Spagnolo, A., Mani, E., Meazza, L., Bertollini, R. & Segni, G. (1988) Birth defects in the Seveso area after TCDD contamination. *J. Am. med. Assoc.*, **259**, 1668–1672

Masuda, Y. (1994) The Yusho rice oil poisoning incident. In: Schecter, A., ed., *Dioxins and Health*, New York, Plenum Press, pp. 633–659

Masuda, Y. (1996) Approach to risk assessment of chlorinated dioxins from Yusho PCB poiso-ning. *Chemosphere*, **32**, 583–594

Masuda, Y., Kuroki, H., Haraguchi, K. & Nagayama, J. (1985) PCB and PCDF congeners in the blood and tissues of Yusho and Yu-Cheng patients. *Environ. Health Perspectives*, **59**, 53–58

Matsuda, M., Funeno, H., Quynh, H.T., Cau, H.D. & Wakimoto, T. (1994) PCDDs/DFs pollu-tion in Vietnam soils. *Organohalogen Compounds*, **20**, 41–45

Matsumoto, M. & Ando, M. (1991) Mutagenicity of 3-chlorodibenzofuran and its metabolic activation. *Environ. mol. Mutag.*, **17**, 104–111

Matsumura, F. (1994) How important is the protein phosphorylation pathway in the toxic expression of dioxin-type chemicals? *Biochem. Pharmacol.*, **48**, 215–224

Matsumura, T., Ito, H., Yamamoto, T. & Morita, M. (1994) Development of pre-concentration system for PCDDs and PCDFs in seawater. *Organohalogen Compounds*, **19**, 109–112

Matsumura, T., Fukaumi, M., Tsubota, H., Tsutsumi, K., Kuramoto, K., Ito, H., Yamamoto, T. & Morita, M. (1995) PCDDs concentration in open-ocean water. *Organohalogen Com-pounds*, **24**, 353

Matsushita, N., Sogawa, K., Ema, M., Yoshida, A. & Fujii-Kuriyama, Y. (1993) A factor binding to the xenobiotic responsive element (XRE) of P-450IA1 gene consists of at least two helix-loop-helix proteins, Ah receptor and Arnt. *J. biol. Chem.*, **268**, 21002–21006

May, G. (1973) Chloracne from the accidental production of tetrachlorodibenzo-dioxin. *Br. J. ind. Med,*. **30**, 276–283

May, G. (1982) Tetrachlorodibenzodioxin: a survey of subjects ten years after exposure. *Br. J. ind. Med.*, **39**, 128–135

McConnell, E.E. (1980) Acute and chronic toxicity, carcinogenesis, reproduction, teratogenesis and mutagenesis in animals. In: Kimbrough, R.D., ed., *Halogenated Biphenyls, Terphenyls, Naphtalenes, Dibenzodioxins, and Related Products*, Amsterdam, Elsevier, pp. 109–150

McConnell, E.E., Moore, J.A., Haseman, J.K. & Harris, M.W. (1978a) The comparative toxicity of chlorinated dibenzo-*p*-dioxins in mice and guinea pigs. *Toxicol. appl. Pharmacol.*, **44**, 335–356

McConnell, E.E., Moore, J.A. & Dalgard, D.W. (1978b) Toxicity of 2,3,7,8-tetrachlorodibenzo-*p*-dioxin in rhesus monkey (*Macaca mulatta*) following a single oral dose. *Toxicol. appl. Pharmacol.*, **43**, 175–187

McGregor, D.B., Brown, A.G., Howgate, S., McBride, D., Riach, C. & Caspary, W.J. (1991) Responses to the L5178Y mouse lymphoma cell forward mutation assay: V. 27 coded chemicals. *Environ. mol. Mutag.*, **17**, 196–219

McGuire, J., Whitelaw, M.L., Pongratz, I., Gustafsson, J.-Å. & Poellinger, L. (1994) A cellular factor stimulates ligand-dependent release of hsp90 from the basic helix-loop-helix dioxin receptor. *Mol. cell. Biol.*, **14**, 2438–2446

McKinney, J.D., Chae, K., Oatley, S.J. & Blake, C.C. (1985) Molecular interactions of toxic chlorinated dibenzo-*p*-dioxins and dibenzofurans with thyroxine binding prealbumin. *J. med. Chem.*, **28**, 375–381

McLachlan, M.S. & Hutzinger, O. (1990) Concentrations of PCDD/F in air and particulate at a rural site in West Germany. *Organohalogen Compounds*, **1**, 441–444

McLachlan, M.S. & Reissinger, M. (1990) The influence of sewage sludge fertilization on the PCDD/F concentration in soil. An example from northeastern Bavaria. *Organohalogen Compounds*, **1**, 577–582

McLachlan, M.S, Thoma, H., Reissinger, M. & Hutzinger, O. (1990) PCDD/F in an agriculturral food chain. 1. PCDD/F mass balance of a lactating cow. *Chemosphere*, **20**, 1013

McLaughlin, D.L., Pearson, R.G. & Clement, R.E. (1989) Concentrations of chlorinated dibenzo-p-dioxins (CDD) and dibenzofurans (CDF) in soil from the vicinity of a large refuse incinerator in Hamilton, Ontario. *Chemosphere*, **18**, 851–854

McMichael, A.J. (1976) Standardized mortality ratios and the 'healthy worker effect': scratching beneath the surface. *J. occup. Med.*, **18**, 128–131

McNulty, W.P. (1975) Toxicity and fetotoxicity of TCDD, TCDF, and PCB isomers in rhesus macaques (*Macaca mulatta*). *Environ. Health Perspectives*, **60**, 77–88

McNulty, W.P. (1977) Toxicity of 2,3,7,8-tetrachlorodibenzo-*p*-dioxin for rhesus monkeys: brief report. *Bull. environ. Contam. Toxicol.*, **18**, 108–109

McNulty, W.P. (1984) Fetotoxicity of 2,3,7,8-tetrachlorodibenzo-*p*-dioxin (TCDD) for rhesus macaques (*Macaca mulatta*). *Am. J. Primatol.*, **6**, 41–47

McNulty, W.P. (1985) Toxicity and fetotoxicity of TCDD, TCDF and PCB isomers in rhesus macaques (*Macaca mulatta*). *Environ. Health Perspectives*, **60**, 77–88

Melnick, R.L. (1992) Does chemically induced hepatocyte proliferation predict liver carcinogenesis ? *Fed. Am. Soc. exp. Biol. J.*, **6**, 2698–2706

Menzel, H.M., Turcer, E., Bienfait, H.G., Albracht, A., Päpke, O., Ball, M. & Bolm-Audorff, U. (1996) Exposure to PCDDs and PCDFs during welding, cutting and burning of metals. *Organohalogen Compounds*, **30**, 70–75

Messerer, P., Zober, A. & Becher, H. (1996) Blood lipid concentrations of PCDD and PCDF in a smaple of BASF-employees who are included in the IARC Register of workers exposed to phenoxy acid herbicides and/or chlorophenols. In: *International Symposium: Dioxins and Furans. Epidemiologic Assessment of Cancer Risks and Other Human Health Effects, (Abstract), 7–8 November 1996*, Heidelberg, Deutsches Krebsforschungszentrum

Meyer, C., O'Keefe, P., Hilker, D., Rafferty, L., Wilson, L., Connor, S. & Aldous, K. (1989) A survey of twenty community water systems in New York State for PCDDs and PCDFs. *Chemosphere*, **19**, 21–26

Meyne, J., Allison, D.C., Bose, K., Jordan, S.W., Ridolpho, P.F. & Smith, J. (1985) Hepatotoxic doses of dioxin do not damage mouse bone marrow chromosomes. *Mutat. Res.*, **157**, 63–69

Michalek, J.E., Wolfe, W.H. & Miner, J.C. (1990) Health status of Air Force veterans occupationally exposed to herbicides in Vietnam. II. Mortality. *J. Am. med. Assoc.*, **264**, 1832–1836

Michalek, J.E., Pirkle, J.L., Caudill, S.P., Tripathi, R.C., Patterson, D.G., Jr & Needham, L.L. (1996) Pharmacokinetics of TCDD in veterans of Operation Ranch Hand: 10-year follow-up. *J. Toxicol. environ. Health*, **47**, 209–220

Miles, W.F., Singh, J., Gurprasad, N.P. & Malis, G.P. (1985) Isomer specific determination of hexachlorodioxins in technical pentachlorophenol (PCP) and its sodium salt. *Chemosphere*, **14**, 807–810

Ministry of Agriculture, Fisheries and Food (1992) *Dioxins in Food* (Food Surveillance Paper No. 31), London, Her Majesty's Stationery Office

Ministry of Agriculture, Fisheries and Food (1995) *Dioxins in Foods — UK Dietary Intakes* (Food Surveillance Information Sheet No 71), London

Missouri Dioxin Health Studies Progress Report (1983) *Missouri Division of Health*, Centers for Disease Control, St. Joseph's Hospital of Kirkwood, St. Louis University Hospital

Mitchum, R.K. & Donnelly, J.R. (1991) Quality assurance/quality control procedures for the determination of polychlorinated dibenzodioxins, dibenzofurans and biphenyls. In: Rappe, C., Buser, H.-R., Dodet, B. & O'Neill, I.K., eds, *Environmental Carcinogens: Methods of Analysis and Exposure Measurement. Vol. 11: Polychlorinated Dioxins and Dibenzofurans* (IARC Scientific Publications No. 108), Lyon, IARC, pp. 161-174

Miyata, H., Kashimoto, T. & Kunita, N. (1977) Detection and determination of polychlorodibenzofurans in normal human tissues and Kanemi rice oil caused 'Kanemi Yusho'. *J. Food Hyg. Soc.*, **19**, 260–265

Miyata, H., Ohta, S. & Aozasa, O. (1992) Levels of PCDDs, PCDFs and non-ortho coplanar PCBs in drinking water in Japan. *Organohalogen Compounds*, **9**, 151–154

Miyata, H., Aozasa, O., Ohta, S., Chang, T. & Yasuda, Y. (1993) Estimated daily intakes of PCDDs, PCDFs and non-ortho coplanar PCBs via drinking water in Japan. *Chemosphere*, **26**, 1527–1536

Mocarelli, P., Marocchi, A., Brambilla, P., Gerthoux, P.M., Young, D.S. & Mantel, N. (1986) Clinical laboratory manifestations of exposure to dioxin in children. A six year study of the effects of an environmental disaster near Seveso, Italy. *J. Am. med. Assoc.*, **256**, 2687–2695

Mocarelli, P., Pocchiari, F. & Nelson, N. (1988) Preliminary report: 2,3,7,8-tetrachlorodibenzo-*p*-dioxin. Exposure to humans — Seveso, Italy. *Morbid. Mortal. Wkly Rep.*, **37**, 733–736

Mocarelli, P., Patterson, D.G., Jr, Marocchi, A. & Needham, L.L. (1990) Pilot study (phase II) for determining polychlorinated dibenzo-*p*-dioxin (PCDD) and polychlorinated dibenzofuran (PCDF) levels in serum of Seveso, Italy residents collected at the time of exposure: future plans. *Chemosphere*, **20**, 967–974

Mocarelli, P., Needham, L.L., Marocchi, A., Patterson, D.G., Jr, Brambilla, P., Gerthoux, P.M., Meazza, L. & Carreri, V. (1991) Serum concentrations of 2,3,7,8-tetrachlorodibenzo-*p*-dioxin and test results from selected residents of Seveso, Italy. *J. Toxicol. environ. Health*, **32**, 357–366

Mocarelli, P., Brambilla, P., Gerthoux, P.M., Patterson, D.G., Jr & Needham, L.L. (1996) Change in sex ratio with exposure to dioxin. *Lancet*, **348**, 409

Moche, W. & Thanner, G. (1996a) Ambient air concentrations of dioxins in Austrian conurbations. *Organohalogen Compounds*, **28**, 286–290

Moche, W. & Thanner, G. (1996b) Ambient air concentrations of dioxins during stable weather conditions. *Organohalogen Compounds*, **28**, 291–294

Moore, J.A., McConnell, E.E., Dalgard, D.W. & Harris, M.W. (1979) Comparative toxicity of three halogenated dibenzofurans in guinea pigs, mice, and rhesus monkeys. *Ann. N.Y. Acad. Sci.*, **320**, 151–163

Moore, R.W., Potter, C.L., Theobald, H.M., Robinson, J.A. & Peterson, R.E. (1985) Androgenic deficiency in male rats treated with 2,3,7,8-tetrachlorodibenzo-p-dioxin. *Toxicol. appl. Pharmacol.*, **79**, 99–111

Moore, R.W., Parsons, J.A., Bookstaff, R.C. & Peterson, R.E. (1989) Plasma concentrations of pituitary hormones in 2,3,7,8-tetrachlorodibenzo-p-dioxin-treated male rats. *J. biochem. Toxicol.*, **4**, 165–172

Moore, R.W., Bookstaff, R.C., Mably, R.A. & Peterson, R.E. (1991) Differential effects of 2,3,7,8-tetrachlorodibenzo-*p*-dioxin on responsiveness of male rats to androgens, 17β-estradiol, luteinizing hormone, gonadotropin releasing hormone, and progesterone. In: *Proceedings of Dioxin '91, the 11th International Symposium on Chlorinated Dioxins and Related Compounds*, Research Triangle Park, NC

Moore, M., Narasimhan, T.R., Steinberg, M., Wang, X. & Safe, S. (1993) Potentiation of *CYP1A1* gene expression in MCF-7 human breast cancer cells cotreated with 2,3,7,8-tetrachlorodibenzo-*p*-dioxin and 12-*O*-tetradecanoylphorbol-13-acetate. *Arch. Biochem. Biophys.*, **305**, 483–488

Moore, M., Wang, X., Lu, Y.-F., Wormke, M., Craig, A., Gerlach, J., Burghardt, R. & Safe, S. (1994) Benzo[a]pyrene resistant (BaP[R]) human breast cancer cells: a unique aryl hydrocarbon (Ah)-nonresponsive clone. *J. biol. Chem.*, **269**, 11751–11759

Morgan, J.E. & Whitlock, J.P., Jr (1992) Transcription-dependent and transcription-independent nucleosome disruption induced by dioxin. *Proc. natl Acad. Sci. USA*, **89**, 11622–11626

Morris, D.L. & Holsapple, M.P. (1991) Effect of 2,3,7,8-tetrachlorodibenzo-p-dioxin (TCDD) on humoral immunity: II. B cell activation. *Immunopharmacology*, **21**, 171–182

Morris, D.L., Jordan, S.D. & Holsapple, M.P. (1991) Effects of 2,3,7,8-tetrachlorodibenzo-p-dioxin (TCDD) on humoral activity: I. Similarities to staphylococcus aureus cowan strain I (SAC) in the in vitro T-dependent antibody response. *Immunopharmacology*, **21**, 159–170

Morris, D.L., Snyder, N.K., Gokani, V., Blair, R.E. & Holsapple, M.P. (1992) Enhanced suppression of humoral immunity in DBA/2 mice following subchronic exposure to 2,3,7,8-tetrachlorodibenzo-*p*-dioxin (TCDD). *Toxicol. appl. Pharmacol.*, **112**, 128–132

Morris, D.L., Karras, J.G. & Holsapple, M.P. (1993) Direct effects of 2,3,7,8-tetrachlorodibenzo-*p*-dioxin (TCDD) on responses to lipopolysaccharide (LPS) by isolated murine B-cells. *Immunopharmacology*, **26**, 105–112

Morris, D.L., Jeong, H.G., Stevens, W.D., Chun, Y.J., Karras, J.G. & Holsapple, M.P. (1994) Serum modulation of the effects of TCDD on the in vitro antibody response and on enzyme induction in primary hepatocytes. *Immunopharmacology*, **27**, 93–105

Morris-Brown, L., Blair, A., Gibson, R., Everett, G.D., Cantor, K.P., Schuman, L.M., Burmeister, L.F., Van Lier, S.F. & Dick, F. (1990) Pesticide exposures and other agricultural risk factors for leukemia among men in Iowa and Minnesota. *Cancer Res.*, **50**, 6585–6591

Morris-Brown, L., Burmeister, L.F., Everett, G.D. & Blair, A. (1993) Pesticide exposures and multiple myeloma in Iowa men. *Cancer Causes Control*, **4**, 153–156

Morrison, H., Savitz, D., Semenciw, R., Hulka, B., Mao, Y., Morison, D. & Wigle, D. (1993) Farming and prostate cancer mortality. *Am. J. Epidemiol.*, **137**, 270–80

Morrison, H., Villeneuve, P., Semenciw, R.M. & Wigle, D. (1994) Farming and prostate cancer mortality (Letter to the Editor). *Am. J. Epidemiol.*, **140**, 1057–59

Morrissey, R.E. & Schwetz, B.A. (1989) Reproductive and developmental toxicity in animals. In: Kimbrough, R.D. & Jensen, A.A., eds, *Halogenated Biphenyls, Terphenyls, Naphthalenes, Dibenzodioxins and Related Products*, 2nd Ed., Amsterdam, Elsevier, pp. 195–225

Morse, D.C., Groen, D., Veerman, M., Van Amerongen, C.J., Koëter, H.B.W.M., Smits-van Prooije, A.E., Visser, T.J., Koeman, J.H. & Brouwer, A. (1993) Interference of polychlorinated biphenyls in hepatic and brain thyroid hormone metabolism in fetal and neonatal rats. *Toxicol. appl. Pharmacol.*, **122**, 27–33

Mortelmans, K., Haworth, S., Speck, W. & Zeiger, E. (1984) Mutagenicity testing of Agent Orange components and related compounds. *Toxicol. appl. Pharmacol.*, **75**, 137–146

Moses, M. & Prioleau, P.G. (1985) Cutaneous histologic findings in chemical workers with and without chloracne with past exposure to 2,3,7,8-tetrachlorodibenzo-p-dioxin. *J. Am. Acad. Dermatol.*, **12**, 497–506

Moses, M., Lilis, R., Crow, K.D., Thornton, J., Fischbein, A., Anderson, H.A. & Selikoff, I.J. (1984) Health status of workers with past exposure to 2,3,7,8-tetrachlorodibenzo-p-dioxin in the manufacture of 2,4,5-trichlorophenoxyacetic acid. Comparison of findings with and without chloracne. *Am. J. ind. Med.*, **5**, 161–182

Mouradian, R., Burt, S., Tepper, A. & Hanley, K. (1995) *Boise Cascade, United Paperworkers International Union, Rumford, ME* (HETA 88-0140-2517), Cincinnati, OH, United States National Institute for Occupational Safety and Health

Muir, D.C.G., Pastershank, G.M., Crosley, R., Noton, L., Ramamoorthy, S. & Brownlee, B. (1995) Pathways of accumulation and temporal trends of PCDD/Fs in fishes downstream from a bleached kraft pulp mill on the Athabsca River (Alberta). *Organohalogen Compounds*, **24**, 463–468

Müller, J.F., Hülster, A., Päpke, P., Ball, M. & Marschner, H. (1993) Transfer pathways of PCDD/PCDF to fruits. *Chemosphere*, **27**, 195–201

Münzel, P., Bock-Hennig, B., Schieback, S., Gschaidmeier, H, Beck-Gschaidmeier, S. & Bock, K.W. (1996) Growth modulation of hepatocytes and rat liver epithelial cells (WB-F344) by 2,3,7,8-tetrachlorodibenzo-p-dioxin (TCDD). *Carcinogenesis*, **17**, 197–202

Murai, K., Okamura, K., Tsuji, H., Kajiwara, E., Watanabe, H., Akagi, K. & Fujishima, M. (1987) Thyroid function in 'Yusho' patients exposed to polychlorinated biphenyls (PCB). *Environ. Res.*, **44**, 179–187

Muralidhara, D.V., Matsumara, F. & Blankenship, A. (1994) 2,3,7,8-Tetrachlorodibenzo-*p*-dioxin (TCDD)-induced reduction of adenosine deaminase activity *in vivo* and *in vitro*. *J. biochem. Toxicol.*, **9**, 249–259

Murray, F.J., Smith, F.A., Nitschke, K.D., Humiston, C.G., Kociba, R.J. & Schwetz, B.A. (1979) Three-generation reproduction study of rats given 2,3,7,8-tetrachlorodibenzo-*p*-dioxin in the diet. *Toxicol. appl. Pharmacol.*, **50**, 241–252

Mussalo-Rauhamaa, H. & Lindström, G. (1995) PCDD and PCDF levels in human milk in Estonia and certain Nordic countries. *Organohalogen Compounds*, **26**, 245–248

Muto, H., Shinada, M., Abe, T. & Takizawa, Y. (1991) The tissue distribution of 2,3,7,8-chlorine substituted dibenzo-*p*-dioxins in humans who died of cancer. *Life Sciences*, **48**, 1645–1657

Nagarkatti, P.S., Sweeny, G.D., Gauldie, J. & Clark, D.A. (1984) Sensitivity to suppression of cytotoxic T cell generation by 2,3,7,8-tetrachlorodibenzo-*p*-dioxin (TCDD) is dependent on the Ah genotype of the murine host. *Toxicol. appl. Pharmacol.*, **72**, 169–176

Nagayama, J., Nagayama, M. & Masuda, Y. (1993) Frequency of micronuclei induced in cultured lymphocytes by highly toxic organochlorine congeners. *Fukuoka Acta med.*, **84**, 189–194

Nagayama, J,. Nagayama, M., Iida, T., Hirakawa, H., Matsueda, T. & Masuda, Y. (1994) Effects of highly toxic organochlorine compounds retained in human body on induction of sister chromatid exchanges in cultured human lymphocytes. *Chemosphere*, **29**, 2349–2354

Nagayama, J., Nagayama, M., Haraguchi, K., Kuroki, H. & Masuda, Y. (1995a) Effect of 2,3,4,7,8-pentachlorodibenzofuran and its analogues on induction of sister chromatid exchanges in cultured human lymphocytes. *Fukuoka Acta med.*, **86**, 184–189

Nagayama, J., Nagayama, M., Iida, T., Hirakawa, H., Matsueda, T., Yanagawa, T., Tsuji, H., Sato, K., Hasegawa, M. & Okamoto, Y. (1995b) Concentrations of chlorinated dioxins and related compounds in the blood and their genotoxicity in Japanese young women. *Organohalogen Compounds*, **25**, 117–122

Nagel, S., Berger, J., Flesch-Janys, D., Manz, A. & Ollroge, I. (1994) Mortality and cancer mortality in a cohort of female workers of a herbicide producing plant exposed to polychlorinated dibenzo-*p*-dioxins and furans. *Inform. Biomet. Epidemiol. Med. Biol.*, **25**, 32–38

Nakamura, M., Matsueda. T., Kurokawa, Y., Takada, S. & Fukamachi, K. (1994) Levels and profiles of PCDDs and PCDFs in soils and plants. *Organohalogen Compounds*, **20**, 103–106

Nakanishi, Y., Shigematsu, N., Kurita, Y., Matsuba, K., Kanegae, H., Ishimaru, S. & Kawazoe, Y. (1985) Respiratory involvement and immune status in Yusho patients. *Environ. Health Perspectives*, **59**, 31–36

Nambu, J.R., Lewis, J.O., Wharton, K.A., Jr & Crews, S.T. (1991) The Drosophila single-minded gene encodes a helix-loop-helix protein that acts as a master regulator of CNS midline development. *Cell*, **67**, 1157–1167

Narasimhan, T.R., Craig, A. Arellano, L., Harper, N., Howie, L. Menache, M., Birnbaum, L. & Safe, S. (1994) Relative sensitivities of 2,3,7,8-tetrachlorodibenzo-p-dioxin induced CYP1a-1 and CYP1a-2 gene expression and immunotoxicity in female B6C3F1 mice. *Fundam. appl. Toxicol.*, **23**, 598–607

Nau, H. & Bass, R. (1981) Transfer of 2,3,7,8-tetrachlorodibenzo-*p*-dioxin (TCDD) to the mouse embryo and fetus. *Toxicology*, **20**, 299–308

Nau, H., Bass, R. & Neubert, D. (1986) Transfer of 2,3,7,8-tetrachlorodibenzo-*p*-dioxin (TCDD) via placenta and milk, and postnatal toxicity in the mouse. *Arch. Toxicol.*, **59**, 36–40

Neal, R.A., Beatty, P.W. & Gasiewicz, T.A. (1979) Studies of the mechanisms of toxicity of 2,3,7,8-tetrachlorodibenzo-*p*-dioxin (TCDD). *Ann. N.Y. Acad. Sci.*, **320**, 204–213

Neal, R.A., Olson, J.R., Gasiewicz, T.A. & Geiger, L.E. (1982) The toxicokinetics of 2,3,7,8-tetrachlorodibenzo-*p*-dioxin in mammalian systems. *Drug Metab. Rev.*, **13**, 355–385

Nelson, C.J., Holson, J.F., Green, H.G. & Gaylor, D.W. (1979) Retrospective study of the relationship between agricultural use of 2,4,5-T and cleft palate occurrence in Arkansas. *Teratology*, **19**, 377–384

Nessel, C.S., Amoruso, M.A., Umbreit, T.H., Meeker, R.J. & Gallo, M.A. (1992) Pulmonary bioavailability and fine particle enrichment of 2,3,7,8-tetrachlorodibenzo-*p*-dioxin in respirable soil particles. *Fundam. appl. Toxicol.*, **19**, 279–285

Nestrick, T.J., Lamparski, L.L., Frawley, N.N., Hummel, R.A., Kocher, C.W., Mahle, N.H., McCoy, J.W., Miller, D.L., Peters, T.L., Pillepich, J.L., Smith, W.E. & Tobey, S.W. (1986) Perspectives of a large scale environmental survey for chlorinated dioxins: overview and soil data. *Chemosphere*, **15**, 1453–1460

Neuberger, M., Landvoigt, W. & Derntl, F. (1991) Blood levels of 2,3,7,8-tetrachlorodibenzo-*p*-dioxin in chemical workers after chloracne and in comparison groups. *Int. Arch. occup. environ. Health*, **63**, 325–327

Neubert, D. & Dillman, I. (1972) Embryotoxic effects in mice treated with 2,4,5-trichlorophenoxyacetic acid and 2,3,7,8-tetrachlorodibenzo-*p*-dioxin. *Naunyn-Schmeideberg's Arch. Pharmacol.*, **272**, 243–264

Neubert, D., Wiesmuller, T., Abraham, K., Krowke, R. & Hagenmaier, H. (1990a) Persistence of various polychlorinated dibenzo-*p*-dioxins and dibenzofurans (PCDDs and PCDFs) in hepatic and adipose tissue of marmoset monkeys. *Arch. Toxicol.*, **64**, 431–442

Neubert, R., Jacob-Müller, U., Stahlmann, R., Helge, H. & Neubert, D. (1990b) Polyhalogenated dibenzo-*p*-dioxins and dibenzofurans and the immune system. 1. Effects on peripheral lymphocyte subpopulations of a non-human primate (*Callithrix jacchus*) after treatment with 2,3,7,8-tetrachlorodibenzo-*p*-dioxin (TCDD). *Arch. Toxicol.*, **64**, 345–359

Neubert, R., Jacob-Müller, U., Helge, H., Stahlmann, R. & Neubert, D. (1991) Polyhalogenated dibenzo-*p*-dioxins and dibenzofurans and the immune system. 2. *In vitro* effects of 2,3,7,8-tetrachlorodibenzo-p-dioxin (TCDD) on lymphocytes of venous blood from man and a non-human primate (*Callithrix jacchus*). *Arch. Toxicol.*, **65**, 213–219

Neubert, R., Golor, G., Stahlmann, R., Helge, H. & Neubert, D. (1992a) Polyhalogenated dibenzo-*p*-dioxins and dibenzofurans and the immune system. 4. Effects of multiple-dose treatment with 2,3,7,8-tetrachlorodibenzo-p-dioxin (TCDD) on peripheral lymphocyte subpopulations of a non-human primate (*Callithrix jacchus*). *Arch. Toxicol.*, **66**, 250–259

Neubert, R., Golor, G., Stahlmann, R., Helge, H. & Neubert, D. (1992b) Dose-dependent TCDD-induced increase or decrease in T-lymphocyte subsets in the blood of new world monkeys (*Callithrix jacchus*). *Chemosphere*, **25**, 1201–1206

Neubert, R., Maskow, L., Webb, J., Jacob-Müller, U., Nogueira, A.C., Delgado, I., Helge, H. & Neubert, D. (1993a) Chlorinated dibenzo-*p*-dioxins and dibenzofurans and the human immune system. 1. Blood cell receptors in volunteers with moderately increased body burdens. *Life Sci.*, **53**, 1995–2006

Neubert, R., Stahlmann, R., Korte, M., van Loveren, H., Vos, J.G., Golor, G., Webb, J.R., Helge, H. & Neubert, D. (1993b) Effects of small doses of dioxins on the immune system of marmosets and rats. *Ann. N.Y. Acad. Sci.*, **685**, 662–686

Neubert, R., Maskow, L., Delgado, I., Helge, H. & Neubert, D. (1995) Chlorinated dibenzo-p-dioxins and dibenzofurans and the human immune system. 2. In vitro proliferation of lymphocytes from workers with quantified moderately-increased body burdens. *Life Sci.*, **56**, 421–436

Neuhold, L.A., Shirayoshi, Y., Ozato, K., Jones, J.E. & Nebert, D.W. (1989) Regulation of mouse CYP1A1 gene expression by dioxin: requirement of two *cis*-acting elements during induction. *Mol. cell. Biol.*, **9**, 2378–2386

Neumann, C.M., Oughton, F.A. & Kerkvliet, N.I. (1993) Anti-CD3-induced T-cell activation — II. Effect of 2,3,7,8-tetrachlorodibenzo-*p*-dioxin (TCDD). *Int. J. Immunopharmacol.*, **15**, 543–550

Newsted, J.L. & Giesy, J.P. (1993) Effect of 2,3,7,8-tetrachlorodibenzo-*p*-dioxin (TCDD) on the epidermal growth factor receptor in hepatic plasma membranes of rainbow trout. *Toxicol. appl. Pharmacol.*, **118**, 119–130

Nguyen, T.N.P., Bui, S.H., Dan, Q.V. & Schecter, A. (1989) Dioxin levels in adipose tissues of hospitalized women living in the south of Vietnam in 1984–85 with a brief review of their clinical histories. *Chemosphere*, **19**, 933–936

Nilsson, C.-A., Andersson, K., Rappe, C. & Westermark, S.-O. (1974) Chromatographic evidence for the formation of chlorodioxins from chloro-2-phenoxyphenols. *J. Chromatogr.*, **96**, 137–147

Nisbet, I.C.T. & Paxton, M.B. (1982) Statistical aspects of three-generation studies of the reproductive toxicity of TCDD and 2,4,5-T. *Am. Stat.*, **36**, 290–298

Nishizumi, M. & Masuda, Y. (1986) Enhancing effect of 2,3,4,7,8-pentachlorodibenzofuran and 1,2,3,4,7,8-hexachlorodibenzofuran on diethylnitrosamine hepatocarcinogenesis in the rat. *Cancer Lett.*, **33**, 333–339

Nolan, R.J., Smith, F.A. & Hefner, J.G. (1979) Elimination and tissue distribution of 2,3,7,8-tetrachlorodibenzo-p-dioxin (TCDD) in female guinea pigs following a single oral dose. *Toxicol. appl. Pharmacol.*, **48**, A162

Norback, D.H. & Allen, J.R. (1973) Biological responses of the nonhuman primate, chicken, and rat to chlorinated dibenzo-*p*-dioxin ingestion. *Environ. Health Perspectives*, **6**, 233–240

Norstrom, R.J. & Simon, M. (1991) Method 5: Determination of specific polychlorinated dibenzo-*p*-dioxins and dibenzofurans in biological matrices by gel-permeation — carbon chromatography and gas chromatography-mass spectrometry. In: Rappe, C., Buser, H.-R., Dodet, B. & O'Neill, I.K., eds, *Environmental Carcinogens: Methods of Analysis and Exposure Measurement. Vol. 11: Polychlorinated Dioxins and Dibenzofurans* (IARC Scientific Publications No. 108), Lyon, IARC, pp. 281–297

Nordström, Å., Rappe, C., Lindahl, P. & Buser, H.-R. (1979) Analysis of some older Scandinavian formulations of 2,4-dichlorophenoxy acetic acid and 2,4,5-trichlorophenoxy acetic acid for contents of chlorinated dibenzo-*p*-dioxins and dibenzofurans. *Scand. J. Work Environ. Health*, **5**, 375–378

Nygren, M., Rappe, C., Lindström, G., Hansson, M., Bergqvist, P.A., Marklund, S., Domellöf, L., Hardell, L. & Olsson, M. (1986) Identification of 2,3,7,8-substituted polychlorinated dioxins and dibenzofurans in environmental and human samples. In: Rappe, C., Choudhary, G. & Keith, L.H., eds, *Chlorinated Dioxins and Dibenzofurans in Perspective*, Chelsea, MI, Lewis Publishers, pp. 17–34

Nygren, M., Hansson, M., Sjöström, M., Rappe, C., Kahn, P., Gochfeld, M., Velez, H., Ghent-Guenther, T. & Wilson, W.P. (1988) Development and validation of a method for determination of PCDDs and PCDFs in human blood plasma. A multivariate comparison of blood and adipose tissue levels between Viet Nam veterans and matched controls. *Chemosphere*, **17**, 1663–1692

Öberg, L.G., Glas, B., Swanson, S.-E., Rappe, C. & Paul, K.G. (1990) Peroxidase-catalyzed oxidation of chlorophenols to polychlorinated dibenzo-*p*-dioxins and dibenzofurans. *Arch. environ. Contam. Toxicol.*, **19**, 930–938

Öberg, L.G., Andersson, R. & Rappe, C. (1993) *De novo* formation of hepta- and octachlorodibenzo-*p*-dioxins from pentachlorophenol in municipal sewage sludge. *Organohalogen Compounds*, **9**, 351–354

Oehme, M., Mano, S., Brevik, E.M. & Knutzen, J. (1989) Determination of polychlorinated dibenzofuran (PCDF) and dibenzo-p-dioxin (PCDD) levels and isomer patterns in fish, crustacea, mussel and sediment samples from a fjord region polluted by Mg-production. *Fresenius J. anal. Chem.*, **335**, 987–997

Oehme, M., Larssen, S. & Brevik, E.M. (1991) Emission factors of PCDD and PCDF for road vehicles obtained by tunnel experiment. *Chemosphere*, **23**, 1699–1708

Ogaki, J., Takayama, K., Miyata, H. & Kashimoto, T. (1987) Levels of PCDDs and PCDFs in human tissues and various foodstuffs in Japan. *Chemosphere*, **16**, 2047–2056

Oishi, S., Morita, M. & Fukuda, H. (1978) Comparative toxicity of polychlorinated biphenyls and dibenzofurans in rats. *Toxicol. appl. Pharmacol.*, **43**, 13–22

O'Keefe, P., Meyer, C., Hilker, D., Aldoves, K., Jelus-Tyror, B., Dillon, K., Donnolly, R., Horn, E. & Sloan, R. (1983) Analysis of 2,3,7,8-tetrachlorodibenzo-*p*-dioxin in Great Lakes fish. *Chemosphere*, **12**, 325–332

O'Keefe, P.W., Silkworth, J.B., Gierthy, J.F., Smith, R.M., DeCaprio, A.P., Turner, J.N., Eadon, G., Hilker, D.R., Aldous, K.M., Kaminsky, L.S. & Collins, D.N. (1985) Chemical and biological investigations of a transformer accident at Binghamton, NY. *Environ. Health Perspectives*, **60**, 201–209

Okey, A.B. (1990) Enzyme induction in the cytochrome P-450 system. *Pharmacol. Ther.*, **45**, 241–298

Okey, A.B., Vella, L.M. & Harper, P.A. (1989) Detection and characterization of a low affinity form of cytosolic Ah receptor in livers of mice nonresponsive to the induction of cytochrome P-450 by 3-methylcholanthrene. *Mol. Pharmacol.*, **35**, 823

Okey, A.B., Riddick, D.S. & Harper, P.A. (1994) The Ah receptor: mediator of the toxicity of 2,3,7,8-tetrachlorodibenzo-*p*-dioxin (TCDD) and related compounds. *Toxicol. Lett.*, **70**, 1–22

Okey, A.B., Riddick, D.S. & Harper, P.A. (1995) Ah receptor role in TCDD toxicity: still some mysteries but no myth. *Toxicol. Lett.*, **75**, 249–254

Okino, S.T., Pendurthi, U.R. & Tukey, R.H. (1992) Phorbol esters inhibit the dioxin receptor-mediated transcriptional activation of the mouse Cyp1a-1 and Cyp1a-2 genes by 2,3,7,8-tetrachlorodibenzo-*p*-dioxin. *J. Biol. Chem.*, **267**, 6991–6998

Oku, A., Tomari, K., Kamada, T., Yamada, E., Miyata, H. & Aozasa, O. (1995) Destruction of PCDDs and PCDFs. A convenient method using alkali-metal hydroxide in 1,3-dimethyl-1-imidazolidinone (DMI). *Chemosphere*, **31**, 3873–3878

Olafsson, P.G., Bryan, A.M. & Stone, W. (1988) Polychlorinated biphenyls and polychlorinated dibenzofurans in the tissues of patients with Yusho or Yu-Cheng: total toxicity. *Bull. environ. Contam. Toxicol.*, **41**, 63–70

Olie, K., Vermeulen, P.L. & Hutzinger, O. (1977) Chlorodibenzo-*p*-dioxins and chlorodibenzofurans are trace components of fly ash and flue gas of some municipal incinerators in the Netherlands. *Chemosphere*, **25**, 455–459

Olie, K., Schecter, A. , Constable, J. , Kooke, R.M. , Serne, P., Slot, P.C. & de Vries, P. (1989) Chlorinated dioxin and dibenzofuran levels in food and wildlife samples in the North and South of Vietnam. *Chemosphere*, **19**, 493–496

Oliver, R.M. (1975) Toxic effects of 2,3,7,8-tetrachlorodibenzo-1,4-dioxin in laboratory workers. *Br. J. ind. Med.*, **32**, 49–53

Olshan, A.F. & Mattison, D.R. (1994) *Male-mediated Developmental Toxicity*, New York, Plenum Press

Olson, J.R. (1986) Metabolism and disposition of 2,3,7,8-tetrachlorodibenzo-*p*-dioxin in guinea pigs. *Toxicol. appl. Pharmacol.*, **85**, 263–273

Olson, J.R. (1994) Pharmacokinetics of dioxins and related chemicals. In: Schechter, A., ed., *Dioxins and Health*, New York, Plenum Press, pp. 163–167

Olson, J.R., Holscher, M.A. & Neal, R.A. (1980) Toxicity of 2,3,7,8-tetrachlorodibenzo-*p*-dioxin in the golden Syrian hamster. *Toxicol. appl. Pharmacol.*, **55**, 67–78

Olson, J.R., Gasiewicz, T.A. & Neal, R.A. (1985) Tissue distribution, excretion and metabolism of 2,3,7,8-tetrachloro-*p*-dioxin (TCDD) in the golden Syrian hamster. *Toxicol. appl. Pharmacol.*, **56**, 78–85

Olson, J.R., McGarrigle, B.P., Tonucci, D.A., Schecter, A. & Eichelberger, H. (1990) Developmental toxicity of 2,3,7,8-TCDD in the rat and hamster. *Chemosphere*, **20**, 1117–1124

Olson, J.R., McGarrigle, B.P., Gigliotti, P., Kumar, S. & McReynolds, J.H. (1994) Hepatic uptake and metabolism of 2,3,7,8-tetrachlorodibenzo-*p*-dioxin and 2,3,7,8-tetrachlorodibenzofuran. *Fund. appl. Toxicol.*, **22**, 631–640

Olsson, M. (1994) Appendix I: Additional sampling recommendations for biological samples. *Fresenius J. analyt. Chem.*, **348**, 177–178

Olsson, H. & Brandt, L. (1988) Risk of non-Hodgkin's lymphoma among men occupationally exposed to organic solvents. *Scand. J. Work Environ. Health*, **14**, 246–251

Ono, M., Wakimoto, T., Tatsukawa, R. & Masuda, Y. (1986) Polychlorinated dibenzo-*p*-dioxins and dibenzofurans in human adipose tissues of Japan. *Chemosphere*, **15**, 1629–1634

Ono, M., Kashima, Y. , Wakimoto, T. & Tatsukama, R. (1987) Daily intake of PCDDs and PCDFs by Japanese through food. *Chemosphere*, **16**, 1823–1828

Ordinance on Sewage Sludge (1992) Revised version of 15 April 1992 (BG B1.IS.917), Germany, Ministry of Environment

Osborne, R. & Greenlee, W.F. (1985) 2,3,7,8-Tetrachlorodibenzo-*p*-dioxin (TCDD) enhances terminal differentiation of cultured human epidermal cells. *Toxicol. appl. Pharmacol.*, **77**, 434–443

Osborne, R., Dold, K.M. & Greenlee, W.F. (1987) Evidence that 2,3,7,8-tetrachlorodibenzo-*p*-dioxin and thyroid hormones act through different mechanisms in human keratinocytes. *Toxicol. appl. Pharmacol.*, *Toxicol. appl. Pharmacol.*, **90**, 522–531

Ott, M.G. & Zober, A. (1996) Cause specific mortality and cancer incidence among employees exposed to 2,3,7,8-TCDD after a 1953 reactor accident. *Occup. environ. Med.*, **53**, 606–612

Ott, M.G., Holder, B.B. & Olson, R.D. (1980) A mortality analysis of employees engaged in the manufacture of 2,4,5-trichlorophenoxyacetic acid. *J. occup. Med.*, **22**, 47–50

Ott, M.G., Olson, R.A., Cook, R.R. & Bond, G.G. (1987) Cohort mortality study of chemical workers with potential exposure to the higher chlorinated dioxins. *J. occup. Med.*, **29**, 422–429

Ott, M.G., Messerer, P. & Zober, A. (1993) Assessment of past occupational exposure to 2,3,7,8-tetrachlorodibenzo-*p*-dioxin using blood lipid analyses. *Int. Arch. occup. environ. Health*, **65**, 1–8

Ott, M.G., Zober, A. & Germann, C. (1994) Laboratory results for selected target organs in 138 individuals occupationally exposed to TCDD. *Chemosphere*, **29**, 2423–2437

Otto, S., Bhattacharyya, K.K. & Jefcoate, C.R. (1992) Polycyclic aromatic hydrocarbon metabolism in rat adrenal, ovary and testis microsomes is catalyzed by the same novel cytochrome P450 (P450RAP). *Endocrinology*, **31**, 3067–3076

Oughton, J.A., Pereira, C.B., DeKrey, G., Collier, J.M., Frank, A.A, & Kerkvliet, N.I. (1995) Phenotypic analysis of spleen, thymus, and peripheral blood cells in aged C57BL/6 mice following long-term exposure to 2,3,7,8-tetrachlorodibenzo-p-dioxin. *Fundam. appl. Toxicol.*, **25**, 60–69

Owens, I.S. (1977) Genetic regulation of UDP-glucuronosyl transferase induction by polycyclic aromatic compounds in mice. Co-segregation with aryl hydrocarbon (benzo[a]pyrene) hydroxylase induction. *J. biol. Chem.*, **252**, 2827–2833

Ozvacic, V. (1986) A review of stack sampling methodology for PCDDs/PCDFs. *Chemosphere*, **15**, 1173–1178

Päpke, O., Ball, M., Lis, A. & Scheunert, K. (1989a) PCDD and PCDF in indoor air of kindergartens in northern W. Germany. *Chemosphere*, **18**, 617–626

Päpke, O., Ball, M., Lis, Z.A. & Scheunert, K. (1989b) PCDD/PCDF in whole blood samples of unexposed persons. *Chemosphere*, **19**, 941–948

Päpke, O., Ball, M. & Lis, A. (1992) Various PCDD/PCDF patterns in human blood resulting from different occupational exposures. *Chemosphere*, **25**, 1101–1108

Päpke, O., Ball, M. & Lis, A. (1993a) Potential occupational exposure of municipal waste incinerator workers with PCDD/PCDF. *Chemosphere*, **27**, 203–209

Päpke, O., Ball, M. & Lis, A. (1993b) PCDD/PCDF in humans — an update of background data. *Organohalogen Compounds*, **13**, 81–84

Päpke, O., Ball, M., Lis, A., Menzel, H.M., Murzen, R., Turcer, E. & Bolm-Audorff, U. (1994a) Occupational exposure of chemical waste incinerators workers to PCDD/PCDF. *Organohalogen Compounds*, **21**, 105–110

Päpke, O., Ball, M. & Lis, A. (1994b) PCDD/PCDF in humans, a 1993-update of background data. *Chemosphere*, **29**, 2355–2360

Päpke, O., Ball, M., Lis, A. & Wuthe, J. (1996) PCDD/PCDFs in humans, follow-up of background data for Germany, 1994. *Chemosphere*, **32**, 575–582

Paroli, L., Lee, C. & Rifkind, A.B. (1994) Identification of hepatocytes as the major locus of 2,3,7,8-tetrachlorodibenzo-*p*-dioxin-induced Cyp1-related P450s, TCDD$_{AA}$ and TCDD$_{AHH}$, in chick embryo liver. *Drug Metab. Dispos.*, **22**, 962–968

Patterson, D.G., Jr, Holler, J.S., Lapeza, C.R., Alexander, L.R., Groce, D.F., O'Connor, R.C., Smith, S.J., Liddle, J.A. & Needham, L.L. (1986a) High-resolution gas chromatography/high-resolution mass spectrometric analysis of human adipose tissue for 2,3,7,8-tetrachlorodibenzo-*p*-dioxin. *Anal. Chem.*, **58**, 705–713

Patterson, D.G., Jr, Hoffman, R.E., Needham, L.L., Roberts, D.W., Bagby, J.R., Pirkle, J.L., Falk, H., Sampson, E.J. & Houk, V.N. (1986b) 2,3,7,8-Tetrachlorodibenzo-*p*-dioxin levels in adipose tissue of exposed and control persons in Missouri. *J. Am. med. Assoc.*, **256**, 2683–2686

Patterson, D.G., Jr, Holler, J.S., Smith, S.J., Liddle, J.A., Sampson, E.J. & Needham, L.L. (1986c) Human adipose data for 2,3,7,8-tetrachlorodibenzo-*p*-dioxin in certain US samples. *Chemosphere*, **15**, 2055–2060

Patterson, D.G., Jr, Needham, L.L., Pirkle, J.L., Roberts, D.W., Bagby, J., Garrett, W.A., Andrews, J.S., Jr, Falk, H., Bernert, J.T., Sampson, E.J. & Houk, V.N. (1988) Correlation between serum and adipose tissue levels of 2,3,7,8-tetrachlorodibenzo-p-dioxin in 50 persons from Missouri. *Arch. environ. Contam. Toxicol.*, **17**, 139–143

Patterson, D.G., Jr, Furst, P., Henderson, L.O., Isaacs, S.G., Alexander, L.R., Turner, W.E., Needham, L.L. & Hannon, H. (1989) Partitioning of in vivo bound PCDD/PCDFs among various compartments in whole blood. *Chemosphere*, **19**, 135

Patterson, D.G., Jr, Turner, W.E., Isaacs, S.G. & Alexander, L.R. (1990) A method performance evaluation and lessons learned after analyzing more than 5,000 human adipose tissue, serum, and breast milk samples for polychlorinated dibenzo-*p*-dioxins (PCDDs) and dibenzofurans (PCDFs). *Chemosphere*, **20**, 829–836

Patterson, D.G., Jr, Isaacs, S.G., Alexander, L.R., Turner, W.E., Hampton, L., Bernert, J.T. & Needham, L.L. (1991) Method 6: determination of specific polychlorinated dibenzo-*p*-dioxins and dibenzofurans in blood and adipose tissue by isotope dilution — high-resolution mass spectrometry. In: Rappe, C., Buser, H.-R., Dodet, B. & O'Neill, I.K., eds, *Environmental Carcinogens: Methods of Analysis and Exposure Measurement. Vol. 11: Polychlorinated Dioxins and Dibenzofurans* (IARC Scientific Publications No. 108), Lyon, IARC, pp. 299–342

Patterson, D.G., Jr, Todd, G.D., Turner, W.E., Maggio, V., Alexander, L.R. & Needham, L.L. (1994) Levels of non-*ortho*-substituted (coplanar), mono- and di-*ortho*-substituted polychlorinated biphenyls, dibenzo-*p*-dioxins, and dibenzofurans in human serum and adipose tissue. *Environ. Health Perspectives*, **102** (Suppl. 1), 195–204

Paulson, K.E., Darnell, J.E., Jr, Rushmore, T. & Pickett, C.B. (1990) Analysis of the upstream elements of the xenobiotic compound-inducible and positionally regulated glutathione *S*-transferase Ya gene. *Mol. cell. Biol.*, **10**, 1841–1852

Paustenbach, D.J., Sarlos, T.T., Lau, V., Finley, B.L., Jeffrey, D.A. & Ungs, M.J. (1991) The potential inhalation hazard posed by dioxin contaminated soil. *J. Air Waste Manag. Assoc.*, **41**, 1334–1340

Paustenbach, D.J., Wnning, R.J., Lau, V., Harrington, N.W., Rennix, D.K. & Parsons, A.H. (1992) Recent developments on the hazards posed by 2,3,7,8-tetrachlorodibenzo-p-dioxin in soil: implications for setting risk-based cleanup levels at residential and industrial sites. *J. Toxicol. environ. Health*, **36**, 103–149

Paustenbach, D.J., Wenning, R.J. & Mathur, D. (1996) PCDD/PCDFs in urban stormwater discharged to San Francisco Bay, California USA. *Organohalogen Compounds*, **28**, 111

Pazdernik, T.L. & Rozman, K.K. (1985) Effect of thyroidectomy and thyroxine on 2,3,7,8-tetrachlorodibenzo-*p*-dioxin-induced immunotoxicity. *Life Sci.*, **36**, 695–703

Pazderova-Vejlupkova, J., Nemcova, M., Pickova, J., Jirasek, L. & Lukas, E. (1981) The development and prognosis of chronic intoxication by tetrachlorodibenzo-*p*-dioxin in man. *Arch. environ. Health*, **36**, 5–11

Pearce, N. (1989) Phenoxy herbicides and non-Hodgkin's lymphoma in New Zealand: frequency and duration of herbicide use (Letter to the Editor). *Br. J. ind. Med.*, **46**, 143–144

Pearce, N.E., Smith, A.H., Howard, J.K., Sheppard, R.A., Giles, H.J. & Teague, C.A. (1986) Non-Hodgkin's lymphoma and exposure to phenoxy herbicides, chlorophenols, fencing work, and meat works employment: a case–control study. *Br. J. ind. Med.*, **43**, 75–83

Pearce, N.E., Sheppard, R.A., Smith, A.H. & Teague, C.A. (1987) Non-Hodgkin's lymphoma and farming: an expanded case-control study. *Int. J. Cancer*, **39**, 155–161

Pearson, R.G., McLaughlin, D.L. & McIlveen, W.D. (1990) Concentrations of PCDD and PCDF in Ontario soils from the vicinity of refuse and sewage sludge incinerators and remote rural and urban locations. *Chemosphere*, **20**, 1543–1548

Pendurthi, U.R., Okino, S.T. & Tukey, R.H. (1993) Accumulation of the nuclear dioxin (Ah) receptor and transcriptional activation of the mouse *Cyp1a-1* and *Cyp1a-2* genes. *Arch. Biochem. Biophys.*, **306**, 65–69

Perdew, G.H. (1988) Association of the Ah receptor with the 90 kD heat shock protein. *J. biol. Chem.*, **263**, 13802–13805

Perdew, G.H. (1992) Chemical cross-linking of the cytosolic and nuclear forms of the Ah receptor in hepatoma cell line 1c1c7. *Biochem. biophys. Res. Commun.*, **182**, 55–62

Pervunina, R.I., Samsonov, D.P. & Rakhmanova, T.V. (1992) 2,3,7,8-Tetrachlorodibenzo-*p*-dioxin in Russian environmental samples. *Organohalogen Compounds*, **9**, 173–176

Pesatori, A.C., Consonni, D., Tironi, A., Zocchetti, C., Fini, A. & Bertazzi, P.A. (1993) Cancer in a young population in a dioxin-contaminated area. *Int. J. Epidemiol.*, **22**, 1010–1013

Peters, J.M. & Wiley, L.M. (1995) Evidence that murine preimplantation embryos express aryl hydrocarbon receptor. *Toxicol. appl. Pharmacol.*, **134**, 214–221

Peterson, R. & Milicic, F. (1992) Chemical treatment of dioxin residues from wastewater processing. *Chemosphere*, **25**, 1565–1568

Peterson, R.E., Theobald, H. M. & Kimmel, G.L. (1993) Developmental and reproductive toxi-city of dioxins and related compounds: cross-species comparisons. *Crit. Rev. Toxicol.*, **23**, 283–335

Petreas, M., Hooper, K., She, J., Visita, P., Winkler, J., McKinney, M., Mok, M., Sy, F. , Garcha, J., Gill, M., Stephens, R., Chuvakova, T., Paltusheva, T., Sharmanov, T. & Semenova, G. (1996) Analysis of human breast milk to assess exposure to chlorinated conta-minants in Kazakhstan. *Organohalogen Compounds*, **30**, 20–23

Phillipps, L.J. & Birchard, G.F. (1991) Regional variations in human toxics exposure in the USA: an analysis based on the national human adipose tissue survey. *Arch. environ. Contam. Toxicol.*, **21**, 159–168

Phillips, M., Enan, E., Liu, P.C.C. & Matsumura, F. (1995) Inhibition of 3T3-L1 adipose diffe-rentiation by 2,3,7,8-tetrachlorodibenzo-*p*-dioxin. *J. Cell Sci.*, **108**, 395–402

Piacitelli, L.A., Haring Sweeney, M., Fingerhut, M.A., Patterson, D.G., Jr, Turner, W.E., Connally, L.B., Wille, K.K. & Tompkins, B. (1992) Serum levels of PCDDs and PCDFs among workers exposed to 2,3,7,8-TCDD contaminated chemicals. *Chemosphere*, **25**, 251–254

Pimental, R.A., Liang, B., Yee, G.K., Wilhelmsson, A., Poellinger, L. & Paulson, K.E. (1993) Dioxin receptor and C/EBP regulate the function of the glutathione S-transferase Ya gene xenobiotic response element. *Mol. cell. Biol.*, **13**, 4365–4373

Piper, W.N., Rose, J.Q. & Gehring, P.J. (1973) Excretion and tissue distribution of 2,3,7,8-tetra-chlorodibenzo-*p*-dioxin in the rat. *Environ. Health Perspectives*, **5**, 241–244

Pirkle, J.L., Wolfe, W.H., Patterson, D.G., Jr, Needham, L.L., Michalek, J.E., Miner, J.C., Peterson, M.R. & Phillips, D.L. (1989) Estimates of the half-life of 2,3,7,8-TCDD Vietnam veterans of Operation Ranch Hand. *J. Toxicol. environ. Health*, **27**, 165–171

Pitot, H.C., Goldsworthy, T., Campbell, H.A. & Poland, A. (1980) Quantitative evaluation of the promotion by 2,3,7,8-tetrachlorodibenzo-*p*-dioxin of hepatocarcinogenesis from diethyl-nitrosamine. *Cancer Res.*, **40**, 3616–3620

Pitot, H.C., Goldsworthy, T.L., Moran, S., Kennan, W., Glauert, H.P., Maronpot, R.R. & Campbell, H.A. (1987) A method to quantitate the relative initiating and promoting potencies of hepatocarcinogenic agents in their dose-response relationships to altered hepatic foci. *Carcinogenesis*, **8**, 1491–1499

Pluim, H.J., Koppe, J.G., Olie, K., van der Slikke, J.W., Kok, J.H., Vulsma, T., Van Tijn, D. & De Vijlder, J.J.M. (1992) Effects of dioxins on thyroid function in newborn babies. Letter to the Editor. *Lancet*, **339**, 1303

Pluim, H.J., Wever, J., Koppe, J.G., van der Slikke, J.W. & Olie, K. (1993a) Intake and faecal excretion of chlorinated dioxins and dibenzofurans in breast-fed infants at different ages. *Chemosphere*, **26**, 1947–1952

Pluim, H.J., Kramer, I., van der Slikke, J.W., Koppe, J.G. & Olie, K. (1993b) Levels of PCDDs and PCDFs in human milk: dependence on several parameters and dietary habits. *Chemo-sphere*, **26**, 1889–1895

Pluim, H.J., de Vijlder, J.J.M., Olie, K., Kok, J.H., Vulsma, T., van Tijn, D.A., van der Slikke, J.W. & Koppe, J.G. (1993c) Effects of pre- and postnatal exposure to chlorinated dioxins and furans on human neonatal thyroid hormone concentrations. *Environ. Health Perspectives*, **101**, 504–508

Pluim, H.J., Boersma, E.R., Kramer, I., Olie, K., van der Slikke, J.W. & Koppe, J.G. (1994a) Influence of short-term dietary measures on dioxin concentrations in human milk. *Environ. Health Perspectives*, **102**, 968–971

Pluim, H.J., Koppe, J.G., Olie, K., van der Slikke, J.W., Slot, P.C. & van Boxtel, C.J. (1994b) Clinical laboratory manifestations of exposure to background levels of dioxins in the perinatal period. *Acta paediatr.*, **83**, 583–587

Plüss, N., Poiger, H., Schlatter, C. & Buser, H.R. (1987) The metabolism of some pentachloro-dibenzofurans in the rat. *Xenobiotica*, **17**, 209–216

Plüss, N., Poiger, H., Hohbach, C., Suter, M. & Schlatter, C. (1988a) Subchronic toxicity of 2,3,4,7,8-pentachlorodibenzofuran (PeCDF) in rats. *Chemosphere*, **17**, 1099–1110

Plüss, N., Poiger, H., Hohbach, C. & Schlatter, C. (1988b) Subchronic toxicity of some chlorinated dibenzofurans (PCDFs) and a mixture of PCDFs and chlorinated dibenzodioxins (PCDDs) in rats. *Chemosphere*, **5**, 973–984

Pocchiari, F. (1980) *Accidental TCDD Contamination in Seveso (Italy): Epidemiological Aspects* (FIFRA Docket No. 415, Exhibit 1469)

Pocchiari, F., Silvano, V., Zampieri, A. & Zampieri, A. (1979) Human health effects from accidental release of tetrachlorodibenzo-*p*-dioxin (TCDD) at Seveso, Italy. *Ann. N.Y. Acad. Sci.*, **77**, 311–320

Pocchiari, F., Silano, V. & Zampieri, A. (1980) *Human Health Effects from Accidental Release of TCDD at Seveso (Italy)* (FIFRA Docket No. 415, Exhibit 1470)

Poellinger, L. (1995) Mechanism of signal transduction by the basic helix-loop-helix dioxin receptor. In: Baeuerle, P.A., ed., *Inducible Gene Expression*, Vol. 1, Birkhäuser, Boston, pp. 177–205

Poellinger, L., Göttlicher, M. & Gustafsson, J.-Å. (1992) The dioxin and peroxisome proliferator-activated receptors: nuclear receptors in search of endogenous ligands. *Trends pharm. Sci.*, **13**, 241–245

Pohjanvirta, R. (1990) TCDD resistance is inherited as an autosomal dominant trait in the rat. *Toxicol. Lett.*, **50**, 49–56

Pohjanvirta, R. & Tuomisto, J. (1987) Han/Wistar rats are exceptionally resistant to TCDD. *Arch. Toxicol.*, **11**, 344–347

Pohjanvirta, R. & Tuomisto, J. (1990a) Letter to the editor. *Toxicol. appl. Pharmacol.*, **105**, 508–509

Pohjanvirta, R. & Tuomisto, J. (1990b) Remarkable residual alterations in responses to feeding regulatory challenges in Han/Wistar rats after recovery from the acute toxicity of 2,3,7,8-tetrachlorodibenzo-*p*-dioxin (TCDD). *Food chem. Toxicol.*, **28**, 677–686

Pohjanvirta, R. & Tuomisto, J. (1990c) 2,3,7,8-Tetrachlorodibenzo-*p*-dioxin enhances responsiveness to post-ingestive satiety signals. *Toxicology*, **63**, 285–299

Pohjanvirta, R., Tuomisto, J., Vartiainen, T. & Rozman, K. (1987) Han/Wistar rats are exceptionally resistant to TCDD. I. *Pharmacol. Toxicol.*, **60**, 145–150

Pohjanvirta, R., Juvonen, R., Kärenlampi, S., Raunio, H. & Tuomisto, J. (1988) Hepatic Ah-receptor levels and the effect of 2,3,7,8-tetrachlorodibenzo-*p*-dioxin (TCDD) on hepatic microsomal monooxygenase activity in a TCDD-susceptible and -resistant rat strain. *Toxicol. appl. Pharmacol.*, **92**, 131–140

Pohjanvirta, R., Kulju, T., Morselt, A.F.W., Tuominen, R., Juvonen, R., Rozman, K., Männistö, P., Collan, Y., Sainio, E.-L. & Tuomisto, J. (1989a) Target tissue morphology and serum biochemistry following 2,3,7,8-tetrachlorodibenzo-*p*-dioxin (TCDD) exposure in a TCDD-susceptible and a TCDD-resistant rat strain. *Fundam. appl. Toxicol.*, **12**, 698–712

Pohjanvirta, R., Tuomisto, L. & Tuomisto, J. (1989b) The central nervous system may be involved in TCDD toxicity. *Toxicology*, **58**, 167–174

Pohjanvirta, R., Tuomisto, J., Linden, J. & Laitinen, J. (1989c) TCDD reduces serum melatonin levels in Long-Evans rats. *Pharmacol. Toxicol.*, **65**, 239–240

Pohjanvirta, R., Vartiainen, T., Uusi-Rauva, A., Monkkonen, J. & Tuomisto, J. (1990a) Tissue distribution, metabolism, and excretion of ^{14}C-TCDD in a TCDD-susceptible and a TCDD-resistant rat strain. *Pharmacol. Toxicol.*, **66**, 93–100

Pohjanvirta, R., Håkansson, H., Juvonen, R. & Tuomisto, J. (1990b) Effects of TCDD on vitamin A status and liver microsomal enzyme activities in a TCDD-susceptible and a TCDD-resistant rat strain. *Food Chem. Toxicol.*, **28**, 197–203

Pohjanvirta, R., Sankari, S., Kulju, T., Naukkarinen, A., Ylinen, M. & Tuomisto, J. (1990c) Studies on the role of lipid peroxidation in the acute toxicity of TCDD in rats. *Pharmacol Toxicol.*, **66**, 399–408

Pohjanvirta, R., Unkila, M. & Tuomisto, J. (1991a) Characterization of the enhanced responsiveness to postingestive satiety signals in 2,3,7,8-tetrachlorodibenzo-*p*-dioxin (TCDD)-treated Han/Wistar rats. *Pharmacol. Toxicol.*, **69**, 433–441

Pohjanvirta, R., Unkila, M. & Tuomisto, J. (1991b) The loss of glucoprivic feeding is an early-stage alteration in TCDD-treated Han/Wistar rats. *Pharmacol. Toxicol.*, **68**, 441–443

Pohjanvirta, R., Unkila, M. & Tuomisto, J. (1993) Comparative acute lethality of 2,3,7,8-tetrachlorodibenzo-*p*-dioxin (TCDD), 1,2,3,7,8-pentachlorodibenzo-*p*-dioxin and 1,2,3,4,7,8-hexachlorodibenzo-*p*-dioxin in the most TCDD-susceptible and the most TCDD-resistant rat strain. *Pharmacol. Toxicol.*, **73**, 52–56

Pohjanvirta, R., Unkila, M. & Tuomisto, J. (1994a) TCDD-induced hypophagia is not explained by nausea. *Pharmacol. biochem. Behav.*, **47**, 273–282

Pohjanvirta, R., Hirvonen, M.R., Unkila, M., Savolainen, K. & Tuomisto, J. (1994b) TCDD decreases brain inositol concentrations in the rat. *Toxicol. Lett.*, **70**, 363–372

Pohjanvirta, R., Laitinen, J.T., Vakkuri, O., Linden, J., Kokkola, T., Unkila, M. & Tuomisto, J. (1996) Mechanism by which 2,3,7,8-tetrachlorodibenzo-*p*-dioxin (TCDD) reduces circulating melatonin levels in the rat. *Toxicology*, **107**, 85–97

Poiger, H. & Buser, H.R. (1984) The metabolism of TCDD in the dog and rat. In: Poland, A. & Kimbrough, R.D., eds, *Biological Mechanisms of Dioxin Action* (Banbury Report 18), Cold Spring Harbor Laboratory, CHS Press, pp. 39–47

Poiger, H. & Schlatter, C. (1979) Biological degradation of TCDD in rats. *Nature*, **281**, 706–707

Poiger, H. & Schlatter, C. (1986) Pharmacokinetics of 2,3,7,8-TCDD in man. *Chemosphere*, **15**, 1489–1494

Poiger, H., Pluess, N. & Buser, H.R. (1989) The metabolism of selected PCDFs in the rat. *Chemosphere*, **18**, 259–264

Poland, A. & Glover, E. (1979) 2,3,7,8-Tetrachlorodibenzo-*p*-dioxin: segregation of toxicity with the Ah locus. *Mol. Pharmacol.*, **17**, 86–94

Poland, A. & Knutson, J.C. (1982) 2,3,7,8-Tetrachlorodibenzo-*p*-dioxin and related halogenated aromatic hydrocarbons: examination of the mechanism of toxicity. *Ann. Rev. Pharmacol. Toxicol.*, **22**, 517–554

Poland, A.P., Smith, D., Metter, G. & Possick, P. (1971) A health survey of workers in a 2,4-D and 2,4,5-T plant. *Arch. environ. Health*, **22**, 316–327

Poland, A., Palen, D. & Glover, E. (1982) Tumour promotion by TCDD in skin of HRS/J hairless mice. *Nature*, **300**, 271–273

Poland, A., Teitelbaum, P. & Glover, E. (1989a) [^{125}I]2-Iodo-3,7,8-trichlorodibenzo-*p*-dioxin binding species in mouse liver induced by agonists for the Ah receptor: characterization and identification. *Mol. Pharmacol.*, **36**, 113–120

Poland, A., Teitelbaum, P., Glover, E. & Kende, A. (1989b) Stimulation of in vivo hepatic uptake and in vitro hepatic binding of [^{125}I]2-iodo-3,7,8-trichlorodibenzo-*p*-dioxin by the administration of agonist for the Ah receptor. *Mol. Pharmacol.*, **36**, 121–172

Polder, A., Becher, G., Savinova, T.N. & Skaare, J.U. (1996) Dioxins, PCBs and some chlorinated pesticides in human milk from the Kola Peninsula, Russia. *Organohalogen Compounds*, **30**, 158–161

Pollenz, R.S., Sattler, C.A. & Poland, A. (1994) The aryl hydrocarbon receptor and aryl hydrocarbon receptor nuclear translocator protein show distinct subcellular localizations in Hepa 1c1c7 cells by immunofluorescence microscopy. *Mol. Pharmacol.*, **45**, 428–438

Pomazanov, V., Kuntsevich, A., Vengerov, Y., Dmitriyeva, L. & Asadova, L. (1992) The conception of gas-chromatographic and chromato-mass-spectrometric detection of polychlorinated dibenzo-*p*-dioxins and dibenzofurans in drinking water. *Organohalogen Compounds*, **9**, 177–181

Pongratz, I., Mason, G.G.F. & Poellinger, L. (1992) Dual roles of the 90 kDa heat shock protein in modulating functional activities of the dioxin receptor. *J. biol. Chem.*, **267**, 13728–13734

Poole, C. (1993) Potential confounding of associations involving occupational exposure to 2,3,7,8-tetrachlorodibenzo-*p*-dioxin (letter). *Epidemiology*, **4**, 483

Porterfield, S.P. & Hendrich, C.E. (1993) The role of thyroid hormones in perinatal and neonatal neurological development — current perspectives. *Endocrinol. Rev.*, **14**, 94–106

Portier, C.J., Sherman, C.D., Kohn, M., Edler, L., Kopp Schneider, A., Maronpot, R.M. & Lucier, G. (1996) Modeling the number and size of hepatic focal lesions following exposure to 2,3,7,8-TCDD. *Toxicol. appl. Pharmacol.*, **138**, 20–30

Pottenger, L.H. & Jefcoate, C.R. (1990) Characterization of a novel cytochrome P450 from the transformable cell line, C3H/10T1/2. *Carcinogenesis*, **11**, 321–327

Pottenger, L.H., Christou, M. & Jefcoate, C.R. (1991) Purification and immunological characterisation of a novel cytochrome P450 from C3H/10T1/2 cells. *Arch. Biochem. Biophys.*, **286**, 488–497

Potter, C.L., Sipes, G.I. & Russel, H.D. (1983) Hypothyroxinemia and hypothermia in rats in response to 2,3,7,8-tetrachlorodibenzo-*p*-dioxin administration. *Toxicol. appl. Pharmacol.*, **69**, 89–95

Potter, C.L., Moore, R.W., Inhorn, S.L., Hagen, T.C. & Peterson, R.E. (1986) Thyroid status and thermogenesis in rats treated with 2,3,7,8-tetrachlorodibenzo-*p*-dioxin. *Toxicol. appl. Pharmacol.*, **84**, 45–55

Pratt, R.M. (1985) Receptor-dependent mechanisms of glucocorticoid and dioxin-induced cleft palate. *Environ. Health Perspectives*, **61**, 35–40

Pratt, R.M. Dencker, L. & Diewert, V.M. (1984) 2,3,7,8-tetrachlorodibenzo-*p*-dioxin-induced cleft palate in the mouse: evidence for alterations in palatal shelf fusion. *Teratog. Carcinog. Mutag.*, **4**, 427–436

Prinz, B ., Krause, G.H.M. & Radermacher, L. (1990) Criteria for the evaluation of dioxins in vegetable plants and soils. In: *Proceedings of the 10th International Conference on Organohalogen Compounds*

Probst, M.R., Reisz-Porszasz, S. Agbunag, R.V., Ong, M.S. & Hankinson, O. (1993) Role of the aryl hydrocarbon receptor nuclear translocator protein in aryl hydrocarbon (dioxin) receptor action. *Mol. Pharmacol.*, **44**, 511–518

Puga, A., Raychaudhuri, B. & Nebert, D.W. (1992) Transcriptional derepression of the murine Cyp 121 gene by mevinolin. *FASE J.*, **6**, 777–785

Puhvel, S.M. & Sakamoto, M. (1988) Effect of 2,3,7,8-tetrachlorodibenzo-*p*-dioxin on murine skin. *J. invest. Dermatol.*, **90**, 354–358

Puhvel, S.M., Sakamoto, M., Ertl, D.C. & Reisner, R.M. (1982) Hairless mice as models for chloracne: a study of cutaneous changes induced by topical application of established chloracnegens. *Toxicol. appl. Pharmacol.*, **64**, 492–503

Puhvel, S.M., Connor, M.J. & Sakamoto, M. (1991) Vitamin A deficiency and the induction of cutaneous toxicity in murine skin by TCDD. *Toxicol. appl. Pharmacol.*, **107**, 106–116

Quattrochi, L.C. & Tukey, R.H. (1989) The human cytochrome *CYP1A2* gene contains regulatory elements responsive to 3-methylcholanthrene. *Mol. Pharmacol.*, **36**, 66–71

Quattrochi, L.C., Vu, T. & Tukey, R.H. (1994) The human *CYP1A2* gene and induction by 3-methylcholanthrene: a region of DNA that supports Ah-receptor binding and promoter-specific induction. *J. biol. Chem.*, **269**, 6949–6954

Rabl, P., Dumler-Gradl, R., Thoma, H. & Vierle, O. (1996) PCDD/F emission measurements in different distances from a emission source. *Organohalogen Compounds*, **28**, 300–303

Ramlow, J.M., Spadecene, N.W., Hoag, S.R., Stafford, B.A., Cartmill, J.B. & Lerner, P.J. (1996) Mortality in a cohort of pentachlorophenol manufacturing owrkers, 1940–1989. *Am. J. ind. Med.*, **30**, 180–194

Ramos, L., Eljarrat, E., Hernández, L.M., Alonso, L., Rivera, J. & González, M.J. (1996) Levels of PCDDs and PCDFs in farm cow's milk located near potential contaminant sources in Asturias (Spain). Comparison with levels found in control points and commercial pasteurized cow's milk. *Organohalogen Compounds*, **28**, 304–307

Ramsey, J.C., Hefner, J.G., Karbowski, R.J., Braun, R.J. & Gehring, P.J. (1982) The in vivo biotransformation of 2,3,7,8-tetrachlorodibenzo-p-dioxin (TCDD) in the rat. *Toxicol. appl. Pharmacol.,* **65**, 280–184

Randerath, K., Putman, K.L., Randerath, E., Mason, G., Kelley, M. & Safe, S. (1988) Organspecific effects of long term feeding of 2,3,7,8-tetrachlorodibenzo-*p*-dioxin and 1,2,3,7,8-pentachlorodibenzo-*p*-dioxin on I-compounds in hepatic and renal DNA of female Sprague-Dawley rats. *Carcinogenesis,* **9**, 2285-2289

Randerath, K., Putman, K.L., Randerath, E., Zacharewski, T., Harris, M. & Safe, S. (1990) Effects of 2,3,7,8-tetrachlorodibenzo-*p*-dioxin on I-compounds in hepatic DNA of Sprague-Dawley rats: sex-specific effects and structure–activity relationships. *Toxicol. appl. Pharmacol.*, **103**, 271–280

Randerath, E., Randerath, K., Reddy, R., Narasimhan, T.R., Wang, X. & Safe, S. (1993) Effects of polychlorinated dibenzofurans on I-compounds in hepatic DNA of female Sprague-Dawley rats: structure dependence and mechanistic considerations. *Chem.-biol. Interactions*, **88**, 175–190

Rao, M.S., Subbarao, V., Prasad, J. & Scarpelli, D. (1988) Carcinogenicity of 2,3,7,8-tetrachlorodibenzo-*p*-dioxin in the Syrian golden hamster. *Carcinogenesis*, **9**, 1677–1679

Rao, G.N., Haseman, J.K., Grumbein, S., Crawford, D.D. & Eustis, S.L. (1990) Growth, body weight, survival, and tumor trends in F344/N rats during an eleven -year period. *Toxicol. Pathol.*, **18**, 61–70

Rappe, C. (1983) *Public Health Risks of the Dioxins: Chemical Analyses of Adipose Tissue*, The Rockefeller University

Rappe, C. (1984a) Analysis of polychlorinated dioxins and furans. *Environ. Sci. Technol.*, **18**, 78A–90A

Rappe, C. (1984b) Chemical analyses of adipose tissues. In: Lowrance, W.W., ed., *Public Health Risks of the Dioxins*, Proceedings of a symposium held on October 19–20, 1983 at the Rockefeller University, New York City, Los Altos, CA, William Kaufmann

Rappe, C. (1992) Dietary exposure and human levels of PCDDs and PCDFs. *Chemosphere*, **25**, 231–234

Rappe, C. (1994) Dioxin, patterns and source identification. *Fresenius J. anal. Chem.*, **348**, 63–75

Rappe, C. & Andersson, R. (1992) Analyses of PCDDs and PCDFs in wastewater from dish washers and washing machines. *Organohalogen Compounds*, **9**, 191–194

Rappe, C. & Buser, H.R. (1981) Occupational exposure to polychlorinated dioxins and dibenzofurans. In: Choudhary, G., ed., *Chemical Hazards in the Workplace — Measurement and Control (ACS Symposium Series No. 149)*, Washington DC, American Chemical Society, pp. 319–342

Rappe, C. & Wågman, N. (1995) Trace analysis of PCDDs and PCDFs in unbleached and bleached pulp samples. *Organohalogen Compounds*, **23**, 377–381

Rappe, C., Buser, H.-R. & Bosshardt, H.-P. (1978a) Identification and quantification of polychlorinated dibenzo-*p*-dioxins (PCDDs) and dibenzofurans (PCDFs) in 2,4,5-T-ester formulations and herbicide Orange. *Chemosphere*, **7**, 431–438

Rappe, C., Garå, A. & Buser, H.-R. (1978b) Identification of polychlorinated dibenzofurans (PCDFs) in commercial chlorophenol formulations. *Chemosphere*, **12**, 981–991

Rappe, C., Buser, H.R. & Bosshardt, H.P. (1979a) Dioxins, dibenzofurans and other polyhalogenated aromatics: production, use, formation, and destruction. Part I. Production, chemistry, and distribution. *Ann. N.Y. Acad. Sci.*, **320**, 1–18

Rappe, C., Nuser, H.R., Kuroki, H. & Masuda, Y. (1979b) Identification of polychlorinated dibenzofurans (PCDFs) retained in patients with Yusho. *Chemosphere*, **4**, 259–266

Rappe, C., Ngyren, M. & Gustafsson, G. (1983) *Human Exposure to Polychlorinated Dibenzo-p-Dioxins and Dibenzofurans*. In: Choudhary, G., Keith, L. & Rappe, C., eds, *Chlorinated Dioxins and Dibenzofurans in the Total Environment, Kansas City, 1982*, Boston, M.A., Butterworths, pp. 355–365

Rappe, C., Kjeller, L.-O. & Marklund, S. (1985a) PCDF isomers and isomer levels found in PCBs. In: Komai, R.Y. & Addis, G., eds, *Proceedings of a Workshop on PCB By-product Formation, Palo Alto, California, 4–6 December 1984*, Palo Alto, CA, Electrical Power Research Institute, pp. 20–23

Rappe, C., Marklund, S., Kjeller, L.-O., Bergqvist, P.-A. & Hansson, M. (1985b) Strategies and techniques for sample collection and analysis: experience from the Swedish PCB accidents. *Environ. Health Perspectives*, **60**, 279–292

Rappe, C., Ngyren, M., Lindström, G. & Hansson, M. (1986a) Dioxins and dibenzofurans in biological samples of European origin. *Chemosphere*, **15**, 1635–1639

Rappe, C., Kjeller, L.-O., Marklund, S. & Nygren, M. (1986b) Electrical PCB accidents, an update. *Chemosphere*, **15**, 1291–1295

Rappe, C., Andersson, R., Bergqvist, P.-A., Brohede, C., Hansson, M., Kjeller, L.-O., Lindström, G., Marklund, S., Nygren, M., Swanson, S.E., Tysklind, M. & Wiberg, K. (1987a) Overview of environmental fate of chlorinated dioxins and dibenzofurans. Sources, levels and isomeric pattern in various matrices. *Chemosphere*, **16**, 1603–1618

Rappe, C., Nygren, M., Lindström, G., Buser, H.R., Blaser, O. & Wüthrich, C. (1987b) Polychlorinated dibenzofurans and dibenzo-*p*-dioxins and other chlorinated contaminants in cow milk from various locations in Switzerland. *Environ. Sci. Technol.*, **21**, 964–970

Rappe, C., Kjeller, L.-O., Bruckmann, P. & Hackhe, K.-H. (1988) Identification and quantification of PCDDs and PCDFs in urban air. *Chemosphere*, **17**, 3–20

Rappe, C., Marklund, S. & Kjeller, L.-O. (1989a) Long-range transport of PCDDs and PCDFs on airborne particles. *Chemosphere*, **18**, 1283-1290

Rappe, C., Kjeller, L.-O. & Andersson, R. (1989b) Analyses of PCDDs ad PCDFs in sludge and water samples. *Chemosphere*, **19**, 13–20

Rappe, C., Tarkowski, S. & Yrjänheikki, E. (1989c) The WHO/EURO quality control study on PCDDs and PCDFs in human milk. *Chemosphere*, **18**, 883–889

Rappe, C., Bergqvist, P.-A. & Kjeller, L.-O. (1989d) Levels, trends and patterns of PCDDs and PCDFs in Scandinavian environmental samples. *Chemosphere*, **18**, 651–658

Rappe, C., Kjeller, L.-O. & Kulp, S.E. (1990a) Sampling and analysis of PCDDs and PCDFs in surface water and drinking water at 0.001 ppq levels. *Organohalogen Compounds*, **2**, 207–210

Rappe, C., Lindström, G., Glas, B., Lundström, K. & Borgström, S. (1990b) Levels of PCDDs and PCDFs in milk cartons and in commercial milk. *Chemosphere*, **20**, 1649-1656

Rappe, C., Buser, H.-R., Dodet, B. & O'Neill, I.K., eds (1991a) *Environmental Carcinogens — Methods of Analysis and Exposure Measurement. Vol. 11: Polychlorinated Dioxins and Dibenzofurans* (IARC Scientific Publications No. 108), Lyon, IARC

Rappe, C., Kjeller, L.-O., Kulp, S.-E., de Wit, C., Hasselsten, I. & Palm, O. (1991b) Levels, profile and pattern of PCDDs and PCDFs in samples related to the production and use of chlorine. *Chemosphere*, **23**, 1629–1636

Rappe, C., Lindström, G., Hansson, M., Andersson, K. & Andersson, R. (1992) Levels of PCDDs and PCDFs in cow's milk and worker's blood collected in connection with a hazardous waste incinerator in Sweden. *Organohalogen Compounds*, **9**, 199–202

Rappe, C., Marklund, S., Fängmark, I. & van Bavel, B. (1993) Sampling and analysis of dioxins, dibenzofurans and PCBs from incinerators. In: Weijnen, M.P.C. & Drinkenburg, A.A.H., eds, *Precision Process Technology*, Dordrecht, Kluwer Academic Publishers, pp. 517–531

Rappe, C., Andersson, R., Kulp, S.-E., Cooper, K., Fiedler, H., Lau, C., Howell, F. & Bonner, M. (1995) Concentrations of PCDDs and PCDFs in soil samples from southern Mississippi, USA. *Organohalogen Compounds*, **24**, 345–348

Reed, L.W., Hunt, G.T., Maisel, B.E., Hoyt, M., Keefe, D. & Hackney, P. (1990) Baseline assessment of PCDDs/PCDFs in the vicinity of the Elk River, Minnesota generating station. *Chemosphere*, **21**, 159–171

Reggiani, G. (1978) Medical problems raised by the TCDD contamination in Seveso, Italy. *Arch. Toxicol.*, **40**, 161–188

Reggiani, G. (1980) Acute human exposure to TCDD in Seveso, Italy. *J. Toxicol. environ. Health*, **6**, 27–43

Rehder, H., Sanchioni, L., Cefis, F. & Gropp, A. (1978) Pathological-embryological investigations in cases of abortion related to the Seveso accident. *Schweiz. med. Wschr.*, **108**, 1617–1625 (in German)

Reiner, E.J., Gizyn, W.I., Khurana, V., Kolic, T.M., MacPherson, K.A., Waddell, D.S. & Bell, R.W. (1995) Environmental impact of polychlorinated dibenzo-*p*-dioxins and dibenzofurans from a cement kiln. *Organohalogen Compounds*, **23**, 419–423

Reiners, J.J., Cantu, A.R. & Scholler, A. (1992) Phorbol ester-mediated suppression cytochrome P450 Cyp1a-1 induction in murine skin: involvement of protein kinase C. *Biochem. biophys. Res. Commun.*, **186**, 970–976

Reiners, J.J., Jr, Scholler, A., Bischer, P., Cantu, A.R. & Pavone, A. (1993) Suppression of cytochrome P450 *Cyp1a-1* induction in murine hepatoma 1c1c7 cells by 12-*O*-tetradecanoyl-phorbol-13-acetate and inhibitors of protein kinase C. *Arch. Biochem. Biophys.*, **301**, 449–454

Reischl, A., Reissinger, M., Thoma, H. & Hutzinger, O. (1989) Uptake and accumulation of PCDD/F in terrestial plants: basic considerations. *Chemosphere*, **19**, 467–474

Reyes, H., Reisz-Porszasz, S. & Hankinson, O. (1992) Identification of the Ah receptor nuclear translocator protein (Arnt) as a component of the DNA binding form of the Ah receptor. *Science*, **256**, 1193–1195

Rhile, M.J., Nagarkatti, M. & Nagarkatti, P.S. (1996) Role of Fas apoptosis and MHC genes in 2,3,7,8-tetrachlorodibenzo-*p*-dioxin (TCDD)-induced immunotoxicity of T-cells. *Toxicology*, **110**, 153–167

Rice, C.D., Merchant, R.E., Jeong, T.C., Karras, J.B. & Holsapple, M.P. (1995) The effects of acute exposure to 2,3,7,8-tetrachlorodibenzo-*p*-dioxin on glioma-specific cytotoxic T-cell activity in Fischer 344 rats. *Toxicology*, **95**, 177–185

Richter, E., Hunder, G. & Forth, W. (1992) Inhibition of intestinal glucose absorption in rats treated with 2,3,7,8-tetrachlorodibenzo-*p*-dioxin. *Vet. hum. Toxicol.* **34**, 123–126

Rier, S.E., Martin, D.C., Bowman, R.E., Dmowski, W.P. & Becker, J.L. (1993) Endometriosis in rhesus monkeys (macaca mulatta) following chronic exposure to 2,3,7,8-tetrachloro-dibenzo-p-dioxin. *Fundam. appl. Toxicol.*, **21**, 433–441

Rifkind, A.B., Hattori, Y., Levi, R., Hughes, M.J, Quilley, C. & Alonson, D.R. (1984) The chick embryo as a model for PCB and dioxin toxicity: evidence for cardiotoxicity and increased prostaglandin synthesis. In: Poland, A. & Kimbrough, R.B., eds, *Biological Mechanisms of Dioxin Action* (Banbury Report 18), Cold Spring Harbor Laboratory, CSH Press, pp. 255–266

Riggs, K.B., Roth, A., Kelly, T.J. & Schrock, M.E. (1996) Ambient PCDD/PCDF levels in Montgomery County, Ohio: comparison to previous data and source attribution. *Organohalogen Compounds*, **28**, 128–133

Riihimäki, V., Asp, S. & Hernberg, S. (1982) Mortality of 2,4-dichlorophenoxyacetic acid and 2,4,5-trichlorophenoxyacetic acid herbicide applicators in Finland. *Scand. J. Work Environ. Health*, **8**, 37–42

Riss, A., Hagenmaier, H., Weberruss, U., Schlatter, C. & Wacker, R. (1990) Comparison of PCDD/PCDF levels in soil, grass, cow's milk, human blood and spruce needles in an area of PCDD/PCDF contamination through emissions from a metal reclamation plant. *Chemosphere*, **21**, 1451–1456

Rivera, J., Eljarrat, E., Espadaler, I., Martrat, M.G. & Caixach, J. (1995) Determination of PCDF/PCDD in sludges from drinking water treatment plant. Influence of chlorination treatment. *Organohalogen Compounds*, **24**, 91–93

Roberts, E.A., Golas, C.L. & Okey, A.B. (1986) Ah receptor mediating induction of aryl hydrocarbon hydroxylase: detection in human lung by binding of 2,3,7,8-[^{3}H]tetrachlorodibenzo-*p*-dioxin. *Cancer Res.*, **46**, 3739–3743

Roegner, R.H., Grubbs, W.D., Lustik, M.B., Brockman, A.S., Henderson, S.C., Williams, D.E., Wolfe, W.H., Michalek, J.E. & Miner, J.C. (1991) *Air Force Health Study: An Epidemiologic Investigation of Health Effects in Air Force Personnel Following Exposure to Herbicides. Serum Dioxin Analysis of 1987 Examination Results* (NTIS# AD A-237-516 through AD A-237-524), Washington DC, National Technical Information Service

Rogan, W.J. (1982) PCBs and cola-colored babies: Japan 1968 and Taiwan 1979. *Teratology*, **26**, 259–261

Rogan, W. (1989) Yu-Cheng. In: Kimbrough, R.D. & Jensen, A.A., eds, *Halogenated Biphenyls, Terphenyls, Naphthalenes, Dibenzodioxins and Related Products*, 2nd Ed., New York, Elsevier, pp. 401–415

Rogan, W.J., Gladen, B.C., Hung, K.-L., Koong, S.L., Shih, L.Y., Taylor, J.S., Wu, Y.C., Yang, D., Ragen, N.B. & Hsu, C.C. (1988) Congenital poisoning by polychlorinated biphenyls and their contaminants in Taiwan. *Science*, **241**, 334–336

Rogers, A.M., Andersen, M.E. & Back, K.C. (1982) Mutagenicity of 2,3,7,8-tetrachlorodibenzo-*p*-dioxin and perfluoro-*n*-decanoic acid in L5178Y mouse-lymphoma cells. *Mutat. Res.*, **105**, 445–449

Roman, B.L., Sommer, R.J., Shinomiya, K. & Peterson, R.E. (1995) In utero and lactational exposure of the male rat to 2,3,7,8-tetrachlorodibenzo-*p*-dioxin: impaired prostate growth and development without inhibited androgen production. *Toxicol. appl. Pharmacol.*, **134**, 241–250

Romkes, M. & Safe, S. (1988) Comparative activities of 2,3,7,8-tetrachlorodibenzo-*p*-dioxin and progesterone as antiestrogens in the female rat uterus. *Toxicol. appl. Pharmacol.*, **92**, 368–380

Romkes, M., Piskorska Pliszczynska, J. & Safe, S. (1987) Effects of 2,3,7,8-tetrachlorodibenzo-*p*-dioxin on hepatic and uterine estrogen receptor levels in rats. *Toxicol. appl. Pharmacol.*, **87**, 306–314

Rordorf, B.F. (1987) Prediction of vapor pressures, boiling points, and enthalpies of fusion for twenty-nine halogenated dibenzo-*p*-dioxins. *Thermochim. Acta*, **112**, 117–122

Rordorf, B.F. (1989) Prediction of vapor pressures, boiling points, and enthalpies of fusion for twenty-nine halogenated dibenzo-*p*-dioxins and fifty-five dibenzofurans by a vapor pressure correlation method. *Chemosphere*, **18**, 183–788

Rose, J.Q., Ramsey, J.C., Wentzler, T.H., Hummel, R.A. & Gehring, P.J. (1976) The fate of 2,3,7,8-tetrachlorodibenzo-p-dioxin following single and repeated oral doses to the rat. *Toxicol. appl. Pharmacol.*, **36**, 209–226

Rosenberg, C., Kontsas, H., Tornaeus, J., Mutanen, P., Jäppinen, P., Patterson, D.G., Jr, Needham, L.L. & Vainio, H. (1994) PCDD/PCDF levels in the blood of workers in a pulp and paper mill. *Organohalogen Compounds*, **21**, 101–104

Rosenberg, C., Kontsas, H., Tornaeus, J., Mutanen, P., Jäppinen, P., Vainio, H., Patterson, D.G., Jr & Needham, L.L. (1995) PCDD/PCDF levels in the blood of workers at a pulp and paper mill. *Chemosphere*, **31**, 3933–3944

Rosenthal, G.J., Lebetkin, E., Thigpen, J.E., Wilson, R., Tucker, A.N. & Luster, M.I. (1989) Characteristics of 2,3,7,8-tetrachlorodibenzo-*p*-dioxin induced endotoxin hypersensitivity: association with hepatoxicity. *Toxicology*, **56**, 239–251

Rotard, W., Christmann, W., Lattner, A., Mann, W., Reichert, A., Reiss, S. & Schinz, V. (1987) Occurrence of PCDD and PCDF in motor oils, rerefined oils and contaminated soils. *Chemosphere*, **16**, 1847–1849

Rotard, W., Christmann, W. & Knoth, W. (1994) Background levels of PCDD/F in soils of Germany. *Chemosphere*, **29**, 2193–2200

Roth, W., Voorman, R. & Aust, S.D. (1988) Activity of thyroid hormone-inducible enzymes following treatment with 2,3,7,8-tetrachlorodibenzo-*p*-dioxin. *Toxicol. appl. Pharmacol.*, **92**, 65–74

Rozman, K. (1984) Hexadecane increases the toxicity of 2,3,7,8-tetrachlorodibenzo-*p*-dioxin (TCDD): is brown adipose tissue the primary target in TCDD-induced wasting syndrome? *Biochem. biophys. Res. Commun.*, **125**, 996–1004

Rozman, K., Rozman, T. & Greim, H. (1984) Effect of thyroidectomy and thyroxine on 2,3,7,8-tetrachlorodibenzo-*p*-dioxin (TCDD) induced toxicity. *Toxicol. appl. Pharmacol.*, **72**, 372–376

Rozman, K., Rozman, T., Scheufler, E., Pazdernik, T. & Greim H. (1985a) Thyroid hormones modulate the toxicity of 2,3,7,8-tetrachlorodibenzo-*p*-dioxin (TCDD). *J. Toxicol. environ. Health*, **16**, 481–491

Rozman, K., Hazelton, G. A., Klaassen, C.D., Arlotto, M.P. & Parkinson, A. (1985b) Effect of thyroid hormones on liver microsomal enzyme induction in rats exposed to 2,3,7,8-tetrachlorodibenzo-*p*-dioxin. *Toxicology*, **37**, 51–63

Rozman, K., Strassle, B. & Iatropoulos, M.J. (1986) Brown adipose tissue is a target tissue in 2,3,7,8-tetrachlorodibenzo-*p*-dioxin (TCDD) induced toxicity. *Arch. Toxicol.*, **9** (Suppl.), 356–360

Rozman, K., Gorski, J.R., Dutton, D. & Parkinson, A. (1987) Effects of vitamin A and/or thyroidectomy on liver microsomal enzymes and their induction in 2,3,7,8-tetrachloro-dibenzo-p-dioxin-treated rats. *Toxicology*, **46**, 107–117

Rozman, K., Pfeifer, B., Kerecsen, L. & Alper, R.H. (1991) Is a serotonergic mechanism involved in 2,3,7,8- tetrachlorodibenzo-p-dioxin (TCDD)-induced appetite suppression in the Sprague Dawley rat? *Arch. Toxicol.*, **65**, 124–128

Rozman, K., Roth, W.L., Greim, H., Stahl, B.U. & Doull, J. (1993) Relative potency of chlori-nated dibenzo-p-dioxins (CDDs) in acute, subchronic and chronic (carcinogenicity) toxicity studies: implications for risk assessment of chemical mixtures. *Toxicology*, **77**, 39–50

Ruangwies, S., Bestervelt, L.L., Piper, D.W., Nolan, C.J. & Piper, W.N. (1991) Human cho-rionic gonadotropin treatment prevents depressed 17-α-hydroxylase/C17-20 lyase activities and serum testosterone concentrations in 2,3,7,8-tetrachlorodibenzo-p-dioxin-treated rats. *Biol. Reprod.*, **45**, 143–150

Rushmore, T.H. & Pickett, C.B. (1993) Glutathione S-transferases, structure, regulation, and therapeutic implications. *J. biol. Chem.*, **268**, 11475–11478

Rushmore, T.H., King, R.G., Paulson, K.E. & Pickett, C.B. (1990) Regulation of glutathione S-transferase Ya subunit gene expression: identification of a unique xenobiotic-responsive element controlling inductible expression by planar aromatic compounds. *Proc. natl Acad. Sci. USA*, **87**, 3826–3830

Ryan, J.J. (1986) Variation of dioxins and furans in human tissue. *Chemosphere*, **15**, 1585–1593

Ryan, J.J. (1991) Method 1: sampling of drinking-waters containing low suspended solids. In: Rappe, C., Buser, H.-R., Dodet, B. & O'Neill, I.K., eds, *Environmental Carcinogens: Methods of Analysis and Exposure Measurement. Vol. 11: Polychlorinated Dioxins and Dibenzofurans* (IARC Scientific Publications No. 108), Lyon, IARC, pp. 199–203

Ryan, J.J., Lau, P.-Y., Pilon, J.C. & Lewis, D. (1983) 2,3,7,8-Tetrachlorodibenzo-p-dioxin and 2,3,7,8-tetrachlorodibenzofuran residues in great lakes commercial and sport fish. In: Choudhary, G., Keith, L.H. & Rappe, C., eds, *Chlorinated Dioxins and Dibenzofurans in the Total Environment*, Boston, Buttersworth Publishers, pp. 87–97

Ryan, J.J., Lizotte, R., Sakuma, T. & Mori, B. (1985a) Chlorinated dibenzo-p-dioxins, chlori-nated dibenzofurans, and pentachlorophenol in Canadian chicken and pork samples. *J. agric. Food Chem.*, **33**, 1021–1026

Ryan, J.J., Williams, D.T., Lau, B.P.-Y. & Sakuma, T. (1985b) Analysis of human fat tissue for 2,3,7,8-tetrachlorodibenzo-p-dioxin and chlorinated dibenzofuran residues. In: Keith, L.H., Rappe, C. & Choudhary, G., eds, *Chlorinated Dioxins and Dibenzofurans in the Total Envi-ronment*, Vol. II, Stoneham, M.A., Butterworth, pp. 205–214

Ryan, J.J., Lizotte, R. & Lau, B.P.-Y. (1985c) Chlorinated dibenzo-p-dioxins and chlorinated dibenzofurans in Canadian human adipose tissue. *Chemosphere*, **14**, 697–706

Ryan, J.J., Schecter, A., Sun, W.-F. & Lizotte, R. (1986) Distribution of chlorinated dibenzo-p-dioxins and chlorinated dibenzofurans in human tissues from the general population. In: Rappe, C., Choudhary, G. & Keith, L.H., eds, *Chlorinated Dioxins and Dibenzofurans in Perspective*, Michigan, Lewis Publishers, pp. 3–16

Ryan, J.J., Schecter, A., Masuda, Y. & Kikuchi, M. (1987) Comparison of PCDDs and PCDFs in the tissues of Yusho Patients with those from the general population in Japan and China. *Chemosphere*, **16**, 2017–2025

Ryan, J.J., Lizotte, R., Panopio, L.G. & Lau, B. P.-Y. (1989a) The effect of strong alkali on the determination of polychlorinated dibenzo-*p*-dioxins (PCDDs). *Chemosphere*, **18**, 149–154

Ryan, R.P., Sunahara, G.I., Lucier, G.W., Birnbaum, L.S. & Nelson, K.G. (1989b) Decreased ligand binding to the hepatic glucocorticoid and epidermal growth factor receptors after 2,3,4,7,8-pentachlorodibenzofuran and 1,2,3,4,7,8-hexachlorodibenzofuran treatment of pregnant mice. *Toxicol. appl. Pharmacol.*, **98**, 454–464

Ryan, J.J., Panopio, L.G., Lewis, D.A., Weber, D.F. & Conacher, H.B.S. (1990) PCDDs/PCDFs in 22 categories of food collected from six Canadian cities between 1985 and 1988. *Organohalogen Compounds*, **1**, 495–500

Ryan, J.J., Panopio, L.G., Lewis, D.A. & Weber, D.F. (1991) Polychlorinated dibenzo-*p*-dioxins and polychlorinated dibenzofurans in cows' milk packaged in plastic-coated bleached paperboard containers. *J. agric. Food Chem.*, **39**, 218–223

Ryan, J.J., Levesque, D., Panopio, L.G., Sun, W.F., Masuda, Y. & Kuroki, H. (1993) Elimination of polychlorinated dibenzofurans (PCDFs) and polychlorinated biphenyls (PCBs) from human blood in the Yusho and Yu-Cheng rice oil poisonings. *Arch. environ. Contam. Toxicol.*, **24**, 504–512

Ryan, J.J., Hsu, C.-C., Boyle, M.J. & Guo, Y.-L.L. (1994) Blood serum levels of PCDFs and PCBs in Yu-Cheng children perinatally exposed to a toxic rice oil. *Chemosphere*, **29**, 1263–1278

Rylander, L. & Hagmar, L. (1995) Mortality and cancer incidence among women with a high consumption of fatty fish contaminated with persistent organochlorine compounds. *Scand. J. Work. Environ. Health*, **21**, 419–426

Ryu, B.W., Roy, S., Sparrow, B.R., Selivonchick, D.P. & Schaup, H.W. (1995) Ah receptor involvement in mediation of pyruvate carboxylase levels and activity in mice given 2,3,7,8-tetrachlorodibenzo-*p*-dioxin. *J. biochem. Toxicol.*, **10**, 103–109

Sadek, C.M. & Allen-Hoffman, B.L. (1994a) Cytochrome P450IA1 is rapidly induced in normal human keratinocytes in the absence of xenobiotics. *J. biol. Chem.*, **269**, 16067–16074

Sadek, C.M. & Allen-Hoffmann, B.L. (1994b) Suspension-mediated induction of Hepa 1c1c7 *Cyp1a-1* expression is dependent on the Ah receptor signal transduction pathway. *J. biol. Chem.*, **269**, 31505–31509

Safe, S.H. (1986) Comparative toxicology and mechanism of action of polychlorinated dibenzo-*p*-dioxins and dibenzofurans. *Ann. Rev. Pharmacol. Toxicol.*, **26**, 371–399

Safe, S. (1990) Polychlorinated biphenyls (PCBs), dibenzo-*p*-dioxins (PCDDs), dibenzofurans (PCDFs) and related compounds: environmental and mechanistic considerations which support the development of toxic equivalency factors (TEFs). *CRC crit. Rev. Toxicol.*, **21**, 51–88

Safe, S. (1995) Modulation of gene expression and endocrine response pathways by 2,3,7,8-tetrachlorodibenzo-*p*-dioxin and related compounds. *Pharmacol. Ther.*, **67**, 247–281

Safe, S., Astroff, B., Harris, M. Zacharewski, T., Dickerson, R., Romkes, M. & Biegel, L. (1991) 2,3,7,8-Tetrachlorodibenzo-*p*-dioxin (TCDD) and related compounds as antiestrogens: characterization and mechanism of action. *Pharmacol. Toxicol.*, **69**, 400–409

Sagunski, H., Csicsaky, M., Fertmann, R., Roller, M. & Schümann, M. (1993) Regressing levels of PCDD/PCDF in human blood samples on age: a new look on reference values. *Chemosphere*, **27**, 227–232

Sandalls, J., Berryman, B., Bennett, L., Newstead, S. & Fox, A. (1996) Dioxins on land around a chemicals waste incinerator and assignment of source. *Organohalogen Compounds*, **28**, 25–30

Sandell, E. & Tuominen, J. (1993) Polychlorinated dioxin and furan levels in sawmill soils. *Organohalogen Compounds*, **12**, 251–254

Santostefano, M.J., Johnson, K.L., Whisnant, N.A., Richardson, V.M., DeVito, M.J., Diliberto, J.J. & Birnbaum, L.S. (1996) Subcellular localization of TCDD differs between the liver, lungs and kidneys after acute and subchronic exposure: species/dose comparisons and possible mechanism. *Fundam. appl. Toxicol.*, **34**, 265-275

Saracci, R., Kogevinas, M., Bertazzi P.A., Bueno de Mesquita, H.B., Coggon, D., Green, L.M., Kauppinen, T., L'Abbé, K. A., Littorin, M., Lynge, E., Mathews, J.D., Neuberger, M., Osman, J., Pearce, N. & Winkelman, R. (1991) Cancer mortality in workers exposed to chlorophenoxy herbicides and chlorophenols. *Lancet*, **338**, 1027–1032

Sauer, P.J.J., Huisman, M., Koopman-Esseboom, C., Morse, D.C., Smits-van Prooije, A.E., van de Berg, K.J., Tuinstra, L.G.M.Th., van der Paauw, C.G., Boersma, E.R., Weisglas-Kuperus, N., Lammers, J.H.C.M., Kulig, B.M. & Brouwer, A. (1994) Effects of polychlorinated biphenyls (PCBs) and dioxins on growth and development. *Hum. exp. Toxicol.*, **13**, 900–906

Savas, U., Bhattacharyya, K.K., Christou, M., Alexander, D.L. & Jefcoate, C.R. (1994) Mouse cytochrome P-450EF, representative of a new 1B subfamily of cytochrome P-450s. Cloning, sequence determination, and tissue expression. *J. biol. Chem.*, **269**, 14905–14911

Schafer, M.W., Madhukar, B.V., Swanson, H.I., Tullis, K. & Denison, M.S. (1993) Protein kinase C is not involved in Ah receptor transformation and DNA binding. *Arch. Biochem. Biophys.* **307**, 267–271

Schantz, S.L. & Bowman, R.E. (1989) Learning in monkeys exposed perinatally to 2,3,7,8-tetra-chlorodibenzo-*p*-dioxin(TCDD). *Neurotoxicol. Teratol.*, **11**, 13–19

Schantz, S.L., Barsotti, D.A. & Allen, J.R. (1979) Toxicological effects produced in nonhuman primates chronically exposed to fifty parts per trillion 2,3,7,8-tetrachlorodibenzo-*p*-dioxin (TCDD). *Toxicol. appl. Pharmacol.*, **48**, A180

Schantz, S.L., Ferguson, S.A. & Bowman, R.E. (1992) Effects of 2,3,7,8-tetrachlorodibenzo-*p*-dioxin on behavior of monkeys in peer groups. *Neurotoxicol. Teratol.*, **14**, 433–446

Schatowitz, B., Brandt, G., Gafner, F., Schlumpf, E., Bühler, R., Hasler, P. & Nussbaumer, T. (1994) Dioxin emissions from wood combustion. *Chemosphere*, **29**, 2005–2013

Schecter, A. (1986) The Binghamton State Office Building PCB, dioxin and dibenzofuran electrical transformer incident: 1981–1986. *Chemosphere*, **15**, 1273–1280

Schecter, A. (1994) *Exposure Assessment Measurement of Dioxins and Related Chemicals in Human Tissues*, In: Schecter, A., ed., *Dioxins and Health*, New York, Plenum Press, pp. 449–485

Schecter, A. & Charles, K. (1991) The Binghamton State Office building transformer incident after one decade. *Chemosphere*, **23**, 1307–1321

Schecter, A., Ryan, J.J., Lizotte, R., Sun, W.-F., Miller, L., Gitlitz, G. & Bogdasarian, M. (1985a) Chlorinated dibenzodioxins and dibenzofurans in human adipose tissue from exposed and control New York State patients. *Chemosphere*, **14**, 933–937

Schecter, A., Tiernan, T., Schaffner, F., Taylor, M., Gitlitz, G., Van Ness, G.F., Garrett, J.H. & Wagel, D.J. (1985b) Patient fat biopsies for chemical analysis and liver biopsies for ultrastructural characterization after exposure to polychlorinated dioxins, furans and PCBs. *Environ. Health Perspectives*, **60**, 241–254

Schecter, A., Ryan, J.J. & Gitlitz, G. (1986a) Chlorinated dioxin and dibenzofuran levels in human adipose tissues from exposed and control populations. In: *Chlorinated Dioxins and Dibenzofurans in Perspective*, Miami Beach, FL, Lewis Publishers, pp. 51–65

Schecter, A.J., Ryan, J.J., Gross, M., Weerasinghe, N.C.A. & Constable, J.D. (1986b) Chlorinated dioxins and dibenzofurans in human tissues from Vietnam, 1983–84. *Chlorinated Dioxins and Dibenzofurans in Perspective*, Miami Beach, FL, Lewis Publishers, pp. 35–50

Schecter, A.J., Ryan, J.J. & Constable, J.D. (1986c) Chlorinated dibenzo-*p*-dioxin and dibenzofuran levels in human adipose tissue and milk samples from the north and south of Vietnam. *Chemosphere*, **15**, 1613–1620

Schecter, A., Ryan, J.J. & Constable, J.D. (1987) Polychlorinated dibenzo-*p*-dioxin and polychlorinated dibenzofuran levels in human breast milk from Vietnam compared with cow's milk and human breast milk from the North American continent. *Chemosphere*, **16**, 2003–2016

Schecter, A., Kooke, R., Serne, P., Olie, K., Do 'Quang Huy, Nguyen Hue & Constable, J. (1989a) Chlorinated dioxin and dibenzofuran levels in food samples collected between 1985–87 in the North and South of Vietnam. *Chemosphere*, **18**, 627–634

Schecter, A., Mes, J. & Davies, D. (1989b) Polychlorinated biphenyl (PCB), DDT, DDE and hexachlorobenzene (HCB) and PCDD/F isomer levels in various organs in autopsy tissue from North American patients. *Chemosphere*, **18**, 811–818

Schecter, A., Dan Vu, Tong, H.Y., Monson, S.J., Gross, M.L. & Constable, J.D. (1989c) Levels of 2,3,7,8-TCDD and 2,3,7,8-TCDF in human adipose tissue from hospitalized persons in the North and South of Vietnam 1984–88. *Chemosphere*, **19**, 1001–1004

Schecter, A., Fürst, P., Ryan, J.J., Fürst, C., Meemken, H.-A., Groebel, W., Constable, J. & Vu, D. (1989d) Polychlorinated dioxin and dibenzofuran levels from human milk from several locations in the United States, Germany and Vietnam. *Chemosphere*, **19**, 979–984

Schecter A., Fürst P., Krüger C., Meemken H.-A., Groebel, W. & Constable, J.D. (1989e) Levels of polychlorinated dibenzofurans, dibenzodioxins, PCBs, DDT and DDE, hexachlorobenzene, dieldrin, hexachlorocyclohexanes and oxychlordane in human breast milk from the United States, Thailand, Vietnam, and Germany. *Chemosphere*, **18**, 445–454

Schecter, A., Fürst, P., Fürst, C., Groebel, W., Constable, J.D., Kolesnikov, S., Beim, A., Boldonov, A., Trubitsun, E., Vaslov, B., Hoang, D.C., Le, C.D. & Hoang, T.Q. (1990a) Levels of chlorinated dioxins, dibenzofurans and other chlorinated xenobiotics in food from the Soviet Union and the South of Vietnam. *Chemosphere*, **20**, 799–806

Schecter, A., Ryan, J.J., Päpke, O. & Ball, M. (1990b) Comparison of dioxin and dibenzofuran levels in whole blood, blood plasma and adipose tissue, on a lipid basis. *Organohalogen Compounds*, **1**, 279–281

Schecter, A., Tong, H.Y., Monson, S.J., Gross, M.L., Raisanen, S., Karhunen, T., Österlund, E.K., Constable, J.D., Hoang, D.C., Le, C.D., Hoang, T.Q., Ton, D.L., Nguyen, T.N.P., Phan, H.P. & Dan, V. (1990c) Human adipose tissue dioxin and dibenzofuran levels and 'dioxin toxic equivalents' in patients from the North and South of Vietnam. *Chemosphere*, **20**, 943–950

Schecter, A., Päpke, O. & Ball, M. (1990d) Evidence for transplacental transfer of dioxins from mother to fetus: chlorinated dioxin and dibenzofuran levels in the livers of stillborn infants. *Chemosphere*, **21**, 1017–1022

Schecter, A., Startin, J.R., Rose, M., Wright, C., Parker, I., Woods, D. & Hansen, H. (1990e) Chlorinated dioxin and dibenzofuran levels in human milk from Africa, Pakistan, Southern Vietnam, the Southern U.S. and England. *Chemosphere*, **20**, 919–925

Schecter, A., Fürst, P., Fürst, C., Groebel, W., Kolesnikov, S., Savchenkov, M, Beim, A., Boldonov, A., Trubitsun, E. & Vlasov, B. (1990f) Levels of dioxins, dibenzofurans and other chlorinated xenobiotics in human milk from the Soviet Union. *Chemosphere*, **20**, 927–934

Schecter, A., Fürst, P., Fürst, C. & Groebel, W. (1990g) Human milk dioxin and dibenzofuran levels and levels of other chlorinated chemicals from various countries, including Vietnam and Cambodia as compared to the Soviet Union, Germany, and United States. *Organohalogen Compounds*, **1**, 267–270

Schecter, A., Ryan, J.J., Constable, J.D., Baughman, R., Bangert, J., Fürst, P., Wilmers, K. & Oates, R.D. (1990h) Partitioning of 2,3,7,8-chlorinated dibenzo-*p*-dioxins and dibenzofurans between adipose tissue and plasma lipid of 20 Massachusetts Vietnam veterans. *Chemosphere*, **20**, 951–958

Schecter, A., Päpke, O., Ball, M. & Ryan, J.J. (1991a) Partitioning of dioxins and dibenzofurans: whole blood, blood plasma and adipose tissue. *Chemosphere*, **23**, 1913–1919

Schecter, A., Fürst, P., Fürst, C., Päpke, O., Ball, M., Le, C.D., Hoang, T.Q., Nguyen, T.N.P., Beim, A., Vlasov, B., Chongchet, V., Constable, J.D. & Charles, K. (1991b) Dioxins, dibenzofurans and selected chlorinated organic compounds in human milk and blood from Cambodia, Germany, Thailand, the U.S.A., the U.S.S.R., and Viet Nam. *Chemosphere*, **23**, 1903–1912

Schecter, A., Päpke, O., Ball, M., Grachev, M., Beim, A., Koptug, V., Hoang, D.C., Le, C.D., Hoang, T.Q., Nguyen, N.T.P. & Huynh, K.C. (1992) Dioxin and dibenzofuran levels in human blood samples from Guam, Russia, Germany, Vietnam and the USA. *Chemosphere*, **25**, 1129–1134

Schecter, A., Päpke, O., Lis, A. & Ball, M. (1993a) Chlorinated dioxin and dibenzofuran content in 2,4-D amine salt from Ufa, Russia. In: Fiedler, H., Frank, H., Hutzinger, O., Parzefall, W., Riss, A. & Safe, S., eds, *Dioxin 1993, 13th International Symposium on Chlorinated Dioxins and Related Compounds, Vienna, September 1993*, pp. 325–328

Schecter, A., Ryan, J.J., Päpke, O., Ball, M. & Lis, A. (1993b) Elevated dioxin levels in the blood of male and female Russian workers with and without chloracne 25 years after phenoxyherbicide exposure: The UFA 'Khimprom' incident. *Chemosphere*, **27**, 253–258

Schecter, A., Startin, J., Wright, C., Kelly, M., Päpke O., Lis, A., Ball, M. & Olson, J.R. (1994a) Congener-specific levels of dioxins and dibenzofurans in US food and estimated daily dioxin toxic equivalent intake. *Environ. Health Perspectives*, **102**, 962–966

Schecter, A., Päpke, O., Lis, A. & Ball, M. (1994b) Chlorinated dioxin and dibenzofuran levels in U.S. human placentas and fetal tissue in comparison with U.S. adult population dioxin levels. *Organohalogen Compounds*, **21**, 63–66

Schecter, A., Le, C.D., Le, T.B.T., Hoang, T.Q., Dinh, Q.M., Hoang, D.C., Constable, J.D., Baughman, R., Päpke, O., Ryan, J.J., Fürst, P. & Räisänen, S. (1995) Agent Orange and the Vietnamese: the persistence of elevated dioxin levels in human tissues. *Am. J. public Health*, **85**, 516–522

Schecter, A., Cramer, P., Boggess, K., Stanley, J., Olson, J.R. & Kessler, H. (1996a) Dioxin intake from U.S. food: results from a new nationwide food survey. *Organohalogen Compounds*, **28**, 320–324

Shecter, A., Startin, J., Wright, C., Päpke, O., Ball, M. & Lis, A. (1996b) Concentrations of polychlorinated dibenzo-*p*-dioxins and dibenzofurans in human placental and fetal tissues from the U.S. and in placentas from Yu-Cheng exposed mothers. *Chemosphere*, **32**, 551–557

Schecter, A., Kassis, I. & Päpke, O. (1996c) Partitioning of PCDDs, PDCFs, and coplanar PCBs in human maternal tissues: blood, milk, adipose tissue and placenta. *Organohalogen Compounds*, **30**, 33–36

Schecter, A., Päpke, O. & Fürst, P. (1996d) Is there a decrease in general population dioxin body burden? A review of German and American data. *Organohalogen Compounds*, **30**, 57–60

Schiller, C.M., King, M.W. & Walden, R. (1986) Alterations in lipid parameters associated with changes in 2,3,7,8-tetrachlorodibenzo-*p*-dioxin (TCDD)-induced mortality in rats. In: Rappe, C., Choudhary, G. & Keith, L.H., eds, *Chlorinated Dioxins and Dibenzofurans in Perspective*, Chelsea, MI, Lewis Publishers, pp. 285–302

Schimmel, H., Griepink, B., Maier, E.A., Kramer, G.N., Roos, A.H. & Tuinstra, L.G.M.T. (1994) Intercomparison study on milk powder fortified with PCDD and PCDF. *Fresenius J. analyt. Chem.*, **348**, 37–46

Schlabach, M., Biseth, A. & Gundersen, H. (1996) Sampling and measurement of PCDD/PCDF and non-ortho PCB in arctic air at Ny-Alesund, Spitsbergen. *Organohalogen Compounds*, **28**, 325–329

Schlatter, C. (1991) Data on kinetics of PCDDs and PCDFs as a prerequisite for human risk assessment. In: Gallo, M.A., Scheuplein, R.J. & van der Heijden, K.A., eds, *Biological Basis for Risk Assessment of Dioxins and Related Compounds* (Banbury Report 35), Cold Spring Harbor Laboratory, NY, CSH Press, pp. 215–228

Schlesing, Dr. H. (1989) Analytical program for the risk assessment of a closed herbicide plant in Germany. *Chemosphere*, **18**, 903–912

Schmid, P. & Schlatter, C. (1992) Polychlorinated dibenzo-*p*-dioxins (PCDDs) and polychlorinated dibenzofurans (PCDFs) in cow's milk from Switzerland. *Chemosphere*, **24**, 1013–1030

Schmidt, A., Stroh, H.-J., Korte, M. & Stahlmann, R. (1992) 2,3,7,8-Tetrachlorodibenzo-*p*-dioxin does not influence the cell proliferation in popliteal lymph nodes after foot pad injection of cellular and non-cellular antigens in mice. *Chemosphere*, **25**, 985–990

Schmidt, J.V., Su, G.H.-T., Reddy, J.K., Simon, M.C. & Bradfield, C.A. (1996) Characterization of a murine Ahr null allele: involvement of the Ah receptor in hepatic growth and development. *Proc. natl Acad. Sci. USA*, **93**, 6731–6736

Schrenk, D., Karger, A., Lipp, H.-P. & Bock, K.W. (1992) 2,3,7,8-Tetrachlorodibenzo-*p*-dioxin and ethinylestradiol as co-mitogens in cultured rat hepatocytes. *Carcinogenesis*, **13**, 453–456

Schrenk, D., Buchmann, A., Dietz, K., Lipp, H.-P., Brunner, H., Sirma, H., Münzel, P., Hagenmaier, H., Gebhardt, R. & Bock, K.W. (1994a) Promotion of preneoplastic foci in rat liver with 2,3,7,8-tetrachlorodibenzo-*p*-dioxin, 1,2,3,4,6,7,8-heptachlorodibenzo-*p*-dioxin and a defined mixture of 49 polychlorinated dibenzo-*p*-dioxins. *Carcinogenesis*, **15**, 509–515

Schrenk, D., Schäfer, S. & Bock, K.W. (1994b) 2,3,7,8-Tetrachlorodibenzo-*p*-dioxin as growth modulator in mouse hepatocytes with high and low affinity Ah receptor. *Carcinogenesis*, **15**, 27–31

Schrenk, D., Stuven, T., Gohl, G., Viebahn, R. & Bock, K.W. (1995) Induction of CYP1A and glutathione S-transferase activities by 2,3,7,8-tetrachlorodibenzo-*p*-dioxin in human hepatocyte cultures. *Carcinogenesis*, **16**, 943–946

Schrey, P., Wittsiepe, J., Ewers, U., Exner, M. & Selenka, F. (1992) Age-related increase of PCDD/F-levels in human blood - a study with 95 unexposed persons from Germany. *Organohalogen Compounds*, **9**, 261–267

Schuhmacher, M., Granero, S., Domingo, J.L., Rivera, J. & Eljarrat, E. (1996) Levels of PCDD/F in soil samples in the vicinity of a municipal solid waste incinerator. *Organohalogen Compounds*, **28**, 330–334

Schwetz, B.A., Norris, J.M., Sparschu, G.L., Rowe, V.K., Gehring, P.J., Emerson, JL. & Gerbid, C.G. (1973) Toxicology of chlorinated dibenzo-*p*-dioxins. *Environ. Health Perspectives*, **5**, 87–99

Seefeld, M.D. & Peterson, R.E. (1984) Digestible energy and efficiency of feed utilization in rats treated with 2,3,7,8-tetrachlorodibenzo-*p*-dioxin *Toxicol. appl. Pharmacol.*, **74**, 214–222

Seefeld, M.D., Albrecht, R.M. & Peterson, R.E. (1979) Effects of 2,3,7,8-tetrachlorodibenzo-*p*-dioxin on indocyanine green blood clearance in rhesus monkeys. *Toxicology*, **14**, 263–272

Seefeld, M.D., Corbett, S.W., Keesey, R.E. & Peterson, R.E. (1984a) Characterization of the wasting syndrome in rats treated with 2,3,7,8-tetrachlorodibenzo-*p*-dioxin. *Toxicol. appl. Pharmacol.*, **73**, 311–322

Seefeld, M.D., Keesey, R.E. & Peterson, R.E. (1984b) Body weight regulation in rats treated with 2,3,7,8-tetrachlorodibenzo-*p*-dioxin. *Toxicol. appl. Pharmacol.*, **76**, 526–536

Seegal, R.F. & Schantz, S.L. (1994) Neurochemical and behavioral sequelae of exposure to dioxins and PCBs. In: Schecter, A., ed., *Dioxins and Health*, New York, Plenum Press, pp. 409–447

Seo, B.-W., Li, M-H., Hansen, L.G., Moore, R.W., Peterson, R.E. & Schantz, S. (1995) Effects of gestational and lactational exposure to coplanar polychlorinated biphenyl PCB) congeners or 2,3,7,8-tetrachlorodibenzo-*p*-dioxin (TCDD) on thyroid hormone concentrations in weanling rats. *Toxicol. Lett.*, **78**, 253–262

Sewall, C.H., Lucier, G.W., Tritscher, A.M., and Clark, G.C. (1993) TCDD-mediated changes in hepatic epidermal growth factor receptor may be a critical event in the hepatocarcinogenic action of TCDD. *Carcinogenesis*, **14**, 1885–1893

Sewall, C.H., Flagler, N., Vanden Heuvel, J.P., Clark, G.C., Tritscher, A.M., Maronpot, R.M. & Lucier, G.W. (1995) Alterations in thyroid function in female Sprague-Dawley rats following chronic treatment with 2,3,7,8-tetrachlorodibenzo-*p*-dioxin. *Toxicol. appl. Pharmacol.*, **132**, 237–244

Shaw, P.M., Reiss, A., Adesnik, M., Nebert, D.W., Schembri, J. & Jaiswal, A.K. (1991) The human dioxin-inducible NAD(P)H:quinone oxidoreductase cDNA-encoded protein expressed in COS-1 cells is identical to diaphorase 4. *Eur. J. Biochem.*, **195**, 161–171

She, J. & Hagenmaier, H. (1996) Levels and fate of PCDD/Fs in soil around Rastatt in Southwest Germany. *Organohalogen Compounds*, **28**, 31–34

Shen, E.S., Gutman, S.I. & Olson, J.R. (1991) comparison of 2,3,7,8-tetrachlorodibenzo-*p*-dioxin-mediated hepatotoxicity in C57BL/6J and DBA/2J mice. *J. Toxicol. environ. Health*, **32**, 367–381

Shen, Z., Liu, J., Wells, R.L. & Elkind, M.M. (1994a) cDNA cloning, sequence analysis, and induction by aryl hydrocarbons of a murine cytochrome P450 gene, *Cyp1B1*. *DNA Cell Biol.*, **13**, 763–769

Shen, Z., Wells, R.L. & Elkind, M.M.(1994b) Enhanced cytochrome P450 (*Cyp1B1*) expression, aryl hydrocarbon hydroxylase activity, cytotoxicity, and transformation of C3H 10T1/2 cells by dimethylbenz(*a*)anthracene in conditioned medium. *Cancer Res.*, **54**, 4052–4056

Shimada, T., Hayes, C.L., Yamazaki, H., Amin, S., Hecht, S.S., Guengerich, F.P. & Sutter, T.R. (1996) Activation of chemically diverse procarcinogens by human cytochrome P-450 1B1. *Cancer Res.*, **56**, 2979–2984

Shiverick, K.T. & Muther, T.F. (1983) 2,3,7,8-tetrachlorodibenzo-p-dioxin (TCDD) effects on hepatic microsomal steroid metabolism and serum estradiol of pregnant rats. *Biochem. Pharmacol.*, **32**, 991–995

Shu, H.P., Paustenbach, D.J. & Murray, F.J. (1987) A critical evaluation of the use of mutagenesis, carcinogenesis, and tumor promotion data in a cancer risk assessment of 2,3,7,8-tetrachlorodibenzo-*p*-dioxin. *Regul. Toxicol. Pharmacol.*, **7**, 57–88

Shuler, C.T., Halpern, D.E., Guo, Y. & Sank, A.C. (1992) Medial edge epithelium fate traced by cell lineage analysis during epithelial-mesenchymal transformation *in vivo*. *Dev. Biol.*, **154**, 318–330

Sievers, S., Reich, T. & Schwörer, R. (1993) Contents of PCDD/F in soil and atmospheric deposition in an agricultural area of an urban region (Hamburg, FRG). *Organohalogen Compounds*, **12**, 275–278

Sijm, D.T.H.M., Wever, H., de Vries, P.J. & Opperhuizen, A. (1989) Octan-1-ol/water partition coefficients of polychlorinated dibenzo-*p*-dioxins and dibenzofurans: experimental values determined with a stirring method. *Chemosphere*, **19**, 263–266

Sills, R.C., Goldsworthy, T.L. & Sleight, S.D. (1994) Tumor-promoting effects of 2,3,7,8-tetrachlorodibenzo-*p*-dioxin and phenobarbital in initiated weanling Sprague-Dawley rats: a quantitative, phenotypic, and *ras* p21 protein study. *Toxicol. Pathol.*, **22**, 270–281

Silver, G. & Krauter, K.S. (1988) Expression of cytochromes P-450c and P-450d mRNAs in cultured rat hepatocytes. 3-Methylcholanthrene induction is regulated primarily at the post-transcriptional level. *J. biol. Chem.*, **263**, 11802–11807

Silverstone, A.E., Frazier, D.E., Fiore, N.C., Soults, J.A. & Gasiewicz, T.A. (1994a) Dexamethasone, 17β-estradiol, and 2,3,7,8-tetrachlorodibenzo-*p*-dioxin elicit thymic atrophy through different cellular targets. *Toxicol. appl. Pharmacol.*, **126**, 248–259

Silverstone, A.E., Frazier, D.E. & Gasiewicz, T.A. (1994b) Alternate immunsystem targets for TCDD: lymphocyte stem cells and extrathymic T-cells development. *Exp. clin. Immunogenet.*, **11**, 94–101

Singh, S.S. & Perdew, G.H. (1993) Effect of staurosporine on the Ah receptor levels in Hepa 1 cells. *Toxicologist*, **13**, 14

Sirkka, U., Pohjanvirta, R., Nieminen, S.A., Tuomisto, J. & Ylitalo, P. (1992) Acute neurobehavioural effects of 2,3,7,8-tetrachlorodibenzo-*p*-dioxin (TCDD) in Han/Wistar rats. *Pharmacol. Toxicol.*, **71**, 284–288

Slob, W., Olling, M., Derks, H.J.G.M. & Dejong, A.P.J.M. (1995) Congener-specific bioavailability of PCDD/Fs and coplanar PCBs in cows: Laboratory and field measurements.. *Chemosphere*, **31**, 3827–3838

Smialowicz, R.J., Riddle, M.M., Willams, W.C. & Diliberto, J.J. (1994) Effects of 2,3,7,8-tetra-chlorodibenzo-*p*-dioxin (TCDD) on humoral immunity and lymphocyte subpopulations: Differences between mice and rat. *Toxicol. appl. Pharmacol.*, **124**, 248–256

Smialowicz, R.J., Williams, W.C. & Riddle, M. (1996) Comparison of the T cell-independent antibody response of mice and rats exposed to 2,3,7,8-tetrachloro-dibenzo-*p*-dioxin. *Fundam. appl. Toxicol.*, **32**, 293–297

Smirnov, A.D., Schecter, A., Päpke, O. & Beljak, A.A. (1996) Conclusions from Ufa, Russia, drinking water dioxin cleanup experiments involving different treatment technologies. *Chemosphere*, **32**, 479–489

Smith, A.H. & Pearce, N.E. (1986) Update on soft tissue sarcoma and phenoxy herbicides in New Zealand. *Chemosphere*, **15**, 1795–1799

Smith, J.G. & Christophers, A.J. (1992) Phenoxy herbicides and chlorophenols: a case control study on soft tissue sarcoma and malignant lymphoma. *Br. J. Cancer*, **65**, 442–448

Smith, A.G., Francis, J.E., Kay, S.J.E. & Greig, J.B. (1981) Hepatic toxicity and uroporphyri-nogen decarboxylase activity following a single dose of 2,3,7,8-tetrachloro-dibenzo-*p*-dioxin to mice. *Biochem. Pharmacol.*, **30**, 2825–2830

Smith, A.H., Fisher, D.O., Pearce, N.E., Teague, C.A. (1982a) Do agricultural chemicals cause soft tissue sarcoma ? Initial findings of a case–control study in New Zealand. *Commun. Health Stud.*, **6**, 114–119

Smith, A.H., Fisher, D.O., Pearce, N. & Chapman, C.J. (1982b) Congenital defects and mis-carriages among New Zealand 2,4,5-T sprayers. *Arch. environ. Health*, **37**, 197–200

Smith, A.H., Fisher, D.O., Giles, H.J. & Pearce, N.E. (1983) The New Zealand soft tissue sarcoma case–control study: Interview findings concerning phenoxyacetic acid exposure. *Chemosphere*, **12**, 565–571

Smith, L.M., Stalling, D.L. & Johnson, J.L. (1984a) Determination of part-per-trillion levels of polychlorinated dibenzofurans and dioxins in environmental samples. *Anal. Chem.*, **56**, 1830–1842

Smith, A.H., Pearce, N.E., Fisher, D.O., Giles, H.J., Teague, C.A. & Howard, J.K. (1984b) Soft tissue sarcoma and exposure to phenoxy herbicides and chlorophenols in New Zealand. *J. natl Cancer Inst.*, **73**, 1111–1117

Smith, R.M., O'Keefe, P.W., Hilker, D.R. & Aldous, K.M. (1989) Ambient air and incinerator testing for chlorinated dibenzofurans and dioxins by low resolution mass spectrometry. *Chemosphere*, **18**, 585–592

Smith, R.M., O'Keefe, P.W., Briggs, R., Valente, H. & Connor, S. (1990a) Continuous ambient air monitoring for CDFs and CDDs: Niagara Falls New York, 1988–1989. *Organohalogen Compounds*, **4**, 233–236

Smith, R.M., O'Keefe, P.W., Aldous, K. & Connor, S. (1990b) Continuous atmospheric studies of chlorinated dibenzofurans and dioxins in New York State. *Chemosphere*, **20**, 1447–1453

Smith, A.H., Patterson, D.G., Jr, Warner, M.L., MacKenzie, R. & Needham, L.L. (1992a) Serum 2,3,7,8-tetrachlorodibenzo-*p*-dioxin levels of New Zealand pesticide applicators and their implications for cancer hypotheses. *J. Natl Cancer Inst*, **84**, 104–108

Smith, R.M., O'Keefe, P.W., Aldous, K., Briggs, R., Hilker, D. & Connor, S. (1992b) Measure-ments of PCDFs and PCDDs in air samples and lake sediments at several locations in upstate New York. *Chemosphere*, **25**, 95–108

Smits-van Prooije, A.E., Lammers, J.H.C.M., Waalkens-Berendsen, D.H. & Kulig, B.M. (1992) Effects of 3,4,5,3′,4′,5′-hexachlorobiphenyl alone and in combination with 3,4,3′,4′-tetra-chlorobiphenyl on the reproduction capacity of rats. *Organohalogen Compounds*, **10**, 217–219

Snyder, N.K., Kramer, C.M., Dooley, R.K. & Holsapple, M.P. (1993) Characterization of protein phosphorylation by 2,3,7,8-tetrachlorodibenzo-*p*-dioxin in murine lymphocytes: indirect evidence for a role in the suppression of humoral immunity. *Drug. chem. Toxicol.*, **16**, 135–163

Sogawa, K., Fujisawa-Sehara, A., Yamane, M. & Fujii-Kuriyama, Y. (1986) Location of regu-latory elements responsible for drug induction in the rat cytochrome P-450c gene. *Proc. natl Acad. Sci. USA*, **83**, 8044–8048

Solch, J.G., Ferguson, G.L., Tiernan, T.O., Van Ness, B.F., Garrett, J. H., Wagel, D.J. & Taylor, M.L. (1985) Analytical methodology for determination of 2,3,7,8-tetrachlorodibenzo-*p*-dioxin in soils. In: Keith, L.H., Rappe, C. & Choudhary, G., eds, *Chlorinated Dioxins and Dibenzofurans in the Total Environment II*, Boston, Butterworth, pp. 377–397

Soong, D.-K. & Ling, Y.-C. (1996) Dioxin in soil samples at a chlorophenol manufacturing site in Taiwan. *Organohalogen Compounds*, **28**, 335–339

Sparrow, B.R., Thompson, C.S., Ryu, B., Selevonchick, D.P. & Schaup, H.W. (1994) 2,3,7,8-Tetrachlorodibenzo-*p*-dioxin induced alterations of pyruvate carboxylase levels and lactate dehydrogenase isozyme shifts in C57BL/6J male mice. *J. biochem. Toxicol.*, **9**, 329–335

Sparschu, G.L., Dunn, F.L. & Rowe, V.K. (1971) Study of the teratogenicity of 2,3,7,8-tetra-chlorodibenzo-*p*-dioxin in the rat. *Fd Cosmet. Toxicol.*, **9**, 405–412

Spink, D.C., Lincoln, D.W., II, Dickerman, H.W. & Gierthy, J.F. (1990) 2,3,7,8-Tetrachloro-dibenzo-*p*-dioxin causes an extensive alteration of 17β-estradiol metabolism in MCF-7 breast tumor cells. *Proc. natl Acad. Sci. USA*, **87**, 6917–6921

Spink, D.C., Eugster, H.-P., Lincoln, D.W., Schuetz, J.D., Schuetz, E.G., Johnson, J.A., Kaminsky, L.S. & Gierthy, J.F. (1992) 17beta-Estradiol hydroxylation catalysed by human cytochrome P450 1A1: a comparison of the activities induced by 2,3,7,8-tetrachlorobenzo-p-dioxin in MCF-7 cells with those from heterologous expression of the cDNA. *Arch. Bio-chem. Biophys.*, **293**, 342–348

Spink, D.C., Hayes, C.L., Young, N.R., Christou, M., Sutter, T.R., Jefcoate, C.R. & Gierthy, J.F. (1994) The effects of 2,3,7,8-tetrachlorodibenzo-*p*-dioxin on estrogen metabolism in MCF-7 breast cancer cells: evidence for induction of a novel 17β-estradiol 4-hydroxylase. *J. steroid Biochem. mol. Biol.*, **51**, 251–258

Stahl, B.U. & Rozman, K. (1990) 2,3,7,8-Tetrachlorodibenzo-*p*-dioxin (TCDD)-induced appe-tite suppression in the Sprague-Dawley rat is not a direct effect on feed intake regulation in the brain. *Toxicol. appl. Pharmacol.*, **106**, 158–162

Stahl, B.U., Alper, R.H. & Rozman, K. (1991) Depletion of brain serotonin does not alter 2,3,7,8-tetrachlorodibenzo-para-dioxin (TCDD)-induced starvation syndrome in the rat. *Toxicol. Lett.*, **59**, 65–72

Stahl, B.U., Kettrup, A. & Rozman, K. (1992a) Comparative toxicity of four chlorinated dibenzo-*p*-dioxins (CDDs) and their mixture. Part I: Acute toxicity and toxic equivalency factors (TEFs). *Arch. Toxicol.*, **66**, 471–477

Stahl, B.U., Beer, D.G., Weber, L.W., Lebofsky, M. & Rozman, K. (1992b) Decreased hepatic phosphoenolpyruvate carboxykinase gene expression after 2,3,7,8-tetrachlorodibenzo-*p*-dioxin treatment: implications for the acute toxicity of chlorinated dibenzo-p-dioxins in the rat. *Arch. Toxicol.*, **15** (Suppl.), 151-5–151-155

Stahl, B.U., Beer, D.G., Weber, L.W.D. & Rozman, K. (1993) Reduction of hepatic phos-phoenolpyruvate carboxykinase (PEPCK) activity by 2,3,7,8-tetrachlorodibenzo-*p*-dioxin (TCDD) is due to decreased mRNA levels. *Toxicology*, **79**, 81–95

Stalling, D.L., Smith, L.M., Petty, J.D., Hogan, J.W., Johnson, J.L., Rappe, C. & Buser, H.R. (1983) Residues of polychlorinated dibenzo-*p*-dioxins and dibenzofurans in laurentian great lakes fish. In: Tucker, R.E., Young, A.L. & Gray, A.P., eds, *Human and environmental risks of chlorinated dioxins and related compounds*, New York, Plenum Press, pp. 221–240

Stanley, J.S. & Bauer, K.M. (1989) *Chlorinated Dibenzo-p-dioxin and Dibenzofuran Residue Levels in Food* (Report No. 8922-A), Missouri, Midwest Research Institute

Stanley, J.S., Going, J.E., Redford, D.P., Kutz, F.W. & Young, A.L. (1985) A survey of ana-lytical methods for measurement of polychlorinated dibenzo-*p*-dioxins (PCDD) and poly-chlorinated dibenzofurans (PCDF) in human adipose tissues. In: Keith, L.H., Rappe, C. & Choudhary, G., eds, *Chlorinated Dioxins and Dibenzofurans in the Total Environment II*, Boston, Butterworth, pp. 181–195

Stanley, J.S., Boggess, K.E., Onstot, J. & Sack, T.M. (1986) PCDDs and PCDFs in human adipose tissue from the EPA FY82 NHATS (National Human Adipose Tissue Survey) repo-sitory. *Chemosphere*, **15**, 1605–1612

Stanley, J.S., Ayling, R.E., Cramer, P.H., Thornburg, K.R., Remmers, J.C., Breen, J.J., Schwemberger, J., Kang, H.K. & Watanabe, K. (1990) Polychlorinated dibenzo-*p*-dioxin and dibenzofuran concentration levels in human adipose tissue samples from the continental United States collected from 1971 through 1987. *Chemosphere*, **20**, 895–901

Startin, J.R. (1996) *Analysis of PCDDs, PCDFs and PCBs in Total Diet Study Samples from the Basque region of Spain* (Report COM/BE42/1), Norwich, Central Science Laboratory

Startin, J.R., Rose, M. & Offen, C. (1989) Analysis of PCDDs and PCDFs in human milk from the UK. *Chemosphere*, **19**, 985–988

Startin, J.R., Rose, M., Wright, C., Parker, I. & Gilbert, J. (1990) Surveillance of British foods for PCDDs and PCDFs. *Chemosphere*, **20**, 793–798

Steer, P., Tashiro, C., McIlveen, W., Buonocore, N., Dobroff, F. & Thompson, T. (1990a) Occurrence of dioxins and furans in air and vegetation samples from a tire fire in Ontario, Canada. *Organohalogen Compounds*, **3**, 421–424

Steer, P., Tashiro, C., Clement, R., Lusis, M. & Reiner, E. (1990b) Ambient air sampling of polychlorinated dibenzo-p-dioxins and dibenzofurans in Ontario: preliminary results. *Chemosphere*, **20**, 1431–1437

Stehr, P.A., Stein, G., Falk, H., Samson, E., Smith, S.J., Steinberg, K., Webb, K., Ayres, S., Schramm, W., Donnell, H.D. & Gedney, W.B. (1986) A pilot epidemiologic study of possible health effects associated with 2,3,7,8-tetrachlorodibenzo-*p*-dioxin contaminations in Missouri. *Arch. environ. Health*, **41**, 16–22

Stellman, S.D., Stellman, J.M. & Sommer J.F. (1988) Health and reproductive outcomes among American legionnaires in relation to combat and herbicide exposure in Vietnam. *Environ. Res.*, **47**, 150–174

Stenhouse, I.A. & Badsha, K.S. (1990) PCB, PCDD and PCDF concentrations in soils from the Kirk/Sandall/Edenthorpe/Barnby Dun area. *Chemosphere*, **21**, 563–573

Stephens, R.D., Rappe, C., Hayward, D.G., Nygren, M., Startin, J., Esbøll, A., Carlé, J. & Yrjänheikki, E.J. (1992) World Health Organization international intercalibration study on dioxins and furans in human milk and blood. *Analyt. Chem.*, **64**, 3109–3117

Stephens, R.D., Petreas, M.X. & Hayward, D.G. (1995) Biotransfer and bioaccumulation of dioxins and furans from soil: chickens as a model for foraging animals. *Sci. Total Environ.*, **175**, 253–273

Sterling, T.D. & Arundel, A. (1986) Review of recent Vietnamese studies on the carcinogenic and teratogenic effects of phenoxy herbicide exposure. *Int. J. Health Serv.*, **16**, 265–278

Stinchcombe, S., Buchmann, A., Bock, K.W. & Schwarz, M. (1995) Inhibition of apoptosis during 2,3,7,8-tetrachlorodibenzo-*p*-dioxin mediated tumour promotion in rat liver. *Carcinogenesis*, **16**, 1271–1275

Stockbauer, J.W., Hoffman, R.E., Schramm, W.F. & Edmonds, L.D. (1988) Reproductive outcomes of mothers with potential exposure to 2,3,7,8-tetrachlorodibenzo-*p*-dioxin. *Am. J. Epidemiol.*, **128**, 410–419

Stohs, S.J. (1990) Oxidative stress induced by 2,3,7,8-tetrachlorodibenzo-p-dioxin (TCDD). *Free. Rad. Biol. Med.*, **9**, 79–90

Stohs, S.J., Hasan, M.Q. & Murray, W.J. (1984) Effects of BHA, *d*-α-tocopherol and retinol acetate on TCDD-mediated changes in lipid peroxidation, glutathione peroxidase activity and survival. *Xenobiotica*, **14**, 533–537

Stohs, S.J., Shara, M.A., Alsharif, N.Z., Wahba, Z.Z. & al-Bayati, Z.A. (1990) 2,3,7,8-Tetrachlorodibenzo-*p*-dioxin-induced oxidative stress in female rats. *Toxicol. appl. Pharmacol.*, **106**, 126–135

Strik, J.J.T.W.A. (1979) The occurrence of chronic-hepatic porphyria in man caused by halogenated hydrocarbons. In: Strik, J.J.T.W.A. & Koeman, J.H., eds, *Chemical Porphyria in Man*, New York, Elsevier/North-Holland, pp. 3–9

Stringer, R.L., Costner, P. & Johnston, P.A. (1995) PVC manufacture as a source of PCDD/Fs. *Organohalogen Compounds*, **24**, 119–123

Stroh, H.-J., Schmidt, A., Korte, M. & Stahlmann, R. (1992) Effects of 2,3,7,8-Tetrachlorodibenzo-*p*-dioxin on liver, thymus and cell proliferation in popliteal lymph nodes after foot pad injection of streptozotocin in rats. *Chemosphere*, **25**, 1221–1226

Sugita, K., Asada, S., Yokochi, T., Ono, M. & Okazawa, T. (1993) Polychlorinated dibenzo-*p*-dioxins, dibenzofurans, co-planar PCBs and mono-ortho PCBs in urban air. *Organohalogen Compounds*, **12**, 127–130

Sugita, K., Asada, S., Yokochi, T, Okazawa, T. Ono, M. & Goto, S. (1994) Survey of polychlorinated dibenzo-*p*-dioxins, polychlorinated dibenzofurans and polychlorinated biphenyls in urban air. *Chemosphere*, **29**, 2215–2221

Sunahara, G.I., Nelson, K.G., Wong, T.K. & Lucier, G.W. (1987) Decreased human birth weights after *in utero* exposure to PCBs and PCDFs are associated with decreased placental EGF-stimulated receptor autophosphorylation capacity. *Mol. Pharmacol.*, **32**, 572–578

Sund, K.G., Carlo, G.L., Crouch, R.L. & Senefelder, B.C. (1993) Background soil concentrations of phenolic compounds, chlorinated herbicides, PCDDs and PCDFs in the Melbourne metropolitan area. *Austr. J. public Health*, **17**, 157–161

Suruda, A.J,. Ward, E.M. & Fingerhut, M.A. (1993) Identification of soft tissue sarcoma deaths in cohorts exposed to dioxin and chlorinated naphthalenes. *Epidemiology*, **4**, 14–19

Suskind, R.R. (1985) Chloracne, 'the hallmark of dioxin intoxication'. *Scand. J. Work Environ. Health*, **11**, 165–171

Suskind, R.R. & Hertzberg, V.S. (1984) Human health effects of 2,4,5-T and its toxic contaminants. *J. Am. med. Assoc.*, **251**, 2372–2380

Sutter, T.R., Guzman, K., Dold, K.M. & Greenlee, W.F. (1991) Targets for dioxin: genes for plasminogen activator inhibitor-2 and interleukin-1b. *Science*, **254**, 415–418

Sutter, T.R., Tang, Y.M., Hayes, C.L., Wo, Y.-Y.P., Jabs, E.W., Li, X., Ying, H., Cody, C.W. & Greenlee, W.F. (1994) Complete cDNA sequence of a human dioxin-inducible mRNA identifies a new gene subfamily of cytochrome P450 that maps to chromosome 2. *J. biol. Chem.*, **269**, 13092–13099

Sutter, T.R., Cody, C.W., Gastel, J.A., Hayes, C.L., Li, Y.L., Walker, N.J. & Yin, H. (1995) Receptor mediated toxicity: the dioxin receptor as an example of biological complexity and experimental approaches. In: Galli, C.L., Goldberg, A.M. & Marinovich, M., eds, *Modulation of Cellular Responses in Toxicity*, Berlin, Springer Verlag, pp. 21–35

Svensson, B.-G., Nilsson, A., Hansson, M., Rappe, C., Åkesson, B. & Skerfving, S. (1991) Exposure to dioxins and dibenzofurans through the consumption of fish. *New Engl. J. Med.*, **324**, 8–12

Svensson, B.G., Barregård, L., Sällsten, G., Nilsson, A., Hansson, M. & Rappe, C. (1993) Exposure to polychlorinated dioxins (PCDD) and dibenzofurans (PCDF) from graphite electrodes in a chloralkali plant. *Chemosphere*, **27**, 259–262

Svensson, B.-G., Nilsson, A., Jonsson, E., Schütz, A., Åkesson, B. & Hagmar, L. (1995a) Fish consumption and exposure to persistent organochlorine compunds, mercury, selenium and methylamines among Swedish fishermen. *Scand. J. Work Environ. Health*, **21**, 96–105

Svensson, B.-G., Mikoczy, Z., Strömberg, U. & Hagmar, L. (1995b) Mortality and cancer incidence among Swedish fishermen with a high dietary intake of persistent organochlorine compounds. *Scand. J. Work Environ. Health*, **21**, 106–115

Swanson, H.I. & Bradfield, C.A. (1993) The Ah receptor: genetics, structure and function. *Pharmacogenetics*, **3**, 213–230

Sweeney, G.D. (1986) Porphyria cutanea tarda, or the uroporphyrinogen decarboxylase deficiency disease. *Clin. Biochem.*, **19**, 3–15

Sweeney, M.H., Fingerhut, M.A., Connally, L.B., Halperin, W.E., Moody, P.L. & Marlowe, D.A. (1989) Progress of the NIOSH cross-sectional medical study of workers occupationally exposed to chemicals contaminated with 2,3,7,8-TCDD. *Chemosphere*, **19**, 973–977

Sweeney, M.H., Fingerhut, M.A., Patterson, D.G., Connally, L.B., Piacitelli, L.A., Morris, J.A., Greife, A.L., Hornung, R.W., Marlow, D.A., Dugle, J.E., Halperin, W.E. & Needham, L.L. (1990) Comparison of serum levels of 2,3,7,8-TCDD in TCP production workers and in an unexposed comparison group. *Chemosphere*, **20**, 993–1000

Sweeney, M.H., Fingerhut, M.A., Arezzo, J.C., Hornung, R.W. & Connally, L.B. (1993) Peripheral neuropathy after occupational exposure to 2,3,7,8-tetrachlorodibenzo-*p*-dioxin (TCDD). *Am. J. ind. Med.*, **23**, 845–858

Swerev, M., Nordsieck, H., Pawlik, V. & Hutzinger, O. (1996) Impact of emissions of modern municipal waste incinerators on atmospheric concentrations of PCDD and PCDF. *Organohalogen Compounds*, **28**, 134–139

Swift, L.L., Gasiewicz, T.A., Dewey Dunn, G., Soule, P.D. & Neal, R.A. (1981) Characterization of the hyperlipemia in guinea pigs induced by 2,3,7,8-tetrachlorodibenzo-*p*-dioxin. *Toxicol. appl. Pharmacol.*, **59**, 489–499

Tai, H.L., McReynolds, J.H., Goldstein, J.A., Eugster H.P., Sengstag, C., Alworth, W.L. & Olson, J.R. (1993) Cytochrome P4501A1 mediates the metabolism of 2,3,7,8-tetrachlorodibenzofuran in the rat and human. *Toxicol. appl. Pharmacol.*, **123**, 34–42

Takahashi, J.S. (1992) Circadian clock genes are ticking. *Science*, **258**, 238–240

Takayama, K., Miyata, H., Mimura, M. & Kashimoto, T. (1991) PCDDs, PCDFs and coplanar PCBs in coastal and marketing fishes in Japan. *Jpn. J. Toxicol. environ. Health*, **37**, 125–131

Takimoto, K., Lindahl, R. & Pitot, H.C. (1991) Superinduction of 2,3,7,8-tetrachlorodibenzo-para-dioxin-inducible expression of aldehyde dehydrogenase by the inhibition of protein synthesis. *Biochem. biophys. Res. Commun.*, **180**, 953–959

Takimoto, K., Lindahl, R. & Pitot, H.C. (1992) Regulation of 2,3,7,8-tetrachlorodibenzo-*p*-dioxin-inducible expression of aldehyde dehydrogenase in hepatoma cells. *Arch. Biochem. Biophys.*, **298**, 493–497

Takimoto, K., Lindahl, R., Dunn, T.J. & Pitot, H.C. (1994) Structure of the 5' flanking region of class 3 aldehyde dehydrogenase in the rat. *Arch. Biochem. Biophys.*, **312**, 539–546

Takizawa, Y. & Muto, H. (1987) PCDDs and PCDFs carried to the human body from the diet. *Chemosphere*, **16**, 1971–1976

Tanaka, N., Nettesheim, P., Gray, T., Nelson, K. & Barrett, J.C. (1989) 2,3,7,8-Tetrachlorodibenzo-p-dioxin enhancement of N-methyl-N'-nitro-N-nitrosoguanidine-induced transformation of rat tracheal epithelial cells in culture. *Cancer Res.*, **49**, 2703–2708

Taucher, J.A., Buckland, S.J., Lister, A.R. & Porter, L.J. (1992) Levels of polychlorinated dibenzo-*p*-dioxins and polychlorinated dibenzofurans in ambient urban air in Sydney, Australia. *Chemosphere*, **25**, 1361–1365

Taylor, J.S. (1979) Environmental chloracne: update and overview. *Ann. N.Y. Acad. Sci.*, **320**, 295–407

Taylor, M.J., Lucier, G.W., Mahler, J.F., Thompson, M., Lockhart, A.C. & Clark, G.C. (1992) Inhibition of acute TCDD toxicity by treatment with anti-tumor necrosis factor antibody or dexamethasone. *Toxicol. appl. Pharmacol.*, **117**, 126–132

Tenchini, M.L., Crimaudo, C., Pacchetti, G., Mottura, A., Agosti, S. & DeCarli, L. (1983) A comparative cytogenetic study on cases of induced abortions in TCDD-exposed and non-exposed women. *Environ. Mutag.*, **5**, 73–85

Teschke, K., Kelly, S.J., Wiens, M., Hertzman, C., Dimich-Ward, H., Ward, J.E.H. & Van Oostdam, J.C. (1992) Dioxins and furans in residents of a forest industry region of Canada. *Chemosphere*, **25**, 1741–1751

Theelen, R.M.C., Liem, A.K.D., Slob, W. & van Wijnen, J.H. (1993) Intake of 2,3,7,8 chlorine substituted dioxins, furans, and planar PCBs from food in the Netherlands: median and distribution. *Chemosphere*, **27**, 1625–1635

Theisen, J., Maulshagen, A. & Fuchs, J. (1993) Organic and inorganic substances in the copper slag 'Kieselrot'. *Chemosphere*, **26**, 881–896

Theobald, H.M. & Peterson, R.E. (1994) Developmental and reproductive toxicity of dioxins and Ah-receptor agonists. In: Schecter, A., Constable, J.D. & Bangers, J.V., eds, *Dioxins and Health*, New York, Plenum Press, pp. 309–346.

Theobald, H.M., Moore, R.W., Katz, L.B., Pieper, R.O., & Peterson (1983) Enhancement of carrageenan and dextran-induced edemas by 2,3,7,8-tetrachlorodibenzo-*p*-dioxin and related compounds. *J. Pharmacol. exp. Ther.*, **225**, 576–583

Theobald, H.M., Ingall, G.B., Mably, T.A. & Peterson, R.E. (1991) Response of the antral mucosa of the rat stomach to 2,3,7,8-tetrachlorodibenzo-*p*-dioxin. *Toxicol. appl. Pharmacol.*, **108**, 167–179

Thiel, R., Koch, E., Ulbrich, B. & Chahoud, I. (1994) Peri- and postnatal exposure to 2,3,7,8-tetrachlorodibenzo-*p*-dioxin: effects on physiological development, reflexes, locomotor activity and learning behaviour in Wistar rats. *Arch. Toxicol.*, **69**, 79–86

Thiess, A.M., Frentzel-Beyme, R. & Link, R. (1982) Mortality study of persons exposed to dioxin in a trichlorophenol-process accident that occurred in the BASF AG on November 17, 1953. *Am. J. ind. Med.*, **3**, 179–189

Thigpen, J.E., Faith, R.E., McConnell, E.E. & Moore, J.A. (1975) Increased susceptibility to bacterial infection as a sequela of exposure to 2,3,7,8-tetrachlorodibenzo-p-dioxin. *Infect. Immun.*, **12**, 1319–1324

Thoma, H., Mücke, W. & Kretschmer, E. (1989) Concentrations of PCDD and PCDF in human fat and liver samples. *Chemosphere*, **18**, 491–498

Thoma, H., Mücke, W. & Kauert, G. (1990) Comparison of the polychlorinated dibenzo-*p*-dioxin and dibenzofuran in human tissue and human liver. *Chemosphere*, **20**, 433–442

Thomas, H.F. (1980) 2,4,5-T use and congenital malformation rates in Hungary. *Lancet*, **ii**, 214–215

Thomas, P.T. & Hinsdill, R.D. (1979) The effect of perinatal exposure to tetrachloro-dibenzo-*p*-dioxin on the immune response of young mice. *Drug chem. Toxicol.*, **2**, 77–98

Thomas, T.L. & Kang, H.K. (1990) Mortality and morbidity among Army Chemical Corps Vietnam veterans: a preliminary report. *Am. J. ind. Med.*, **18**, 665–673

Thomas, V.M. & Spiro, T.G. (1995) An estimation of dioxin emissions in the United States. *Toxicol. Environ. Chem.*, **50**, 1–37

Thu, T.X., Bocharov, B., Klujev, N., Jilnikov, V., Brodsky, E. & Quan, N.C.Q. (1992) Determination of PCDD/PCDF in soil and water samples from South Vietnam regions sprayed with Agent Orange by GC-MS. *Organohalogen Compounds*, **4**, 289–290

Thunberg, T. & Håkansson, H. (1983) Vitamin A (retinol) status in the Gunn rat. The effect of 2,3,7,8-tetrachlorodibenzo-*p*-dioxin. *Arch. Toxicol.*, **53**, 225–233

Thunberg, T., Ahlborg, U.G., Håkansson, H., Krantz, C. & Monier, M. (1980) Effect of 2,3,7,8-tetrachlorodibenzo-*p*-dioxin on the hepatic storage of retinol in rats with different dietary supplies of vitamin A (retinol). *Arch. Toxicol.*, **45**, 273–285

Tian, H., McKnight, S.L. & Russell, D.W. (1997) Endothelial PAS domain protein 1 (EPAS1), a transcription factor selectively expressed in endothelial cells. *Genes Dev.*, **11**, 72–82

Tiernan, T.O., Wagel, D.J., Vanness, G.F., Garrett, J.H., Solch, J.G. & Harden, L.A. (1989) PCDD/PCDF in the ambient air of a metropolitan area in the US. *Chemosphere*, **19**, 541–546

Tomar, R.S. & Kerkvliet, N.I. (1991) Reduced T-helper cell function in mice exposed to 2,3,7,8-tetrachlorodibenzo-*p*-dioxin (TCDD). *Toxicol. Lett.*, **57**, 55–64

Tondeur, Y. & Beckert, W.F. (1991) Method 3: determination of polychlorinated dibenzo-*p*-dioxins and polychlorinated dibenzofurans in various environmental matrices by high-resolution gas chromatography-high resolution mass spectrometry. In: Rappe, C., Buser, H.-R., Dodet, B. & O'Neill, I.K., eds, *Environmental Carcinogens: Methods of Analysis and Exposure Measurement. Vol. 11: Polychlorinated Dioxins and Dibenzofurans* (IARC Scientific Publications No. 108), Lyon, IARC, pp. 211–249

Tondeur, Y., Chu, M. & Hass, J.R. (1991) Method 9: determination of polychlorinated dibenzodioxins and dibenzofurans in ambient air and airborne dust samples by high-resolution gas chromatography-high resolution mass spectrometry. In: Rappe, C., Buser, H.-R., Dodet, B. & O'Neill, I.K., eds, *Environmental Carcinogens: Methods of Analysis and Exposure Measurement. Vol. 11: Polychlorinated Dioxins and Dibenzofurans* (IARC Scientific Publications No. 108), Lyon, IARC, pp. 377–398

Tonn, T., Esser, C., Schneider, E.M., Steinmann-Steiner-Haldenstätt, W. & Gleichmann, E. (1996) Persistence of decreased T-helper cell function in industrial workers 20 years after exposure to 2,3,7,8-tetrachlorodibenzo-*p*-dioxin. *Environ. Health Perspectives*, **104**, 422–426

Tóth, K., Somfai-Relle, S., Sugár, J. & Bence, J. (1979) Carcinogenicity testing of herbicide 2,4,5-trichlorophenoxyethanol containing dioxin and of pure dioxin in Swiss mice. *Nature*, **278**, 548–549

Towara, J., Kaupp, H. & McLachlan, M.S. (1993) Distribution of airborne PCDD/F in relation to particle size. *Organohalogen Compounds*, **12**, 115–119

Townsend, J.C., Bodner, K.M., van Peenen, P.F.D., Olson, R.D. & Cook, R.R. (1982) Survey of reproductive events of wives of employees exposed to chlorinated dioxins. *Am. J. Epidemiol.*, **115**, 695–713.

Travis, C.C. & Hattemer-Frey, H.A. (1991) Human exposure to dioxin. *Sci. total Environ.*, **104**, 97–127

Triebig, G. , Werle, E., Päpke, O., Heim, G. & Broding, M.C. (1996) Effects of dioxins and furans on liver function, lipid metabolism and thyroid parameters in former thermal metal recycling workers. In: *25th International Congress on Occupational Health, Stockholm, Sweden, 15–20 September 1996*

Tritscher, A.M., Goldstein, J.A., Portier, C.J., McCoy, Z., Clark, G.C. & Lucier, G.W. (1992) Dose-response relationships for chronic exposure to 2,3,7,8-tetrachlorodibenzo-*p*-dioxin in a rat tumor promotion model: quantification and immunolocalization of CYP1A1 and CYP1A2 in the liver. *Cancer Res.*, **52**, 3436–3442

Tritscher, A.M., Clark, G.C., Sewall, C., Sills, R.C., Maronpot, R. & Lucier, G.W. (1995) Persistence of TCDD-induced hepatic cell proliferation and growth of enzyme altered foci after chronic exposure followed by cessation of treatment in DEN initiated female rats. *Carcinogenesis*, **16**, 2807–2811

Tritscher, A.M., Seacat, A.M., Yager, J.D., Groopman, J.D., Miller, B.D., Bell, D., Sutter, T.R. & Lucier, G.W. (1996) Increased oxidative DNA damage in livers of 2,3,7,8-tetrachlorodibenzo-*p*-dioxin treated intact but not ovariectomized rats. *Cancer Lett.*, **98**, 219–225

Tucker, A.N., Vore, S.J. & Luster, M.I. (1986) Suppression of B cell differentiation by 2,3,7,8-tetrachloro-dibenzo-*p*-dioxin (TCDD). *Mol. Pharmacol.*, **29**, 372–377

Tuinstra, L.G.M.T., Huisman, M. & Boersma, E.R. (1994) The Dutch PCB/dioxin study contents of dioxins, planar and other PCBs in human milk from the Rotterdam and Groningen area. *Chemosphere*, **29**, 2267–2277

Tuinstra, L.G.M.T., Huisman, M., Boersma, E.R., Koopman-Esseboom, C. & Sauer, P.J.J. (1995) Contents of dioxins, planar and other PCBs in 168 Dutch human milk samples. *Organohalogen Compounds*, **26**, 255–256

Tukey, R.H., Hannah, R.R., Negishi, M., Nebert, D.W. & Eisen, H.J. (1982) The Ah locus: correlation of intranuclear appearance of inducer-receptor complex with induction of cyto-chrome P-450 mRNA. *Cell*, **31**, 275–284

Tulp, M.T.M. & Hutzinger, O. (1978) Rat metabolism of polychlorinated dibenzo-*p*-dioxins. *Chemosphere*, 9, 761–768

Tuomisto, J. & Pohjanvirta, R. (1987) The Long-Evans rat: a prototype of an exteemely TCDD-susceptible strain variant. *Pharmacol. Toxicol.*, **60**, 72

Tuomisto, J., Pohjanvirta, R., MacDonald, E. & Tuomisto, L. (1990) Changes in rat brain mono-amines, monoamine metabolites and histamine after a single administration of 2,3,7,8-tetra-chlorodibenzo-*p*-dioxin (TCDD). *Pharmacol. Toxicol.*, **67**, 260–265

Tuomisto, J.T., Unkila, M., Pohjanvirta, R., Koulu, M. & Tuomisto, L. (1991) Effect of a single dose of TCDD on the level of histamine in discrete nuclei in rat brain. *Agents Actions*, **33**, 154–156

Tuomisto, J., Adrzejewski, W., Unkila, M., Pohjanvirta, R., Linden, J., Vartiainen, T. & Tuomisto, L. (1995) Modulation of TCDD-induced wasting syndrome by portocaval anasto-mosis and vagotomy in Long-Evans and Han/Wistar rats. *Eur. J. Pharmacol.*, **292**, 277–285

Turner, J.N. & Collins, D.N. (1983) Liver morphology in guinea pigs administered either pyrolysis products of a polychlorinated biphenyl transformer fluid or 2,3,7,8-tetrachloro-dibenzo-*p*-dioxin. *Toxicol. appl. Pharmacol.*, **67**, 417–429

Turner, W.E., Isaacs, S.G., Patterson, D.G., Jr & Needham, L.L. (1991) Method 7: enrichment of biological samples by the semi-automated Smith, Stalling and Johnson method: human serum and adipose tissue. In: Rappe, C., Buser, H.R., Dodet, B. & O'Neill, I.K., eds, *Environmental Carcinogens: Methods of Analysis and Exposure Measurement. Vol. 11: Polychlorinated Dioxins and Dibenzofurans* (IARC Scientific Publications No. 108), Lyon, IARC, pp. 343–355

Turteltaub, K.W., Felton, J.S., Gledhill, B.L., Vogel, J.S., Southon, J.R., Caffee, M.W., Finkel, R.C., Nelson, D.E., Proctor, I.D. & Davis, J.C. (1990) Accelerator mass spectrometry in bio-medical dosimetry: relationship between low-level exposure and covalent binding of heterocyclic amine carcinogens to DNA. *Proc. natl Acad. Sci. USA*, **87**, 5288–5292

Tyskling, M., Carey, A.E., Rappe, C. & Miller, G.C. (1992) Photolysis of OCDF and OCDD on soil. *Organohalogen Compounds*, **6**, 293

Tysklind, M., Fängmark, I., Marklund, S., Lindskog, A., Thaning, L. & Rappe, C. (1993) Atmospheric transport and transformation of polychlorinated dibenzo-*p*-dioxins and dibenzo-furans. *Environ. Sci. Technol.*, **27**, 2190–2197

Umbreit, T.H. & Gallo, M A. (1988) Physiological implications of estrogen receptor modulation by 2,3,7,8-tetrachlorodibenzo-*p*-dioxin. *Toxicol. Lett.*, **42**, 5–14

Umbreit, T.H., Hesse, E.J., MacDonald, G.J. & Gallo, M.A. (1988) Effects of TCDD-estradiol interactions in three strains of mice. *Toxicol. Lett.*, **40**, 1–9

Umbreit, T.H., Scala, P.L., MacKenzie, S.A. & Gallo, M.A. (1989) Alteration of the acute toxicity of 2,3,7,8-tetrachlorodibenzo-*p*-dioxin (TCDD) by estradiol and tamoxifen. *Toxicology*, **59**, 163–169

Unger, H.-J. & Prinz, D. (1991) Traffic PCDD/PCDF-emissions in soils near roads in Baden-Württemberg. *Organohalogen Compounds*, **7**, 335–346 (in German)

United States Environmental Protection Agency (1986) Method 8280 — The analysis of polychlorinated dibenzo-*p*-dioxins and polychlorinated dibenzofurans. In: *Test Methods for Evaluating Solid Waste. Vol. 1B: Laboratory Manual — Physical/Chemical Methods*, Research Triangle Park, NC, pp. 8280-1–8280-33 and appendices

United States Environmental Protection Agency (1994) *Estimating Exposure to Dioxin-like Compounds* (EPA/600/6-88/005Cb), Washington DC

United States Environmental Protection Agency (1995) Method 23 — Determination of polychlorinated dibenzo-*p*-dioxins and polychlorinated dibenzofurans from stationary sources. *Ch. 1, Part 60, App. A*, pp. 834–847

United States Environmental Protection Agency (1996a) Method 613 — 2,3,7,8-Tetrachlorodibenzo-*para*-dioxins. *Code fed. Regul.*, **40**, 179–188

United States Environmental Protection Agency (1996b) *Drinking Water Regulations and Health Advisories (USEPA Report No. EPA-822/B-96-002), Washington, DC, Office of Water*

United States National Institute for Occupational Safety and Health (1994) *Pocket Guide to Chemical Hazards*, Research Triangle Park, NC, pp. 298–299, 342

United States National Toxicology Program (1979a) *Bioassay of Dibenzo-p-dioxin (CAS No. 262-12-4) for Possible Carcinogenicity* (Tech. Rep. Series No. 122), Bethesda, MD, National Cancer Institute

United States National Toxicology Program (1979b) *Bioassay of 2,7-Dichlorodibenzo-p-dioxin (DCDD) (CAS No. 33857-26-0) for Possible Carcinogenicity* (Tech. Rep. Series No. 123; DHEW Publication No. (NIH) 79–1378), Bethesda, MD, National Cancer Institute

United States National Toxicology Program (1980a) *Bioassay of a Mixture of 1,2,3,6,7,8-Hexachlorodibenzo-p-dioxin and 1,2,3,7,8,9-Hexachlorodibenzo-p-dioxin (CAS No. 57653-85-7 and CAS No. 19408-74-3) for Possible Carcinogenicity (Gavage Study)* (Tech. Rep. Series No. 198; DHHS Publication No. (NIH) 80–1754), Bethesda, MD, National Cancer Institute

United States National Toxicology Program (1980b) *Bioassay of a Mixture of 1,2,3,6,7,8-Hexachlorodibenzo-p-dioxin and 1,2,3,7,8,9-Hexachlorodibenzo-p-dioxin (CAS No. 57653-85-7 and CAS No. 19408-74-3) for Possible Carcinogenicity (Dermal Study)* (Tech. Rep. Series No. 202;NIH Publication No. 80-1758), Bethesda, MD, National Cancer Institute

United States National Toxicology Program (1982a) *Carcinogenesis Bioassay of 2,3,7,8-Tetrachlorodibenzo-p-dioxin (CAS No. 1746-01-6) in Osborne-Mendel Rats and B6C3F1 Mice (Gavage Study)* (Tech. Rep. Series No. 209; DHEW Publication No. (NIH) 82-1765), Research Triangle Park, NC

United States National Toxicology Program (1982b) *Carcinogenesis Bioassay of 2,3,7,8-Tetrachlorodibenzo-p-dioxin (CAS No. 1746-01-6) in Swiss-Webster Mice (Dermal Study)* (Technical Report No. 201; DHEW Publication No. (NIH) 82-1757), Research Triangle Park, NC

Unkila, M., Tuomisto, J.T., Pohjanvirta, R., MacDonald, E., Tuomisto, L., Kuolu, M. & Tuomisto, J. (1993a) Effect of a single lethal dose of TCDD on the levels of monoamines, their metabolites and tryptophan in discrete brain nuclei and peripheral tissues of Long-Evans rats. *Pharmacol. Toxicol.*, **72**, 279–285

Unkila, M., Pohjanvirta, R., Honkakoski, P., Torronen, R. & Tuomisto, J. (1993b) 2,3,7,8-Tetra-chlorodibenzo-*p*-dioxin (TCDD) induced ethoxyresorufin-*O*-deethylase (EROD) and aldehyde dehydrogenase (ALDH3) activities in the brain and liver. A comparison between the most TCDD-susceptible and the most TCDD-resistant rat strain. *Biochem. Pharmacol.*, **46**, 651–659

Unkila, M., Pohjanvirta, R., MacDonald, E. & Tuomisto, J. (1994) Characterization of 2,3,7,8-tetrachlorodibenzo-*p*-dioxin-induced brain serotonin metabolism in the rat. *Eur. J. Pharma-col.*, **270**, 157–166

Unkila, M., Ruotsalainen, M., Pohjanvirta, R., Viluksela, M., MacDonald, E., Tuomisto, J. T., Rozman, K. & Tuomisto, J. (1995) Effect of 2,3,7,8-tetrachlorodibenzo-*p*-dioxin (TCDD) on tryptophan and glucose homeostasis in the most TCDD-susceptible and the most TCDD-resistant species, guinea pigs and hamsters. *Arch. Toxicol.*, **69**, 677–683

Urabe, H. & Asahi, M. (1985) Past and current dermatological status of Yusho patients. *Envi-ron. Health Perspectives*, **59**, 11–15

Van Cleuvenbergen, R., Schoeters, J., Wevers, M., De Fré, R. & Rymen, T. (1993) Soil conta-mination with PCDDs and PCDFs at some typical locations in Flanders. *Organohalogen Compounds*, **12**, 243–246

Van den Berg, M., van der Wielen, F.W.M., Olie, K. & van Boxtel, C.J. (1986a) The presence of PCDDs and PCDFs in human breast milk from the Netherlands. *Chemosphere*, **15**, 693–706

Van den Berg, M., DeVroom, E., Olie, K. & Hutzinger, O. (1986b) Bioavailability of PCDDs and PCDFs on fly ash after semi-chronic oral ingestion by guinea pig and Syrian golden hamster. *Chemosphere*, **15**, 519

Van den Berg, M., Meerman, L., Olie, K. & Hutzinger, O. (1986c) Retention of PCDDs and PCDFs in the liver of the rat and hamster after oral administration of a municipal incinerator fly ash extract. *Toxicol. environ. Chem.*, **12**, 267

Van den Berg, M., Heeremans, C., Veenhoven, E. & Olie, K. (1987) Transfer of polychlorinated dibenzodioxins and dibenzofurans to fetal and neonatal rats. *Fundam. appl. Toxicol.*, **9**, 635–644

Van den Berg, M., van-Wijnen, J., Wever, H. & Seinen, W. (1989a) Selective retention of toxic polychlorinated dibenzo-p-dioxins and dibenzofurans in the liver of the rat after intravenous administration of a mixture. *Toxicology*, **55**, 173–182

Van den Berg, M., de Jongh, J., Eckhart, P. & Van der Wielen, F.W. (1989b) Disposition and elimination of three polychlorinated dibenzofurans in the liver of the rat. *Fundam. appl. Toxicol.*, **12**, 738–747

Van den Berg, M., De Jongh, J., Poiger, H. & Olson, J.R. (1994) The toxicokinetics and meta-bolism of polychlorinated dibenzo-*p*-dioxins (PCDDs) and dibenzofurans (PCDFs) and their relevance for toxicity. *Crit. Reviews Toxicol.*, **24**, 1–74

Van den Heuvel, J.P. & Lucier, G. (1993) Environmental toxicity of polychlorinated dibenzo-*p*-dioxins and polychlorinated dibenzofurans. *Environ. Health Perspectives*, **100**, 189–200

Van Miller, J.P., Marlar, R.J. & Allen, J.R. (1976) Tissue distribution and excretion of tritiated tetrachlorodibenzo-*p*-dioxin in non-human primates and rats. *Food Cosmet. Toxicol.*, **14**, 31–34

Van Miller, J.P., Lalich, J.J. & Allen, J.R. (1977) Increased incidence of neoplasma in rats exposed to low levels of 2,3,7,8-tetrachlorodibenzo-*p*-dioxin. *Chemosphere*, **9**, 537–544

Van der Molen, G.W., Kooijman, S.A.L.M. & Slob, W. (1996) A generic toxicokinetic model for persistent lipophilic compounds in humans: an application to TCDD. *Fundam. appl. Toxicol.*, **31**, 83–94

Vannier, B. & Raynaud, J.P. (1980) Long term effects of prenatal estrogen treatment on genital morphology and reproductive function in the rat. *J. Reprod. Fert.*, **59**, 43–49

Vecchi, A., Mantovani, A., Sironi, M., Liuini, W., Cairo, M. & Garattini, S. (1980) Effect of acute exposure to 2,3,7,8-tetrachlordibenzo-*p*-dioxin on humoral antibody production mice. *Chem.-biol. Interactions*, **30**, 337–342

Vecchi, A,., Sironi, M., Canegrati, M.A., Recchia, M. & Garattini, S. (1983) Immuno-suppressive effects of 2,3,7,8-tetrachlorodibenzo-*p*-dioxin in strains of mice with different susceptibility to induction of aryl hydrocarbon hydroxylase. *Toxicol. appl. Pharmacol.*, **68**, 434–441

Veerkamp, W., Wever, J. & Hutzinger, O. (1981) The metabolism of some polychlorinated dibenzofurans by rats. *Chemosphere*, **10**, 397

Vikelsoe, J., Madsen, H. & Hansen, K. (1994) Emission of dioxins from Danish wood-stoves. *Chemosphere*, **29**, 2019–2027

Villanueva, E.C., Jennings, R.W., Burse, V.M. & Kimbrough, R.D. (1974) Evidence of chloro-dibenzo-*p*-dioxin and chlorodibenzofuran in hexachlorobenzene. *J. agric. Food Chem.*, **22**, 916–917

Vineis, P., Terracini, B., Ciccone, G., Cignetti, A., Colombo, E., Donna, A., Maffi, L., Pisa, R., Ricci, P., Zanini, E. & Comba, P. (1986) Phenoxy herbicides and soft tissue sarcomas in female rice weeders: a population-based case-referent study. *Scand. J. Work Environ. Health*, **13**, 9–17

Viswanathan, T.S. & Kleopfer, R.D., eds (1985) *The Presence of Hexachloroxanthene at Missouri Dioxin Sites*, Miami Beach, FL, Lewis Publishers, pp. 201–210

Vogel, C., Döhr, O. & Abel, J. (1994) Transforming growth factor-b[1] inhibits TCDD-induced cytochrome P450IA1 expression in human lung cancer A549 cells. *Arch. Toxicol.*, **68**, 303–307

Vollmuth, S. & Niessner, R. (1995) Degradation of PCDD, PCDF, PAH, PCB and chlorinated phenols during the destruction-treatment of landfill seepage water in laboratory model reactor (UV, ozone and UV/ozone). *Chemosphere*, **30**, 2317–2331

Vollmuth, S., Zajc, A. & Niessner, R. (1994) Formation of polychlorinated dibenzo-*p*-dioxins and polychlorinated dibenzofurans during the photolysis of pentachlorophenol-containing water. *Environ. Sci. Technol.*, **28**, 1145–1149

Voorman, R. & Aust, S. (1987) Specific binding of polyhalogenated aromatic hydrocarbon inducers of cytochrome P-450d to the cytochrome and inhibition of its estradiol 2-hydroxy-lase activity. *Toxicol. appl. Pharmacol.*, **90**, 69–78

Voorman, R. & Aust, S.D. (1989) TCDD (2,3,7,8-tetrachlorodibenzo-p-dioxin) is a tight binding inhibitor of cytochrome P-450d. *J. biochem. Toxicol.*, **4**, 105–109

Vos, J.G. & Koeman, J.H. (1970) Comparative toxicologic study with polychlorinated biphenyls in chickens with special reference to porphyria, edema formation, liver necrosis, and tissue residues. *Toxicol. appl. Pharmacol.*, **17**, 656–668

Vos, J. G. & Beems, R.B. (1971) Dermal toxicity studies of technical polychlorinated biphenyls and fractions thereof in rabbits. *Toxicol. appl. Pharmacol.*, **19**, 617–633

Vos, J.G. & Luster, M.I. (1989) Immune alterations. In: Kimbrough, R.D. & Jensen, S., eds, *Halogenated Biphenyls, Terphenyls, Naphthalenes, Dibenzodioxins and Related Products*, Amsterdam, Elsevier, pp. 295–322

Vos, J.G. & Moore, J.A. (1974) Suppression of cellular immunity in rats and mice by maternal treatment with 2,3,7,8-tetrachlorodibenzo-*p*-dioxin. *Int. Arch. Allergy*, **47**, 777–794

Vos, J.G., Koeman, J.H., van der Maas, H.L., ten Noever de Brauw, M.C. & de Vos, R.H. (1970) Identification and toxicological evaluation of chlorinated dibenzofuran and chlorinated naphthalene in two commercial polychlorinated biphenyls. *Food Cosmet. Toxicol.*, **8**, 625–633

Vos, J.G., Moore, J.A. & Zinkl, J.G. (1973) Effect of 2,3,7,8-tetrachlorodibenzo-*p*-dioxin on the immune system of laboratory animals. *Environ. Health Perspect.*, **5**, 149–162

Vos, J.G., Moore, J.A. & Zinkl, J.G. (1974) Toxicity of 2,3,7,8-tetrachloro-dibenzo-*p*-dioxin (TCDD) in C57Bl/6 mice. *Toxicol. appl. Pharmacol.*, **29**, 229–241

Vos, J.G., Kreeftenberg, J.G., Engel, H.W.B., Minderhoud, A. & van Noorle Jansen, L.M. (1978) Studies on 2,3,7,8-tetrachlorodibenzo-*p*-dioxin induced immune suppression and decreased resistance to infection: endotoxin hypersensitivity, serum zinc concentrations and effect of thymosin treatment. *Toxicology*, **9**, 75–86

Vos, J.G., van Loveren, H. & Schuurman, H.-J. (1991) Immunotoxicity of dioxin: immune function and host resistance in laboratory animals and humans. In: Gallo, M.A., Scheuplein, R.J. & van der Heijden, C.A., *Biological Basis for Risk Assessment of Dioxins and Related Compounds* (Banbury Report 35), Cold Spring Harbor, NY, Cold Spring Harbor Press

de Waal, E.J., Schuurman, H.-J., Loeber, G., Van Loveren, H. & Vos, J.G. (1992) Alteration in the cortical thymic epithelium of rats after in vivo exposure to 2,3,7,8-tetrachlorodibenzo-*p*-dioxin (TCDD): an (immuno)histological study. *Toxicol. appl. Pharmacol.*, **115**, 80–88

de Waal, E., Rademakers, L.H.P.M., Schuurman, H.-J., Van Loveren H. & Vos J.G. (1993) Ultrastructure of the cortical epithelium of the rat thymus after in vivo exposure to 2,3,7,8-tetrachlorodibenzo-*p*-dioxin (TCDD). *Arch. Toxicol.*, **67**, 558–564

Waalkens-Berendsen, I.D.H., Smits-van Prooije, A.E.S-V., Bouwman, C.A. & Van Den Berg, M. (1996) Reproductive effects in F1-generation rats perinatally exposed to PCB126, PCB118, PCB153 or 2,3,4,7,8-PnCDF. *Organohalogen Compounds*, **29**, 190–194

Wacker, R., Poiger, H. & Schlatter, C. (1986) Pharmacokinetics and metabolism of 1,2,3,7,8-pentachlorodibenzopdioxin in the rat. *Chemosphere*, **15**, 1473

Wacker, R., Poiger, H. & Schlatter, C. (1990) Levels of 2,3,7,8-substituted polychlorinated dibenzo-p-dioxins and dibenzofurans (PCDD/PCDF) in human liver and adipose tissue. *Organohalogen Compounds*, **4**, 155–158

Waern, F., Flodström, S., Busk, L., Kronevi, T., Nordgren, I. & Ahlborg, U.G. (1991) Relative liver tumour promoting activity and toxicity of some polychlorinated dibenzo-*p*-dioxin- and dibenzofuran-congeners in female Sprague-Dawley rats. *Pharmacol. Toxicol.*, **69**, 450–458

Wahba, Z.Z., Lawson, T.A. & Stohs, S.J. (1988) Induction of hepatic DNA single strand breaks in rats by 2,3,7,8-tetrachlorodibenzo-*p*-dioxin (TCDD). *Cancer Lett.*, **39**, 281–286

Wahba, Z.Z., Lawson, T.W., Murray, W.J. & Stohs, S.J. (1989) Factors influencing the induction of DNA single strand breaks in rats by 2,3,7,8-tetrachlorodibenzo-*p*-dioxin. *Toxicology*, **58**, 57–69

Wahba, Z.Z., Murray, W.J. & Stohs, S.J. (1990) Desferrioxamine-induced alterations in hepatic iron distribution, DNA damage and lipid peroxidation in control and 2,3,7,8-tetrachlorodibenzo-*p*-dioxin-treated rats. *J. appl. Toxicol.*, **10**, 119–124

Walden, R. & Schiller, C.M. (1985) Comparative toxicity of 2,3,7,8-tetrachlorodibenzo-*p*-dioxin (TCDD) in four (sub)strains of adult male rats. *Toxicol. appl. Pharmacol.*, **77**, 490–495

Walker, A.E. & Martin, J.V. (1979) Lipid profiles in dioxin-exposed workers [letter]. *Lancet*, **i**, 446–447

Walker, N.J., Gastel, J.A., Costa, L.T., Clark, G.C., Lucier, G.W. & Sutter, T.R. (1995) Rat CYP1B1: an adrenal cytochrome P450 that exhibits sex-dependent expression in livers and kidneys of TCDD-treated animals. *Carcinogenesis*, **16**, 1319–1327

Wallenhorst, T., Krauss, P. & Hagenmaier, H. (1995) PCDD/F in ambient air and deposition in Baden-Württemberg, Germany. *Organohalogen Compounds*, **24**, 157–161

Walsh, P.J.J., Brimblecombe, P., Creaser, C.S. & Olphert, R. (1994) Biomass burning and polychlorinated dibenzo-p-dioxins and furans in soil. *Organohalogen Compounds*, **20**, 283–287

Wang, X., Porter, W., Krishnan, V., Narasimhan, T.R. & Safe, S. (1993) Mechanism of 2,3,7,8-tetrachlorodibenzo-*p*-dioxin (TCDD)-mediated decrease of the nuclear estrogen receptor in MCF-7 human breast cancer cells. *Mol. cell. Endocrinol.*, **96**, 159–166

Wang, G.L., Jiang, B.H., Rue, E.A. & Semenza, G.L. (1995) Hypoxia-inducible factor 1 is a basic-helix-loop-helix-PAS heterodimer regulated by cellular O_2 tension. *Proc. natl Acad. Sci. USA*, **92**, 5510–5514

Wanner, R., Brömmer, S., Czarnetzki, B.M., and Rosenbach, T. (1995) The differentiation-related upregulation of aryl hydrocarbon receptor transcript levels is suppressed by retinoic acid. *Biochem. biophys. Res. Commun.*, **209**, 706–711

Watson, A.J. & Hankinson, O. (1992) Dioxin-dependent and Ah receptor-dependent protein binding to xenobiotic responsive elements and G-rich DNA studied by *in vivo* footprinting. *J. biol. Chem.*, **267**, 6874–6878

Watson, A.J., Weir-Brown, K.I., Bannister, R.M., Chu, F., Reisz-Porszasz, S., Fujii-Kuriyama, Y., Sogawa, K. & Hankinson, O. (1992) Mechanism of action of a repressor of dioxin-dependent induction of *Cyp1a1* gene transcription. *Mol. cell. Biol.*, **12**, 2115–2123

Watson, M.A., Devereux, T.R., Malarkey, D.E., Anderson, M.W. & Maronpot, R.R. (1995) H-*ras* oncogene mutation spectra in B6C3F1 and C57BL/6 mouse liver tumors provide evidence for TCDD promotion of spontaneous and vinyl carbamate-initiated liver cells. *Carcinogenesis*, **16**, 1705–1710

Wearne, S.J., Harrison, N., Gem, M.G. de M., Startin, J.R., Wright, C., Kelly, M., Robinson, C., White, S., Hardy, D. & Edinburgh, V. (1996) Time trends in human dietary exposure to PCDDs, PCDFs and PCBs in the UK. *Organohalogen Compounds*, **31**, 1–6

Webb, K.B., Evans, R.G., Knudsen, A.P. & Roodman, S.T. (1989) Medical evaluation of subjects with known body levels of 2,3,7,8-tetrachlorodibenzo-*p*-dioxin. *J. Toxicol. environ. Health*, **28**, 183–193

Weber, H. & Birnbaum, L. (1985) 2,3,7,8-Tetrachlorodibenzo-*p*-dioxin (TCDD) and 2,3,7,8-tetrachlorodibenzofuran (TCDF) in pregnant C57BL/6N mice: distribution to the embryo and excretion. *Arch. Toxicol.*, **57**, 159–162

Weber, L.D.W. & Rozman, K. (1993) Dose-responses and structure-activity relationship of decreased tryptophan 2,3-dioxygenase activity after exposure of rats to chlorinated dibenzo-*p*-dioxins. *Toxicologist*, **13**, 199

Weber, L.W., Zesch, A. & Rozman, K. (1991a) Penetration, distribution and kinetics of 2,3,7,8-tetrachlorodibenzo-p-dioxin in human skin *in vitro*. *Arch. Toxicol.*, **65**, 421–428

Weber, L.W., Lebofsky, M., Greim, H. & Rozman, K. (1991b) Key enzymes of gluconeogenesis are dose-dependently reduced in 2,3,7,8-tetrachlorodibenzo-*p*-dioxin (TCDD)-treated rats. *Arch. Toxicol.*, **65**, 119–123

Weber, L.W., Lebofsky, M., Stahl, B.U., Gorski, J.R., Muzi, G. & Rozman, K. (1991c) Reduced activities of key enzymes of gluconeogenesis as possible cause of acute toxicity of 2,3,7,8-tetrachlorodibenzo-*p*-dioxin (TCDD) in rats. *Toxicology*, **66**, 133–144

Weber, L.W., Palmer, C.D. & Rozman, K. (1994) Reduced activity of tryptophan 2,3-dioxygenase in the liver of rats treated with chlorinated dibenzo-*p*-dioxins (CDDs): dose-responses and structure-activity relationship. *Toxicology*, **86**, 63–69

Weber, R., Kühn, T., Schrenk, D., Häfelinger, G. & Hagenmaier, H. (1996) Quantum chemical and metabolic studies towards an explanation of the exceptional status of the 2,3,7,8-positions in dibenzodioxin. *Organohalogen Compounds*, **29**, 489–494

Webster, G.R.B., Muldrew, D.H., Graham, J.J., Sarna, L.P. & Muir, D.C.G. (1986) Dissolved organic matter mediated aquatic transport of chlorinated dioxins. *Chemosphere*, **15**, 1379–1386

Weintraub, H. (1993) The MyoD family and myogenesis: redundancy, networks, and thresholds. *Cell*, **75**, 1241–1244

Weisglas-Kuperus, N., Sas, T.C.J., Koopman-Esseboom, C., Van der Zwan, C.W., de Ridder, M.A.J., Beishuizen, A., Hooijkaas, H. & Sauer, P.J. (1995) Immunologic effects of background prenatal and postnatal exposure to dioxins and polychlorinated biphenyls in Dutch infants. *Pediatr. Res.*, **38**, 404–410

Weiß, C., Kolluri, S.K., Kiefer, F. & Göttlicher, M. (1996) Complementation of Ah receptor deficiency in hepatoma cells: negative feedback regulation and cell cycle control by the Ah receptor. *Exp. Cell Res.*, **226**, 154–163

Weiss, P., Gschmeidler, E. & Schentz, H. (1993) Multivariate statistical survey of PCDD/F-profiles and PCB-patterns of soil samples from an industrialized urban area (Linz, Upper Austria). *Organohalogen Compounds*, **12**, 259–263

Weiss, P., Riss, A., Gschmeidler, E. & Schentz, H. (1994) Investigation of heavy metal, PAH, PCB patterns and PCDD/F profiles of soil samples from an industrialized urban area (Linz, Upper Austria) with multivariate statistical methods. *Chemosphere*, **29**, 2223–2236

Welge, P., Wittsiepe, J., Schrey, P., Ewers, U., Exner, M. & Selenka, F. (1993) PCDD/F-levels in human blood of vegetarians compared to those of non-vegetarians. *Organohalogen Compounds*, **12**, 13–17

Wendling, J.M., Orth, R.G., Poiger, H. & Hileman, F.D. (1990a) Methodology for the analysis of 2,3,7,8-tetrachlorodibenzo-*p*-dioxin in feces. *Chemosphere*, **20**, 343–347

Wendling, J.M., Orth, R.G. & Poiger, H. (1990b) Determination of [^{3}H]-2,3,7,8-tetrachloro-dibenzo-*p*-dioxin in human feces to ascertain its relative metabolism in man. *Anal. Chem.*, **62**, 796–800

Weston, W. M., Nugent, P. & Greene, R.M. (1995) Inhibition of retinoic-acid-induced gene expression by 2,3,7,8-tetrachlorodibenzo-*p*-dioxin. *Biochem. Biophys. Res. Commun.*, **207**, 690–694

Wevers, M., de Fré, R. & Rymen, T. (1992) Dioxins and dibenzofurans in tunnel air. *Organohalogen Compounds*, **9**, 321–324

Wevers, M., de Fré, R., Van Cleuvenbergen, R. & Rymen, T. (1993) Concentrations of PCDDs and PCDFs in ambient air at selected locations in Flanders. *Organohalogen Compounds*, **12**, 123–126

White, K.L., Jr, Lysy, H.H., McCay, J.A. & Anderson, A.C. (1986) Modulation of serum complement levels following exposure to polychlorinated dibenzo-p-dioxins. *Toxicol. appl. Pharm.*, **84**, 209–219

White, T.E.K., Rucci, G., Liu, Z. & Gasiewicz, T.A. (1995) Weanling female Sprague-Dawley rats are not sensitive to the antiestrogenic effects of 2,3,7,8-tetrachlorodibenzo-*p*-dioxin (TCDD). *Toxicol. appl. Pharmacol.*, **133**, 313–320

Whitelaw, M.L., Pongratz, I., Wilhelmsson, A., Gustafsson, J.-Å. & Poellinger, L. (1993a) Ligand-dependent recruitment of the Arnt coregulator determines DNA recognition by the dioxin receptor. *Mol. cell. Biol.*, **13**, 2504–2514

Whitelaw, M.L., Göttlicher, M., Gustafsson, J.-Å. & Poellinger, L. (1993b) Definition of a novel ligand binding domain of a nuclear bHLH receptor: co-localization of ligand and hsp90 binding activities within the regulable inactivation domain of the dioxin receptor. *EMBO J.*, **12**, 4169–4179

Whitelaw, M.L., Gustafsson, J.-Å. & Poellinger, L. (1994) Identification of transactivation and repression functions of the dioxin receptor and its basic helix-loop-helix/PAS partner factor Arnt: inducible versus constitutive modes of regulation. *Mol. cell. Biol.*, **14**, 8343–8355

Whitelaw, M.L., McGuire, J., Picard, D., Gustafsson, J.Å. & Poellinger, L. (1995) Heat shock protein hsp90 regulates dioxin receptor function in vivo. *Proc. Natl. Acad. Sci. USA*, **92**, 4437–4441

Whitlock, J.P. (1986) The regulation of cytochrome P-450 gene expression. *Ann. Rev. Pharmacol. Toxicol.*, **26**, 333–369

Whitlock, J.P., Jr (1987) The regulation of gene expression of 2,3,7,8-tetrachlorodibenzo-*p*-dioxin. *Pharmacol. Rev.*, **39**, 147–161

Whitlock, J.P., Jr (1990) Genetic and molecular aspects of 2,3,7,8-tetrachlorodibenzo-*p*-dioxin action. *Ann. Rev. Pharmacol. Toxicol.*, **30**, 251–277

Whitlock, J.P., Jr (1993) Mechanistic aspects of dioxin action. *Chem. Res. Toxicol.*, **6**, 754–763

Whitlock, J.P., Jr (1994) The aromatic hydrocarbon receptor, dioxin action, and endocrine homeostasis. *Trends Endocrinol. Metab.*, **5**, 183–188

Whysner, J. & Williams, G.M. (1996) 2,3,7,8-tetrachlorodibenzo-p-dioxin mechanistic data and risk assessment: gene regulation, cytotoxicity, enhanced cell proliferation and tumor promotion. *Pharmacol. Ther.*, **71**, 193–223

Wichmann, H., Lorenz, W. & Bahadir, M. (1995) Release of PCDD/F and PAH during vehicle fires in traffic tunnels. *Chemosphere*, **31**, 2755–2766

Wiebel, F.J., Klose, U. & Kiefer, F. (1991) Toxicity of 2,3,7,8-tetrachlorodibenzo-*p*-dioxin in vitro: H4IIEC3-derived 5L hepatoma cells as a model system. *Toxicol. Lett.*, **55**, 161–169

Wigle, D.T., Semenciw, R.M., Wilkins, K., Riedel, D., Ritter, L., Morrison, H.I. & Mao, Y. (1990) Mortality study of Canadian male farm operators: non-Hodgkin's lymphoma mortality and agricultural practices in Saskatchewan. *J. natl Cancer Inst.*, **82**, 575–82

van Wijnen, J., van Bavel, B., Lindström, G., Koppe, J.G. & Olie, K. (1990) Placental transport of PCDDs and PCDFs in humans. *Organohalogen Compounds*, **1**, 47–50

van Wijnen, J.H., Liem, A.K.D., Olie, K. & van Zorge, J.A. (1992) Soil contamination with PCDDs and PCDFs of small (illegal) scrap wire and scrap car incineration sites. *Chemosphere*, **24**, 127–134

Wiklund, K. & Holm, L.E. (1986) Soft-tissue sarcoma risk in Swedish agricultural and forestry workers. *J. natl Cancer Inst.*, **76**, 229–234

Wiklund, K., Dich, J. & Holm, L.-E. (1987) Risk of malignant lymphoma in Swedish pesticide applicators. *Br. J. Cancer*, **56**, 505–508

Wiklund, K., Dich, J. & Holm, L.-E. (1988) Soft-tissue sarcoma risk in Swedish licensed pesticide applicators. *J. occup. Med.*, **30**, 801–804

Wiklund, K., Dich, J., Holm, L.-E. & Eklund G. (1989) Risk of cancer in pesticide applicators in Swedish agriculture. *Br. J. ind. Med.*, **46**, 809–814

Wikström, E., Löfvenius, G., Rappe, C. & Marklund, S. (1996) Influence of level and form of chlorine on the formation of chlorinated dioxins, dibenzofurans and benzenes during combustion of an artificial fuel in a laboratory reactor. *Environ. Sci. Technol.*, **30**, 1637–1644

Wilfe, D., Becker, E. & Schmutte, C. (1993) Growth stimulation of primary rat hepatocytes by 2,3,7,8-tetrachlorodibenzo-*p*-dioxin. *Cell. Biol. Toxicol.*, **9**, 15–31

Wilhelmsson, A., Cuthill, S., Denis, M., Wikström, A.-C., Gustafsson, J.-Å. & Poellinger, L. (1990) The specific DNA binding activity of the dioxin receptor is modulated by the 90 kD heat shock protein. *EMBO J.*, **9**, 69–76

Wilk, R.I., Weizman, I. & Shilo, B.-Z. (1996) Trachealess encodes a bHLH-PAS protein that is an inducer of tracheal cell fates in Drosophila. *Genes Dev.*, **10**, 93–102

Wilker, C.E., Welsh, T.H., Jr, Safe, S.H., Narasimhan, T.R. & Johnson, L. (1995) Human chorionic gonadotropin protects Leydig cell function against 2,3,7,8-tetrachlorodibenzo-*p*-dioxin in adult rats: role of Leydig cell cytoplasmic volume. *Toxicol.*, **95**, 93–102

Williams, D.T., LeBel, G.L. & Benoit, F.M. (1992) Polychlorodibenzodioxins and polychlorodibenzofurans in dioxazine dyes and pigments. *Chemosphere*, **24**, 169–180

Wipf, H.-K., Homberger, E., Neuner, N., Ranalder, U.B., Vetter, W. & Vuilleumier, J.P. (1982) TCDD-levels in soil and plant samples from the Seveso area. In: Hutzinger, O., Frei, R.W., Merian, E. & Pocchiari, F., eds, *Chlorinated Dioxins and Related Compounds: Impact on the Environment*, Oxford, Pergamon Press, pp. 115–126

de Wit, C., Jansson, B., Strandell, M., Olsson, M., Bergek, S., Boström, M., Bergqvist, P.-A., Rappe, C. & Andersson, Ö. (1990) Polychlorinated dibenzo-*p*-dioxin and dibenzofuran levels and patterns in fish samples analyzed within the Swedish dioxin survey. *Organohalogen Compounds*, **1**, 471–474

Wittsiepe, J., Ewers, U., Schrey, P., Kramer, M., Exner, M., Selenka, F., Beine, W., Kemper, K., Schmeer, D. & Weber, H. (1993) PCDD/F in blood fat of subjects from Marsberg. *Z. Umweltchem. Ökotox.*, **5**, 206–215 (in German)

Wolfe, W.H., Michalek, J.E., Miner, J.C. & Peterson, M.R. (1988) Serum 2,3,7,8-tetrachlorodibenzo-*p*-dioxin levels in Air Force Health Study personnel. *Morbid. Mortal. Wkly Rep.*, **37**, 309–311

Wolfe, W.H., Michalek, J.E., Miner, J.C., Rahe, A.R., Silva, J., Thomas, W.F., Grubbs, W.D., Lustik, M.B., Karrison, T.G., Roegner, R.H. & Williams, D.E. (1990) Health status of Air force veterans occupationally exposed to herbicides in Vietnam 1. Physical health. *J. Am. med. Assoc.*, **264**, 1824–1831

Wolfe, W.H., Michalek, J.E. & Miner, J.C. (1992) Diabetes versus dioxin body burden in veterans of Operation Ranch Hand. In: *Proceedings of the 12th International Symposium on Chlorinated Dioxins, August 24-28, Tampere, Finland*

Wolfe, W.H., Michalek, J.E. & Miner, J.C. (1994) Determinants of TCDD half-life in veterans of operation ranch hand. *J. Toxicol. environ. Health*, **41**, 481–488

Wolfe, W.H., Michalek, J.E., Miner, J.C., Rahe, A.J., Moore, C.A., Needham, L.L. & Patterson, D.G., Jr (1995) Paternal serum dioxin and reproductive outcomes among veterans of operation Ranch Hand. *Epidemiology*, **6**, 17–22

Wölfle, D. & Marquardt, H. (1996) Antioxidants inhibit the enhancement of malignant cell transformation induced by 2,3,7,8-tetrachlorodibenzo-p-dioxin. *Carcinogenesis*, **17**, 1273–1278

Wölfle, D., Schmutte, C. & Marquardt, H. (1993) Effects of 2,3,7,8-tetrachlorodibenzo-*p*-dioxin on protein kinase C and inositol phosphate metabolism in primary cultures of rat hepatocytes. *Carcinogenesis*, **14**, 2283–2287

Wood, S.C. & Holsapple, M.P. (1993) Short communication. Direct suppression of superantigen-induced IgM secretion in human lymphocytes by 2,3,7,8-TCDD. *Toxicol. appl. Pharmacol.*, **122**, 308–313

Wood, S.C., Karras, J.G. & Holsapple, M.P. (1992) Integration of the human lymphocyte into immunotoxicological investigations. *Fundam. appl. Toxicol.*, **18**, 450–459

Wood, S.C., Jeong, H.G., Morris, D.L. & Holsapple, M.P. (1993) Direct effects of 2,3,7,8-tetrachlorodibenzo-*p*-dioxin (TCDD) on human tonsillar lymphocytes. *Toxicology*, **81**, 131–143

Woods, J.S. & Polissar, L. (1989) Non-Hodgkin's lymphoma among phenoxy herbicide-exposed farm workers in western Washington State. *Chemosphere*, **18**, 401–406

Woods, J.S., Polissar, L., Severson, R.K., Heuser, L.S. & Kulander, B.G. (1987) Soft tissue sarcoma and non-Hodgkin's lymphoma in relation to phenoxy herbicide and chlorinated phenol exposure in western Washington. *J. natl Cancer Inst.*, **78**, 899–910

World Health Organization (WHO) (1989) *Polychlorinated Dibenzo-para-dioxins and Dibenzofurans* (Environmental Health Criteria 88), Geneva

World Health Organization (WHO) (1991) *Consultation on Tolerable Daily Intake from Food of PCDDs and* PCDFs (EUR/ICP/PCS 030(s)), Copenhagen, World Health Organization Regional Office for Europe

World Health Organization (WHO) (1993) *Polychlorinated Biphenyls and Terphenyls* (Environmental Health Criteria 140), Geneva

World Health Organization (WHO) (1996) *Levels of PCBs, PCDDs and PCDFs in Human Milk* (Environmental Health in Europe No. 3), Bilthoven, WHO European Centre for Environment and Health

World Health Organization/Regional Office for Europe WHO/EURO) (1987) *Dioxins and Furans from Municipal Incinerators* (Environmental Health Series 17), Copenhagen

Wörner, W. & Schrenk, D. (1996) Influence of liver tumor promoters on apoptosis in rat hepatocytes induced by 2-acetylaminofluorene, ultraviolet light, or transforming growth factor $\beta 1$. *Cancer Res.*, **56**, 1272–1278

Wright, C. & Startin, J.R. (1995) *Concentrations of PCDDs and PCDFs in Total Diet Study Samples from 1982 and 1992* (Report FD 94/200), Norwich, UK, Central Science Laboratory

Wroblewski, V.J. & Olson, J.R. (1985) Hepatic metabolism of 2,3,7,8-tetrachlorodibenzo-*p*-dioxin (TCDD) in the rat and guinea pig. *Toxicol. appl. Pharmacol.*, **81**, 231–240

Wu, L. & Whitlock, J.P., Jr (1992) Mechanism of dioxin action: Ah receptor-mediated increase in promoter accessibility *in vivo. Proc. natl Acad. Sci. USA*, **89**, 4811–4815

Wu, L. & Whitlock, J.P., Jr (1993) Mechanism of dioxin action: receptor-enhancer interactions in intact cells. *Nucleic Acids Res.*, **21**, 119–125

Wu, W.Z., Schramm, K.-W., Henkelmann, B., Xu, Y., Zhang, Y.Y. & Kettrup, A. (1995) PCDD/Fs, PCBs, HCHs and HCB in sediments and soils of Ya-Er Lake area in China: results on residual levels and correlation to the organic carbon and the particle size. *Organohalogen Compounds*, **24**, 329–332

Wuthe, J., Klett, M., Hagenmaier, H., Päpke, O., Gugel, L. & Siefert, D. (1990) PCDD/PCDF levels in human blood of people living in a highly PCDD/PCDF contaminated area next to a metal reclamation plant. *Organohalogen Compounds*, **1**, 615–620

Wuthe, J., Link, B., Walther, J., Päpke, O., Hagenmaier, H., Frommberger, R., Lillich, W. & Rack, J. (1993) Dioxin and furan (PCDD/PCDF) levels in human blood from persons living in a contaminated area. *Chemosphere*, **27**, 287–293

Yager, J.D. & Liehr, J.G. (1996) Molecular mechanisms of estrogen carcinogenesis. *Ann. Rev. Pharmacol. Toxicol.*, **36**, 203–232

Yamagishi, T., Miyazaki, T., Akiyama, K., Morita, M., Nakagawa, J., Horii, S. & Kaneko, S. (1981) Polychlorinated dibenzo-p-dioxins and dibenzofurans in commercial diphenyl ether herbicides and in freshwater fish collected from the application area. *Chemosphere*, **10**, 1137–1144

Yamashita, F. & Hayashi, M. (1985) Fetal PCB syndrome: clinical features, intrauterine growth retardation and possible alteration in calcium metabolism. *Environ. Health Perspectives*, **59**, 41–45

Yanagida, A., Sogawa, K., Yasumoto, K. I. & Fujii-Kuriyama, Y. (1990) A novel *cis*-acting DNA element required for a high level of inducible expression of the rat P-450$_c$ gene. *Mol. cell. Biol.*, **10**, 1470–1475

Yang, K.H., Croft, W.A. & Peterson, R.E. (1977) Effects of 2,3,7,8-tetrachlorodibenzo-*p*-dioxin on plasma disappearance and biliary excretion of foreign compounds in rats. *Toxicol. appl. Pharmacol.*, **40**, 485–496

Yang, J.-H., Thraves, P., Dritschilo, A. & Rhim, J.S. (1992) Neoplastic transformation of immortalized human keratinocytes by 2,3,7,8-tetrachlorodibenzo-*p*-dioxin. *Cancer Res.*, **52**, 3478–3482

Yang, G.Y., Lebrec, H. & Burleson, G.R. (1994) Effect of 2,3,7,8-tetrachlorodibenzo-*p*-dioxin (TCDD) on pulmonary influenza virus titer and natural killer (NK) activity in rats. *Fundam. appl. Toxicol.*, **23**, 125–131

Yao, C. & Safe, S. (1989) 2,3,7,8-Tetrachlorodibenzo-*p*-dioxin-induced porphyria in genetically inbred mice: partial antagonism and mechanistic studies. *Toxicol. appl. Pharmacol.*, **100**, 208–216

Yoshimura, H., Kuroki, J., Koga, N., Kuroki, H., Masuda, Y., Fukasaku, N. & Hasegawa, M. (1984) High accumulation of 2,3,4,7,8-pentachlorodibenzofuran to hepatic microsomes of rats. *J. Pharmacobiodyn.*, **7**, 414

Yoshimura, Y., Kamimura, H., Oguri, K., Honda, Y. & Nakano, M. (1986) Stimulating effect of activated charcoal beads on fecal excretion of 2,3,4,7,8-pentachlorodibenzofuran in rats. *Chemosphere*, **15**, 219

Yoshimura, H., Kuroki, J. & Koga, N. (1987) Unique features of subcellular distribution of 2,3,4,7,8-pentachlorodibenzofuran in rat liver. *Chemosphere*, **16**, 1695

Young, A.L. (1983) Long-term studies on the persistence and movement of TCDD in a natural ecosystem. In: Tucker, R.E., Young, A.L. & Gray, P., eds, *Human and Environmental Risks of Chlorinated Dioxins and Related Compounds*, New York, Plenum Press, pp. 173–190

Young, A.L., Calcagni, J.A., Thalken, C.E. & Tremblay, J.W. (1978) *The Toxicology, Environmental Fate, and Human Risk of Herbicide Orange and Its Associated Dioxin (US AF Technical Report OEHL TR-78-92)*, Air Force Base, TX, US Air Force, Occupational and Environmental Health Laboratory

Yrjänheikki, E.J., ed. (1989) *Levels of PCBs, PCDDs and PCDFs in Breast Milk; Results of WHO Coordinated Interlaboratory Quality Control Studies and Analytical Field Studies* (Environmental Health 34), Copenhagen, FADL Publishers

Yu, M.-L., Hsu, C.C., Gladen, B.C. & Rogan, W.J. (1991) In utero PCB/PCDF exposure: relation of developmental delay to dysmorphology and dose. *Neurotoxicol. Teratol.*, **13**, 195–202

Yu, M.-L., Guo, Y.-L.L., Hsu, C.-C. & Rogan, W.J. (1997) Increased mortality from chronic liver disease and cirrhosis 13 years after the Taiwan Yucheng ('oil disease') incident. *Am. J. ind. Med.*, **31**, 172–175

Zacharewski, T., Harris, M. & Safe, S. (1989) Induction of cytochrome P-450-dependent monooxygenase activities in rat hepatoma H-4II E cells in culture by 2,3,7,8-tetrachlorodibenzo-*p*-dioxin and related compounds: mechanistic studies using radiolabeled congeners. *Arch. Biochem. Biophys.*, **272**, 344–355

Zacharewski, T., Harris, M. & Safe, S. (1991) Evidence for the mechanism of action of the 2,3,7,8-tetrachlorodibenzo-p-dioxin-mediated decrease of nuclear estrogen receptor levels in wild-type and mutant mouse Hepa 1c1c7 cells. *Biochem. Pharmacol.*, **41**, 1931–1939

Zacharewski, T., Harris, M., Biegel, L., Morrison, V., Merchant, M. & Safe, S. (1992) 6-Methyl-1,3,8-trichlorodibenzofuran (MCDF) as an antiestrogen in human and rodent cancer cell lines: evidence for the role of the Ah receptor. *Toxicol. appl. Pharmacol.*, **113**, 311–318

Zacharewski, T., Bondy, K., McDonell, P. & Wu, Z. F. (1994) Antiestrogenic effects of 2,3,7,8-tetrachlorodibenzo-*p*-dioxin on 17β-estradiol-induced pS2 expression. *Cancer Res.*, **54**, 2707–2713

Zack, J.A. & Gaffey, W.R. (1983) A mortality study of workers employed at the Monsanto Company plant in Nitro, West Virginia. In: Tucker, R., Young, A. & Grey, A., eds, *Human and Environmental Risks of Chlorinated Dioxins and Related Compounds*, New York, Plenum Press, pp. 575–591

Zack, J.A. & Suskind, R.R. (1980) The mortality experience of workers exposed to tetrachlorodibenzodioxin in a trichlorophenol process accident. *J. occup. Med.*, **22**, 11–14

Zeiger, E., Anderson, B., Haworth, S., Lawlor, T. & Mortelmans, K. (1988) *Salmonella* mutagenicity tests: IV. Results from the testing of 300 chemicals. *Environ. mol. Mutag.*, **11** (Suppl. 12), 1–158

Zemek, A. & Kocan, A. (1991) 2,3,7,8-Tetrachlorodibenzo-p-dioxin in soil samples from a trichlorophenol-producing plant. *Chemosphere*, **23**, 1769–1776

Zinkl, J.F., Vos, J.G., Moore, J.A. & Gupta, B.N. (1973) Hematologic and clinical chemistry effects of 2,3,7,8-tetrachlorodibenzo-*p*-dioxin in laboratory animals. *Environ. Health Perspectives*, **5**, 111–118

Zober, A. & Päpke, O. (1993) Concentrations of PCDDs and PCDFs in human tissue 36 years after accidental dioxin exposure. *Chemosphere*, **27**, 413–418

Zober, A., Messerer, P. & Huber, P. (1990) Thirty-four-year mortality follow-up of BASF employees exposed to 2,3,7,8-TCDD after the 1953 accident. *Int. Arch. occup. environ. Health*, **62**, 139–157

Zober, M.A., Ott, M.G., Päpke, O., Senft, K. & Germann, C. (1992) Morbidity study of extruder personnel with potential exposure to brominated dioxins and furans. I. Results of blood monitoring and immunological tests. *Br. J. ind. Med.*, **49**, 532–544

Zober, A., Ott, M.G., Fleig, I. & Heidemann, A. (1993) Cytogenetic studies in lymphocytes of workers exposed to 2,3,7,8-TCDD. *Int. Arch. occup. environ. Health*, **65**, 157–161

Zober, A., Ott, M.G. & Messerer, P. (1994) Morbidity follow up study of BASF employees exposed to 2,3,7,8-tetrachlorodibenzo-p-dioxin (TCDD) after a 1953 chemical reactor incident. *Occup. environ. Med.*, **51**, 479–486

Zook, D.R. & Rappe, C. (1994) Environmental sources, distribution, and fate of polychlorinated dibenzodioxins, dibenzofurans, and related organochlorines. In: Schecter, A., ed., *Dioxins and Health*, New York, Plenum Press, pp. 79–113

Zorn, N. E., Russell, D. H., Buckley, A. R. & Sauro, M. D. (1995) Alterations in splenocyte protein kinase C (PKC) activity by 2,3,7,8-tetrachlorodibenzo-*p*-dioxin *in vivo*. *Toxicol. Lett.*, **78**, 93–100

SUMMARY OF FINAL EVALUATIONS

Agent	Degree of evidence of carcinogenicity		Overall evaluation of carcinogenicity to humans
	Human	Animal	
Dibenzo-*para*-dioxin	ND	ESL	3
Polychlorinated dibenzo-*para*-dioxins	ND		3
(other than 2,3,7,8-tetrachlorodibenzodioxin)			
2,7-DCDD		I	
1,2,3,7,8-PeCDD		I	
1,2,3,6,7,8-/1,2,3,7,8,9-HxCDD		L	
1,2,3,4,6,7,8-HpCDD		I	
Polychlorinated dibenzofurans	I		3
2,3,7,8-TCDF		I	
2,3,4,7,8-PeCDF		L	
1,2,3,4,7,8-HxCDF		L	
2,3,7,8-Tetrachlorodibenzo-*para*-dioxin	L	S	1[a]

ND, no adequate data; ESL, evidence suggesting lack of carcinogenicity; S, sufficient evidence; L, limited evidence; I, inadequate evidence; 3, group 3: not classifiable as to its carcinogenicity to humans; 1, group 1: carcinogenic to humans; for definitions of criteria for degrees of evidence and groups, see preamble, pp. 23–27.

[a] Mechanism data taken into account in making the overall evaluation

ABBREVIATIONS

ADI	Acceptable daily intake
Ah	Aryl hydrocarbon
Ah^b/Ah^b	Low-affinity Ah receptor
Ah^d/Ah^d	Mild-type high-affinity Ah receptor
ALT	Alanine aminotransferase = SGPT
Arnt	Ah receptor nuclear translocator
AST	Aspartate aminotransferase = SGOT
ATPase	Adenosine triphosphatase
bHLH	Basic helix-loop-helix
CNP	1,3,4-Trichloro-2-(4-nitrophenoxy)benzene
CFP	Chemical fertilizer plant
CRR	Conditional risk ratio
CTL	Cytotoxic T-lymphocyte
CWI	Clinical waste incinerator
Cx	Connexon
2,4-D	2,4-Dichlorophenoxyacetic acid
DCDD	Dichlorodibenzo-*para*-dioxin
DGA	D-glutaric acid
DN	Double negative
DP	Double positive
DNP	Dinitrophenyl
ECD	Electron capture detection
ECF	Elemental chlorine-free
ECOD	7-Ethoxycoumarin-*O*-deethylase
EC_{50}	50% Effective concentration
ED_{50}	50% Effective dose
EEG	Electroencephalogram
EGF	Epidermal growth factor
EROD	7-Ethoxyresorufin *O*-deethylase
FEV_1	Forced expiratory volume in 1 second
FSH	Follicle-stimulating hormone
FTI	Free thyroxine index
FT4	Free thyroxine
FVC	Forced vital capacity
GC	Gas chromatography
GGT	γ-Glutamyl transferase
GJIC	Gap-junctional intercellular communication

GLUT	Glucose transporter
GnRH	Gonadotropin-releasing hormone
GST	Glutathione S-transferase
GSTP	Glutathione *S*-transferase P
GT	Glucuronosyl transferase
HDDV	Heavy-duty (diesel) vehicle
HIF	Hypoxia-inducible factor
HOMO	Highest occupied molecular orbital
HpCDD	Heptachlorodibenzo-*para*-dioxin
HpCDF	Heptachlorodibenzofuran
HPLC	High-performance liquid chromatography
hr	Hairless
A=HRGC	High-resolution gas chromatography
B=HRMS	High-resolution mass spectrometry
hsp	Heat shock protein
HxCDD	Hexachlorodibenzo-*para*-dioxin
HxCDF	Hexachlorodibenzofuran
I	Isomer-specific polar column
IC (ID)	Inhibition concentration (dose)
IG	Immunoglobulin
IL	Interleukin
IRR	Incidence rate ratio
I-TEQ	International toxic equivalent
IWI	Industrial waste incinerator
LH	Luteinizing hormone
LDV	Light-duty vehicle
LOEL	Lowest observed effect level
LPS	Lipopolysaccharide
a=LRGC	Low-resolution gas chromatography
C=LRMS	Low-resolution mass spectrometry
MCPA	4-Chloro-2-methylphenoxyacetic acid
MCPP	2-(4-Chloro-2-methylphenoxy)propanoic acid (mecoprop)
MNNG	*N*-Methyl-*N'*-nitro-*N*-nitrosoguanidine
MS	Mass spectrometry
MSS	Municipal sewage sludge
MSW	Municipal solid waste
MWI	Municipal solid waste incinerator
MWTP	Municipal water treatment plant
N	No information
NDEA	*N*-Nitrosodiethylamine
NHATS	(United States Environmental Protection Agency) National Human Adipose Tissue Survey
NIOSH	(United States) National Institute for Occupational Safety and Health
NIP	2,4-Dichloro-1-(4-nitrophenoxy)benzene; nitrofen

NK	Natural killer
NOEL	No observed effect level
O	Other than isomer-specific nonpolar column
OCDD	Octachlorodibenzo-*para*-dioxin
OCDF	Octachlorodibenzofuran
8-OH-dG	8-Hydroxydeoxyguanine
PAI	Plasminogen-activator inhibitor
PAS	Per-Arnt-Sim
PCB	Polychlorinated biphenyl
PCDD	Polychlorinated dibenzo-*para*-dioxin
PCDF	Polychlorinated dibenzofuran
PCQ	Polychlorinated terphenyl
PCP	Pentachlorophenol
PCT	Porphyria cutanea tarda
PeCDD	Pentachlorodibenzo-*para*-dioxin
PeCDF	Pentachlorodibenzofuran
PEPCK	Phosphoenol pyruvate carboxykinase
Per	Period
PFC	Plaque-forming cell
PGHS	Prostaglandin endoperoxide H synthase
PMN	Polymorphonuclear neutrophils
R	Reduced clean-up
RAG	Recombinase activating gene
RDF	Refuse-derived fuel incinerator
RR	Relative risk
S	Sophisticated clean-up
SCID	Severe combined immunodeficient
SFE	Supercritical fluid extraction
Sim	Single-minded
SIR	Standardized incidence ratio
SMR	Standardized mortality ratio
SRBC	Spleen anti-sheep red blood cell
SSI	Sewage sludge incinerator
T4	Thyroxine
TBG	Thyroxine-binding globulin
TCDD	Tetrachlorodibenzo-*para*-dioxin
TCDF	Tetrachlorodibenzofuran
TCF	Total chlorine-free
TCP	2,4,5-Trichlorophenol
TCR	T-cell receptor
TDI	Tolerable daily intake
TdT	Terminal deoxynucleotidyl transferase
2,4,5-T	2,4,5-Trichlorophenoxyacetic acid
2,4,6-TCP	2,4,6-Trichlorophenol

T3	Triiodothyronine
TEF	Toxic equivalency factor
TEQ	Toxic equivalent
TGF	Transforming growth factor
TNFα	Tumour necrosis factor α
TNP	Trinitrophenyl
TPA	12-*O*-Tetradecanoylphorbol 13-acetate
TRK	German occupational technical exposure limit
TSH	Thyroid-stimulating hormone
UDP-GT	Uridine diphosphate-glucuronosyl transferase
W	WHO-accepted laboratory
WCOT	Wall-coated open-tubular
X-52	chlomethoxynil; 2,4-dichloro-1-(3-methoxy-4-nitrophenoxy)benzene
XRE	Xenobiotic-responsive enhancer = DRE (dioxin-responsive enhancer)

SUPPLEMENTARY CORRIGENDA TO VOLUMES 1–69

Volume 60

p. 513, last para before References, '*Environmental Health Research and Testing Inc.*' should be replaced by '*Integrated Laboratory System*' and '*EHRT*' should be replaced by '*ILS*'.

Volume 62

p. 370, para above Fig. 1,
　　8th line: '100 000 mg/ml' should be replaced by '100 000 µg/ml'
　　last line: '10 mg/ml' should be replaced by '10 µg/ml'
p. 371, (*b*), '10^3 mg/ml' should be replaced by '10^3 µg/ml'
p. 373, last para above References, '*Environmental Health Research and Testing Inc.*' should be replaced by '*Integrated Laboratory System*' and '*EHRT*' should be replaced by '*ILS*'.

Volume 63

p. 500, para above Fig. 1,
　　8th line: '100 000 mg/ml' should be replaced by '100 000 µg/ml'
　　last line: '10 mg/ml' should be replaced by '10 µg/ml'
p. 501, (*b*), '10^3 mg/ml' should be replaced by '10^3 µg/ml'
p. 503, last para above References, '*Environmental Health Research and Testing Inc.*' should be replaced by '*Integrated Laboratory System*' and '*EHRT*' should be replaced by '*ILS*'.

Volume 65

p. 524, para above Fig. 1,
　　8th line: '100 000 mg/ml' should be replaced by '100 000 µg/ml'
　　last line: '10 mg/ml' should be replaced by '10 µg/ml'
p. 525, (*b*), '10^3 mg/ml' should be replaced by '10^3 µg/ml'
p. 527, last para above References, '*Environmental Health Research and Testing Inc.*' should be replaced by '*Integrated Laboratory System*' and '*EHRT*' should be replaced by '*ILS*'.

Volume 66

p. 468, para above Fig. 1,

8th line: '100 000 mg/ml' should be replaced by '100 000 µg/ml'

last line: '10 mg/ml' should be replaced by '10 µg/ml'

p. 469, (*b*), '10^3 mg/ml' should be replaced by '10^3 µg/ml'

p. 471, last para above References, '*Environmental Health Research and Testing Inc.*' should be replaced by '*Integrated Laboratory System*' and '*EHRT*' should be replaced by '*ILS*'.

Volume 68

p. 464, para above Fig. 1,

8th line: '100 000 mg/ml' should be replaced by '100 000 µg/ml'

last line: '10 mg/ml' should be replaced by '10 µg/ml'

p. 465, (*b*), '10^3 mg/ml' should be replaced by '10^3 µg/ml'

p. 467, last para above References, '*Environmental Health Research and Testing Inc.*' should be replaced by '*Integrated Laboratory System*' and '*EHRT*' should be replaced by '*ILS*'.

CUMULATIVE CROSS INDEX TO *IARC MONOGRAPHS ON THE EVALUATION OF CARCINOGENIC RISKS TO HUMANS*

The volume, page and year of publication are given. References to corrigenda are given in parentheses.

A

A-α-C	*40*, 245 (1986); *Suppl. 7*, 56 (1987)
Acetaldehyde	*36*, 101 (1985) (*corr. 42*, 263); *Suppl. 7*, 77 (1987)
Acetaldehyde formylmethylhydrazone (*see* Gyromitrin)	
Acetamide	*7*, 197 (1974); *Suppl. 7*, 389 (1987)
Acetaminophen (*see* Paracetamol)	
Acridine orange	*16*, 145 (1978); *Suppl. 7*, 56 (1987)
Acriflavinium chloride	*13*, 31 (1977); *Suppl. 7*, 56 (1987)
Acrolein	*19*, 479 (1979); *36*, 133 (1985); *Suppl. 7*, 78 (1987); *63*, 337 (1995) (*corr. 65*, 549)
Acrylamide	*39*, 41 (1986); *Suppl. 7*, 56 (1987); *60*, 389 (1994)
Acrylic acid	*19*, 47 (1979); *Suppl. 7*, 56 (1987)
Acrylic fibres	*19*, 86 (1979); *Suppl. 7*, 56 (1987)
Acrylonitrile	*19*, 73 (1979); *Suppl. 7*, 79 (1987)
Acrylonitrile-butadiene-styrene copolymers	*19*, 91 (1979); *Suppl. 7*, 56 (1987)
Actinolite (*see* Asbestos)	
Actinomycins	*10*, 29 (1976) (*corr. 42*, 255); *Suppl. 7*, 80 (1987)
Adriamycin	*10*, 43 (1976); *Suppl. 7*, 82 (1987)
AF-2	*31*, 47 (1983); *Suppl. 7*, 56 (1987)
Aflatoxins	*1*, 145 (1972) (*corr. 42*, 251); *10*, 51 (1976); *Suppl. 7*, 83 (1987); *56*, 245 (1993)
Aflatoxin B₁ (*see* Aflatoxins)	
Aflatoxin B₂ (*see* Aflatoxins)	
Aflatoxin G₁ (*see* Aflatoxins)	
Aflatoxin G₂ (*see* Aflatoxins)	
Aflatoxin M₁ (*see* Aflatoxins)	
Agaritine	*31*, 63 (1983); *Suppl. 7*, 56 (1987)
Alcohol drinking	*44* (1988)
Aldicarb	*53*, 93 (1991)
Aldrin	*5*, 25 (1974); *Suppl. 7*, 88 (1987)
Allyl chloride	*36*, 39 (1985); *Suppl. 7*, 56 (1987)
Allyl isothiocyanate	*36*, 55 (1985); *Suppl. 7*, 56 (1987)
Allyl isovalerate	*36*, 69 (1985); *Suppl. 7*, 56 (1987)
Aluminium production	*34*, 37 (1984); *Suppl. 7*, 89 (1987)

Benzofuran	*63*, 431 (1995)
Benzo[*ghi*]perylene	*32*, 195 (1983); *Suppl. 7*, 58 (1987)
Benzo[*c*]phenanthrene	*32*, 205 (1983); *Suppl. 7*, 58 (1987)
Benzo[*a*]pyrene	*3*, 91 (1973); *32*, 211 (1983)
	(*corr. 68*, 477); *Suppl. 7*, 58 (1987)
Benzo[*e*]pyrene	*3*, 137 (1973); *32*, 225 (1983);
	Suppl. 7, 58 (1987)
para-Benzoquinone dioxime	*29*, 185 (1982); *Suppl. 7*, 58 (1987)
Benzotrichloride (*see also* α-Chlorinated toluenes)	*29*, 73 (1982); *Suppl. 7*, 148 (1987)
Benzoyl chloride	*29*, 83 (1982) (*corr. 42*, 261);
	Suppl. 7, 126 (1987)
Benzoyl peroxide	*36*, 267 (1985); *Suppl. 7*, 58 (1987)
Benzyl acetate	*40*, 109 (1986); *Suppl. 7*, 58 (1987)
Benzyl chloride (*see also* α-Chlorinated toluenes)	*11*, 217 (1976) (*corr. 42*, 256); *29*,
	49 (1982); *Suppl. 7*, 148 (1987)
Benzyl violet 4B	*16*, 153 (1978); *Suppl. 7*, 58 (1987)
Bertrandite (*see* Beryllium and beryllium compounds)	
Beryllium and beryllium compounds	*1*, 17 (1972); *23*, 143 (1980)
	(*corr. 42*, 260); *Suppl. 7*, 127
	(1987); *58*, 41 (1993)
Beryllium acetate (*see* Beryllium and beryllium compounds)	
Beryllium acetate, basic (*see* Beryllium and beryllium compounds)	
Beryllium-aluminium alloy (*see* Beryllium and beryllium compounds)	
Beryllium carbonate (*see* Beryllium and beryllium compounds)	
Beryllium chloride (*see* Beryllium and beryllium compounds)	
Beryllium-copper alloy (*see* Beryllium and beryllium compounds)	
Beryllium-copper-cobalt alloy (*see* Beryllium and beryllium compounds)	
Beryllium fluoride (*see* Beryllium and beryllium compounds)	
Beryllium hydroxide (*see* Beryllium and beryllium compounds)	
Beryllium-nickel alloy (*see* Beryllium and beryllium compounds)	
Beryllium oxide (*see* Beryllium and beryllium compounds)	
Beryllium phosphate (*see* Beryllium and beryllium compounds)	
Beryllium silicate (*see* Beryllium and beryllium compounds)	
Beryllium sulfate (*see* Beryllium and beryllium compounds)	
Beryl ore (*see* Beryllium and beryllium compounds)	
Betel quid	*37*, 141 (1985); *Suppl. 7*, 128 (1987)
Betel-quid chewing (*see* Betel quid)	
BHA (*see* Butylated hydroxyanisole)	
BHT (*see* Butylated hydroxytoluene)	
Bis(1-aziridinyl)morpholinophosphine sulfide	*9*, 55 (1975); *Suppl. 7*, 58 (1987)
Bis(2-chloroethyl)ether	*9*, 117 (1975); *Suppl. 7*, 58 (1987)
N,N-Bis(2-chloroethyl)-2-naphthylamine	*4*, 119 (1974) (*corr. 42*, 253);
	Suppl. 7, 130 (1987)
Bischloroethyl nitrosourea (see also Chloroethyl nitrosoureas)	*26*, 79 (1981); *Suppl. 7*, 150 (1987)
1,2-Bis(chloromethoxy)ethane	*15*, 31 (1977); *Suppl. 7*, 58 (1987)
1,4-Bis(chloromethoxymethyl)benzene	*15*, 37 (1977); *Suppl. 7*, 58 (1987)
Bis(chloromethyl)ether	*4*, 231 (1974) (*corr. 42*, 253);
	Suppl. 7, 131 (1987)
Bis(2-chloro-1-methylethyl)ether	*41*, 149 (1986); *Suppl. 7*, 59 (1987)
Bis(2,3-epoxycyclopentyl)ether	*47*, 231 (1989)
Bisphenol A diglycidyl ether (*see* Glycidyl ethers)	
Bisulfites (see Sulfur dioxide and some sulfites, bisulfites and metabisulfites)	
Bitumens	*35*, 39 (1985); *Suppl. 7*, 133 (1987)
Bleomycins	*26*, 97 (1981); *Suppl. 7*, 134 (1987)
Blue VRS	*16*, 163 (1978); *Suppl. 7*, 59 (1987)

Cobalt-chromium-molybdenum alloys (*see* Cobalt and cobalt compounds)
Cobalt metal powder (*see* Cobalt and cobalt compounds)
Cobalt naphthenate (*see* Cobalt and cobalt compounds)
Cobalt[II] oxide (*see* Cobalt and cobalt compounds)
Cobalt[II,III] oxide (*see* Cobalt and cobalt compounds)
Cobalt[II] sulfide (*see* Cobalt and cobalt compounds)

Coffee	*51*, 41 (1991) (*corr. 52*, 513)
Coke production	*34*, 101 (1984); *Suppl. 7*, 176 (1987)
Combined oral contraceptives (*see also* Oestrogens, progestins and combinations)	*Suppl. 7*, 297 (1987)
Conjugated oestrogens (*see also* Steroidal oestrogens)	*21*, 147 (1979)
Contraceptives, oral (*see* Combined oral contraceptives; Sequential oral contraceptives)	
Copper 8-hydroxyquinoline	*15*, 103 (1977); *Suppl. 7*, 61 (1987)
Coronene	*32*, 263 (1983); *Suppl. 7*, 61 (1987)
Coumarin	*10*, 113 (1976); *Suppl. 7*, 61 (1987)
Creosotes (*see also* Coal-tars)	*35*, 83 (1985); *Suppl. 7*, 177 (1987)
meta-Cresidine	*27*, 91 (1982); *Suppl. 7*, 61 (1987)
para-Cresidine	*27*, 92 (1982); *Suppl. 7*, 61 (1987)
Cristobalite (*see* Crystalline silica)	
Crocidolite (*see* Asbestos)	
Crotonaldehyde	*63*, 373 (1995) (*corr. 65*, 549)
Crude oil	*45*, 119 (1989)
Crystalline silica (*see also* Silica)	*42*, 39 (1987); *Suppl. 7*, 341 (1987); *68*, 41 (1997)
Cycasin	*1*, 157 (1972) (*corr. 42*, 251); *10*, 121 (1976); *Suppl. 7*, 61 (1987)
Cyclamates	*22*, 55 (1980); *Suppl. 7*, 178 (1987)
Cyclamic acid (*see* Cyclamates)	
Cyclochlorotine	*10*, 139 (1976); *Suppl. 7*, 61 (1987)
Cyclohexanone	*47*, 157 (1989)
Cyclohexylamine (*see* Cyclamates)	
Cyclopenta[*cd*]pyrene	*32*, 269 (1983); *Suppl. 7*, 61 (1987)
Cyclopropane (*see* Anaesthetics, volatile)	
Cyclophosphamide	*9*, 135 (1975); *26*, 165 (1981); *Suppl. 7*, 182 (1987)

D

2,4-D (*see also* Chlorophenoxy herbicides; Chlorophenoxy herbicides, occupational exposures to)	*15*, 111 (1977)
Dacarbazine	*26*, 203 (1981); *Suppl. 7*, 184 (1987)
Dantron	*50*, 265 (1990) (*corr. 59*, 257)
D&C Red No. 9	*8*, 107 (1975); *Suppl. 7*, 61 (1987); *57*, 203 (1993)
Dapsone	*24*, 59 (1980); *Suppl. 7*, 185 (1987)
Daunomycin	*10*, 145 (1976); *Suppl. 7*, 61 (1987)
DDD (*see* DDT)	
DDE (*see* DDT)	
DDT	*5*, 83 (1974) (*corr. 42*, 253); *Suppl. 7*, 186 (1987); *53*, 179 (1991)
Decabromodiphenyl oxide	*48*, 73 (1990)
Deltamethrin	*53*, 251 (1991)
Deoxynivalenol (*see* Toxins derived from *Fusarium graminearum*, *F. culmorum* and *F. crookwellense*)	

trans-1,4-Dichlorobutene	15, 149 (1977); Suppl. 7, 62 (1987)
3,3'-Dichloro-4,4'-diaminodiphenyl ether	16, 309 (1978); Suppl. 7, 62 (1987)
1,2-Dichloroethane	20, 429 (1979); Suppl. 7, 62 (1987)
Dichloromethane	20, 449 (1979); 41, 43 (1986); Suppl. 7, 194 (1987)
2,4-Dichlorophenol (see Chlorophenols; Chlorophenols, occupational exposures to)	
(2,4-Dichlorophenoxy)acetic acid (see 2,4-D)	
2,6-Dichloro-para-phenylenediamine	39, 325 (1986); Suppl. 7, 62 (1987)
1,2-Dichloropropane	41, 131 (1986); Suppl. 7, 62 (1987)
1,3-Dichloropropene (technical-grade)	41, 113 (1986); Suppl. 7, 195 (1987)
Dichlorvos	20, 97 (1979); Suppl. 7, 62 (1987); 53, 267 (1991)
Dicofol	30, 87 (1983); Suppl. 7, 62 (1987)
Dicyclohexylamine (see Cyclamates)	
Dieldrin	5, 125 (1974); Suppl. 7, 196 (1987)
Dienoestrol (see also Nonsteroidal oestrogens)	21, 161 (1979)
Diepoxybutane	11, 115 (1976) (corr. 42, 255); Suppl. 7, 62 (1987)
Diesel and gasoline engine exhausts	46, 41 (1989)
Diesel fuels	45, 219 (1989) (corr. 47, 505)
Diethyl ether (see Anaesthetics, volatile)	
Di(2-ethylhexyl)adipate	29, 257 (1982); Suppl. 7, 62 (1987)
Di(2-ethylhexyl)phthalate	29, 269 (1982) (corr. 42, 261); Suppl. 7, 62 (1987)
1,2-Diethylhydrazine	4, 153 (1974); Suppl. 7, 62 (1987)
Diethylstilboestrol	6, 55 (1974); 21, 173 (1979) (corr. 42, 259); Suppl. 7, 273 (1987)
Diethylstilboestrol dipropionate (see Diethylstilboestrol)	
Diethyl sulfate	4, 277 (1974); Suppl. 7, 198 (1987); 54, 213 (1992)
Diglycidyl resorcinol ether	11, 125 (1976); 36, 181 (1985); Suppl. 7, 62 (1987)
Dihydrosafrole	1, 170 (1972); 10, 233 (1976) Suppl. 7, 62 (1987)
1,8-Dihydroxyanthraquinone (see Dantron)	
Dihydroxybenzenes (see Catechol; Hydroquinone; Resorcinol)	
Dihydroxymethylfuratrizine	24, 77 (1980); Suppl. 7, 62 (1987)
Diisopropyl sulfate	54, 229 (1992)
Dimethisterone (see also Progestins; Sequential oral contraceptives	6, 167 (1974); 21, 377 (1979))
Dimethoxane	15, 177 (1977); Suppl. 7, 62 (1987)
3,3'-Dimethoxybenzidine	4, 41 (1974); Suppl. 7, 198 (1987)
3,3'-Dimethoxybenzidine-4,4'-diisocyanate	39, 279 (1986); Suppl. 7, 62 (1987)
para-Dimethylaminoazobenzene	8, 125 (1975); Suppl. 7, 62 (1987)
para-Dimethylaminoazobenzenediazo sodium sulfonate	8, 147 (1975); Suppl. 7, 62 (1987)
trans-2-[(Dimethylamino)methylimino]-5-[2-(5-nitro-2-furyl)-vinyl]-1,3,4-oxadiazole	7, 147 (1974) (corr. 42, 253); Suppl. 7, 62 (1987)
4,4'-Dimethylangelicin plus ultraviolet radiation (see also Angelicin and some synthetic derivatives)	Suppl. 7, 57 (1987)
4,5'-Dimethylangelicin plus ultraviolet radiation (see also Angelicin and some synthetic derivatives)	Suppl. 7, 57 (1987)
2,6-Dimethylaniline	57, 323 (1993)
N,N-Dimethylaniline	57, 337 (1993)
Dimethylarsinic acid (see Arsenic and arsenic compounds)	
3,3'-Dimethylbenzidine	1, 87 (1972); Suppl. 7, 62 (1987)

Ethylene dibromide   *15*, 195 (1977); *Suppl. 7*, 204 (1987)
Ethylene oxide   *11*, 157 (1976); *36*, 189 (1985)
                                                                  (*corr. 42*, 263); *Suppl. 7*, 205
                                                                  (1987); *60*, 73 (1994)
Ethylene sulfide   *11*, 257 (1976); *Suppl. 7*, 63 (1987)
Ethylene thiourea   *7*, 45 (1974); *Suppl. 7*, 207 (1987)
2-Ethylhexyl acrylate   *60*, 475 (1994)
Ethyl methanesulfonate   *7*, 245 (1974); *Suppl. 7*, 63 (1987)
N-Ethyl-*N*-nitrosourea   *1*, 135 (1972); *17*, 191 (1978);
                                                                  Suppl. 7, 63 (1987)
Ethyl selenac (*see also* Selenium and selenium compounds)   *12*, 107 (1976); *Suppl. 7*, 63 (1987)
Ethyl tellurac   *12*, 115 (1976); *Suppl. 7*, 63 (1987)
Ethynodiol diacetate (*see also* Progestins; Combined oral   *6*, 173 (1974); *21*, 387 (1979)
    contraceptives)
Eugenol   *36*, 75 (1985); *Suppl. 7*, 63 (1987)
Evans blue   *8*, 151 (1975); *Suppl. 7*, 63 (1987)

F

Fast Green FCF   *16*, 187 (1978); *Suppl. 7*, 63 (1987)
Fenvalerate   *53*, 309 (1991)
Ferbam   *12*, 121 (1976) (*corr. 42*, 256);
                                                                  Suppl. 7, 63 (1987)
Ferric oxide   *1*, 29 (1972); *Suppl. 7*, 216 (1987)
Ferrochromium (*see* Chromium and chromium compounds)
Fluometuron   *30*, 245 (1983); *Suppl. 7*, 63 (1987)
Fluoranthene   *32*, 355 (1983); *Suppl. 7*, 63 (1987)
Fluorene   *32*, 365 (1983); *Suppl. 7*, 63 (1987)
Fluorescent lighting (exposure to) (*see* Ultraviolet radiation)
Fluorides (inorganic, used in drinking-water)   *27*, 237 (1982); *Suppl. 7*, 208 (1987)
5-Fluorouracil   *26*, 217 (1981); *Suppl. 7*, 210 (1987)
Fluorspar (*see* Fluorides)
Fluosilicic acid (*see* Fluorides)
Fluroxene (*see* Anaesthetics, volatile)
Formaldehyde   *29*, 345 (1982); *Suppl. 7*, 211 (1987);
                                                                  62, 217 (1995) (*corr. 65*, 549;
                                                                  corr. 66, 485)
2-(2-Formylhydrazino)-4-(5-nitro-2-furyl)thiazole   *7*, 151 (1974) (*corr. 42*, 253);
                                                                  Suppl. 7, 63 (1987)
Frusemide (*see* Furosemide)
Fuel oils (heating oils)   *45*, 239 (1989) (*corr. 47*, 505)
Fumonisin B$_1$ (*see* Toxins derived from Fusarium moniliforme)
Fumonisin B$_2$ (*see* Toxins derived from Fusarium moniliforme)
Furan   *63*, 393 (1995)
Furazolidone   *31*, 141 (1983); *Suppl. 7*, 63 (1987)
Furfural   *63*, 409 (1995)
Furniture and cabinet-making   *25*, 99 (1981); *Suppl. 7*, 380 (1987)
Furosemide   *50*, 277 (1990)
2-(2-Furyl)-3-(5-nitro-2-furyl)acrylamide (*see* AF-2)
Fusarenon-X (*see* Toxins derived from *Fusarium graminearum*,
    F. culmorum and *F. crookwellense*)
Fusarenone-X (*see* Toxins derived from *Fusarium graminearum*,
    F. culmorum and *F. crookwellense*)
Fusarin C (*see* Toxins derived from *Fusarium moniliforme*)

G

H

K

Kaempferol — *31*, 171 (1983); *Suppl. 7*, 65 (1987)
Kepone (*see* Chlordecone)

L

Lasiocarpine — *10*, 281 (1976); *Suppl. 7*, 65 (1987)
Lauroyl peroxide — *36*, 315 (1985); *Suppl. 7*, 65 (1987)
Lead acetate (*see* Lead and lead compounds)
Lead and lead compounds — *1*, 40 (1972) (*corr. 42*, 251); *2*, 52, 150 (1973); *12*, 131 (1976); *23*, 40, 208, 209, 325 (1980); *Suppl. 7*, 230 (1987)

Lead arsenate (*see* Arsenic and arsenic compounds)
Lead carbonate (*see* Lead and lead compounds)
Lead chloride (*see* Lead and lead compounds)
Lead chromate (*see* Chromium and chromium compounds)
Lead chromate oxide (*see* Chromium and chromium compounds)
Lead naphthenate (*see* Lead and lead compounds)
Lead nitrate (*see* Lead and lead compounds)
Lead oxide (*see* Lead and lead compounds)
Lead phosphate (*see* Lead and lead compounds)
Lead subacetate (*see* Lead and lead compounds)
Lead tetroxide (*see* Lead and lead compounds)
Leather goods manufacture — *25*, 279 (1981); *Suppl. 7*, 235 (1987)
Leather industries — *25*, 199 (1981); *Suppl. 7*, 232 (1987)
Leather tanning and processing — *25*, 201 (1981); *Suppl. 7*, 236 (1987)
Ledate (*see also* Lead and lead compounds) — *12*, 131 (1976)
Light Green SF — *16*, 209 (1978); *Suppl. 7*, 65 (1987)
d-Limonene — *56*, 135 (1993)
Lindane (*see* Hexachlorocyclohexanes)
Liver flukes (*see Clonorchis sinensis, Opisthorchis felineus* and
    Opisthorchis viverrini)
Lumber and sawmill industries (including logging) — *25*, 49 (1981); *Suppl. 7*, 383 (1987)
Luteoskyrin — *10*, 163 (1976); *Suppl. 7*, 65 (1987)
Lynoestrenol (*see also* Progestins; Combined oral contraceptives) — *21*, 407 (1979)

M

Magenta — *4*, 57 (1974) (*corr. 42*, 252); *Suppl. 7*, 238 (1987); *57*, 215 (1993)
Magenta, manufacture of (*see also* Magenta) — *Suppl. 7*, 238 (1987); *57*, 215 (1993)
Malathion — *30*, 103 (1983); *Suppl. 7*, 65 (1987)
Maleic hydrazide — *4*, 173 (1974) (*corr. 42*, 253); *Suppl. 7*, 65 (1987)
Malonaldehyde — *36*, 163 (1985); *Suppl. 7*, 65 (1987)
Maneb — *12*, 137 (1976); *Suppl. 7*, 65 (1987)
Man-made mineral fibres — *43*, 39 (1988)
Mannomustine — *9*, 157 (1975); *Suppl. 7*, 65 (1987)
Mate — *51*, 273 (1991)
MCPA (*see also* Chlorophenoxy herbicides; Chlorophenoxy — *30*, 255 (1983)
    herbicides, occupational exposures to)

MeA-α-C   *40*, 253 (1986); *Suppl. 7*, 65 (1987)
Medphalan   *9*, 168 (1975); *Suppl. 7*, 65 (1987)
Medroxyprogesterone acetate   *6*, 157 (1974); *21*, 417 (1979)
    (*corr. 42*, 259); *Suppl. 7*, 289 (1987)

Megestrol acetate (*see also* Progestins; Combined oral contraceptives)
MeIQ   *40*, 275 (1986); *Suppl. 7*, 65 (1987);
    56, 197 (1993)

MeIQx   *40*, 283 (1986); *Suppl. 7*, 65 (1987)
    56, 211 (1993)

Melamine   *39*, 333 (1986); *Suppl. 7*, 65 (1987)
Melphalan   *9*, 167 (1975); *Suppl. 7*, 239 (1987)
6-Mercaptopurine   *26*, 249 (1981); *Suppl. 7*, 240 (1987)
Mercuric chloride (*see* Mercury and mercury compounds)
Mercury and mercury compounds   *58*, 239 (1993)
Merphalan   *9*, 169 (1975); *Suppl. 7*, 65 (1987)
Mestranol (*see also* Steroidal oestrogens)   *6*, 87 (1974); *21*, 257 (1979)
    (*corr. 42*, 259)

Metabisulfites (*see* Sulfur dioxide and some sulfites, bisulfites
    and metabisulfites)
Metallic mercury (*see* Mercury and mercury compounds)
Methanearsonic acid, disodium salt (*see* Arsenic and arsenic compounds)
Methanearsonic acid, monosodium salt (*see* Arsenic and arsenic
    compounds
Methotrexate   *26*, 267 (1981); *Suppl. 7*, 241 (1987)
Methoxsalen (*see* 8-Methoxypsoralen)
Methoxychlor   *5*, 193 (1974); *20*, 259 (1979);
    Suppl. 7, 66 (1987)

Methoxyflurane (*see* Anaesthetics, volatile)
5-Methoxypsoralen   *40*, 327 (1986); *Suppl. 7*, 242 (1987)
8-Methoxypsoralen (*see also* 8-Methoxypsoralen plus ultraviolet   *24*, 101 (1980)
    radiation)
8-Methoxypsoralen plus ultraviolet radiation   *Suppl. 7*, 243 (1987)
Methyl acrylate   *19*, 52 (1979); *39*, 99 (1986);
    Suppl. 7, 66 (1987)

5-Methylangelicin plus ultraviolet radiation (*see also* Angelicin
    and some synthetic derivatives)   *Suppl. 7*, 57 (1987)
2-Methylaziridine   *9*, 61 (1975); *Suppl. 7*, 66 (1987)
Methylazoxymethanol acetate   *1*, 164 (1972); *10*, 131 (1976);
    Suppl. 7, 66 (1987)

Methyl bromide   *41*, 187 (1986) (*corr. 45*, 283);
    Suppl. 7, 245 (1987)

Methyl carbamate   *12*, 151 (1976); *Suppl. 7*, 66 (1987)
Methyl-CCNU [*see* 1-(2-Chloroethyl)-3-(4-methylcyclohexyl)-
    1-nitrosourea]
Methyl chloride   *41*, 161 (1986); *Suppl. 7*, 246 (1987)
1-, 2-, 3-, 4-, 5- and 6-Methylchrysenes   *32*, 379 (1983); *Suppl. 7*, 66 (1987)
N-Methyl-*N*,4-dinitrosoaniline   *1*, 141 (1972); *Suppl. 7*, 66 (1987)
4,4′-Methylene bis(2-chloroaniline)   *4*, 65 (1974) (*corr. 42*, 252);
    Suppl. 7, 246 (1987); *57*, 271 (1993)
4,4′-Methylene bis(*N,N*-dimethyl)benzenamine   *27*, 119 (1982); *Suppl. 7*, 66 (1987)
4,4′-Methylene bis(2-methylaniline)   *4*, 73 (1974); *Suppl. 7*, 248 (1987)
4,4′-Methylenedianiline   *4*, 79 (1974) (*corr. 42*, 252);
    39, 347 (1986); *Suppl. 7*, 66 (1987)
4,4′-Methylenediphenyl diisocyanate   *19*, 314 (1979); *Suppl. 7*, 66 (1987)
2-Methylfluoranthene   *32*, 399 (1983); *Suppl. 7*, 66 (1987)

N

Nafenopin	*24*, 125 (1980); *Suppl. 7*, 67 (1987)
1,5-Naphthalenediamine	*27*, 127 (1982); *Suppl. 7*, 67 (1987)
1,5-Naphthalene diisocyanate	*19*, 311 (1979); *Suppl. 7*, 67 (1987)
1-Naphthylamine	*4*, 87 (1974) (*corr. 42*, 253);
	Suppl. 7, 260 (1987)
2-Naphthylamine	*4*, 97 (1974); *Suppl. 7*, 261 (1987)
1-Naphthylthiourea	*30*, 347 (1983); *Suppl. 7*, 263 (1987)
Nickel acetate (*see* Nickel and nickel compounds)	
Nickel ammonium sulfate (*see* Nickel and nickel compounds)	
Nickel and nickel compounds	*2*, 126 (1973) (*corr. 42*, 252); *11*, 75
	(1976); *Suppl. 7*, 264 (1987)
	(*corr. 45*, 283); *49*, 257 (1990)
Nickel carbonate (*see* Nickel and nickel compounds)	
Nickel carbonyl (*see* Nickel and nickel compounds)	
Nickel chloride (*see* Nickel and nickel compounds)	
Nickel-gallium alloy (*see* Nickel and nickel compounds)	
Nickel hydroxide (*see* Nickel and nickel compounds)	
Nickelocene (*see* Nickel and nickel compounds)	
Nickel oxide (*see* Nickel and nickel compounds)	
Nickel subsulfide (*see* Nickel and nickel compounds)	
Nickel sulfate (*see* Nickel and nickel compounds)	
Niridazole	*13*, 123 (1977); *Suppl. 7*, 67 (1987)
Nithiazide	*31*, 179 (1983); *Suppl. 7*, 67 (1987)
Nitrilotriacetic acid and its salts	*48*, 181 (1990)
5-Nitroacenaphthene	*16*, 319 (1978); *Suppl. 7*, 67 (1987)
5-Nitro-*ortho*-anisidine	*27*, 133 (1982); *Suppl. 7*, 67 (1987)
2-Nitroanisole	*65*, 369 (1996)
9-Nitroanthracene	*33*, 179 (1984); *Suppl. 7*, 67 (1987)
7-Nitrobenz[*a*]anthracene	*46*, 247 (1989)
Nitrobenzene	*65*, 381 (1996)
6-Nitrobenzo[*a*]pyrene	*33*, 187 (1984); *Suppl. 7*, 67 (1987);
	46, 255 (1989)
4-Nitrobiphenyl	*4*, 113 (1974); *Suppl. 7*, 67 (1987)
6-Nitrochrysene	*33*, 195 (1984); *Suppl. 7*, 67 (1987);
	46, 267 (1989)
Nitrofen (technical-grade)	*30*, 271 (1983); *Suppl. 7*, 67 (1987)
3-Nitrofluoranthene	*33*, 201 (1984); *Suppl. 7*, 67 (1987)
2-Nitrofluorene	*46*, 277 (1989)
Nitrofural	*7*, 171 (1974); *Suppl. 7*, 67 (1987);
	50, 195 (1990)
5-Nitro-2-furaldehyde semicarbazone (*see* Nitrofural)	
Nitrofurantoin	*50*, 211 (1990)
Nitrofurazone (*see* Nitrofural)	
1-[(5-Nitrofurfurylidene)amino]-2-imidazolidinone	*7*, 181 (1974); *Suppl. 7*, 67 (1987)
N-[4-(5-Nitro-2-furyl)-2-thiazolyl]acetamide	*1*, 181 (1972); *7*, 185 (1974);
	Suppl. 7, 67 (1987)
Nitrogen mustard	*9*, 193 (1975); *Suppl. 7*, 269 (1987)
Nitrogen mustard *N*-oxide	*9*, 209 (1975); *Suppl. 7*, 67 (1987)
1-Nitronaphthalene	*46*, 291 (1989)
2-Nitronaphthalene	*46*, 303 (1989)
3-Nitroperylene	*46*, 313 (1989)
2-Nitro-*para*-phenylenediamine (*see* 1,4-Diamino-2-nitrobenzene)	
2-Nitropropane	*29*, 331 (1982); *Suppl. 7*, 67 (1987)

Norethynodrel (*see also* Progestins; Combined oral contraceptives   6, 191 (1974); 21, 461 (1979)
(corr. 42, 259)
Norgestrel (*see also* Progestins, Combined oral contraceptives)   6, 201 (1974); 21, 479 (1979)
Nylon 6   19, 120 (1979); *Suppl. 7*, 68 (1987)

O

Ochratoxin A   10, 191 (1976); 31, 191 (1983)
(corr. 42, 262); *Suppl. 7*, 271
(1987); 56, 489 (1993)
Oestradiol-17β (*see also* Steroidal oestrogens)   6, 99 (1974); 21, 279 (1979)
Oestradiol 3-benzoate (*see* Oestradiol-17β)
Oestradiol dipropionate (*see* Oestradiol-17β)
Oestradiol mustard   9, 217 (1975); *Suppl. 7*, 68 (1987)
Oestradiol-17β-valerate (*see* Oestradiol-17β)
Oestriol (*see also* Steroidal oestrogens)   6, 117 (1974); 21, 327 (1979);
Suppl. 7, 285 (1987)
Oestrogen-progestin combinations (*see* Oestrogens, progestins
   and combinations)
Oestrogen-progestin replacement therapy (*see also* Oestrogens,   *Suppl. 7*, 308 (1987)
   progestins and combinations)
Oestrogen replacement therapy (*see also* Oestrogens, progestins   *Suppl. 7*, 280 (1987)
   and combinations)
Oestrogens (*see* Oestrogens, progestins and combinations)
Oestrogens, conjugated (*see* Conjugated oestrogens)
Oestrogens, nonsteroidal (*see* Nonsteroidal oestrogens)
Oestrogens, progestins and combinations   6 (1974); 21 (1979);
Suppl. 7, 272 (1987)
Oestrogens, steroidal (*see* Steroidal oestrogens)
Oestrone (*see* also Steroidal oestrogens)   6, 123 (1974); 21, 343 (1979)
(corr. 42, 259)
Oestrone benzoate (*see* Oestrone)
Oil Orange SS   8, 165 (1975); *Suppl. 7*, 69 (1987)
Opisthorchis felineus (infection with)   61, 121 (1994)
Opisthorchis viverrini (infection with)   61, 121 (1994)
Oral contraceptives, combined (*see* Combined oral contraceptives)
Oral contraceptives, investigational (*see* Combined oral contraceptives)
Oral contraceptives, sequential (*see* Sequential oral contraceptives)
Orange I   8, 173 (1975); *Suppl. 7*, 69 (1987)
Orange G   8, 181 (1975); *Suppl. 7*, 69 (1987)
Organolead compounds (*see also* Lead and lead compounds)   *Suppl. 7*, 230 (1987)
Oxazepam   13, 58 (1977); *Suppl. 7*, 69 (1987);
66, 115 (1996)
Oxymetholone [*see also* Androgenic (anabolic) steroids]   13, 131 (1977)
Oxyphenbutazone   13, 185 (1977); *Suppl. 7*, 69 (1987)

P

Paint manufacture and painting (occupational exposures in)   47, 329 (1989)
Palygorskite   42, 159 (1987); *Suppl. 7*, 117 (1987);
68, 245 (1997)
Panfuran S (*see also* Dihydroxymethylfuratrizine)   24, 77 (1980); *Suppl. 7*, 69 (1987)
Paper manufacture (*see* Pulp and paper manufacture)

Polychloroprene	*19*, 141 (1979); *Suppl. 7*, 70 (1987)
Polyethylene	*19*, 164 (1979); *Suppl. 7*, 70 (1987)
Polymethylene polyphenyl isocyanate	*19*, 314 (1979); *Suppl. 7*, 70 (1987)
Polymethyl methacrylate	*19*, 195 (1979); *Suppl. 7*, 70 (1987)
Polyoestradiol phosphate (*see* Oestradiol-17β)	
Polypropylene	*19*, 218 (1979); *Suppl. 7*, 70 (1987)
Polystyrene	*19*, 245 (1979); *Suppl. 7*, 70 (1987)
Polytetrafluoroethylene	*19*, 288 (1979); *Suppl. 7*, 70 (1987)
Polyurethane foams	*19*, 320 (1979); *Suppl. 7*, 70 (1987)
Polyvinyl acetate	*19*, 346 (1979); *Suppl. 7*, 70 (1987)
Polyvinyl alcohol	*19*, 351 (1979); *Suppl. 7*, 70 (1987)
Polyvinyl chloride	*7*, 306 (1974); *19*, 402 (1979); *Suppl. 7*, 70 (1987)
Polyvinyl pyrrolidone	*19*, 463 (1979); *Suppl. 7*, 70 (1987)
Ponceau MX	*8*, 189 (1975); *Suppl. 7*, 70 (1987)
Ponceau 3R	*8*, 199 (1975); *Suppl. 7*, 70 (1987)
Ponceau SX	*8*, 207 (1975); *Suppl. 7*, 70 (1987)
Potassium arsenate (*see* Arsenic and arsenic compounds)	
Potassium arsenite (*see* Arsenic and arsenic compounds)	
Potassium bis(2-hydroxyethyl)dithiocarbamate	*12*, 183 (1976); *Suppl. 7*, 70 (1987)
Potassium bromate	*40*, 207 (1986); *Suppl. 7*, 70 (1987)
Potassium chromate (*see* Chromium and chromium compounds)	
Potassium dichromate (*see* Chromium and chromium compounds)	
Prazepam	*66*, 143 (1996)
Prednimustine	*50*, 115 (1990)
Prednisone	*26*, 293 (1981); *Suppl. 7*, 326 (1987)
Printing processes and printing inks	*65*, 33 (1996)
Procarbazine hydrochloride	*26*, 311 (1981); *Suppl. 7*, 327 (1987)
Proflavine salts	*24*, 195 (1980); *Suppl. 7*, 70 (1987)
Progesterone (*see also* Progestins; Combined oral contraceptives)	*6*, 135 (1974); *21*, 491 (1979) (*corr. 42*, 259)
Progestins (*see also* Oestrogens, progestins and combinations)	*Suppl. 7*, 289 (1987)
Pronetalol hydrochloride	*13*, 227 (1977) (*corr. 42*, 256); *Suppl. 7*, 70 (1987)
1,3-Propane sultone	*4*, 253 (1974) (*corr. 42*, 253); *Suppl. 7*, 70 (1987)
Propham	*12*, 189 (1976); *Suppl. 7*, 70 (1987)
β-Propiolactone	*4*, 259 (1974) (*corr. 42*, 253); *Suppl. 7*, 70 (1987)
n-Propyl carbamate	*12*, 201 (1976); *Suppl. 7*, 70 (1987)
Propylene	*19*, 213 (1979); *Suppl. 7*, 71 (1987); *60*, 161 (1994)
Propylene oxide	*11*, 191 (1976); *36*, 227 (1985) (*corr. 42*, 263); *Suppl. 7*, 328 (1987); *60*, 181 (1994)
Propylthiouracil	*7*, 67 (1974); *Suppl. 7*, 329 (1987)
Ptaquiloside (*see also* Bracken fern)	*40*, 55 (1986); *Suppl. 7*, 71 (1987)
Pulp and paper manufacture	*25*, 157 (1981); *Suppl. 7*, 385 (1987)
Pyrene	*32*, 431 (1983); *Suppl. 7*, 71 (1987)
Pyrido[3,4-*c*]psoralen	*40*, 349 (1986); *Suppl. 7*, 71 (1987)
Pyrimethamine	*13*, 233 (1977); *Suppl. 7*, 71 (1987)
Pyrrolizidine alkaloids (*see* Hydroxysenkirkine; Isatidine; Jacobine; Lasiocarpine; Monocrotaline; Retrorsine; Riddelliine; Seneciphylline; Senkirkine)	

Q

R

S

N-Vinyl-2-pyrrolidone	*19*, 461 (1979); *Suppl. 7*, 73 (1987)
Vinyl toluene	*60*, 373 (1994)

W

Welding	*49*, 447 (1990) (*corr. 52*, 513)
Wollastonite	*42*, 145 (1987); *Suppl. 7*, 377 (1987); *68*, 283 (1997)
Wood dust	*62*, 35 (1995)
Wood industries	*25* (1981); *Suppl. 7*, 378 (1987)

X

Xylene	*47*, 125 (1989)
2,4-Xylidine	*16*, 367 (1978); *Suppl. 7*, 74 (1987)
2,5-Xylidine	*16*, 377 (1978); *Suppl. 7*, 74 (1987)
2,6-Xylidine (*see* 2,6-Dimethylaniline)	

Y

Yellow AB	*8*, 279 (1975); *Suppl. 7*, 74 (1987)
Yellow OB	*8*, 287 (1975); *Suppl. 7*, 74 (1987)

Z

Zearalenone (*see* Toxins derived from *Fusarium graminearum, F. culmorum* and *F. crookwellense*)	
Zectran	*12*, 237 (1976); *Suppl. 7*, 74 (1987)
Zeolites other than erionite	*68*, 307 (1997)
Zinc beryllium silicate (*see* Beryllium and beryllium compounds)	
Zinc chromate (*see* Chromium and chromium compounds)	
Zinc chromate hydroxide (*see* Chromium and chromium compounds)	
Zinc potassium chromate (*see* Chromium and chromium compounds)	
Zinc yellow (*see* Chromium and chromium compounds)	
Zineb	*12*, 245 (1976); *Suppl. 7*, 74 (1987)
Ziram	*12*, 259 (1976); *Suppl. 7*, 74 (1987); *53*, 423 (1991)

IARC Monographs on the Evaluation of Carcinogenic Risks to Humans

Supplement No. 3
Cross Index of Synonyms and Trade Names in Volumes 1 to 26
1982; 199 pages; ISBN 92 832 1405 6
(out of print)

Supplement No.4
Chemicals, Industrial Processes and Industries Associated with Cancer in Humans (Volumes 1 to 29)
1982; 292 pages; ISBN 92 832 1407 2
(out of print)

Supplement No. 5
Cross Index of Synonyms and Trade Names in Volumes 1 to 36
1985; 259 pages; ISBN 92 832 1408 0
(out of print)

Supplement No. 6
Genetic and Related Effects: An Updating of Selected IARC Monographs from Volumes 1 to 42
1987; 729 pages; ISBN 92 832 1409 9

Supplement No. 7
Overall Evaluations of Carcinogenicity: An Updating of IARC Monographs Volumes 1 to 42
1987; 440 pages; ISBN 92 832 1411 0

Supplement No. 8
Cross Index of Synonyms and Trade Names in Volumes 1 to 46
1989; 346 pages; ISBN 92 832 1417 X

IARC Scientific Publications

No. 1
Liver Cancer
1971; 176 pages; ISBN 0 19 723000 8

No. 2
Oncogenesis and Herpesviruses
Edited by P.M. Biggs, G. de Thé and L.N. Payne
1972; 515 pages; ISBN 0 19 723001 6

No. 3
N-Nitroso Compounds: Analysis and Formation
Edited by P. Bogovski, R. Preussman and E.A. Walker
1972; 140 pages; ISBN 0 19 723002 4

No. 4
Transplacental Carcinogenesis
Edited by L. Tomatis and U. Mohr
1973; 181 pages; ISBN 0 19 723003 2

No. 5/6
Pathology of Tumours in Laboratory Animals. Volume 1: Tumours of the Rat
Edited by V.S. Turusov
1973/1976; 533 pages; ISBN 92 832 1410 2

No. 7
Host Environment Interactions in the Etiology of Cancer in Man
Edited by R. Doll and I. Vodopija
1973; 464 pages; ISBN 0 19 723006 7

No. 8
Biological Effects of Asbestos
Edited by P. Bogovski, J.C. Gilson, V. Timbrell and J.C. Wagner
1973; 346 pages; ISBN 0 19 723007 5

No. 9
N-Nitroso Compounds in the Environment
Edited by P. Bogovski and E.A. Walker
1974; 243 pages; ISBN 0 19 723008 3

No. 10
Chemical Carcinogenesis Essays
Edited by R. Montesano and L. Tomatis
1974; 230 pages; ISBN 0 19 723009 1

No. 11
Oncogenesis and Herpes-viruses II
Edited by G. de-Thé, M.A. Epstein and H. zur Hausen
1975; Two volumes, 511 pages and 403 pages; ISBN 0 19 723010 5

No. 12
Screening Tests in Chemical Carcinogenesis
Edited by R. Montesano, H. Bartsch and L. Tomatis
1976; 666 pages; ISBN 0 19 723051 2

No. 13
Environmental Pollution and Carcinogenic Risks
Edited by C. Rosenfeld and W. Davis
1975; 441 pages; ISBN 0 19 723012 1

No. 14
Environmental N-Nitroso Compounds. Analysis and Formation
Edited by E.A. Walker, P. Bogovski and L. Griciute
1976; 512 pages; ISBN 0 19 723013 X

No. 15
Cancer Incidence in Five Continents, Volume III
Edited by J.A.H. Waterhouse, C. Muir, P. Correa and J. Powell
1976; 584 pages; ISBN 0 19 723014 8

No. 16
Air Pollution and Cancer in Man
Edited by U. Mohr, D. Schmähl and L. Tomatis
1977; 328 pages; ISBN 0 19 723015 6

No. 17
Directory of On-Going Research in Cancer Epidemiology 1977
Edited by C.S. Muir and G. Wagner
1977; 599 pages; ISBN 92 832 1117 0
(out of print)

No. 18
Environmental Carcinogens. Selected Methods of Analysis. Volume 1: Analysis of Volatile Nitrosamines in Food
Editor-in-Chief: H. Egan
1978; 212 pages; ISBN 0 19 723017 2

No. 19
Environmental Aspects of N-Nitroso Compounds
Edited by E.A. Walker, M. Castegnaro, L. Griciute and R.E. Lyle
1978; 561 pages; ISBN 0 19 723018 0

No. 20
Nasopharyngeal Carcinoma: Etiology and Control
Edited by G. de Thé and Y. Ito
1978; 606 pages; ISBN 0 19 723019 9

No. 21
Cancer Registration and its Techniques
Edited by R. MacLennan, C. Muir, R. Steinitz and A. Winkler
1978; 235 pages; ISBN 0 19 723020 2

No. 22
Environmental Carcinogens: Selected Methods of Analysis. Volume 2: Methods for the Measurement of Vinyl Chloride in Poly(vinyl chloride), Air, Water and Foodstuffs
Editor-in-Chief: H. Egan
1978; 142 pages; ISBN 0 19 723021 0

No. 23
Pathology of Tumours in Laboratory Animals. Volume II: Tumours of the Mouse
Editor-in-Chief: V.S. Turusov
1979; 669 pages; ISBN 0 19 723022 9

No. 24
Oncogenesis and Herpesviruses III
Edited by G. de-Thé, W. Henle and F. Rapp
1978; Part I: 580 pages, Part II: 512 pages; ISBN 0 19 723023 7

IARC Technical Reports

H. Sriplung, K. Chindavijak, S. Sontipong,
S. Sriamporn, D.M. Parkin and J. Ferlay
1993; 164 pages; ISBN 92 832 1430 7

No. 18
Intervention Trials for Cancer Prevention
By E. Buiatti
1994; 52 pages; ISBN 92 832 1432 3

No. 19
**Comparability and Quality Control in
Cancer Registration**
By D.M. Parkin, V.W. Chen, J. Ferlay,
J. Galceran, H.H. Storm and S.L. Whelan
1994; 110 pages plus diskette;
ISBN 92 832 1433 1

No. 20
**Epidémiologie du cancer
dans les pays de langue
latine**
1994; 346 pages; ISBN 92 832 1434 X

No. 21
ICD Conversion Programs for Cancer
By J. Ferlay
1994; 24 pages plus diskette;
ISBN 92 832 1435 8

No. 22
Cancer in Tianjin
By Q.S. Wang, P. Boffetta,
M. Kogevinas and D.M. Parkin
1994; 96 pages; ISBN 92 832 1433 1

No. 23
**An Evaluation Programme for Cancer
Preventive Agents**
By Bernard W. Stewart
1995; 40 pages; ISBN 92 832 1438 2

No. 24
**Peroxisome Proliferation and its Role
in Carcinogenesis**
1995; 85 pages; ISBN 92 832 1439 0

No. 25
**Combined Analysis of Cancer
Mortality in Nuclear Workers in
Canada, the United Kingdom and the
United States of America**
By E. Cardis, E.S. Gilbert, L.
Carpenter, G. Howe, I. Kato, J. Fix, L.
Salmon, G. Cowper, B.K. Armstrong,
V. Beral, A. Douglas, S.A. Fry, J. Kaldor,
C. Lavé, P.G. Smith, G. Voelz and
L. Wiggs

1995; 160 pages; ISBN 92 832 1440 4

No. 26
**Mortalité par Cancer des Imigrés en
France, 1979-1985**
By C. Bouchardy, M. Khlat, P. Wanner
and D.M. Parkin
1997; 150 pages; ISBN 92 832 2404 3

No. 27
**Cancer in Three Generations of Young
Israelis**
By J. Iscovich and D.M. Parkin
1997; 150 pages; ISBN 92 832 2441 2

No. 29
**International Classification of Childhood
Cancer 1996**
By E. Kramarova, C.A. Stiller, J. Ferlay,
D.M. Parkin, G.J. Draper, J.Michaelis, J.
Neglia and S. Qurechi
1997; 48 pages + diskette; ISBN 92 832
1443 9

IARC CancerBase

No. 1
**EUCAN90: Cancer in the European
Union** (Electronic Database with Graphic
Display)
By J. Ferlay, R.J. Black, P. Pisani, M.T.
Valdivieso and D.M. Parkin
1996; Computer software on 3.5" IBM
diskette + user's guide (50 pages);
ISBN 92 832 1450 1

All IARC Publications are available directly from
IARCPress, 150 Cours Albert Thomas, F-69372 Lyon cedex 08, France
(Fax: +33 4 72 73 83 02; E-mail: press@iarc.fr).

IARC Monographs and Technical Reports are also available from the
World Health Organization Distribution and Sales, CH-1211 Geneva 27
(Fax: +41 22 791 4857)
and from WHO Sales Agents worldwide.

IARC Scientific Publications are also available from
Oxford University Press, Walton Street, Oxford, UK OX2 6DP
(Fax: +44 1865 267782).